DATE DUE

AUG 2 2 2011	

Play in Occupational Therapy for Children

Play in Occupational Therapy for Children

Second Edition

Edited by

L. Diane Parham, PhD, OTR/L, FAOTA
Professor, Department of Pediatrics
Chief, Division of Occupational Therapy
Director, Occupational Therapy Graduate Program
University of New Mexico
Albuquerque, New Mexico

Linda S. Fazio, PhD, OTR/L, FAOTA
Professor of Clinical Occupational Therapy
Department of Occupational Science
and Occupational Therapy
University of Southern California
Los Angeles, California

Primary photographer: Shay McAtee

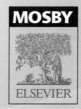

MOSBY

ELSEVIER

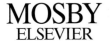

11830 Westline Industrial Drive
St. Louis, Missouri 63146

PLAY IN OCCUPATIONAL THERAPY FOR CHILDREN
Second Edition
Copyright © 2008, 1997 by Mosby, Inc., an affiliate of Elsevier Inc.

ISBN: 978-0-323-02954-4

Notice

Neither the Publisher nor the Editors/ assume any responsibility for any loss or injury and/or damage to persons or property arising out of or related to any use of the material contained in this book. It is the responsibility of the treating practitioner, relying on independent expertise and knowledge of the patient, to determine the best treatment and method of application for the patient.

The Publisher

Library of Congress Control Number 2007938341

Vice President and Publisher: Linda Duncan
Senior Editor: Kathy Falk
Senior Developmental Editor: Melissa Kuster Deutsch
Publishing Services Manager: Patricia Tannian
Design Direction: Andrea Lutes

Printed in the United States of America

Last digit is the print number: 9 8 7 6 5 4 3 2 1

Contributors

ERNA IMPERATORE BLANCHE, PHD, OTR/L, FAOTA
Assistant Professor
Department of Occupational Science and Occupational Therapy
University of Southern California
Los Angeles, California

KIMBERLY C. BRYZE, PHD, OTR/L
Director and Associate Professor
Occupational Therapy Programs
Midwestern University
Downers Grove, Illinois

ANITA C. BUNDY, SCD, FAOTA, OTR
Professor, Chair, and Head
School of Occupation and Leisure Sciences
University of Sydney
New South Wales, Australia

JANICE POSATERY BURKE, PHD, OTR/L, FAOTA
Professor and Chair
Department of Occupational Therapy
Jefferson College of Health Professions
Philadelphia, Pennsylvania

SHARON CERMAK, EDD, OTR/L, FAOTA
Professor
Department of Occupational Therapy and Rehabilitation Counseling
Sargent College of Health and Rehabilitation Sciences
Boston University
Boston, Massachusetts

LISA A. DAUNHAUER, SCD, OTR
Assistant Professor
Department of Occupational Therapy
Colorado State University
Fort Collins, Colorado

JEAN CROSETTO DEITZ, PHD, OTR/L, FAOTA
Professor and Graduate Program Coordinator
Department of Rehabilitation Medicine
University of Washington
Seattle, Washington

LINDA L. FLOREY, PhD, OTR/L, FAOTA
Chief, Rehabilitation Services
Resnick Neuropsychiatric Institute at UCLA
Los Angeles, California

SANDRA GREENE, MA, OTR/L
Principal
Sandra Greene & Associates
Santa Monica, California

T. BRIANNA LOMBA HALL, MS, OTR/L
Pediatric Occupational Therapist
Children's Therapy Center
Gilroy, California

ALEXIS HENRY, SCD, OTR/L
Research Assistant Professor of Psychiatry
Center for Health Policy and Research
University of Massachusetts Medical School
Worcester, Massachusetts

JIM HINOJOSA, PhD, OT, FAOTA
Professor and Chair
Department of Occupational Therapy
New York University
New York, New York

ELISE HOLLOWAY, MPH, OTR/L
Occupational Therapy Clinical Specialist, Neonatology
Huntington Memorial Hospital
Pasadena, California
Occupational Therapy Consultant, Early Start Program
Eastern Los Angeles Regional Center for Developmental Disabilities
Alhambra, California

SUSAN KNOX, PhD, OTR, FAOTA
Private Practice
Los Angeles, California

PAULA KRAMER, PhD, OTR/L, FAOTA
Chair and Professor
Department of Occupational Therapy
University of the Sciences in Philadelphia
Philadelphia, Pennsylvania

SHELLY J. LANE, PhD, OTR/L, FAOTA
Professor and Chair
Department of Occupational Therapy
VCU Health Systems
Richmond, Virginia

ZOE MAILLOUX, MA, OTR, FAOTA
Director of Administration
Pediatric Therapy Network
Torrance, California

SUSAN MISTRETT, MS Ed
Let's Play! Research Project, PI
AT Training Online (ATTO) Project, Project Director
AT in the Schools Project, AT Consultant/Trainer
Center for Assistive Technology
School of Public Health and Health Professions
University at Buffalo, State University of New York
Buffalo, New York

VERONIQUE MUNIER
Endowed Chair Research Coordinator
Department of Occupational Therapy
Eastern Kentucky University
Richmond, Kentucky

CHRISTINE TEETERS MYERS, MHS, OTR/L
Assistant Professor
Department of Occupational Therapy
Eastern Kentucky University
Richmond, Kentucky

DORIS PIERCE, PhD, OTR/L, FAOTA
Professor and Endowed Chair
Department of Occupational Therapy
Eastern Kentucky University
Richmond, Kentucky

ROSEANN C. SCHAAF, PhD, OTR/L, FAOTA
Vice Chairman, Instructor, and Director of Graduate
Programs
Department of Occupational Therapy
Jefferson College of Health Professions
Philadelphia, Pennsylvania

GEVA SKARD, MS, OTR
Occupational Therapist and Special Needs Education
Counselor
SVT
Drammen, Norway

SUSAN L. SPITZER, PhD, OTR/L
Adjunct Assistant Professor of Clinical Occupational
Therapy
Department of Occupational Science and Therapy
University of Southern California
Los Angeles, California
Private Practice
Pasadena, California

YVONNE SWINTH, PhD, OTR/L, FAOTA
Associate Professor
School of Occupational Therapy and Physical Therapy
University of Puget Sound
Tacoma, Washington
Occupational Therapist
University Place School District
University Place, Washington

KARI J. TANTA, PhD, OTR/L
Clinical Assistant Professor
Department of Rehabilitation Medicine
University of Washington
Seattle, Washington
Program Coordinator
Children's Therapy
Valley Medical Center
Renton, Washington

To the spirit of play in our daughters
April, Holly, and Dorothy Helen

Foreword

A revolution is occurring that promises to transform occupational therapy in the twenty-first century. Its impetus has come from scholars, researchers, educators, and practitioners who do not wish to see the profession's commitment to occupation irretrievably lost in the turbulence of global upheaval. These courageous individuals are generating scholarly papers, developing intervention models, and producing research that powerfully address the linkages of occupation to health. They are giving us hope, in the midst of the more depressing aspects of massive political and economic changes, that occupational therapy will be able to continue safeguarding the public good, not by abrogating its traditional focus, but instead by expanding its knowledge base on occupation and the applications of occupation to health care.

The seemingly overwhelming pressures of economic challenges on a multinational scale, coupled with the fear that occupation may vanish from health care, appear to have stimulated the American Occupational Therapy Association to revitalize its mission and focus its resources on ensuring that the profession of occupation is poised to vitally serve societal needs in the twenty-first century. This refocusing of priorities is evidenced by the Centennial Vision of the association, which targets six critical areas in which occupational therapy is uniquely situated to make important contributions to the health and participation of people facing adverse and unpredictable life challenges (Baum, 2006).

Diane Parham, Linda Fazio, and their contributors are to be commended for creating a book that is well suited to propel the profession toward realization of the Centennial Vision. First of all, the focus of the entire book is on play, the primary occupation in which children engage, and therefore targets one of the six critical areas around which the profession is rallying: *Children and Youth*. Some chapters focus on the well-being of children and youth by examining how occupational therapists can use play to support children's success in school (Swinth & Tanta), their engagement with families and communities (Burke, Schaaf, and Lomba Hall; Hinojosa and Kramer; Holloway), and their acquisition of skills that will contribute to competence and productivity in adulthood (Munier, Myers, and Pierce; Mailloux and Burke). Other chapters specifically address *Mental Health*, another critical area. For example, Florey and Greene discuss play in relation to the social participation of children with psychiatric conditions in middle childhood,

whereas Spitzer describes highly original, research-based strategies to increase play engagement of children with autism spectrum disorders. Most of the chapters are relevant to *Rehabilitation, Disabilities, and Participation*, a third area identified by the Centennial Vision as critical. In particular, the work contributed by Blanche, by Deitz and Swinth, and by Lane and Mistrett provides information on use of therapeutic strategies, assistive technology, and universal design to promote play engagement among children with physical or developmental disabilities. The critical area of *Health and Wellness* is also addressed by some authors, such as Fazio, who discusses storytelling as a way to help children find solutions to life challenges, and Parham, who asserts that play is a vital ingredient of health and quality of life. In addition, the play assessment tools presented by Bryze, Skard and Bundy, Henry, and Knox are tailored to assist therapists in evaluating the contributions of play to the health and participation of children who may have disabilities or are at risk for chronic conditions affecting mental or physical health.

In this second edition of *Play in Occupational Therapy for Children*, play continues to be addressed in a manner that is in sharp contrast to traditional approaches, which understood play through the theoretical lenses of psychologists and play theorists from other disciplines and which employed play in treatment contexts that were prescriptive and deficit oriented. The content of this book successfully challenges these conventional notions and approaches. Play theories and assessments imported from other disciplines are carefully presented; alongside them, however, we are introduced to the unique theories and assessments that have resulted from research conducted by occupational therapists and occupational scientists and have led to new conceptualizations of practice. The book's numerous case studies reveal a detailed picture of how pediatric occupational therapy (1) is shaped when it is guided by state-of-the-art occupational therapy theory on play, (2) is context sensitive, and (3) is nonprescriptive.

It is fascinating that so many of the chapters in this book ultimately deal with the situatedness of play. They are thematically unified by their emphasis on context, though this concern takes on a variety of appearances. The new chapter by Daunhauer and Cermak describes in vivid and heartbreaking detail how the day-to-day caregiving routines of impoverished institutions may create deprivation conditions that have profound effects on child development. They describe how educating institutional caregivers to play with the children can be a powerful tool for ameliorating the adverse developmental sequelae of institutionalization. The intervention strategies they recommend are highly specific to the conditions and culture in which the caregiver-child interactions take place. In the chapter by Holloway, we are provoked to think about whether playfulness should be addressed with medically fragile infants in neonatal intensive care units. Holloway not only justifies the need to do so, but provides illustrations in case examples of how this is done, despite the constraints of the highly technological and threatening hospital context. Munier, Myers, and Pierce, on the other hand, force us to acknowledge the limitations of clinic-based occupational therapy through the elaboration of a practice theory that can guide therapists in harnessing sources of therapeutic power that are indigenous to home settings. Swinth and Tanta call our attention to the often neglected, but potentially powerful and multifaceted, uses of play in the school environment. In their chapter Hinojosa and Kramer present a compelling argument that it is insufficient to address a child's play in isolation from his family's play patterns. They describe the therapeutic benefits of including the child with a disability in family play and, conversely, family members in the play of the child with disabilities. Just as Marjorie Devault (1991), in her acclaimed ethnography, demonstrated that feeding the family was essential to the social construction of a family "as family," so too do Hinojosa and Kramer convince us of the absolute necessity of including family play in intervention that claims to meet the needs of the family.

Although the focus of this book is clearly on play and context, it is not surprising that most of the chapters also address the therapeutic relationship between the parent, the child with disability, and the therapist. It seems that the contributors believe that a prescriptive, deficit-focused, directive approach will inevitably undermine play-focused interventions. Holloway, for example, advocates embracing a nonprescriptive stance in which parents are sensitized to the infant's adaptive capacities rather than informed about deficits or dysfunction. Burke, Schaaf, and Lomba Hall suggest storytelling as an approach for building connective knowing in which the therapist's assessment can be tied to the parent's concern. Bryze discusses how parents and therapists can work together to find shared meaning in the child's play. Fazio recommends storytelling as a playful occupation through which the therapist can develop a keener understanding of the life world of the child. All of these methods, it would seem, cast parent, therapist, and child as collaborators in a fluid, spontaneous, and improvisational relationship, the kind of relationship that seems particularly well suited for interventions centered on play.

It is hard for me to imagine a better example of the kind of books occupational therapy needs to enrich and secure its place in serving the public good. We are much in debt to the editors and contributors for demonstrating how the time-honored occupational therapy focus on play, illuminated through state-of-the-art theory and research, can be reforged to meet the health care challenges of these times.

REFERENCES

Baum, M. C. (2006). Presidential address, 2006: Centennial challenges, millennium opportunities. *American Journal of Occupational Therapy, 60,* 609-616.

DeVault, M. L. (1991). *Feeding the family.* Chicago, IL: University of Chicago Press.

FLORENCE CLARK, PhD, OTR, FAOTA
Professor and Associate Dean
Chair, Division of Occupational Science and
Occupational Therapy at the School of Dentistry
University of Southern California
Los Angeles, California

Preface

*We dance around in a ring and suppose but the
secret sits in the middle and knows.*
ROBERT FROST

Play is a secret that occupational therapists have danced around for many years. Since the early twentieth century, the profession has declared that play is essential to a healthy lifestyle (Meyer, 1922). It has long been part of the profession's clinical folk knowledge that play confers a nearly magical power to open up human potentials constrained by disability, disadvantage, or chronic illness. Yet for many years, play was kept a secret by occupational therapists, in part because of its low status within the scientific and medical establishments and in part because, until relatively recently, so little was understood by any discipline regarding the nature of play.

The secret of play's power remained shrouded in mystery as long as therapists were embarrassed by it. Afraid of being dismissed as frivolous or trivial through association with play, mid–twentieth century occupational therapists turned their efforts in professional development toward more clearly scientific endeavors, and the problems of play—what it is, why it works, and how to assess and apply it systematically in clinical practice—remained unexamined.

It was not until Mary Reilly published *Play as Exploratory Learning* in 1974 that the problem of play became a focus of serious study and theory-based clinical applications in the profession. That work became a stimulus for a new generation of clinicians and scholars who were intrigued by play's power and who, building on the foundation laid by Reilly and her students, were no longer embarrassed to claim play as both a therapeutic agent and a critical outcome of intervention. Today, poised at the beginning of the twenty-first century, the profession identifies play as a primary domain of concern in official documents (e.g., American Occupational Therapy Association, 2002). Thanks to the work of scholars and clinicians over the past few decades, contemporary occupational therapists have at hand a variety of theoretical interpretations, assessment approaches, and treatment models that support innovative and effective applications of play in occupational therapy.

This book was designed to present an overview of current research and practice related to play in pediatric occupational therapy. In addition, it provides clinicians and researchers with several specific instruments for measuring play and

playfulness of children and offers guidelines for clinical evaluation and intervention that build on research evidence and expert clinical experience.

As in the first edition, the second edition of this book is divided into four main sections. The four sections are organizational devices that call the reader's attention to different angles on the topic of play and its clinical applications, but the sections are not entirely discrete and their boundaries are not rigid.

Section I, Introduction to Play and Occupational Therapy, provides an historical and conceptual backdrop for the rest of the book. It consists of one chapter that offers an extensive review of multidisciplinary play theories and rhetorics, an historical overview of play in occupational therapy practice, and a discussion of current streams of research and practice concerning play in occupational therapy. New topics discussed include research on play and disability, evidence-based practice, culture and play, and implications for occupational justice. The remaining sections of the book focus on ideas and guidelines for clinical assessment and treatment that are grounded in theory and research, as well as in clinical experience.

Section II, Assessment of Play, presents specific assessment instruments and discussions of how to incorporate a family-centered, narrative approach into the assessment process. Several new instruments, collectively named the Pediatric Interest Profiles, are featured in this section. In addition, the Test of Environmental Supports (TOES) is introduced in the revised chapter on assessment of playfulness.

Section III, Play as a Means for Enhancing Development and Skill Acquisition, addresses play as a means to an end. Chapters in this section focus on play as a tool to promote perceptual, motor, cognitive, self-care, and social skills; environmental negotiation in space and time; sensory integrative development; social participation; and school success. New material in this section includes a chapter addressing the design of play-based assessment and intervention to improve the developmental outcomes of children living with deprivation because of institutionalization, as well as a chapter focusing on play as a tool for occupational therapists working in school systems.

Section IV, Play as a Goal of Intervention, focuses on play as an end in itself. Chapters in this section describe ways to expand the child's play life by making it more accessible, satisfying, and meaningful. Authors discuss strategies for facilitating play within the context of the family and within the contexts of specialized areas of practice. New chapters address how to help children with autism to have richer, more expanded play experiences and how to use universal design to support the play of children in early intervention programs.

This book is intended to meet the needs of several audiences. First, it is intended to be used in the entry-level professional occupational therapy curriculum at the master's degree level. Chapter 1 provides important theoretical background on play for entry-level students, and additional chapters provide extensive assessment and treatment guidelines to demonstrate clearly how theory may be put into practice. The inclusion of ample case illustrations will be particularly useful in helping the student or novice clinician to visualize what assessment or treatment may look like in a clinical situation. Although most occupational therapy curricula do not include a specific course on play, this book gives faculty a tool with which to infuse play concepts throughout the curriculum. Because the chapters can stand alone as individual readings, separate chapters may be assigned in courses on occupational development, pediatric practice, assessment, interventions for psychosocial or physical dysfunctions, and practice skills. For example, the chapters on assistive technology and universal design would be an excellent way to relate this topic to occupation in a course on interventions for physical dysfunction.

This book is also intended to be used by postprofessional graduate students (i.e., enrolled in postprofessional master's, OTD, PhD, or other doctoral degree programs). The extensive literature reviewed, the original ideas presented, and the guidelines for assessment and treatment described in many of the chapters may serve as a springboard for seminar discussions, clinical and community program development, policy projects, research, and scholarship.

Experienced occupational therapists who work with children may find this book valuable as a reference. For those who did not receive adequate theoretical preparation regarding play in their formal professional education or who wish to refresh or update their knowledge, this book can become the basis of a self-study process. We hope that even clinicians who are known experts on play will discover much that is stimulating within its covers.

Scholars and clinicians from other fields who are interested in play may find that the notion of play as occupation puts a new twist on an old topic and thus opens up new avenues for thinking about play. Although many of the instruments and intervention programming ideas presented here were originally conceived for use in occupational therapy, they are appropriate for many interdisciplinary applications.

An important final note: the focus of this book is on applications to children simply because most of the work on play in our profession (and in other disciplines) has been directed to this portion of the lifespan. We do endorse play in occupational therapy for adults, and we hope to see the occupational therapy play literature expand in the coming years to include life after adolescence.

REFERENCES

American Occupational Therapy Association (2002). Occupational therapy practice framework: Domain and process. *American Journal of Occupational Therapy, 56,* 609-639.

Meyer, A. (1922). The philosophy of occupation therapy. *Archives of Occupational Therapy, 1,* 1-10.

Reilly, M. (Ed.) (1974). *Play as exploratory learning.* Beverly Hills, CA: Sage Publications.

L. DIANE PARHAM
LINDA S. FAZIO

Acknowledgments

In this, the second edition of *Play in Occupational Therapy for Children,* we are reminded of what the wonderful contributors brought to the first edition and now to this one. Chapter authors are some of the finest theoreticians and practitioners in the profession's growing literature on play. We commend them all and are grateful for their willingness to share their time and expertise.

The talent of photographer Shay McAtee continues to grace this edition. Shay's expertise in technique and subject selection contribute greatly to the descriptions and explanations provided by the authors. We also thank the other photographers who contributed to this edition.

We continue to be grateful to colleagues both present and past without whose expertise, guidance, willing discussions, and insights this work would not have come to fruition. We are well aware that we are standing on the shoulders of Mary Reilly and her colleagues, whose work paved the way for us to create a textbook on play in occupational therapy in the 1990s. Her courage and foresight in bringing play out of hiding and into the light as a serious topic of scholarship are honored. The inspiration of occupational therapists who are expert players is also acknowledged. In particular, the memory of A. Jean Ayres, who was a genius at using play to engage a child in therapy, is treasured. The inspiration and leadership of Elizabeth Yerxa, whose vision shaped the doctoral program in occupational science at USC, continue to be tremendously influential. Her legacy as Chair of the Department of Occupational Science and Occupational Therapy has continued in the visionary work of present Chair Florence Clark. Many lectures and discussions of both formal and informal nature with these leaders have greatly benefited this text.

We appreciate the hard work of the editors and managers at Elsevier, especially Kathy Falk, Melissa Kuster, Robin Sutter, and Trish Tannian. Their encouragement and assistance have made the work possible.

And to our families and our colleagues at the University of Southern California and the University of New Mexico, your continued support and understanding … invaluable!

L. DIANE PARHAM
LINDA S. FAZIO

Contents

Play in Occupational Therapy for Children

I

Introduction to Play and Occupational Therapy

1

Play and Occupational Therapy

L. Diane Parham

Play is a child's way of learning and an outlet for his innate need of activity. It is his business or his career. In it he engages himself with the same attitude and energy that we engage ourselves in our regular work. For each child it is a serious undertaking not to be confused with diversion or idle use of time. Play is not folly. It is purposeful activity.
Norma Alessandrini, in the *American Journal of Occupational Therapy,* 1949

These are the opening lines from an article written nearly 60 years ago by an occupational therapist, Norma Alessandrini. At the time she wrote this, she was Director of Children's Recreation Service at Bellevue Hospital in New York City. Interestingly, the philosophy of play that Alessandrini outlined in this article resounds with a core idea being explored by contemporary occupational therapy leaders: that play is a significant and primary occupation of children.

The purpose of this chapter is to provide the reader with a broad overview of how play is approached in the profession of occupational therapy, particularly in relation to children. The chapter begins with questions regarding the nature of play: how it is defined and how it has been explained from the diverse perspectives of many disciplines. The chapter then moves on to examine how play historically has been viewed and used within the field of occupational therapy. The chapter concludes with a review of contemporary streams of ideas on play in occupational therapy.

A caveat is in order before this discussion of play continues. The focus of this chapter, and of the entire text, is on children's play solely because the topic of play has been addressed in the literature predominantly in relation to childhood. Concepts of play are indeed relevant throughout the lifespan and offer a potentially rich field of knowledge that, for the most part, has not yet been explored or applied by occupational therapists in a systematic manner. Many of the ideas that have sprung from research and clinical work with children may be applicable to adults as well.

WHAT IS PLAY?

"It's child's play." This colloquial expression is used to denote a task so simple that it does not require effort. To scholars, however, the study of child's play is not a simple task. Play is an elusive concept and is difficult (some would say impossible) to define. Before reading further, the reader should try the exercise in Box 1-1.

In everyday use the meaning of "play" seems clear enough, but its boundaries are fuzzy (Garvey, 1990). Even when people easily agree that what they are observing is play, they may struggle to articulate what play is. Scholars over the years have attempted to define it, explain it, suggest criteria for it, and relate it to other types of behaviors, but debate continues over its definition. One reason for this, no doubt, is the wide range of meanings the word "play" takes on in the English language. A cursory dictionary search of *Merriam-Webster Online* (2007) yielded

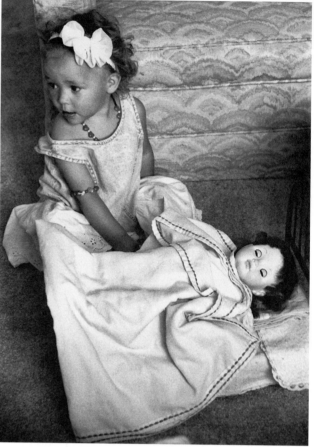

Figure 1-1
Among the dictionary definitions of play are the spontaneous activity of children, to engage in or occupy oneself, and to pretend to engage in an activity. Play is most prevalent among children but occurs throughout the human lifespan. (Courtesy Shay McAtee.)

approximately 23 definitions of play as a noun, such as a recreational activity, the spontaneous activity of children, the absence of serious or harmful intent, and one's turn in a game. In addition, 60 definitions of play as a verb were identified, for example, to engage in sport or recreation, to toy or fiddle around with something, to move or function freely within prescribed limits, to engage in or occupy oneself, and to pretend to engage in an activity (Figure 1-1).

The philosopher Ludwig Wittgenstein dealt with the problem of defining elusive concepts in his discussion of games. His view was that the multifarious activities that people call games have no one thing in common that makes them all games, yet they are related to each other in a variety of ways. The same idea can apply to the diverse occupations that are called play.

> Consider for example the proceedings that we call "games." I mean board games, card-games, ball-games, Olympic games, and so on. What is common to them all?...Look for example at board games....Now pass to card-games; here you find many correspondences with the first group, but many features drop out, and others appear. When we pass next to ball-games, much that is common is retained, but much is lost.—Are they all "amusing"? Compare chess with noughts and crosses. Or is there always winning and losing, or competition between players?...In ball games there is winning and losing; but when a child throws his ball at the wall and catches it again, this feature has disappeared....Think now of games like ring-a-ring-a-roses; here is the element of amusement, but how many other characteristic features have disappeared!...The result of this examination is: we see a complicated network of similarities overlapping and criss-crossing: sometimes overall similarities, sometimes similarities of detail....I can think of no better expression to characterize these similarities than "family resemblances." (Wittgenstein, 1958, pp. 31-32)

Characteristics of the Play Experience

Drawing from Wittgenstein's ideas, we can see that many of the efforts to define play involve an identification of the types of "family resemblances," or groups of related characteristics, that encompass the broad domain of play. Play has been described by various authors as voluntary or internally motivated, process oriented, fun or enjoyable, creative, not performed for a serious (survival-oriented) purpose, and characterized by tension and conflict (Apter & Kerr, 1991; Burghardt, 2005; Huizinga, 1950; Sutton-Smith, 1997). Not all activities that most people think of as play, however, share all of these characteristics. For example, we talk about playing chess, but this game, as well as many other games and sports, imposes strict rules that constrain the player's actions.

Intrinsic motivation is the feature of play that seems to be most often accepted across different theories and definitions of play that address human experience. This means that engagement in play is motivated by the experience of the play itself, not by the promise of rewards that are external to the play (Rubin, Fein, & Vandenberg, 1983). In the play literature the adjective "autotelic" is sometimes used to refer to this quality. This term originates in the Greek words for self (*aut*) and goal (*telos*) and thus conveys that the goal of playing is the play itself.

An idea related to intrinsic motivation is that play emphasizes the *process*, rather than the product, of doing (Caillois, 1961). The term "process flexibility" has been used to emphasize how, in play, the player interacts flexibly with objects, coming up with his or her own ideas for actions, instead of objects' directing the actions that the player will do (Clark & Miller, 1998).

Another criterion of play that seems closely related to intrinsic motivation is *free choice* (Johnson, Christie, & Yawkey, 1999). An activity that is play is chosen freely by the person. In this view, if the activity is performed because it is required or expected by someone else, it is work rather than play.

Enjoyment or pleasure, associated with positive affect, is also often considered one of the defining features of play (Clark & Miller, 1998). Positive affect is not always apparent, however, particularly if the activity requires the player's concentrated attention. Moreover, a variety of emotions, including fear and anxiety, may occur and change during a play session (Sutton-Smith, 2003). For these reasons Burghardt (2005) does not consider positive affect to be a defining criterion of play.

Scholars often disagree on the roles of other features in defining play. Some writers emphasize that play is characterized by self-imposed goals that can change at the whim of the player and therefore carries an element of *spontaneity*. In this view the focus on the *means* of the behavior rather than its ends demarcates play from other intrinsically motivated behaviors with specific, often externally imposed goals, such as work (Rubin et al., 1983).

Another popular concept is that play involves *active engagement*. This factor discriminates between play and passive states of inactivity and boredom. It begs the question, however, of whether daydreaming is a form of play (Sutton-Smith, 1997). It can be argued that this is the case, because in daydreaming a person plays with ideas.

Authors who study the biological aspects of play, particularly in nonhuman animals, often describe play as *noninstrumental*, or not serious. In play, the organism seems to be "fooling around" in ways that under serious conditions would support survival- and reproduction-related goals, such as hunting, fleeing a predator, fighting an enemy or competitor, finding food, or having sexual intercourse. For example, domestic dogs often engage in play fighting, which resembles real fighting but without the serious bites that would cause real injury. A cat might pounce on a toy as if hunting, but instead of trying to eat it, in play the cat might repeatedly fling and catch it. Objects are treated as if they were something else, so play has a pretend quality that distinguishes it from serious behaviors that directly support survival of the organism or species. This concept, when applied to children's play, has been called *nonliterality* and is characteristic of the pretend and sociodramatic play that is prevalent in early childhood (Clark & Miller, 1998).

Taxonomies of Observed Play Behavior

Human play, at its core, is thought to involve experiential characteristics that are not directly observable, such as intrinsic motivation, enjoyment, and active engagement. Performing a clinical assessment of play, or conducting research on play, however, may require that the clinician or researcher make inferences about play based on observations of behavior. To this end, a number of clinicians and scholars have developed observational systems and taxonomies. In this text the Knox Preschool Play Scale (Chapter 3) and Bundy's Test of Playfulness (Chapter 4) are two examples of clinical instruments that use observations of child behavior to draw inferences about the state of the child's play development or playfulness.

One of the best-known taxonomies of children's play behavior is Piaget's (1962) description of play as a developmental sequence of three stages: (1) practice games, (2) symbolic games, and (3) games with rules. Other theorists have defined "play" in terms of categories of behavior, such as play with language, play with motion and interaction, and play with objects (Garvey, 1990), or categories of social interaction, such as onlooker, solitary independent play, parallel play, associative play, and cooperative play (Parten, 1932).

Taxonomies of play are useful because they provide criteria to guide observations of behaviors that often are indicators of play; they lead to the development of narrower categories of play that may be easier to observe, describe, and explain; and they lend themselves to developmental explanations that may be obscured by a focus on psychological dispositions of play (Rubin et al., 1983). It should be remembered, however, that taxonomies often rely on observable behaviors, which ignores the person's experience. This is a problem because an activity that one person experiences as play may be experienced by another person as work or even drudgery. Furthermore, when categories are narrowed to easily documented, observable behaviors (e.g., patterns of manual manipulation or social interaction), the essence of play may be lost, even as the observer gains more detailed knowledge of the particular behaviors examined.

Contexts of Play

The context in which an activity occurs powerfully influences whether the person doing the activity experiences it as play. As noted earlier, a specific activity may be perceived by one person as play, whereas another perceives it as work or obligation. These differences in experience are related to the contexts of the time and place of the activity, the individual's life history, and the larger culture in which the person lives. Consider the activity of playing basketball: a weekend warrior may think of this occupation as enjoyable and lighthearted physical and social play, whereas a professional basketball player who is performing under pressure may see it as obligatory work.

Biologists who study nonhuman animal behavior have identified contexts that are critical to play across many species. These include the provision of a safe environment (physically, socially, and emotionally); the availability of a variety of interesting objects, materials, activities, or other organisms with which to interact; the freedom of choice to play or not, and social sanctions that communicate "This is play" via cues from the environment, especially when the cues come from other animals. Animal research has also shown that play behavior diminishes or does not appear when an animal is fatigued, sick, threatened, or otherwise stressed (Burghardt, 2005) (Figure 1-2).

In clinical practice, a therapist must consider how the context affects the person's experience and performance of an occupation. Although an activity may be classified as "play" in a given culture, this does not mean that every person within the culture experiences the characteristics of play when engaging in that activity. The therapist must analyze the extent to which the activity provides a play experience for the person engaging in it. This involves considering not only the cultural sanctions for the activity as play, but also the person's history with the activity, his or her reasons for doing it, the immediate physical and social contexts in which it is to be done, and the person's perception of safety and well-being when doing it.

Is a Definition of Play Always Necessary?

Why has so much effort gone into attempts to define play? Scholars have devoted a great deal of attention to the definitional problem because, when a concept becomes an object of study, it must be defined clearly enough to enable researchers and consumers of research to agree that they are talking about the same thing (Garvey, 1990; Reynolds, 1971). Furthermore, from the viewpoint of traditional science, precise definitions are desirable because they enable precise measurement, which in turn can be used in research to explore the nature of the phenomenon and its relationships with other phenomena (Reynolds, 1971). According to this reasoning, a good definition of play should enable therapists to develop a good test or

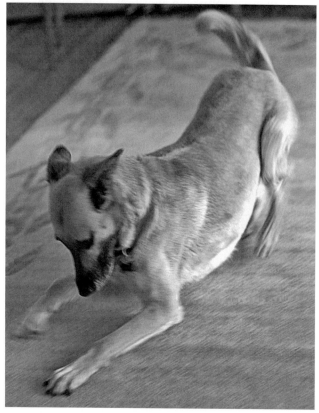

Figure 1-2
Play occurs in an environment that the organism perceives as safe and nonthreatening. This common posture among dogs, called the play bow, signals "Let's play!" The play bow is an example of Bateson's concept of metacommunication. (Courtesy Shay McAtee.)

evaluation of play, which in turn would enable them to do research examining the relationship between play and other capacities or outcomes, such as problem-solving ability or adaptive skills. Despite the many definitions of play that have been generated by scholars over the years, however, no specific definition of play has gained widespread acceptance. As Rubin and associates (1983) point out, no single approach "adequately encompasses the range of plausible perspectives that continue to be germane to an intuitive meaning of play" (p. 698).

The inability to settle on a precise definition of play has led some scientists to abandon the quest to study play in favor of more easily defined constructs (Berlyne, 1969). Experts in the field of occupational therapy, however, have not given up play as a topic worthy of study. Intuitively, play seems to be an important aspect of human experience that is deserving of study. Historically, play has been considered to be so significant to the profession of occupational therapy that it (along with the term "leisure," often used interchangeably with "play") is one of the major categories in taxonomies of occupation or occupational performance that have been generated by occupational therapists (e.g., American Occupational Therapy Association, 2002; Christiansen, 1991; Clark et al., 1991; Kielhofner, 2002; Meyer, 1922; Reilly, 1969; Yerxa et al., 1989). Moreover, from a pragmatic standpoint, play is a powerful concept when applied in clinical practice, and usefulness in the context of practice is crucial in assessing the value of a concept or theory (Hoshmand & Polkinghorne, 1992).

It is interesting to note that Wittgenstein, in his analysis of the problem of definition, asserted that drawing the boundaries of a concept was not necessary for it to be useful in a pragmatic sense: "We can draw a boundary—for a special purpose. Does it take that to make the concept usable? Not at all! (Except for that special purpose.)" (1958, p. 33). This stance leads to the conclusion that, although precise definitions of play may be appropriate for the specific purposes of particular research programs, a concise, all-purpose definition of play to suit the diverse needs of the entire profession may not be necessary, possible, or even desirable.

The complexity of the play concept led Mary Reilly (1974), a prominent occupational therapy theorist, to describe it as a cobweb, an image that evokes Wittgenstein's notion of a "complicated network of similarities overlapping and criss-crossing" (1958, p. 32). Rather than submit to pressures from the scientific community to atomize play into subcomponents that could be easily studied or to compromise its essence by reducing it to an easily operationalized definition, Reilly chose to synthesize a vast terrain of multidisciplinary literature on play to cultivate a full appreciation of its meanings and potential clinical applications. An overview of this literature is presented next to give the reader a background on the diverse theoretical views that have contributed to therapists' understanding of play.

EXPLANATIONS OF PLAY

Many theories of play have been proposed, each contributing its own explanation of play. This chapter reviews some of the most influential theories that are relevant to occupational therapy. Discussed first are classical theories, which originated in the late nineteenth and early twentieth centuries, followed by contemporary theories, which emerged and developed from the mid–twentieth century to the present time.

Classical Theories of Play

This review examines four well-known classical theories: (1) the surplus energy theory (Spencer, 1878/1978), (2) the recreation (Lazarus, 1883) or relaxation theory (Patrick, 1916), (3) the preexercise theory (Groos, 1898/1978), and (4) the recapitulation theory (Hall,

---

Box 1-2 *Exercise 2: Embedded Theories*

Reread the first sentence of this chapter, which is a quotation from an article by Norma Alessandrini (1949). The rudiments of at least two different classical theories of play are implicit in this statement. Which two are they? The core ideas of the classical theories of play seem to be part of the "folk wisdom" of our culture and are often embedded in the offhand comments that people (especially parents) make about children's play, such as, "He needs to go outside and blow off some steam." Can you think of one or two other examples of such comments?

1908/1978). After learning about these four theories, the reader should try Exercise 2 in Box 1-2.

Surplus Energy Theory

The surplus energy theory (sometimes called the Schiller-Spencer theory) is one of the first attempts to explain why play occurs. An early version of this theory was developed by Schiller (1795/1967), an eighteenth-century poet, who related play to the essence of life and beauty (Burghardt, 2005). A more refined version of the theory was developed by Spencer (1878/1978), a nineteenth-century psychologist. The basic idea behind the surplus energy theory is much older, however; it can be traced back to the Aristotelian concept of catharsis (Mellou, 1994). According to this theory, play is a prominent behavior among the young of a species because it results from their surplus energy. Since the young of a species depend on caregivers for maintenance and preservation and do not have to expend energy on these functions, they possess an excess of energy that must be expelled, so they play. In addition, play is more characteristic of "higher" animals because they have more efficient survival strategies than those of lower animals and therefore they have surplus energy available for nonessential activities. The surplus energy theory attempts to explain where the energy in children's play originates, but it has been criticized because it does not explain why children choose to play in the many different ways that they do (Slobin, 1964).

Recreation or Relaxation Theory

In direct contrast to the surplus energy theory stands the recreation or relaxation theory. This theory postulates that play derives not from a surplus of energy but from a deficit of energy. The purpose of play is to replenish spent energy. Play is most likely to be seen in childhood because fatigue builds up in the child in response to energy expenditures in unfamiliar and relatively new tasks (Gilmore, 1971). Lazarus (1883) viewed play as a recreational activity that restores energy, whereas Patrick (1916) saw play as an opportunity for relaxation. Lazarus and Patrick believed that play has no cognitive content or function. Similar to the surplus energy theory of play, the recreation or relaxation theory does not consider the content of play; it simply states that play occurs (Slobin, 1964).

Preexercise Theory

The preexercise theory views play as an instinctive behavior. Play emerges from instincts and exercises these instincts in preparation for their serious use in the future. According to Groos (1898/1978), childhood is a period of immaturity, the purpose of which is to provide the opportunity for instinctive behaviors to be refined into the mature behaviors that are required in adult life. Play is the primary vehicle in which this refinement of instinctive behavior occurs. Groos theorized that the length of the period of immaturity varies according to the complexity of the organism and its place on the phylogenetic scale. As organisms became increasingly complex on an evolutionary scale, longer periods of immaturity were needed for them to practice the complex skills that would be required for survival at maturity. As a result, play is a more prominent behavior among the young of the more complex species. Thus Groos believed that play serves an adaptive purpose in the evolutionary process.

Groos's ideas have been very influential among play theorists throughout the twentieth century to the present. For example, Vandenberg (1978) has continued Groos's line of thinking about the evolutionary function of play. His view is that, with increased complexity along the phylogenetic scale, the young of the species are not born with the skills that will be necessary to survive and flourish in adulthood. They need to construct the adaptive skills they will require throughout life, and they accomplish this in play. Vandenberg (1978) used the term "constructive adaptation" to explain how phylogenetically higher species construct the skills they need to adapt to the environment. As discussed later in the chapter, theorists about play have recently expanded upon this view (Burghardt, 2005).

Recapitulation Theory

The recapitulation theory of play also views play as a product of an evolutionary biological process (Hall, 1908/1978). This theory differs dramatically, however, from the preexercise theory; instead of claiming that play allows the organism to prepare for future demands of life, it posits that play is a carryover of behaviors that were critical for survival in the evolutionary past but are no longer important. The word "recapitulation" captures the idea that the ontogeny of the child reenacts the phylogeny of the human species. In other words, the development of the individual human being follows the evolutionary history of the entire human species. Thus children's play passes through developmental stages of the human race in an evolutionary sequence. According

to the recapitulation theory of Hall (1908/1978), no new skills or abilities can emerge in play because play consists of remnants of the evolutionary past.

Contemporary Theories of Play

The classical theories of play provide a foundation for modern theories of play, which address both the causes and the functions of play. For the purposes of this book, contemporary theories of play are grouped into the following categories: (1) biological, (2) psychodynamic, (3) cognitive developmental, and (4) sociocultural.

Biological Theories of Play
Evolutionary Biology of Play

Why do animals play (Figure 1-3)? This puzzle has intrigued philosophers, biologists, and psychologists for as long as these disciplines have existed. In fact, all of the classical theories of play reviewed previously in this chapter address nonhuman as well as human play, and all of them speak to biological reasons for play, such as energy regulation, ontogeny, and evolutionary function.

Understanding the biology of animal play is an interdisciplinary problem. Burghardt (2005), a biologist and psychologist, recently produced an authoritative volume that has taken a significant step toward solving that problem. He integrated an enormous body of multidisciplinary theory and research on animal (including human) play, culminating in a new synthesis of the whats, whys, and hows of play across many species. In contrast to more traditional animal behavior scholars, Burghardt argued and presented evidence that the primary elements of play are observable not only in mammals, which are famous for their playfulness, but also in birds, in some reptiles and fish, and perhaps (most controversially) even in some insects.

Burghardt specified five required criteria for identifying play across species (including humans):

1. Limited immediate function (includes elements that do not contribute to current survival)
2. Endogenous component (spontaneous, intentional, voluntary, pleasurable, or autotelic)
3. Structural or temporal difference (exaggerated, out of context, fragmented, or incomplete action sequence)
4. Repeated performance (repeated form of action, but not rigidly stereotyped)
5. Relaxed field (occurs when animal is fed, healthy, and free from external threats)

Burghardt (2005) described play as both a product and a cause of evolutionary change. In other words, play involves remnants of prior evolutionary events, but it can also lead to enhanced and even new functions. In this regard Burghardt's orientation resembles an updating and blending of the old surplus energy, preexercise, and recapitulation theories of play. He proposed a "surplus

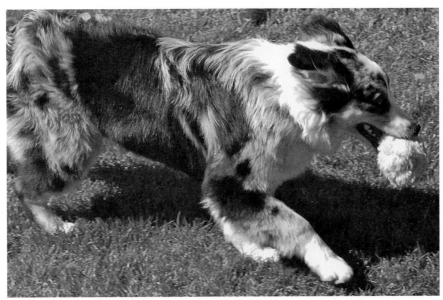

Figure 1-3

The dog's behavior meets Burghardt's criteria for play: (1) not needed for survival; (2) intentional; (3) out of context and fragmented behavioral sequence compared to "serious" activity, which in this case would be hunting and catching prey; (4) repeated form, but not rigidly stereotyped; and (5) occurring in a relaxed, nonthreatening context of well-being. (Courtesy Shay McAtee.)

resource theory" of play (Burghardt, 1984, 2005), in which animal play (including human) is most prevalent when resources exceed the organism's basic needs for survival and physiological, motivational, psychosocial, and ecological systems are favorable for play. Burghardt's theoretical model depicts four main factors that maximize playfulness in a species: energetics (including high metabolic rate and nutritious diet), ecology (e.g., complex habitat, low predation risk, and appropriate climate for the species), psychology and sociality (e.g., need for stimulation to support arousal, diverse motivational resources, flexible social system, and peer availability), and ontogeny (e.g., born immature, long juvenile period, extensive parental care, need for practice and learning).

Burghardt (2005) proposed a hierarchy of three evolutionary types of play: primary, secondary, and tertiary process. Primary process play is most characteristic of animals that rarely play or play at a very simple level, but it may also be seen occasionally in more complex animals, including humans. Play at this level is a side effect of factors that are not inherently related to play, as in conditions where there is excess metabolic energy, or where deprivation conditions lead to lowered thresholds for stimulation. In secondary process play, play actively contributes to the maintenance, refinement, or development of physiological and behavioral capacities such as neural processing, physical fitness, perceptual-motor coordination, and behavioral flexibility. At the tertiary process

Table 1-1
Biological Functions of Play

General Function	*Specific Capacity*
Maintenance	Neural processing
	Behavioral flexibility
	Physical fitness
	Perceptual and motor coordination
Generativity	Neural and behavioral development
	Transformation of physical to mental activity
	Reorganization of behavior patterns
	Social success
	Novel behavior and creativity

Modified from Burghardt, G. M. (2005). *The genesis of animal play.* Cambridge, MA: M. I. T. Press.

level, play becomes a major factor in the generation of new or enhanced abilities. At this level, creativity and innovations emerge from play. The functions of the secondary and tertiary process levels are probably those most relevant to occupational therapy, since they address how play influences adaptation to changing environmental demands. The adaptive functions of play at these levels, as described by Burghardt (2005), are summarized in Table 1-1.

The concept of tertiary play is consistent with Sutton-Smith's (1997) proposal that a primary function of play is adaptive variability. This concept builds on Stephen Jay Gould's (1996) assertion that optimal adaptation involves quirkiness, redundancy, and flexibility. Sutton-Smith suggested that, because play is characterized structurally by these same qualities, a primary biological function of play is to maximize adaptation by maintaining variability in brain functions, as well as behavioral patterns.

Occupational therapists may be especially interested in the association of play with neural processes. Burghardt (2005) suggested that play may be one of the routes through which enriched environments enhance neural development in the brains of many species. This idea is consistent with the findings of Byers and Walker (1995), who proposed that locomotor play functions to support synaptic development in the cerebellum. Their research shows that, across several mammalian species, locomotor play (such as jumping and chasing) begins and peaks in juveniles at the same time that cerebellar synaptic growth peaks.

Interestingly, play does not seem to require that an animal have a neocortex. Grandin and Johnson (2005) suggested that the more dominant the frontal lobes, the more "serious" and less playful the person or animal. They reported anecdotally that parents of children with attention deficit hyperactivity disorder complain that their children lose too much playfulness when taking stimulant medications such as Ritalin, which activates frontal lobe functioning, and that young animals given stimulants also show a reduction in play behavior.

Play seems to be closely tied to the basal ganglia and limbic system, which are the brain systems strongly associated with motivation, activation, and emotion-laden instinctive behavior (Burghardt, 2001). Animal research has shown that the amygdala may be especially critical in social play. The limited animal research on neurotransmitters suggests that dopamine, which is concentrated in the basal ganglia and related structures, is the primary neurotransmitter involved in play (Burghardt, 2005). Dopamine is associated with reward, pleasure, arousal, and motor patterning of motivated behavior. Siviy (1998) suggested that dopamine may be involved in the initiation of play and that increased noradrenergic and opioid activity probably supports focused attention and pleasure during play, while serotonin levels must stay low to sustain play. These neurotransmitters also play a special role in current theories of arousal modulation and play, which are discussed next.

Arousal Modulation

As noted in the preceding discussion of the biology of play, one of the psychosocial factors thought to maximize playfulness is having a nervous system that needs stimulation to support arousal. Over the past two decades, occupational therapists have been increasingly interested in arousal modulation as a critical function for adaptive behavior and have incorporated arousal modulation theories into clinical practice (e.g., Miller, Wilbarger, Stackhouse, Trunnell, & Hanft, 2002; Williams & Shellenberg, 1996).

Arousal modulation theories of play originated in the discipline of psychology. They initially were proposed to account for problems that arose in the drive theories of learning. According to drive theories, play and exploration were seen as secondary to behaviors that serve to reduce basic drives, such as those aimed at reducing hunger, cold, or thirst (Rubin et al., 1983). Research demonstrated, however, that animals would exhibit exploratory or play behaviors in place of drive-reducing behaviors even when the drives were assumed to be strong. For example, rats were observed to explore new features of their environment first before satisfying their hunger (Berlyne, 1966). Findings such as these led researchers to distinguish between external and internal motivation.

Berlyne (1969) developed a theory of intrinsic motivation in which play was associated with exploration and explained in terms of its role in the modulation of arousal states within an organism. In his view, tissue needs, such as hunger, thirst, and sex, lead to externally motivated behavior but central nervous system functions are responsible for intrinsically motivated behavior (Berlyne, 1960, 1966). These self-motivated behaviors directly affect the level of arousal within the central nervous system. Early arousal modulation theories posited that the central nervous system of an organism tries to attain or maintain an optimal arousal level through its interactions with the environment (Berlyne, 1966; Ellis, 1973) According to these theories, when an organism is in a strange or unpredictable environment, it attempts to reduce its level of arousal through exploration of the specific source of arousal. In other words, when faced with novelty, discrepancy, or uncertainty, the organism carefully investigates the situation to reduce the high arousal level that is associated with anxiety. The resulting behaviors are called *specific* exploration (Berlyne, 1966) and are thought to be rewarded by consequent arousal reduction. In contrast, *diversive* exploration occurs when an organism is in a predictable, monotonous environment and consequently seeks out stimuli that have novel, discrepant, complex, or ambiguous properties, not out of curiosity but out of boredom. In diversive exploration the stimulus-seeking behaviors are thought to be rewarded by an increase in arousal (Berlyne, 1971). Building on Berlyne's work, Ellis (1973) reframed diversive exploration as the essence of play. His definition of play was "behavior that is motivated by the need to elevate the level of arousal towards the optimal" (1973, p. 110).

Hutt (1970) also acknowledged that the amount of novelty present in the environment affects the way the organism interacts with the environment. She differentiated between exploration and play in her research on child behavior. In her framework, exploration occurs in a novel situation and involves investigation of a new object or setting. Exploration is characterized by a relaxed, somewhat nonchalant attitude and positive affect. In play the child asks, "What can *I* do with this object?" (Hutt, 1970). Although Hutt (1970) advocated a formal conceptual distinction between exploration and play, this distinction is not always clear or meaningful in the ecology of children's everyday activities (Weisler & McCall, 1976). Nevertheless, it may be useful to remember that although play sometimes includes aspects of exploration, not all curiosity and exploration should be considered play (Burghardt, 2005).

For the past four decades, Zuckerman (1994), another arousal modulation researcher, has led a productive line of inquiry on sensation seeking that is relevant to understanding people's choices of play and leisure activities. His work originated in the classic arousal modulation theories and evolved into a complex model that links biological predispositions and environmental influences to a trait he calls sensation seeking. He defines this as "the seeking of varied, novel, complex, and intense sensations and experiences, and the willingness to take physical, social, legal, and financial risks for the sake of such experience" (Zuckerman, 1994, p. 27). Because he studies sensation seeking as a personality trait, Zuckerman is concerned with individual differences in activity preferences rather than transient changes in arousal in response to environmental stimuli. His review of research on sports indicates that people who are high sensation seekers engage in high-risk sports, such as scuba diving and downhill skiing, as well as body contact sports, more often than low sensation seekers. Furthermore, the data suggest that sensation seekers choose these activities not because they involve risk, but because they are likely to provide the strong arousal that is associated with intense and novel stimuli. Similar findings are apparent in relation to preferences for art, music, drug use, and eating: sensation seekers tend to prefer activities that involve intense, complex, and novel sensory experiences, as in enjoyment of complex abstract art, hard rock music, illegal polydrug use, and exotic or spicy food (Figure 1-4).

Zuckerman presents a strong argument that sensation seeking, combined with impulsivity and sociability traits, constitutes a temperament pattern that is about 40% to 60% genetic in origin. His most recent theoretical model suggests that sensation-seeking traits involve interactions among key neurotransmitters (specifically dopamine, norepinephrine, and serotonin) and that the activities of these neurotransmitters are regulated not only by inherited biological predispositions, but also by the sensation-seeking or -reducing behaviors of the individual. This body of research also indicates that developmental changes occur over adulthood, specifically a significant

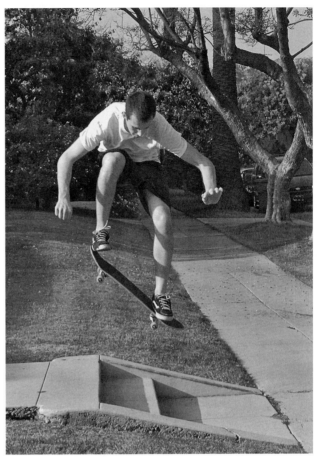

Figure 1-4
Sensation seekers enjoy varied novel, complex, and intense sensations and experiences and are willing to tolerate some degree of risk for such experience. Sensation seeking usually peaks in adolescence and young adulthood and gradually declines thereafter. (Courtesy Shay McAtee.)

reduction in sensation-seeking behavior from young to older adulthood. The research, however, has examined sensation seeking in age groups no younger than the late teens. If sensation seeking truly is an aspect of temperament, some indicators of this trait would be expected to appear in childhood. Perhaps future research will explore how arousal modulation associated with sensation seeking influences play style and play interests across childhood and adolescence. This might provide valuable knowledge to occupational therapists who are committed to supporting healthy lifestyles and preventing health-compromising events, such as accidents or drug abuse, among children and youth.

Psychodynamic Theories of Play
Although Freud (1961) did not develop an articulated theory of play, he referred to play many times throughout his work. Later theorists expanded on his work; therefore

his view of play has made a significant impact on theories of play, especially those that have attempted to explain the role of play in the emotional development of children (Rubin et al., 1983). Freud hypothesized that play serves two functions for children: (1) wish fulfillment, that is, the desire to be big, powerful, or simply in someone else's shoes; and (2) mastery of traumatic events, through which children could take an active role in a situation where they were previously passive victims (Gilmore, 1971; Rubin et al., 1983).

Erikson (1963) used the mastery component of Freud's theory of play to address ego development and the coping effects of play for children. In play, children create situations in which they can deal successfully with anxieties and uncertainty, leading to their ability to master reality. Erikson's work on the mastery aspect of play became the foundation for psychodynamically oriented play therapy, which traditionally is conducted by psychologists and psychiatrists. Through repetition of a traumatic event in play therapy, children with emotional difficulties become active agents with feelings of mastery rather than passive victims overwhelmed by anxiety and helplessness. Thus, by use of Freudian and Eriksonian concepts of mastery through play, children are encouraged in play therapy to "play out" their emotional problems just as adults may "talk out" their problems (Axline, 1969).

Cognitive Developmental Theories of Play

Cognitive developmental theories of play generally describe play as a voluntary activity in which children often interact with objects or toys that are under their control. Play is seen as a cognitive process and is believed to contribute to cognitive development, including problem solving and creativity (Sutton-Smith, 1980). The focus of these theories is usually on children's formation of and manipulation of concepts and symbols.

Play, Creativity, and Adaptation

Some cognitive theories of play emphasize its link to development of novelty and flexibility in human behavior (Rubin et al., 1983). Two theorists in particular, Sutton-Smith (1967) and Bruner (1972), have proposed that play provides a safe context in which ideas and behaviors can be combined in new ways. These new combinations may then be used in other contexts outside of play. In this manner, play contributes to human adaptation.

Sutton-Smith (1967) used the term "as if" to describe symbolic play in which the child uses something or someone "as if" it were something different. Children interact and play with sticks "as if" they are guns or with a sibling "as if" she or he is a cat. Through play, they combine ideas into new forms or alternative symbolic constructions (Rubin et al., 1983). Later on, in "serious," nonplay situations requiring problem solving, these alternative symbolic constructions may be called into action and thus

contribute to adaptation (Sutton-Smith, 1977). Consequences of the "as if" phenomenon for human development include divergent thinking (thought that breaks free from set and restricted modes), role flexibility and reversals, and feelings of autonomy.

In contrast to Sutton-Smith's focus on the manipulation of ideas within play, Bruner (1972) suggested that play provides an opportunity for new combinations of cognitively guided motor behaviors, particularly the manual and handling skills required for tool use. According to Bruner, play in childhood affords a pressure-free environment within which behavioral subroutines of complex skills required for adulthood may be combined and recombined in novel ways without concern for the result or goal of the actions. Children are free to attend to the means of their behavior, not its ends. This behavioral flexibility in play accounts for both children's and the human species' adaptation and development over time (Bruner, 1972).

Common to both Bruner's and Sutton-Smith's theories is the hypothesis that play develops behavioral innovation and flexibility, leading to enhanced problem solving and adaptation. Active experimentation in play results in formation of a repertoire of skills and behaviors needed for future creative and cognitive tasks. Thus these theories suggest that play prepares children for adulthood through its opportunity to generate novel and flexible thinking and behaviors (Mellou, 1994).

Cognitive Development and Play

Some of the best-known descriptions of play as a manifestation of cognitive development can be found in the work of Piaget (1951/1962). Piaget, however, was focused on the study of the emergence of intelligence, not on play per se. In his formal theory of intellectual development, play at its purest is considered to be an expression of the cognitive process of assimilation, that is, the interpreting of experience in light of existing mental structures. In this view play is not the origin of novel problem-solving efforts; rather it is a joyful exercising of existing cognitive abilities through action. The nature of play is viewed as different from imitation, in which actions and their underlying mental structures are modified to correspond to new experiences (a process called accommodation). Piaget's limited view of play contrasts with the theoretical orientation of Sutton-Smith (1967), who considered play to be a powerful vehicle for creative problem solving. According to Sutton-Smith, play is an important source of innovation in culture because of its creative potential, but Piaget's strict definition of play leads to the opposite conclusion, since innovative problem solving would not originate in play. In a well-known debate, Sutton-Smith (1966) challenged Piaget on this important point.

Piaget (1951/1962) discussed the development of play behavior through his classification of games, which has been very influential in shaping child development research. He described three types of games, corresponding to stages of cognitive development: practice games, symbolic games, and games with rules (Piaget, 1951/1962).

Practice games involve the doing of actions purely for the pleasure of practicing them, without elements of make-believe or socially shared rules. An example would be a child jumping into a puddle of water simply for the pleasure of jumping and experiencing the splash. This type of play dominates the first 2 years of infancy but also occurs throughout childhood, whenever new skills are acquired and practiced (Piaget, 1951/1962). The term "sensorimotor play" is often used to apply to this type of play because it is characterized by exploration of sensations and movements (Figure 1-5).

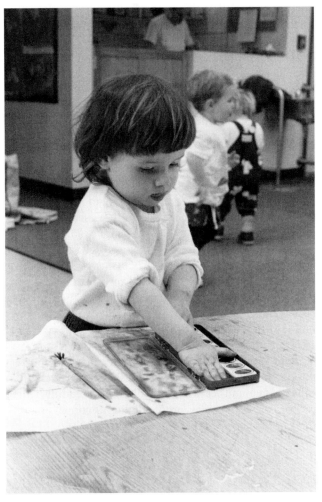

Figure 1-5

The child is exploring the tactile and visual sensations associated with paint, rather than trying to create a picture. This is usually called sensorimotor play. Piaget would call this activity a practice game, whereas Reilly would call it exploratory behavior. (Courtesy Shay McAtee.)

Symbolic games have an imaginative element because they involve make-believe or pretend play. An example would be a child feeding a doll with invisible food or with an object that represents food. Piaget believed that symbolic play is a significant milestone in cognitive development because it marks the child's ability to imagine objects and events that are not present, thus laying the groundwork for abstract problem solving and language development. The term "functional play" is sometimes used to refer to presymbolic games, in which the infant uses an object in a functionally appropriate way in relation to his or her own body (Largo & Howard, 1979), for example, raising an empty cup to the lips. This kind of play typically appears around 12 months of age and evolves into pretend actions directed toward a doll (e.g., giving the doll a drink). When pretend play involves an agent other than the self (e.g., the doll), the term "representational play" is often used (Largo & Howard, 1979), although this term is sometimes used more broadly to include functional play as well. In true symbolic play the child uses an unrealistic or invisible object in pretense, as in giving the doll a drink using a coin or using his or her empty hand as if it held a cup. Such symbolic play is typically seen by 24 months of age (Fein, 1981). Symbolic play becomes increasingly complex in the preschool years, with longer sequences of pretend behaviors evolving into dramatic scenarios with peers, a type of play known as "sociodramatic play."

Games with rules predominate in the play of 7- to 11-year-olds and continue to be a dominant mode of play throughout life (Piaget, 1951/1962). Piaget referred here to explicit rules that are socially constructed and abided by in the cooperative play of at least two individuals. Games with rules may be handed down, as is the case when children learn to participate in games such as jacks or dodgeball, or they may be invented spontaneously, as when a group of several children make up rules for playing with a new object. Piaget (1951/1962) felt that these types of games are important agents of socialization and that they replace functional and symbolic games, which essentially disappear in later childhood. This latter point contrasts with the viewpoints of such authors as Sutton-Smith (1966) and the Singers (Singer & Singer, 1990), who believed that symbolic play, in the form of imagination, does not disappear but goes "underground" in the form of internalized fantasy and plays a critical role in maintaining creativity and emotional health throughout life.

Development of Creativity in Play

Gardner (1982), like Piaget (1951/1962), examined childhood play in relation to cognitive development. Instead of focusing on the child's ability to solve problems or comply with rules, however, Gardner (1982) traced the unfolding of creativity and its expression through the arts.

In the first 2 years of life, children acquire direct knowledge about the physical world and, to some extent, the social world through the use of their senses and the consequences of their actions (Gardner, 1982). Thus their understanding of the world is dependent on their active involvement with the things, people, and space around them. Between the ages of 2 and 7 years, children's knowledge expands to include symbolic forms of information, including speech and language, hand and body gestures, music, numbers, and pictures. Children are now capable of understanding and communicating their experiences through use of the many symbols in their culture (Gardner, 1982). It is at this point in their development that children frequently combine these symbols in unique and striking ways.

Gardner (1982) referred to the preschool years as the "golden age of creativity" (p. 86). Children in this age group exhibit highly imaginative and inventive behaviors. In addition to designing intricate and fascinating structures out of play dough or blocks, preschool-age children create rich, colorful, and beautifully composed drawings and paintings. They sing and dance in a creative fashion. Even their language has a poetic quality (Gardner, 1982). Unfortunately, by elementary school age, children appear to lose this creative approach and their participation in artistic endeavors declines. At this point children have reached what Gardner called "the literal stage," a time of conformity and compliance with convention (1982, p. 88). Children at this age want to be like their peers. Their play is dominated by a desire to follow the rules and not to deviate from the norm. Similarly, their symbolic activities are often riddled with convention; they have little interest in novelty or experimentation. Drawings become copies rather than creations, and many children do not draw at all. The poetic language of the preschool years declines. Gardner believed that this stage of development is essential for development of artistic creativity because it is a time for mastery of rules. Although children may begin to understand and show an interest in artistic works of others in the literal stage of development, it is not until adolescence that a sensitivity to artistic qualities may reemerge.

Sociocultural Theories of Play

Sociocultural theories of play focus on the relationship of play with culture. Contemporary theorists think of play as having a reciprocal relationship with culture, meaning that it both influences and is influenced by culture (Roopnarine & Johnson, 1994).

First, play influences culture: Play contributes to the socialization and enculturation of children because it is the context for children's learning of social norms, values, roles, and behaviors (Schwartzman, 1978). Furthermore, human collective behavior is organized through play (Sutton-Smith, 1980). The Dutch historian Huizinga (1944/1950) went so far as to assert that play was the germinal element that gave rise to civilization itself.

Second, culture influences play: Culture is expressed or embodied in play (Roopnarine & Johnson, 1994). Play is both a type of communication and an interpretation of society (Sutton-Smith, 1980). As such, play mirrors or, indeed, parodies the socialization process of society (Schwartzman, 1978).

Play as Socialization

George Herbert Mead (1934) theorized that children learn social rules and norms through their play in games with other children. As they move between roles within a game, children's perspectives change. To participate in games with rules, each player must understand and be able to take on the perspective of the other players in addition to his or her own role. In so doing, each player is able "to predict what will happen next and adjust his [sic] behavior accordingly" (Slobin, 1964, p. 69). These changes in roles and perspectives lead to the development of a self-identity and of the concept of a "generalized other," that is, the perspective of the collective group. Through the process of developing an awareness of a "generalized other," the player learns social rules and norms that regulate the conduct of members of society (Mead, 1934). Self-identity is formed as the player compares his or her abilities with those of the other players (Slobin, 1964) and as social rules become internalized.

Mead's theory (1934) is an example of what Schwartzman (1978) called the "play as preparation or socialization" school of thought. This school of thought is based on functional analysis, which attempts to explain the stability of a culture or social system in terms of its parts or structures, which function to preserve the sameness of its whole. Thus certain structural systems within a society, such as kinship, religious, or economic systems, are thought to function as mechanisms to maintain the status quo. When functional analysis is extended to the play of children, their seemingly purposeless play becomes "transformed into activities functional for the maintenance and perpetuation of the social order" (Schwartzman, 1978, p. 100). For example, children playing house may be interpreted as imitating adults. In this view the purpose of play is to provide a context within which children can practice and learn socially appropriate adult behaviors or roles. Thus play, according to functional analysis, serves a socialization function. Some sociocultural theorists have challenged this view of play and have suggested that play may, in fact, be a form of communication (Schwartzman, 1978).

Play as Communication

Bateson (1972) was the first theorist to put forth the idea that play is a type of communication (Sutton-Smith, 1980). In the course of exploring the paradoxical and ambiguous nature of communication, he coined the term "metacommunication," that is, communication about communication, within play. The message "This is play," which is universally signaled by players before beginning to play, is a metacommunication (Bateson, 1972). Wrestling or physical fighting, when preceded by the signal "This is play," does not denote the same thing that it would had the play signal not been communicated. The view of play as communication does not separate play from reality; play and reality are related (Rubin et al., 1983; Sutton-Smith, 1980). In contrast to the "play as socialization" school of thought, play is not seen as an agent of socialization, developing skills needed for adulthood. Instead, play itself is the skill required to function within the real world of daily life (Sutton-Smith, 1980). Rather than learning about how to be a parent by taking on the role of a mommy or daddy in play, children are learning about how to frame or reframe roles themselves. Thus "they are not learning about a particular role, but about the concept of roles" (Rubin et al., 1983, p. 712) (Figure 1-6).

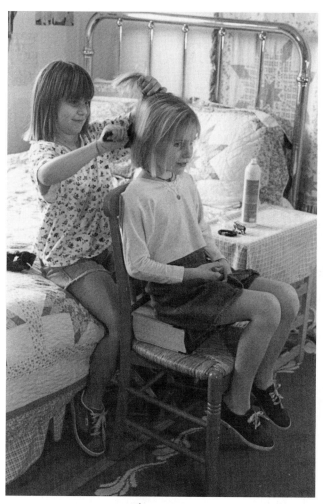

Figure 1-6
In playing beauty shop, these girls are playing with the concept of roles. (Courtesy Shay McAtee.)

Schwartzman (1978), among others, has elaborated on Bateson's notion of play as communication. Children's play frequently consists of parody, satire, or caricature that inverts or even subverts the current social order (Schwartzman, 1978). Many children's games mock and challenge society's authority and power structures in the form of parents, teachers, or police. Schwartzman suggests that, in their play, children may be questioning the assumptions of existing social roles and systems. Thus play, as a form of communication, reflects and interprets culture as seen through the eyes of a child (Sutton-Smith, 1980).

RHETORICS OF PLAY

The scope of play theories, as the preceding discussion demonstrates, covers wide territory and emanates from diverse fields of study, ranging from evolutionary biology to cultural anthropology. This poses a challenge to those who seek a more unified interdisciplinary discourse on play. Toward the end of the twentieth century, Brian Sutton-Smith (1997), an interdisciplinary scholar whose eminent academic career has focused on play, suggested that identifying the rhetorics behind play theories might lead to new insights on how to bridge the gaps between the various disciplines. Because occupational therapists are challenged to integrate knowledge about play from diverse fields of study—from neurobiology to anthropology to spirituality—Sutton-Smith's formulation of play rhetorics may provide a helpful guide to sorting out the myriad ways that play is discussed.

The term "rhetoric," as Sutton-Smith (1997) used it, refers to a "persuasive discourse" or "implicit narrative" employed to convey to others the correctness and value of the speaker's point of view. Rhetoric pervades ordinary conversations, as well as academic and professional ones. Often the speaker using a particular rhetoric is not aware of it and may not be consciously striving to persuade others to think in the same way. It could be viewed as the underground belief system that colors the way a person talks about something.

Sutton-Smith (1997) proposed that seven main cultural rhetorics underlie the assumptions and values that drive the prevalent discourses about play. These rhetorics may either covertly or overtly shape theories and interventions in regard to play. The seven rhetorics are described in the following sections, beginning with the most ancient, which emphasize community relationships, and ending with the modern, which focus on individual experience. The ancient rhetorics predate written history, whereas the modern rhetorics emerged over the past two centuries and perhaps are most evident in westernized cultures. The seven rhetorics overlap to some extent, yet have distinct features.

Ancient Rhetorics

Play as Fate

The rhetoric of play as fate is very old and rests on the assumption that human lives, including play, are controlled by external forces, such as destiny, gods, or luck. This rhetoric is prominent in gambling and games of chance (Figure 1-7). Although it is no longer a dominant rhetoric in Western cultures, it continues to be popular at a grassroots level.

Play as Power

Play as power is an ancient rhetoric applied most often to sports and contests. Play is depicted here as representing conflict and as a way to reinforce the power of those who control the play. The classic work of Huizinga (1944/1950), who defined the essence of play as agonistic, epitomizes this rhetoric (Figure 1-8).

Play as Community Identity

The rhetoric of play as community identity applies to community festivals and celebrations, which serve to reinforce or promote the identity of the participants with a particular group. This rhetoric often goes hand in glove with the rhetoric of power. An example is the festive atmosphere that often surrounds sports events and the way spectators often demonstrate strong identification with their team by wearing certain colors and chanting slogans.

Play as Frivolity

The frivolity rhetoric frames play as worthless and silly (Figure 1-9). In this rhetoric, play is nonsense, yet it may also carry power when it parodies conventional social structures. Cultural figures such as tricksters, jesters, and stand-up comics embody the frivolity rhetoric. They may be considered to be fools, but their foolish behavior often provides a commentary or critique of some established social order.

Modern Rhetorics

Play as Progress

Play as progress is a relatively new rhetoric that assumes that play promotes the development and adaptation of children and other young animals. Therefore, in this rhetoric, play is valued because it promotes progress in the individual's attainment of skills and capacities—not because play involves fun or enjoyment (Figure 1-10). Of the seven rhetorics, play as progress appears to be the most dominant in occupational therapy, particularly in pediatric practice. Therapists often speak of encouraging play to improve fine motor performance, develop social skills, or enhance abilities such as motor planning.

Play as the Imaginary

In the rhetoric of play as the imaginary, play is idealized as a wellspring of creativity manifested in forms such as literature, drama, and other arts. In this rhetorical stance,

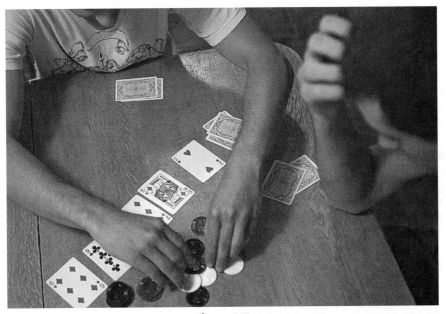

Figure 1-7
The ancient rhetoric of play as fate speaks to the dominance of luck or destiny in human life. Games of chance exemplify this rhetoric, for example, the myriad forms of gambling (as in playing cards or playing the horses). (Courtesy Shay McAtee.)

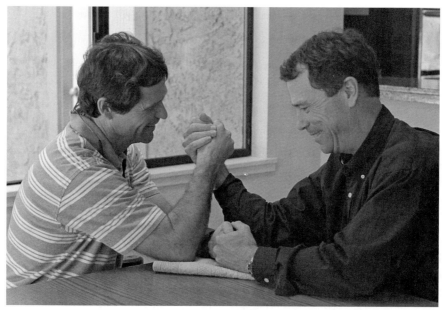

Figure 1-8

In the rhetoric of play as power, conflict or tension between opposing parties is the most salient feature of play. (Courtesy Shay McAtee.)

play has a lighthearted, spontaneous quality that involves imaginative and flexible improvisation. This rhetoric is historically aligned with the Romantic Movement that emerged in the late 1700s. It emphasizes the freedom and originality of the individual player.

Play as Self

The rhetoric of self is perhaps the most recent of the modern play rhetorics. It represents play as intrinsically motivated and desired by the player. Because the emphasis here is on the person's unique, individual experience, play is thought to contribute to the construction of the self (Figure 1-11). This rhetoric is evident in occupational therapy when play is used to support a person's construction or reconstruction of identity.

Rhetorics of Play in Occupational Therapy

Sutton-Smith's (1997) discussion of rhetorics may be useful to occupational therapists because it calls attention to the kinds of rhetorics that therapists habitually use unconsciously—or do not use—when thinking and talking about play. This leads to a consideration of whether there might be a valuable time or place for using alternative rhetorics.

For most American occupational therapists, it seems safe to assume that the most commonly used rhetorics are those of play as progress and play as self, used separately or together. For example, therapists commonly talk about developing motor or social skills through play (play as

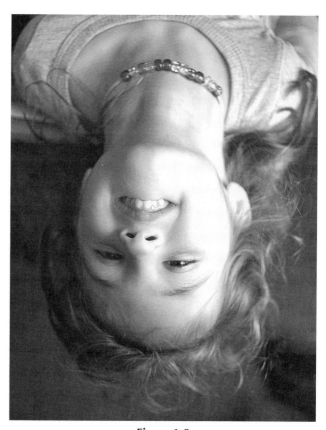

Figure 1-9

The rhetoric of frivolity frames play as silly and nonsensical—although such play may carry power when it parodies serious social conventions. (Courtesy Shay McAtee.)

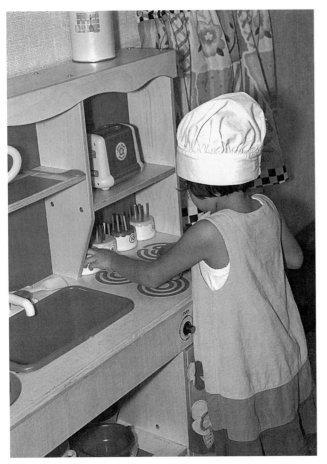

Figure 1-10

The rhetoric of progress might describe this child as developing fine motor, cognitive, language, and social skills through her sociodramatic play in this play kitchen. Progress is the most dominant rhetoric of play in occupational therapy, as well as other fields such as early childhood education and developmental psychology. (Courtesy Shay McAtee.)

progress) or encouraging a parent to let a child explore activities that he or she enjoys (play as self, usually linked to a "play as progress" rationale).

Therapists can then consider whether these rhetorics provide the best fit for the people they serve and for the profession itself. Many (perhaps most) American therapists may decide that progress and self are the most appropriate rhetorics for their clients and their profession, since these rhetorics convey values consistent with the dominant culture, that is, individualism expressed in the desire to "get better," to improve oneself, to be independent, and to invent or reinvent oneself. Other rhetorics, however, can assume an important role at times in occupational therapy, such as when a therapist is working with a person or culture that does not highly value individualism. For instance, the community identity rhetoric might be more powerful and appropriate for an individual to whom identification with a group is extremely important.

This discussion of rhetorics raises the question of whether occupational therapy should create its own rhetoric of play. Because occupational therapy is a health profession, it seems plausible that a rhetoric of play as health would be worth constructing. A well-developed rhetoric of play as health might, for instance, relate occupations experienced as play to a state of health characterized by vibrancy, optimism, and flexibility, regardless of the presence or absence of disability (Figure 1-12). Play, as an index of well-being, then becomes a quality of life issue. This rhetoric would also give rise to questions that could be examined in research in occupational science and occupational therapy, such as: What does play look like, and how is it experienced, as people engage in it? How does play relate to health? What aspects of health are affected by play? When is play the best way to promote health? How can we nurture play in others? What kinds of effects can we expect when play is part of an intervention?

Such a rhetoric of play as health may already be embedded in the occupational therapy literature. The next section examines this literature to trace the concept of play from the founding of the profession to current research.

PLAY IN THE EARLY HISTORY OF OCCUPATIONAL THERAPY

Occupational therapy's interest in play reaches back to the early years of the profession. Founders of occupational therapy in the United States viewed human beings in terms of their occupational nature, which encompassed a rhythmic temporal pattern and dynamic balance of work, rest, play, and sleep. Adolph Meyer (1922) referred to work, rest, play, and sleep as "the big four" rhythms that help shape the "whole of human organization" (p. 641) and that need to be balanced even under difficult circumstances for an individual to adapt to the demands of living in a complex social world. Meyer's philosophy of occupation was influential in the development of early occupational therapy programs for people with physical and psychosocial disabilities (Dunton, 1915; Kidner, 1931; Saunders, 1922; Slagle, 1922; Stevenson, 1932). Writers in the profession spoke of a play spirit that is essential for worthwhile living (Saunders, 1922; Slagle, 1922; Ziegler, 1924). These founders viewed play as a human trait that is as important to health as work.

During the founding years of the profession, play was a highly visible aspect of occupational therapy programming, especially in occupational therapy for children. The association of play with occupational therapy was so strong that the occupational therapist (who typically was a woman) might be called the "play lady" by the children with whom she worked (Whittier, 1922). Nevertheless,

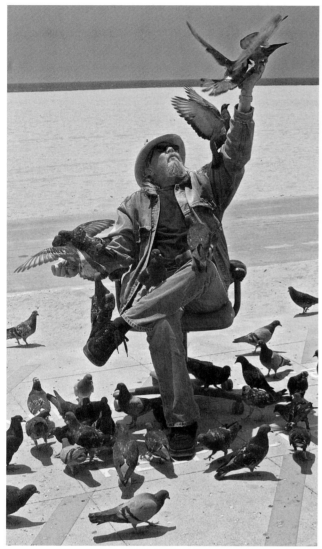

Figure 1-11
The rhetoric of play as self emphasizes the creation and expression of identity through intrinsically motivated and self-selected activities, which may be unique. (Courtesy Shay McAtee.)

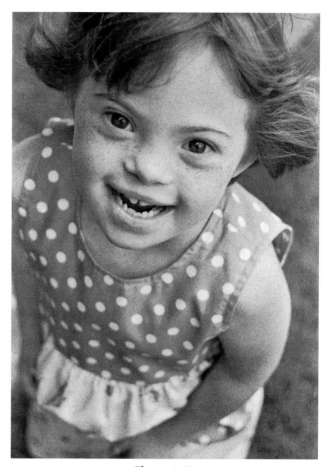

Figure 1-12
A rhetoric of play as health invokes such characteristics as vibrancy, optimism, and flexibility, regardless of whether a disability is present. (Courtesy Shay McAtee.)

putting Meyer's philosophy of occupation into practice in the first few decades of the profession was not a straightforward enterprise.

As Granoff (1995) has pointed out, the literature of the early twentieth century indicates a tremendous amount of inconsistency in how play was incorporated into treatment programs. Economic pressures strongly influenced programming. For example, patients who were capable of working were often placed in industrial settings, such as the laundry or book bindery, where they could make an economic contribution to the institution, whereas patients considered unable to work or produce salable goods were often encouraged to participate in recreation programs (Inch, 1936). Furthermore, it became apparent that the experience of the individual influenced whether a given occupation was play or work; this realization complicated the task of planning group work and play programs. It also became apparent that play and work could be viewed as overlapping constructs, rather than distinct entities, and thus could exist simultaneously in a given activity, making it difficult to evaluate and treat the "balance" of work, rest, and play. The therapeutic goals of play or recreational activities also varied from one setting to another. In some settings recreation was used to render patients more compliant and manageable (Ellis, 1934); in others it was used as a diversion, simply to make patients' lives more pleasant and to keep them busy (Hohman, 1938); and in yet other settings it was used for specific remedial or curative purposes (Slagle, 1934). These practice dilemmas involving economic pressures, conceptual ambiguity, and therapeutic goals in relation to play still confront contemporary practitioners.

Perhaps these pragmatic difficulties contributed to the fact that, by the mid–twentieth century, occupational therapy had drifted away from its original commitment to the occupational nature of its patients. Although the concept of play as occupation still appeared in the profession's literature (Alessandrini, 1949; Smith, 1958), play was eclipsed by more scientifically and technically oriented concerns. In the pediatric occupational therapy literature, such issues as neuromuscular techniques, handedness, adaptive equipment, specific motor and self-care skills, and sensory-perceptual functions became the dominant topics, with little or no reference to occupation (Abbott, 1950; Ayres, 1958; Derse, 1950; Grayson, 1948; Rood, 1956). This shift in focus, according to Kielhofner and Burke (1977), was the result of external pressures on occupational therapy to become more respectable through adoption of a scientific posture. As occupational therapy became more scientifically oriented, the identity of the occupational therapist as "play lady" became an embarrassment and, if still alive at all, was hidden away in the closet.

Mary Reilly is to be credited with bringing the concept of play back into focus as a topic worthy of study in occupational therapy. Her landmark book, *Play as Exploratory Learning* (1974), was the culmination of more than a decade of scholarship that sought to construct a comprehensive conceptual framework for the practice of occupational therapy. This framework was built on a concept called "occupational behavior," which linked play with work in a developmental continuum (Reilly, 1969). Under Reilly's leadership the play lady was taken out of the closet (Florey, 1971) and a new generation of leaders and scholars in the profession was inspired to reclaim play as a fundamental concept in occupational therapy practice and to make it an object of research. Because her work continues to be very influential in the profession today, her ideas are reviewed in more detail in the following section.

THE OCCUPATIONAL BEHAVIOR TRADITION

The occupational behavior frame of reference emerged in the 1960s under the leadership of Mary Reilly (1966, 1969). According to Reilly (1974), play is significant because it is intermeshed with the struggle for mastery within a person's environment, particularly the struggle of people with disabilities to develop skills and competency. The theme of the human struggle for mastery and achievement, regardless of individual circumstances, is a central tenet of the occupational behavior frame of reference. Play and work are viewed as the contexts in which mastery, achievement, and adaptation emerge (Reilly, 1969, 1974). Play in childhood is seen as the primary vehicle for the cultivation of skills, abilities, interests, and habits of competition and cooperation needed for competence in adulthood. Thus childhood play "is the antecedent preparation area for work" (Reilly, 1969, p. 302). Play in adulthood, in the form of recreational behavior, is interpreted as a support to adult work patterns. The entire developmental continuum of play and work is called "occupational behavior" (Reilly, 1969).

Reilly noted that clinical experience had indicated that play had "an organizing effect" on patients who were behaviorally incompetent or disorganized (1974, p. 9). With this clinical legacy in mind, she embarked on a quest to understand why and how play contributes to mastery.

Reilly's Systems Explanation of Play

Reilly (1974) acknowledged that play is complex and can be viewed from the perspective of many different disciplines. To begin to grasp the "cobweb" that is play, she used a general systems approach, integrating the literature on play from the fields of anthropology, evolutionary biology, psychology, and sociology. She chose a systems approach because it enabled her to organize isolated disciplinary constructs into a more comprehensive network of interrelated, hierarchically nested processes. For example, rather than interpreting play as purely a regulator of neurophysiological arousal mechanisms (Ellis, 1973) or as a manifestation of cognitive processes (Piaget, 1951/1962), she developed a view of play in which neurologically based arousal systems give rise to the emergence of cognitive-symbolic systems. She was convinced that play is a multidimensional phenomenon; therefore she advocated an interdisciplinary account of play as "a biosocial phenomenon" (Reilly, 1974, p. 122).

Rule Learning Through Play

Given her assumption that play has an organizing effect on behavior, Reilly believed that it must have an adaptive function. To explain how play serves adaptation, Reilly (1974) used the concept of rule learning. She hypothesized that play is a dimension of the imagination that culminates out of three hierarchical action systems: the neurological subsystem, the symbolization subsystem, and the language subsystem. At the lowest level of the hierarchy the central nervous system selectively takes in and organizes information from the environment. At the next level (the symbolization subsystem), sensory data are transformed into meaning in the form of symbols. These symbols provide a sort of shorthand for experiences, leading to the human capacity to think in a complex, yet economical, manner and to generalize from one situation to another. At the highest level of the hierarchy is the language subsystem. Reilly described the language subsystem as having diverse aspects, one of which deals with play. Play at this level entails the complex use of symbols derived from action on the environment. These action-related symbols are called "rules." Reilly used the term "rules" to refer to mental representations or symbols for how the world and the self operate. These rules, she hypothesized, are generated in play. Thus play deals with "reality problems" and is viewed as "processing or mastering reality" (Reilly, 1974, p. 145).

Through play, children learn sensorimotor rules, rules of objects and of people, and rules of thinking. Once rudimentary rules are generated, complex organizations of rules can be consolidated, and these give rise to the skills needed for the competency of the adult individual and the technology of society. Robinson (1977), one of Reilly's students, elaborated on this idea by describing a rule as a map of reality that guides actions. This is to say that a person's understanding of an object determines the way he or she interacts with it. For example, a ball is a thing that is spherical, and people's rules about spherical objects tell them that they can roll, kick, throw, and possibly bounce the ball, but they are not likely to have much success stacking it on top of another ball. Robinson called these simple rule-driven actions "subroutines" and further posited that subroutines are gradually linked together in a flexible series to form skills that are responsive to changing environmental conditions. For example, a child learning to play soccer would first need to know the rules about how balls work, as well as rules about how her or his body works. These would enable the child to generate subroutines of kicking and stopping the ball with her or his foot. Then, the child would combine these subroutines in a sequence and integrate them with other subroutines, for example, running and kicking at the same time. When the child begins to practice and combine these subroutines while playing with friends, she or he needs to integrate them with subroutines derived from rules of people, particularly those related to reciprocity and communication. Finally, the child would refine the skills of kicking, running and kicking, and stopping the ball while playing under varying conditions, such as with different team members or on different playing surfaces.

Reilly's Developmental Stages of Play

Drawing from Berlyne's work on arousal (Berlyne, 1960), Reilly (1974) linked play with an exploratory drive of curiosity and conflict. As a child interacts with the environment, conflict between the expected and the unexpected and between the known and the unknown arises. This conflict generates curiosity, which serves to energize and motivate play as the child searches for rules to understand how objects, people, ideas, and events work. Building on this idea, Robinson (1977) noted that the optimal situation for learning rules is a safe environment for play in which there is neither too much nor too little challenge: "The right challenge or conflict is necessary for the state of curiosity to exist that will support the individual's play and thus the generating of rules" (pp. 251-252).

According to Reilly, the exploratory drive of curiosity is expressed in three hierarchical stages of play development through which competencies emerge. The three stages occur progressively during childhood. The stages are (1) exploratory behavior, (2) competency behavior, and (3) achievement behavior.

Exploratory behavior occurs in infancy and early childhood play or in novel, unfamiliar situations. It arises from an interest in the environment, and its focus is on the means of behavior, not its ends (Reilly, 1974). Engagement in this behavior is intrinsically motivated. The emphasis is on sensory experience as children test the limits of reality in their search for rules. When children engage in exploratory behavior in a safe environment, hope and trust are generated.

Competency behavior is characterized by effectance motivation (Reilly, 1974), which is an inborn urge toward competence (White, 1959). Competence may be defined as the ability to meet adequately the demands of a particular situation (White, 1971). Effectance motivation produces feelings of efficacy and "joy in being a cause" (White, 1971, p. 273). Children's play in the form of competency behavior is driven by their need to interact with the environment, to have an effect on it, and to receive feedback from their actions on it (Reilly, 1974). The attitude of children engaged in this behavior is one of "I want to do it myself." They display intense concentration and persistence while involved in the activity. Through practice, mastery is achieved and self-confidence and self-reliance are generated (Reilly, 1974).

Achievement behavior is the third stage of play development and incorporates the learning of the first two stages. The concept of achievement is associated with expectations of success or failure and with criteria of winning or losing (Reilly, 1974). Performance is compared to some standard of excellence; achievement behavior is therefore seen as more extrinsically motivated than exploratory and competency behaviors. There is a competitive element here; children compete either with themselves or with others. Engagement in achievement behavior involves risk taking and strategizing with skills. During this stage the hope, trust, self-confidence, and self-reliance generated in the first stages are transformed into courage (Reilly, 1974).

Occupational Role of Player

"Occupational role" is a central organizing concept in the occupational behavior frame of reference. *Role* is conceived as "the expected pattern of behavior associated with occupancy of a distinctive position in society," whereas *occupational role* is the "activity in an individual's life that contributes to society, and thereby, defines the person's societal worth" (Heard, 1977, p. 244). These concepts, imported from the field of social psychology, tie occupational behavior to the individual's capacity to perform services to society and thus to survive economically in a technically complex world (Heard, 1977; Reilly, 1966). Occupations, from this perspective, are activities that fill economically based niches in society. Occupational roles change across the lifespan: An individual is transformed from player and preschooler to student, then to worker or homemaker, and finally to retiree. Each occupational role involves a set of expectations for behavior (Heard, 1977).

The primary occupational role of the infant and young child is that of player (Heard, 1977). The player role, like other occupational roles, comes with a set of expectations, for example, playing in the manner that is expected by caregivers at home or at preschool. Being a player is deemed a legitimate occupational role because it is through play that essential rules, skills, and habits are acquired for competence in later occupational roles (Burke, 1993; Heard, 1977; Robinson, 1977). The term "habit" refers here to skills that have become so routine that they are performed automatically, enabling the individual to attend to the novel demands of a task. Skills and habits generated in childhood play lay the groundwork for the individual's decisions regarding occupational choice in late adolescence or early adulthood (Shannon, 1974) and provide essential ingredients for success as an adult worker (Heard, 1977). Skills of decision making and risk taking are considered particularly important outcomes of play that will contribute to later occupational choice and work performance (Shannon, 1974). (At this point the reader should try the exercise in Box 1-3.)

The child's occupational role as player has been a focal point in the work of influential contemporary writers in occupational therapy. For example, Burke, Heard-Igi, and Kielhofner, all students of Reilly during the 1970s, collaborated to produce the first published version of the Model of Human Occupation, a frame of reference that is built on occupational behavior concepts and has gained considerable international attention in the occupational therapy profession (Kielhofner, Burke, & Igi, 1980). Occupational role is a guiding concept in the Model of Human Occupation, and the young child's major occupational roles are identified as player and family member (Kielhofner, 2002). Janice Burke (1993) describes the occupational role of player as a key construct in the application of occupational therapy assessment and treatment methods in early intervention. This view is discussed in Chapter 6 of this text, in which Burke collaborates with Roseann Schaaf and Brianna Lomba Hall to show how the therapist can use family narratives to construct a story of the child as player.

Cadre of Scholars on Play

Reilly guided many of her graduate students at the University of Southern California during the late 1960s and the 1970s to explore the topic of play in search of insights to guide occupational therapy practice. Thus she systematically developed a cadre of scholars who grappled with play as a form of occupational behavior. Many of these scholars wrote papers that became classic pieces in the occupational behavior literature, and many of their ideas continue to be influential in contemporary practice.

Linda Florey (1971), for example, proposed that the concept of intrinsic motivation be used as an organizing construct for the study of play. She noted that play is a learning process that occurs throughout every child's day; therefore occupational therapists need to attend to children's play outside, as well as inside, the boundaries of treatment programs. Florey (1971) also expressed concern for the potentially aversive effects of illness or disability on children's play: "a child with a reading disability may also have a 'playground disability' or a 'cub scout disability'" (p. 277). She urged occupational therapists to attend to these often overlooked, yet important, aspects of a child's play life. Over the years she has developed an impressive store of pragmatic knowledge regarding how to translate these ideas into practice. In Chapter 10 of this text, she and her colleague Sandra Greene describe the reasoning processes behind the use of play in treatment programs for very challenging children with psychiatric diagnoses.

Grounded in the assumption that play progresses in a predictable developmental fashion, Takata (1974) constructed a taxonomy of six developmental phases of childhood play, which she called "play epochs." These are described in Table 1-2. Takata's taxonomy differs from Reilly's stages of play in that it describes changes in the observable structure of children's play instead of changes in the underlying dynamics of play (Figure 1-13). Using her play epochs as a guide, Takata constructed a Play History instrument to be used as an assessment tool by occupational therapists. This tool was designed to help therapists develop a play diagnosis and play prescription for children with dysfunction. An updated perspective on the Play History is discussed by Kimberly Bryze in Chapter 2.

Another play assessment instrument, the Play Scale, was originally developed by Susan Knox (1974) under Reilly's guidance. The Knox Play Scale has been widely used as a research and clinical tool. Knox reviews the literature on this instrument, including the revised version that was introduced in the first edition of this book, in Chapter 3.

Another influential instrument, the Interest Checklist, was originally designed for use with adults by Janice Matsutsuyu (1969), also a student of Reilly. This instrument inspired many related assessment tools, especially by clinician scholars working with the Model of Human Occupation (MOHO), founded by Reilly's students Gary Kielhofner, Janice Burke, and Cynthia Heard Igi (1980). In Chapter 5 of this book, Alexis Henry presents the Pediatric Interest Profiles, an original group of instruments for clinical assessment of children that was influenced by the occupational behavior and MOHO traditions.

Box 1-3 *Exercise 3: Developing Skills Through Play*

Write down two activities that were favorite play occupations for you when you were a child. These may be the two occupations that you listed in Exercise 1 (Box 1-1) in this chapter. What skills did you develop in the course of practicing those play occupations? In what ways do you use those skills today in your work occupations?

Table 1-2
Takata's Play Epochs

Epoch	Age	Description
Sensorimotor	0-2	Purely autotelic play with sensations and motion in first 18 months: peekaboo, pat-a-cake, hide and chase, and imitation with caregivers; dropping objects; container play; exploration of object properties; practice of new motor skills; simple problem solving
Symbolic and simple constructive	2-4	Symbolic play: beginning make-believe and pretend play; experiences represented in play. Shift from solitary play to parallel play. Builds simple constructions that represent another object or situation. Climbing and running are honed.
Dramatic, complex constructive, and pregame	4-7	Expansion of social participation: shift from parallel to associative play; dramatic role play enacting child's daily experiences, social roles, and fairy tales and myths. Skill in activities requiring hand dexterity. Daredevil activities involving strength and skill outdoors. Constructions are realistic, complex. Verbal humor, creates rhymes.
Game	7-12	Games with rules: fascination with rules; masters established rules and makes up new ones; risk taking in games; concern with peer status; friendship groups important; interest in sports and formal groups (e.g., scouts); cooperative play. Interest in how things work, nature, crafts.
Recreational	12-16	Formal peer group orientation: teamwork and cooperation; respect for rules; games that challenge skills; competitive sports; service clubs. Realistic constructive projects and complex manual skills.

Modified from Takata, N. (1974). Play as a prescription. In M. Reilly (Ed.), *Play as exploratory learning* (pp. 209-246). Beverly Hills, CA: Sage Publications.
Ages are in years and are approximate. The terms "solitary," "parallel," "associative," and "cooperative" are from Parten (1932). Solitary, no peer interaction; parallel, side by side with peer but little or no interaction; associative, participates in group play with shared activity; cooperative, cooperates extensively with peers in highly organized activity.

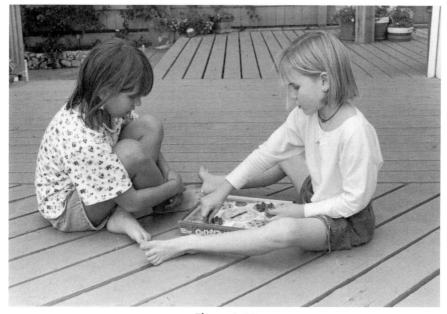

Figure 1-13
These girls are on the threshold of Takata's game epoch, which is dominated by what Piaget called games with rules. They are absorbed in the process of learning to abide by socially agreed upon rules. (Courtesy Shay McAtee.)

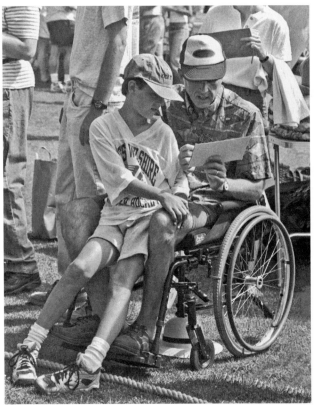

Figure 1-14
Play is an active ingredient of a healthy lifestyle, regardless of age. (Courtesy Shay McAtee.)

Others who were schooled in the occupational behavior perspective also developed instruments for assessing play. Readers interested in exploring these may find it useful to start with the integrative review provided by Florey (1981).

PLAY IN CONTEMPORARY OCCUPATIONAL THERAPY

In the occupational behavior tradition, play in childhood is deemed important because it prepares the child for the student role and, ultimately, for the adult worker role. In adulthood, leisure or recreation is important because it refreshes or prepares the person to return to work (Reilly, 1966). This position is what Parham (1996) has called a functionalist view: that play is important because it is an effective way to develop other functions, such as sensory integrative, motor, social, cognitive, self-care, or work skills. In other words, play is justifiable only because it is a means to an end.

Gaining momentum is an alternative view that play is a legitimate end in itself because it is a critical element of the human experience. Play therefore may be understood as a vehicle of meaning; it reveals what makes life worth living for an individual (Parham, 1996). From this perspective, play becomes a quality of life issue in the here and now. Play promotes health not only because it prepares a person for work at some later time (Reilly, 1969), but also because it is an active ingredient of a healthy lifestyle in the present (Ornstein & Sobel, 1989; Parham, 1996) (Figure 1-14). The exercise in Box 1-4 may help the reader to appreciate this aspect of play.

The valuing of play for its own sake does not preclude adopting a functionalist position; both stances make powerful contributions to clinical practice. It is likely that the functionalist view dominates occupational therapy practice because, by linking play to accepted school- and work-related outcomes, it may make play in therapy easier to justify economically. Acknowledgment that play is important in its own right, however, opens the door to intervention that makes enhancement of the child's play life the goal. This may turn out to be the most efficient way to influence child health in some circumstances.

The scholarship of Anita Bundy (1993) was one of the forces in the 1990s that reenergized research on play in occupational therapy for children and oriented the profession toward treating play as a goal, as well as a means, of therapy. She proposed that occupational therapists are unique in their perspective of play as an occupation. They use play as a tool to create therapeutic situations in which their clients can try out new behaviors and skills with fewer risks and consequences for failure than would normally exist in the clients' daily lives. Thus occupational therapists "make a living by creating 'play' and by enabling others to play" (Bundy, 1991, p. 48). She concluded that occupational therapists must form a precise definition of play simply because it is an important tool of intervention; play must be distinguished from nonplay. If occupational therapists truly believe that the conceptualization of play as an occupation makes a valuable contribution to play theory and research as well as to their clients' lives, they "must take play seriously" (Bundy, 1993, p. 221). Reliable and valid assessments of play must be developed, the process of integrating elements of play into interventions must be examined, and play must be promoted as an explicit and distinct goal of occupational therapy (Bundy, 1993).

With the objectives just described in mind, Bundy developed a model of playfulness (Bundy, 1991) and designed an ingenious assessment tool, the Test of Playfulness (ToP). These are discussed in Chapter 4, where Bundy and her colleague, Geva Skard, provide an overview of research and practice using the ToP to assess a child's playfulness.

Although the work of Bundy was well received in the profession, the assessment and intervention practices actually carried out by occupational therapists in clinical settings continued to reflect a strongly functionalist orientation through the 1990s. In a questionnaire survey of 224 American occupational therapists working clinically with preschoolers (Couch, Deitz, & Kanny, 1998), 91% of respondents indicated that play was very important in motivating a child to participate in therapy and 92% responded that they used play as a means to elicit motor, sensory, or psychosocial outcomes. Only 2%, however, stated that their predominant use of play was as an outcome in itself. Practice setting seemed to be an important factor in whether the therapist performed clinical assessments of play: only 54% of school-based respondents assessed play behaviors, whereas 79% of non-school-based respondents did so. This was probably related to the different roles of occupational therapists in school versus nonschool work settings. The authors of this study speculated that perhaps occupational therapists in school settings relinquish play to other team members and focus their intervention efforts on performance areas such as gross and fine motor skills. Outside of school settings, it is likely that third-party reimbursement and the necessity of medical prescriptions may limit therapists' use of play as an outcome of intervention.

Readers should keep in mind that the study by Couch and associates (1998) was completed about the same time that the first edition of this book was published. In the Couch study, respondents' first year of registration as an occupational therapist ranged from 1957 to 1994. It would be interesting to examine whether any changes have transpired in occupational therapy practices in regard to play with young children since the late 1990s, and what sociopolitical as well as professional trends may be influencing the apparent changes or lack of change.

One potentially powerful influence on practice was the adoption of the Occupational Therapy Practice Framework (OTPF) by the American Occupational Therapy Association (2002). In the OTPF, play is one of seven overarching areas of occupation that are addressed by occupational therapists in practice. In addition, the OTPF specifies that "engagement in occupation to support participation" is the overarching outcome of the occupational therapy process (AOTA, 2002, p. 615). This would imply that, when working with young children, occupational therapists should address play not only as a means to attain therapeutic goals, but also as a primary outcome area. The inclusion of "participation" in this dictum suggests that a primary concern would be the child's engagement in play within the contexts of home, school, and community life.

Time will tell whether the practices of clinicians will eventually shift to address play as both means and ends of occupational therapy for children. Undoubtedly a knowledge base is needed to support the development of play interventions that will serve public health needs. Such development requires knowledge of what play looks like in everyday contexts (including the presence of a disability), of the relationship of play to health and well-being, and of the effectiveness of occupational therapy using play, whether it is a means or a goal of intervention.

The final sections of this chapter survey several key areas of knowledge that may inform and transform the use of play in occupational therapy practice, including evidence-based practice. The chapter concludes with a discussion of play as an occupational justice issue.

Play as Occupation

Play as occupation is a theme on which divergent theorists and clinicians in occupational therapy have been converging over the past two decades. Play is valued as a major class of occupations in which people engage throughout the course of their lives (Christiansen, 1991; Kielhofner, 2002; Primeau, Clark, & Pierce, 1989; Yerxa et al., 1989).

Occupational science is an academic discipline that was designed to generate knowledge about occupation for use by occupational therapists (Clark et al., 1991). This discipline is intended not only to provide a knowledge base for existing practice, but also to lead to innovative clinical practice. By illuminating the nature of occupation and how it influences health, occupational science is expected to stimulate new ideas for intervention (Wood, 1996; Yerxa et al., 1989).

It is important to note that occupation is the central construct for study in occupational science. It is also important to realize that the study of occupation needs an interdisciplinary perspective. A full understanding of occupation requires the integration of knowledge from many disciplines, such as philosophy, biology, psychology, sociology, and anthropology, to produce a new synthesis of knowledge about occupation (Clark et al., 1991;

Yerxa et al., 1989). Therefore the study of play in occupational science requires an interdisciplinary orientation.

A promising strategy for studying occupation is to make it the primary unit of analysis in research (Parham, 1995). In other words, if therapists want to understand play as occupation, they need to study play directly as it occurs in context. This approach differs from more traditional research on play, in which it is assumed that the study of isolated performance skills, such as cognitive, motor, or social skills, will lead to an understanding of occupation. Studying performance skills may be valuable, but at some point it becomes necessary to reframe isolated skills and integrate them into a broader knowledge base that is focused at the level of occupational engagement. One important research strategy toward this goal is to build a rich body of descriptive research on play as it occurs in natural contexts.

The following sections examine several topics that are particularly germane to the study of play as occupation and to the practice of occupational therapists: description of patterns of play in natural settings, play in relation to disability, and play as seen through the lens of culture.

What Does Play Look Like in Everyday Life?

Description of what play looks like when it happens in everyday life is an important goal of research in occupational science. In this vein, researchers study play by observing it as it occurs in natural environments and by garnering information from people regarding their experiences and perceptions of play, so as to provide a description of naturally occurring patterns of play. Blanche (1998) furnished an example of such research by using participant observation, interview, and questionnaire methods to study play experiences of American adults. Her findings provide clues that many occupations enjoyed in adulthood have precursors extending back to early childhood play experiences.

A large body of multidisciplinary research in child development identifies normative patterns of child play related to maturation, gender, and parent-child interactions (e.g., Belsky & Most, 1981; Caldera, Huston, & O'Brien, 1989; Fabes, Martin, & Hanish, 2003; Pellegrini, 2002; Power, 1985). The knowledge provided by this research is valuable in informing occupational therapists about broadly generalizable patterns of child play behavior within the dominant culture. In their day-to-day practice, however, occupational therapists also need to have knowledge about play that illuminates the process and experience of the players within the context of their lives. Research in occupational science often aims to furnish this kind of information. An example follows to help the reader appreciate how this kind of research provides insights that can lead to innovations in occupational therapy.

Loree Primeau et al. (1998) studied the orchestration of parent-child play within the context of daily routines in the home. To identify patterns of parent-child play, she spent extensive amounts of time observing 10 families with preschool children in their homes and conducting intensive interviews of the parents involved. Her occupational science orientation led her to identify some patterns of parent-child play that had not previously been documented in the play literature. Specifically, she found two main types of strategies used by parents to incorporate play into daily routines at home: strategies of segregation and strategies of inclusion. In strategies of segregation the child's play takes place as an entirely separate activity from parental household work, as when parents take a break from work to play with the child or when they work while the child plays independently. In strategies of inclusion the child's play is embedded in the parent's work, as when the parent participates in household work and plays with the child at the same time or when the parent allows the child to participate playfully in the adult work task.

Primeau et al. (1998) found that when a child participated in adult chores, often the parents would structure and support the activity so that the child could perform as much of it as possible; thus the situation becomes one in which the child develops skills under the adult's guidance. For example, the parent may modify the physical environment, provide verbal suggestions, or eliminate unnecessary steps to allow the child to participate maximally. Primeau called this process "occupational scaffolding" because the adult's guidance becomes a scaffold on which the child learns to perform the task (Figure 1-15). Interestingly, she found that children were highly motivated and enthusiastic during situations that involved occupational scaffolding and that most parents interpreted their children's involvement in the task as play, even though conventionally the task itself was viewed as household work. Parents interpreted their own experiences as simultaneously work and play during occupational scaffolding situations. Primeau et al. (1998) suggested that occupational scaffolding may be an important process through which participation in childhood occupations fosters competence in adulthood.

Primeau's study has several implications for the fields of occupational science and occupational therapy. First, it identifies occupational scaffolding as the possible dynamic through which children learn skills for doing household work occupations; it thus addresses the important question of how childhood occupations shape adulthood accomplishments. Second, it calls attention to the fact that work and play are not always separate experiences; it thus calls for a rethinking of the notion of a balance of work, rest, and play. Finally, it is a source of new ideas for intervention. It tells therapists that parents employ a variety of strategies to manage their children's play in the context of daily household routines. This knowledge can be the source of suggestions that therapists can share with families who are struggling to meet the

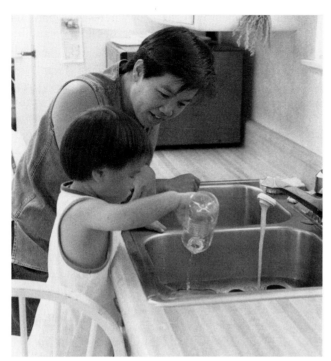

Figure 1-15
Occupational scaffolding. The child is being allowed to participate in a cleanup task, and his mother is structuring the activity by providing verbal cues and a chair at the right height, so that he can do his part of the task successfully. This is play for the child and may be experienced by the mother as both play and work. (Courtesy Shay McAtee.)

demands of household management, work outside the home, and child care, while at the same time valuing opportunities to play with their children. Families who have children with disabilities may especially appreciate hearing about strategies other families have found useful for managing their complex daily occupations.

Disability and Play
Studies of play patterns of people who experience disability are particularly relevant to occupational therapists, who serve these populations. The presence of a disability often presents special challenges to play, although this is certainly not always the case.

Missiuna and Pollock (1991) reviewed the research on play of children with physical disabilities and suggested that such children often suffer from secondary disabilities imposed by deprivation through the imposition of physical, social, personal, and environmental barriers. They urged occupational therapists to be advocates in promoting free, active community play experiences for these children. Their concern was validated by Richardson (2002), who conducted a small qualitative study of children with physical disabilities within the context of school. Results showed that the children were often onlookers because of social barriers, and that when they did participate in

activities, the quality of their occupational engagement was affected.

The powerful influence of environmental context may account for contradictory findings in some studies as to whether differences in playfulness distinguish between children with and without physical disabilities or cerebral palsy (Harkness & Bundy, 2001; Okimoto, Bundy, & Hanzlik, 2000). In a study of children with developmental disabilities, Hamm (2006) found that ToP scores were significantly lower for these children compared with nondisabled children matched for cognitive age. She also found, however, that compared with the nondisabled children, the children with disabilities had a stronger correlation between scores on ToP and on the Test of Environmental Supportiveness, suggesting that the environment played a particularly influential role in this group's observed playfulness. Rigby and Gaik (2007) administered ToP to 16 children with cerebral palsy in three different settings (home, community, and school) and found a significant difference in playfulness across settings, with most playfulness observed at home and least at school. Most of the children had high ToP scores in at least one setting, demonstrating that they had the capacity to be playful. It was evident, however, that their play was supported in some environments more than in others, indicating that external barriers are likely to have a significant impact on the play of these children. The findings of these studies, taken together, point to the potency of the physical and social environments in affecting the play lives of children with physical and developmental disabilities and emphasize the need for research to more closely examine how environments support or interfere with play.

Children with less severe or invisible disabilities may be less likely to experience internal or external barriers to participation, although this probably varies depending on the particular child and the environment. Research on children with sensory integration problems indicates that they often, but not always, have play difficulties (Bundy, 1989; Clifford & Bundy, 1989). Using Knox's Play Scale, Bundy (1989) found that groups of preschool-age boys with and without sensory integrative dysfunction did indeed differ significantly, on the average, in level of play development, with lower play scores characterizing the children with sensory integration problems. About one third of the group of boys with sensory integrative dysfunction, however, had play skills within normal expectations. Furthermore, most preschoolers with sensory integrative dysfunction, like those without dysfunction, were found to express strong preferences for the types of play in which their play skills were strongest (Clifford & Bundy, 1989). In other words, most children seemed to have matched their play preferences with their abilities (Bundy, 1991). This strategy might be adaptive in the short run in that it preserves self-esteem and minimizes disruption to play skills. On the other hand, it is possible that long-range negative effects may occur if the child continues to avoid certain types of play, thereby missing out on some of the opportunities to develop motor and social skills that are available to most children. From this line of research, Bundy (1991) concluded that sensory integration clearly might influence the child's ability to play but is only one of many complex foundations of play. Based on her research and clinical experience, she suggested that assessment of sensory integration alone does not provide an adequate assessment of play and, further, that improving an individual's sensory integrative functioning might not automatically improve his or her play.

Not surprisingly, similar issues arise with respect to children with developmental coordination disorders (DCD), a diagnostic group that overlaps with sensory integration dysfunction. Generally speaking, children with DCD are less physically active and have patterns of social and physical play different from their well-coordinated peers (Poulsen & Ziviani, 2004). Perhaps this is because these children, like those studied by Bundy, tend to match play preferences with ability.

Overall, research on disability indicates that intraindividual characteristics, as well as social and physical environments, are important mediators of an individual child's play characteristics and experiences. Readers should bear this in mind while studying the chapters in this book that focus on the play issues associated with particular disabilities and conditions, including delays associated with early deprivation (Chapter 8), sensory integration problems (Chapter 9), high-risk infants (Chapter 13), autism (Chapter 14), and cerebral palsy (Chapter 15).

Culture and Play

The assumption that play is a child's major occupation may not be a universally held belief (Bazyk, Stalnaker, Llerena, Ekelman, & Bazyk, 2003). It appears to be a culturally dependent viewpoint.

Research by Gaskins (1996, 2000) and Bazyk et al. (2003) with rural, traditional Mayan families provides a powerful illustration of how culture shapes the structure and interpretation of child play. For the most part, the findings of these two participant observation studies were similar in showing that Mayan children's daily activities are structured primarily around adult work, not play, and that children are expected to occupy themselves independently during free time. Gaskins (2000) reported that play activities of Mayan children peak at 3 to 5 years of age, when play comprises approximately 40% of the child's daily activities, mostly in the form of gross motor and object play activities. Between ages 5 and 12 years, play gradually decreases to about 5% of the day and is replaced by gender-based household work, which occupies about 60% of the child's day by age 12. Most Mayan children are independent and competent in self-care by ages 5 to 6 years. By age 6 years, they regularly participate in household chores, errands, and care of younger siblings.

Bazyk et al. (2003) pointed out that the way play is defined can lead to different conclusions about the play of Mayan children. If defined as an activity distinct from work and self-care, play seems to have a very limited role in Mayan child life. If play is viewed as an attitude or style of interaction (i.e., playfulness), however, it appears to be embedded throughout Mayan children's daily lives as manifested by humor, smiling, playful social interactions, and playful approach to tasks (Figure 1-16).

The findings of Bazyk et al. (2003) contrast dramatically with those of Primeau et al. (1998), whose American participants apparently place a high value on play as activity that is developmentally important and should be encouraged in children. As described earlier in this chapter, Primeau found that American parents created strategies of inclusion or segregation to maximize child play in the home. In contrast, Bazyk et al. found that Mayan children, not parents, created strategies for inclusion and segregation of play through the course of the day. Children would engage in play activities when their work was completed (segregation) and would also imbue their work with a playful attitude or activity, for example, making bubbles while washing clothes in the river (inclusion). Interestingly, although the Mayan adults did not structure such play experiences for their children, they often tolerated it by smiling or laughing, that is, if it did not impede the work that needed to be done. They viewed play as simply "what children do" and seemed to place a higher value on the development of work skills to prepare children for adult obligations.

Bazyk et al. (2003) made the critical point that, because most of the existing child play research is on middle-class children in Western contexts, American professionals and researchers may pass negative value judgments on a

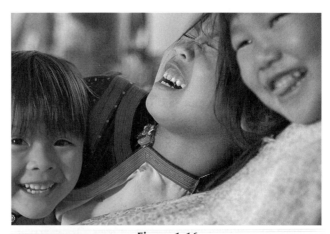

Figure 1-16
Children often embed playfulness into activities, even if the activity would be considered work by an adult. (Courtesy Shay McAtee.)

minority group if its play patterns differ from the American mainstream (Fleer, 1996). As a result, a child or group of children could mistakenly be identified as having a deficit (Fleer, 1996; Göncü, Tuermer, Jain, & Johnson, 1999; Soto & Negron, 1994). Such an interpretation could have damaging consequences, since it might lead to marginalization or inappropriate interventions, when in actuality the behavior in question is meaningful and appropriate for the family's cultural belief system.

A growing body of interdisciplinary research is revealing that adults' assumptions and beliefs about child development are strongly culture bound and that these assumptions pattern the ways child play is manifested and the ways it is managed by adults (Harkness & Super, 1986, 1996). For example, Artin Göncü and his colleagues studied social play of toddlers in four different cultural communities in Guatemala, Turkey, India, and the United States. They found that social play occurred in each of the cultures, but the frequency of play, number of toddlers engaging in various types of play, and their social play partners varied across cultures. Tobin, Wu, and Davidson (1989) contributed a fascinating cross-cultural study of preschools in Japan, China, and the United States, demonstrating that adult beliefs about child development and human nature dictate preschool routines, including when and how play occurs. They also found that when participating preschool teachers viewed videotapes of preschools in the other cultures, they tended to negatively and harshly judge the classroom management styles of the preschool teachers in the other cultures. Within the United States, Farver and Lee-Shin (2000) studied the parenting and play attitudes of Korean immigrant mothers. They found that mothers with an "assimilated" cultural style were more accepting and encouraging of children's creativity and play and reported more parent-child play at home than did mothers who were less assimilitated into mainstream American values regarding parenting. At preschool the children of the more assimilated mothers engaged in pretend play more frequently and were rated by teachers as more difficult behaviorally than the children of less assimilated mothers. These findings indicate that, within one country, important cultural differences can exist between people whose ancestry lies in the same nationality and that these differences influence parental beliefs and practices that, in turn, shape child play.

The body of research regarding culture and play presents difficult challenges for the occupational therapist who is serving families that hold cultural beliefs that differ from the dominant mainstream, a situation that is becoming more familiar throughout the United States and globally. Normative information about play from mainstream or dominant cultural groups will not always be applicable to children living within other cultural groups, whether inside or outside the dominant culture. The earlier discussion of Sutton-Smith's rhetorics of play is a useful reminder that a therapist working with families of different cultural backgrounds may have to reframe play using different rhetorics. The dominant rhetoric of childhood play in the United States is that play is progress—it helps the child to learn many different skills, to become adaptable, and to develop creativity, and therefore time to play should be encouraged. This rhetoric is unlikely to be meaningful or effective with families that do not share this set of beliefs and assumptions. Shifting rhetorics when relating to families does not mean that the therapist relinquishes his or her professional knowledge base. Instead, it means trying a different perspective that will allow the therapist to communicate respectfully and possibly more effectively, opening the possibility that family members will be co-partners in constructing novel solutions to clinical dilemmas.

Play in Evidence-Based Practice

The research reviewed throughout this chapter, and in the other chapters of this book, furnishes evidence about play that therapists can use to inform their practice. For example, research on the biological prerequisites of play in animals (human and nonhuman) shows that for play to emerge and flourish, a child needs to feel physically and emotionally safe and to have an adequate level of physiological stability and metabolic resources. Therefore, to use play in assessment or intervention, the clinician needs to make sure that these conditions are present. The research on developmental progressions in play, such as those proposed by Piaget, describes how play typically appears and changes as children mature in Western cultures, but the research on play in diverse cultures cautions that these normative classifications of play may not always be reflective of what is typical or desirable for children in non-Western or nondominant cultures. Therefore therapists may need to construct new approaches to assessing the play of children in some cultural groups, as well as to reconstruct the rhetorics about play when relating to their families.

Emerging scholarship on children's occupations should be used by the occupational therapist to inform practice. For example, Humphry's work emphasizes the contexts and meanings of activities as critical elements in the child's motivation to engage in them, thereby influencing development (Bober, Humphry, Carswell, & Core, 2001; Humphry & Wakeford, 2006). She advocates simultaneously considering cultural practices, social interactions, and individual engagement patterns in generating multiple therapeutic strategies. Using a case example of a preschooler's play with blocks, she demonstrates how therapeutic strategies addressing the spatial organization of the room, the social resources available (peer and adult interactions), and visual aids to support the child's interest in the activity were created by therapist and teacher collaboratively in the preschool setting, with successful results (Humphry & Wakeford, 2006) (Figure 1-17).

Development of a rhetoric of play as health might lead to use of multidisciplinary research to support and develop innovative individual, group, and community interventions. For instance, research by Hess and Bundy (2003) found that playfulness was strongly related to coping skills among adolescents with severe emotional disturbance, as well as typical adolescents, who were more playful and had better coping. This suggests that interventions using play and playfulness may be useful in improving coping skills in adolescents. Other potentially important areas where play interventions could be developed to support health and minimize health risks might address family routines and community opportunities involving television viewing, computer game usage, outdoor place spaces, and physical activity (Christakis, Ebel, Rivara, & Zimmerman, 2004; Dorman, 1997; Jordan, Hersey, McDivitt, & Heitzler, 2006; Pellegrini & Smith, 1998; Rosenbaum, 1998; Tandy, 1999).

The next section examines recent research related to occupational therapy that directly evaluates interventions that use play or playfulness as either a means or an end goal of intervention (or both) with children. The reader should keep in mind that this is not intended to be an exhaustive review, but a cursory sampling of a few representative studies.

Play as Means of Intervention

Although use of play as a means to obtain nonplay occupational therapy goals is prevalent among pediatric occupational therapists (Couch et al., 1998), few studies have examined outcomes of play-based interventions. Those that exist address diverse outcomes, spanning physiological to psychosocial domains.

Occupational therapists who work with children in burn units traditionally provide interventions to prevent deformity, facilitate recovery of functional skills, and support emotional well-being. Because passive or active movement can cause severe pain, therapists may use play activities to encourage children's participation in therapeutic activities. In a single-subject, randomized, multiple-treatment study, Melchert-McKearnan, Deitz, Engel, and White (2000) compared the effects of purposeful activity (framed as play) and rote exercise on pain perception, distress, completion of range-of-motion goals, and enjoyment of activity in two boys hospitalized for severe upper extremity burn injuries. The play intervention involved games that were identified by the child as activities that he enjoyed doing. For each play session the child was offered a choice of three of the previously identified play activities. Compared with rote exercise, in which the child was instructed to perform a certain number of range-of-motion repetitions, the play intervention yielded better results overall on all outcome measures.

Case-Smith (2000) studied the influence of various occupational therapy intervention activities, including play, on fine motor and functional outcomes in 44 preschoolers, aged 4 to 6 years, with fine motor delays. The children in the study received occupational therapy services for 8 months in a preschool setting. Occupational therapy services were not experimentally manipulated but were conducted as they would ordinarily be delivered in the school setting. Therapists documented the interventions they used in each session with each child, and a research team administered standard evaluations at the beginning and end of the academic year. Interventions included tactile input and motor planning, in-hand manipulation, visual motor integration, bilateral coordination, self-care, play, and peer interaction activities. Outcomes were scores on eight measures of fine motor, visual-perceptual, visual-motor, self-care, and social function. Results of regression analyses, taking into account the frequency with which each intervention was used, revealed that play activities and peer interaction were the only interventions that significantly predicted gains in fine motor skills. Case-Smith speculated that this result may be due to the power of play to motivate and engage children so that they exert more

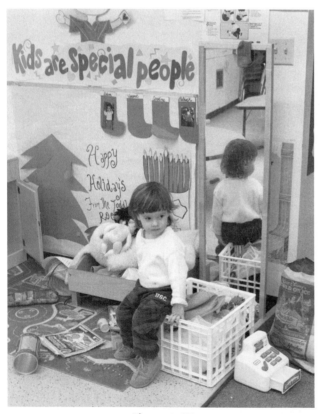

Figure 1-17

Occupational science emphasizes the unique situation of the individual child, addressing intrapersonal characteristics such as temperament and interests, as well as how the environment supports and shapes play. (Courtesy Shay McAtee.)

effort in or attention to fine motor activities. Alternatively, it may be that play activities gave the children an enjoyable context for practicing fine motor skills, or that therapists who reported using play were more skillful and creative in motivating children to engage in activities.

Child abuse and neglect represent another area in which occupational therapists may intervene by using play as a therapeutic modality (Cooper, 2000). A recent metaanalysis of psychologically oriented intervention outcomes for sexually abused children and adolescents indicated that play therapy was most effective for social functioning outcomes (Hetzel-Riggin, Brausch, & Montgomery, 2007). Other interventions (e.g., cognitive-behavioral, abuse-specific, family, or supportive therapy, either in group or in individual formats) were most effective for other outcomes such as behavior problems, psychological distress, and low self-concept. This study therefore targeted social outcomes as an area in which occupational therapists, using play as a means of intervention, might be able to help children suffering from abuse. In Chapter 18 of this book, Linda Fazio provides excellent examples of using such psychologically oriented play therapy methods in occupational therapy to help children who are experiencing a variety of life difficulties.

Play as Goal of Intervention
Roseann Schaaf, with her colleagues, was one of the first researchers in occupational therapy to use an occupational therapy intervention that is not primarily defined as play to produce gains in play behavior. Specifically, using single case description and system design methods, she provided a sensory integration–based occupational therapy program for preschoolers and then documented intervention effectiveness using measurement of play behaviors (Schaaf, 1990; Schaaf, Merrill, & Kinsella, 1987). Case-Smith and Bryan (1999) later used a single-subject, AB design to evaluate outcomes of sensory integration–based occupational therapy with five preschoolers who had autism. During the intervention phase, four children showed decreased frequency of nonengaged behavior and three demonstrated more frequent goal-directed mastery play.

The rationale for using sensory integration–based intervention in the studies is that enhancement of play skills is an expected long-term outcome of this intervention (Parham & Mailloux, 2005). It should be acknowledged, though, that sensory integration intervention involves an element of play by emphasizing pleasurable sensorimotor activities that are chosen and controlled to some extent by the child, with the therapist's guidance (Parham et al., 2007). Perhaps the play ingredient is critical in obtaining gains in child play.

Play as Both Means and Goal
In addition to research in which a nonplay intervention was used to improve play, Schaaf designed intervention research in which play was used as both means and ends of occupational therapy. Her Family-Centered Framework for Early Intervention (Schaaf & Mulrooney, 1989) was based on the Model of Human Occupation (Kielhofner et al., 1980) and was used to design a 10-week program involving direct and consultative occupational therapy in home visits and in the early intervention environments where the children were enrolled. The program was evaluated by use of a single-subject, multiple-baseline design with five preschoolers who had developmental, neuromuscular, and sensory impairments (Schaaf & Mulrooney, 1989). Play was a central concern in assessment, intervention, and measurement of outcomes. Results on the Knox Preschool Play Scale (Knox, 1974) indicated the clearest gains on the Participation score, which reflects primarily social interaction. Material Management improved in two subjects, indicating improvements in object play skills. No gains, however, were found in the Space Management or Imitation dimensions. Although these results are encouraging, it is difficult to sort out whether the positive outcomes were due to the occupational therapy program component or to the early intervention programs in which the children were enrolled.

Another study of preschoolers examined frequency of social interactions when children with social play delays were paired in free play with children of differing developmental levels (Tanta, Deitz, White, & Billingsley, 2005). Five preschoolers with play delays participated in a study with a single-subject alternating treatments design, in which each child was paired with one peer who had lower developmental play skills and with one peer who had higher play skills. Dyads were videotaped in a playroom, and data were coded for frequency of initiation and response to initiation. All five children showed more initiation and more response to initiation in play when paired with higher functioning peers. These results show that occupational therapists working with preschoolers whose goals include improving social play should consider pairing these children with peers who have higher play skills.

Mother-child interaction is another area in which a play intervention has been shown to be effective in improving play participation. A long line of research has found that mother-child interaction is often disrupted when the child has a physical disability such as cerebral palsy (Barrera & Vella, 1987; Brooks-Gunn & Lewis, 1984; Hanzlik, 1989a; Hanzlik & Stevenson, 1986; Kogan & Tyler, 1973). Mothers of these children tend to be more directive and controlling and to engage in more physical contact with the child than mothers of typically developing children. In turn, the children tend to be less responsive and less independent than peers. In an effort to enhance mother-child interactions, Hanzlik (1989b) designed a 1-hour intervention for mothers of children with cerebral palsy. The intervention can be considered play based in that it involved discussing play and modeling play interaction techniques and styles. Mothers were coached on taking turns, imitating child behavior, interacting face to face, decreasing verbal and physical directives during toy play, and matching play-oriented interactions to the child's tempo. Hanzlik (1989b) and Hanzlik and Stevenson (1986) investigated the effectiveness of this intervention by videotaping mother-infant play before and after intervention. Infants with cerebral palsy and developmental delays, along with their mothers, were assigned randomly to either the 1-hour mother-child intervention or a 1-hour neurodevelopmental treatment (NDT) session. In her original analysis, Hanzlik (1989b) found that both mothers and infants who received her intervention improved in their interactions as intended. The videotaped data were reanalyzed in a later study (Okimoto et al., 2000) to examine whether the intervention had resulted in an improvement in infant playfulness as measured by the ToP. Results showed that those who received Hanzlik's intervention, but not those who received the NDT intervention, had significant gains in playfulness. An examination of the long-term effects of this interesting intervention might be valuable, with perhaps repeated contacts with participants to help sustain gains as the children grow and change developmentally.

Play and Occupational Justice

Occupational justice is an emerging concern of occupational therapists who seek to apply their knowledge and energies toward improving the health and well-being of communities and groups, as well as individuals (Wilcock & Townsend, 2000). An offshoot of social justice, occupational justice is concerned with recognizing and providing for the occupational needs of people as part of a fair society (Watson & Swartz, 2004). Leaders in occupational justice call on occupational therapists to become activists for societal change, using their knowledge of occupation to identify social inequities that impede people's opportunities to engage in meaningful activities and advocate for positive change (Kronenberg, Algado, & Pollard, 2005). Occupational justice is a growing movement on a global scale.

Advocates of occupational justice suggest that conditions such as those leading to occupational deprivation—the inability to engage in desired and appropriate occupations because of some external restriction—can be alleviated through social and political activities that aim to change whatever is unfairly impeding a person's or group's occupational engagement (Watson & Swartz, 2004; Whiteford, 2000). Occupational deprivation may stem from economic injustices, but this is not always the case. Examples of occupational deprivation involving play might include children who are regularly excluded from play activities or are not permitted access to playgrounds or other play spaces because of a disability or different-ness, minority status, family background, or environmental dangers.

In countries such as the United States, affluent children may suffer from play deprivation because of cultural pressures for achievement in academics or enrichment activities such as music or athletics. Children may have hurried family lifestyles that leave little room for play or even quiet reflection. Recently the American Academy of Pediatrics released the clinical report "The Importance of Play in Promoting Healthy Child Development and Maintaining Strong Parent-Child Bonds," which was generated out of concern that time for child-driven free play or recess is markedly reduced for some children (Ginsburg et al., 2006). The report encourages pediatricians to advocate for children by helping families, schools, and communities to protect playtime so that children will have balanced lives. This is a prime example of an occupational justice issue.

Another significant occupational justice issue is the case for recess. Recess periods in school provide children with opportunities to structure their own time, play freely, be physically active, or socialize with peers. During recess, students learn how to negotiate social worlds that are important to them (Huecker, 2005). A body of research shows that children benefit academically and behaviorally from recess (Pellegrini, 2005). For example, children have better attention in class on the days they have recess (Jarrett et al., 1998), and longer confinement in class is related to diminishing attention to seat work (Pellegrini & Davis, 1993). Despite this evidence, since 1989, approximately 40% of America's 16,000 school districts have minimized or abolished, or are considering eliminating, recess from elementary schools because of increased pressure to improve academic test scores (Jarrett, 2003). Moreover, a national study of how children spend their time in school indicated that lack of recess is most commonly experienced by minority students, students below the poverty line, those living in urban areas, and those with lower test scores (Roth, Brooks-Gunn, Linver, & Hofferth, 2002). To redress this injustice, educators and parents have become politically active, and to some extent successful, in systematically lobbying legislators to mandate at least one recess break per day (State of Connecticut, 2004; State of Michigan, 2000; State of Virginia, 2000). The case for valuing, protecting, and restoring school recess has been taken up by leaders in early childhood education (e.g., Jarrett, 2003), as well as organizations such as the American Association for the Child's Right to Play (IPA/USA) (American Association for the Child's Right to Play, 2007) and the Council for Physical Education and Children (2001).

The importance of play for child well-being is endorsed by the United Nations in its Declaration of the Rights of the Child (1959), article 7, paragraph 3: "The child shall have full opportunity for play and recreation which should be directed to the same purposes as education; society and the public authorities shall endeavor to promote the enjoyment of this right." This statement is the organizing credo of the International Play Association (IPA), of which the IPA/USA is a branch. The IPA originated in Denmark and is recognized as a nongovernmental organization with consultative status by the United Nations Economic and Social Council, as well as UNICEF. It is devoted to supporting child play and bringing a child's perspective to policy development globally. As such, the IPA and its affiliate organizations are important groups for those interested in play justice.

Occupational therapists are in a position to notice play injustices in their communities. Do all children have access to safe, accessible, and appropriate playgrounds and play spaces? Are families who have children with disabilities provided with information, resources, and support to ensure that their child is able to participate as fully as possible at home, in the community, and at school? Are programs available to increase peer awareness and acceptance of disability? Are children who experience difficulties playing, for physical or psychosocial reasons, identified and provided with appropriate support for playfulness and play activities? Working to correct these injustices, whether through occupational therapy service delivery, advocacy, political action, community activism, or some other route, will contribute to the profession's purpose—to meet societal needs.

SUMMARY AND CONCLUSION

Play is a complex phenomenon that has been examined by many different academic disciplines, from evolutionary biology to anthropology and sociology. Occupational therapists have acknowledged that play is a multidimensional, biopsychosocial phenomenon and in recent years have generated research that builds on their long history of concern with play as an integral part of a healthy lifestyle. Scholarship in occupational therapy and occupational science is concerned particularly with the study of naturally occurring patterns of play in people with and without disabilities, biological and cultural influences on play, measurement of play, and evidence-based practice in which play is the means or the end goal, or both, of intervention. Systematic applications of play principles in practice have developed in the profession, as is demonstrated by the remaining chapters in this text. The emergence of interest in occupational justice may stimulate occupational therapists to collaborate with parents and other professionals to shape public policy affecting the play lives of all children.

The topic of play is usually addressed in occupational therapy in relation to children, but concepts of play are likely to be relevant throughout the lifespan, and applications of play for adults should be explored. For example,

questions arise as to the concept of playfulness and whether it contributes to flexibility, and therefore adaptation, in adulthood. How can playfulness be encouraged in adults, and how may it contribute to intervention? How does play fit into the lives of adults at various life stages? Is it meaningful to separate play from other occupations, such as self-care and work, or would it be more useful to consider play an attitude that can permeate any occupation? Can health-related effects of play be demonstrated, for example, through changes in stress hormones or the immune system? I hope that occupational therapists in the next decade will take play seriously enough to investigate the ways in which play concepts may be applied to benefit all people, regardless of age.

Review Questions

1. Why is play so difficult to define? When is a definition necessary, and when is it not?
2. What are the characteristics of the play experience?
3. How does context influence play?
4. Compare and contrast the four classical theories of play.
5. Name Burghardt's five criteria for identifying play across species.
6. Discuss the biological functions and outcomes of play, including adaptive variability.
7. Identify brain structures and neurotransmitters that are most closely associated with play.
8. Explain arousal modulation theories of play.
9. Describe psychodynamic theories of play.
10. Contrast Sutton-Smith's with Piaget's view of play.
11. Outline and describe the content of the following taxonomies of play development: Piaget's classification of games, Reilly's stages of play development, Takata's play epochs.
12. Discuss sociocultural theories of play, including the concept of metacommunication.
13. Explain Sutton-Smith's rhetorics of play, and identify which are most characteristic of occupational therapists.
14. How did play fit into Meyer's philosophy of occupation?
15. What is the significance of rule learning in the occupational behavior framework?
16. What is meant by "play as means" versus "play as ends"? Provide examples of research that exemplify each of these concepts.
17. Why is it valuable for occupational therapy to build knowledge about how play looks in everyday life?
18. Describe the strategies parents use to incorporate play into daily routines at home. What is occupational scaffolding, and how may it contribute to competence in adulthood?
19. What does the research on play of children with disabilities tell us about the role of environment?

20. In what ways might culture influence child play, and why is culture critical to consider in clinical practice?
21. What kinds of evidence can the occupational therapist use to guide and justify decisions made about employing play in practice?
22. What is occupational justice, and what are some examples of play injustices?

REFERENCES

Abbott, M. (1950). Present day trends in cerebral palsy. *American Journal of Occupational Therapy, 4*, 53-55.

Alessandrini, N. A. (1949). Play—A child's world. *American Journal of Occupational Therapy, 3*, 9-12.

American Association for the Child's Right to Play (IPA/USA). (2007). The case for elementary school recess. Retrieved July 31, 2007 from http://www.ipausa.org/recesshandbook.htm.

American Occupational Therapy Association (1994). Uniform terminology for occupational therapy: Third edition. *American Journal of Occupational Therapy, 48*, 1047-1054.

American Occupational Therapy Association (2002). Occupational therapy practice framework: Domain and process. *American Journal of Occupational Therapy, 56*, 609-639.

Apter, M. J., & Kerr, J. H. (1991). The nature, function and value of play. In J. H. Kerr & M. J. Apter (Eds.), *Adult play: A reversal theory approach* (pp. 163-176). Amsterdam: Swets & Zeitlinger.

Axline, V. (1969). *Play therapy*. New York: Ballantine Books.

Ayres, A. J. (1958). The visual-motor function. *American Journal of Occupational Therapy, 12*, 130-138.

Barrera, M. E., & Vella, D. M. (1987). Disabled and non-disabled infants' interactions with their mothers. *American Journal of Occupational Therapy, 41*, 168-172.

Bateson, G. (1972). *Steps to an ecology of mind*. New York: Ballantine Books.

Bazyk, S., Stalnaker, D., Llerena, M., Ekelman, B., & Bazyk, J. (2003). Play in Mayan children. *American Journal of Occupational Therapy, 57*(3), 273-283.

Belsky, J., & Most, R. K. (1981). From exploration to play: A cross-sectional study of infant free play behavior. *Developmental Psychology, 17*, 630-639.

Berlyne, D. E. (1960). *Conflict, arousal, and curiosity*. New York: McGraw-Hill.

Berlyne, D. E. (1966). Curiosity and exploration. *Science, 153*, 25-33.

Berlyne, D. E. (1969). Laughter, humor, and play. In G. Lindzey & E. Aronson (Eds.), *The handbook of social psychology, Vol. 3.* (pp. 795-852). Reading, MA: Addison-Wesley.

Berlyne, D. E. (1971). *Aesthetics and psychobiology*. New York: Meredith.

Blanche, E. I. (1998). *Play and process: The experience of play in the life of the adult* (Unpublished dissertation. Los Angeles: University of Southern California).

Bober, S. J., Humphry, R., Carswell, H. W., & Core, A. J. (2001). Toddlers' persistence in the emerging occupations of functional play and self-feeding. *American Journal of Occupational Therapy, 55*, 369-376.

Brooks-Gunn, J., & Lewis, M. (1984). Maternal responsivity in interactions with handicapped infants. *Child Development, 55*(3), 782-793.

Bruner, J. S. (1972). Nature and uses of immaturity. *American Psychologist, 27*, 687-708.

Bundy, A. C. (1989). A comparison of the play skills of normal boys and boys with sensory integrative dysfunction. *Occupational Therapy Journal of Research, 9*, 84-100.

Bundy, A. C. (1991). Play theory and sensory integration. In A. G. Fisher, E. A. Murray, & A. C. Bundy (Eds.), *Sensory integration: Theory and practice* (pp. 46-68). Philadelphia: F.A. Davis.

Bundy, A. C. (1993). Assessment of play and leisure: Delineation of the problem. *American Journal of Occupational Therapy, 47*, 217-222.

Burghardt, G. M. (1984). On the origins of play. In P. K. Smith (Ed.), *Play in animals and humans* (pp. 5-41). Oxford: Basil Blackwell.

Burghardt, G. M. (2001). Play: Attributes and neural substrates. In E. M. Blass (Ed.), *Handbook of behavioral neurobiology. Vol. 13. Developmental psychobiology* (pp. 327-366). New York: Plenum.

Burghardt, G. M. (2005). *The genesis of animal play: Testing the limits*. Cambridge, MA: M. I. T. Press.

Burke, J. P. (1993). Play: The life role of the infant and young child. In J. Case-Smith (Ed.), *Pediatric occupational therapy and early intervention* (pp. 198-224). Boston: Andover Medical Publications.

Byers, J. A., & Walker, C. V. (1995). Refining the motor training hypothesis for the evolution of play. *American Naturalist, 146*, 25-40.

Caillois, R. (1961). *Man, play, and games*. Glencoe, IL: Free Press.

Caldera, Y. M., Huston, A. C., & O'Brien, M. (1989). Social interactions and play patterns of parents and toddlers with feminine, masculine, and neutral toys. *Child Development, 60*, 70-76.

Case-Smith, J. (2000). Effects of occupational therapy services on fine motor and functional performance in preschool children. *American Journal of Occupational Therapy, 54*(4), 372-380.

Case-Smith, J., & Bryan, T. (1999). The effects of occupational therapy with sensory integration emphasis on preschool-age children with autism. *American Journal of Occupational Therapy, 53*, 489-497.

Christakis, D. A., Ebel, B. E., Rivara, F. P., & Zimmerman, F. J. (2004). Television, video, and computer game usage in children under 11 years of age. *Journal of Pediatrics, 145*, 652-656.

Christiansen, C. (1991). Occupational therapy: Intervention for life performance. In C. Christiansen & C. Baum (Eds.), *Occupational therapy: Overcoming human performance deficits*. Thorofare, NJ: Slack.

Clark, C. D., & Miller, P. J. (1998). Play. In H. Friedman (Ed.), *Encyclopedia of mental health, Vol. 3.* (pp. 189-197). San Diego: Academic Press.

Clark, F. A., Parham, L. D., Carlson, M. E., Frank, G., Jackson, J., Pierce, D. , et al. (1991). Occupational science: Academic innovation in the service of occupational therapy's future. *American Journal of Occupational Therapy, 45,* 300-310.

Clifford, J. M., & Bundy, A. C. (1989). Play preference and play performance in normal boys and boys with sensory integrative dysfunction. *Occupational Therapy Journal of Research, 9,* 202-217.

Cooper, R. (2000). The impact of child abuse on children's play: A conceptual model. *Occupational Therapy International, 7,* 259-276.

Couch, K. J., Deitz, J. C., & Kanny, E. M. (1998). The role of play in pediatric occupational therapy. *American Journal of Occupational Therapy, 52,* 111-117.

Council on Physical Education and Children. (2001). *Recess in elementary schools: A position paper from the National Association for Sport and Physical Education.* Retrieved July 30, 2007, from www.aahperd.org/naspe/pdf_files/pos_papers/current_res.pdf.

Declaration of the Rights of the Child, G.A. res. 1386 (XIV), 14 U.N. GAOR Supp. (No. 16) at 19, U.N. Doc. A/4354 (1959).

Derse, P. (1950). The emotional problems of behavior in the spastic, athetoid, and ataxic type of cerebral palsied child. *American Journal of Occupational Therapy, 4,* 252-259.

Dorman, S. M. (1997). Video and computer games: Effect on children and implications for health education. *Journal of School Health, 67*(4), 133-138.

Dunton, W. R. (1915). *Occupational therapy: A manual for nurses.* Philadelphia: W.B. Saunders.

Ellis, M. J. (1973). *Why people play.* Englewood Cliffs, NJ: Prentice Hall.

Ellis, W. J. (1934). The importance of occupational therapy in institutional management. *Occupational Therapy and Rehabilitation, 13,* 1-11.

Erikson, E. H. (1963). *Childhood and society.* New York: W.W. Norton.

Fabes, R. A., Martin, C. L., & Hanish, L. D. (2003). Young children's play qualities in same-, other-, and mixed-sex peer groups. *Child Development, 74,* 921-932.

Farver, J. M., & Lee-Shin, Y. (2000). Acculturation and Korean-American children's social and play behavior. *Social Development, 9,* 316-336.

Fein, G. G. (1981). Pretend play in childhood: An integrative review. *Child Development, 52,* 1095-1118.

Fleer, M. (1996). Theories of play: Are they ethnocentric or inclusive? *Australian Journal of Early Childhood, 21,* 12-17.

Florey, L. L. (1971). An approach to play and play development. *American Journal of Occupational Therapy, 25,* 275-280.

Florey, L. L. (1981). Studies of play: Implications for growth, development, and for clinical practice. *American Journal of Occupational Therapy, 35,* 519-524.

Freud, S. (1961). *Beyond the pleasure principle.* New York: W.W. Norton.

Gardner, H. (1982). *Art, mind, and brain: A cognitive approach to creativity.* New York: Basic Books.

Garvey, D. (1990). *Play.* Cambridge, MA: Harvard University Press.

Gaskins, S. (1996). How Mayan parental theories come into play. In S. Harkness & C. Super (Eds.), *Parents' cultural belief systems: Their origins, expressions, and consequences* (pp. 345-363). New York: Guilford Press.

Gaskins, S. (2000). Children's daily activities in a Mayan village: A culturally grounded description. *Cross-Cultural Research, 34*(4), 375-389.

Gilmore, J. B. (1971). Play: A special behavior. In R. E. Herron & B. Sutton-Smith (Eds.), *Child's play* (pp. 311-325). New York: John Wiley & Sons.

Ginsburg, K. R., American Academy of Pediatrics Committee on Communications, & American Academy of Pediatrics Committee on Psychosocial Aspects of Child and Family Health. (2006). The importance of play in promoting healthy child development and maintaining strong parent-child bonds. *Pediatrics 119*(1):182-191.

Göncü, A., Tuermer, U., Jain, J., & Johnson, D. (1999). Children's play as cultural activity. In A. Göncü (Ed.), *Children's engagement in the world: Sociocultural perspectives.* Cambridge, UK: Cambridge University Press.

Gould, S. J. (1996). *Full house: The spread of excellence from Plato to Darwin.* New York: Harmony Books.

Grandin, T., & Johnson, C. (2005). *Animals in translation: Using the mysteries of autism to decode animal behavior.* New York: Scribner.

Granoff, N. (1995). *The evolution and operationalization of the concept of play in early occupational therapy* (Unpublished manuscript, University of Southern California, Los Angeles).

Grayson, E. S. (1948). Handedness testing for cerebral palsied children. *American Journal of Occupational Therapy, 2,* 91-94.

Groos, K. (1978). The value of play for practice and self-realization. In D. Muller-Schwarze (Ed.), *Evolution of play behavior* (pp. 16-23). Stroudsburg, PA: Dowden, Hutchinson, & Ross. (Reprinted from *The play of animals,* pp. 72-81, by K. Groos, trans. by E. L. Baldwin, 1898, D. Appleton & Company.)

Hall, G. S. (1978). Growth of motor power and function. In D. Muller-Schwarze (Ed.), *Evolution of play behavior* (pp. 24-29). Stroudsburg, PA: Dowden, Hutchinson, & Ross. (Reprinted from *Adolescence, its psychology and its relations to physiology, anthropology, sex, crime, religion and education, Vol. 1,* pp. 202-217, by G. S. Hall, 1908, D. Appleton & Company.)

Hamm, E. M. (2006). Playfulness and the environmental support of play in children with and without developmental disabilities. *Occupational Therapy Journal of Research, 26*(3), 88-96.

Hanzlik, J. R. (1989a). Interactions between mothers and their infants with developmental disabilities: Analysis and review. *Physical and Occupational Therapy in Pediatrics, 9*(1), 33-47.

Hanzlik, J. R. (1989b). The effect of intervention on the free-play experience for mothers and their infants with developmental delay and cerebral palsy. *Physical and Occupational Therapy in Pediatrics, 9*(2), 33-51.

Hanzlik, J. R., & Stevenson, M. B. (1986). Interactions of mothers with their infants who are mentally retarded, retarded with cerebral palsy, or non-retarded, *American Journal of Mental Deficiency, 90,* 513-520.

Harkness, L., & Bundy, A. C. (2001). The Test of Playfulness and children with physical disabilities. *Occupational Therapy Journal of Research, 21,* 73-89.

Harkness, S., & Super, C. M. (1986). The cultural structuring of children's play in a rural African community. In K. Blanchard (Ed.), *The many faces of play* (pp. 96-104). Champaign, IL: Human Kinetics Publishers.

Harkness, S., & Super, C. (1996). *Parents' cultural belief systems: Their origins, expressions, and consequences.* New York: Guilford Press.

Heard, C. (1977). Occupational role acquisition: A perspective on the chronically disabled. *American Journal of Occupational Therapy, 31,* 243-247.

Hess, L. M., & Bundy, A. C. (2003). The association between playfulness and coping in adolescents. *Physical and Occupational Therapy in Pediatrics, 23*(2), 5-17.

Hetzel-Riggin, M. D., Brausch, A. M., & Montgomery, B. S. (2007). A meta-analytic investigation of therapy modality outcomes for sexually abused children and adolescents: An exploratory study. *Child Abuse and Neglect, 31*(2), 125-141.

Hohman, L. B. (1938). Difficult children and work habits. *Occupational Therapy and Rehabilitation, 17,* 1-9.

Hoshmand, L. T., & Polkinghorne, D. E. (1992). Redefining the science-practice relationship and professional training. *American Psychologist, 47,* 55-66.

Huecker, E. M. (2005). *Something's happening: Emergence of social worlds on the school playground* (Unpublished dissertation. UMI # 3196819. Los Angeles: University of Southern California).

Huizinga, J. (1950). *Homo ludens.* Boston: Beacon Press. (Original work published in 1944 in German, trans. unknown.)

Humphry, R., & Wakeford, L. (2006). An occupation-centered discussion of development and implications for practice. *American Journal of Occupational Therapy, 60,* 258-267.

Hutt, C. (1970). Specific and diversive exploration. *Advances in Child Development and Behavior, 5,* 119-180.

Inch, C. F. (1936). Therapeutic placement of mental plays in state hospital industries. *Occupational Therapy and Rehabilitation, 15,* 241-248.

Jarrett, O. S. (2003). Recess in elementary school: What does the research say? *ERIC Digest. Retrieved July 31, 2007 from* www.ericdigests.org/2003-2/recess.html.

Jarrett, O. S., Maxwell, D. M., Dickerson, C., Hoge, P., Davies, G., & Yetley, A. (1998). The impact of recess on classroom behavior: Group effects and individual differences. *Journal of Educational Research, 92*(2), 121-126.

Johnson, J. E., Christie, J. F., & Yawkey, T. D. (1999). *Play and early childhood development.* New York: Longman.

Jordan, A. B., Hersey, J. C., McDivitt, J. A., & Heitzler, C. D. (2006). Reducing children's television-viewing time: A qualitative study of parents and their children. *Pediatrics, 118,* 1303-1311.

Kidner, T. B. (1931). Occupational therapy: Its diagnosis, scope, and possibilities. *Archives of Occupational Therapy, 10,* 1-11.

Kielhofner, G. (Ed.). (2002). *A model of human occupation* (3rd ed.) Baltimore: Williams & Wilkins.

Kielhofner, G., & Burke, J. P. (1977). Occupational therapy after 60 years: An account of changing identity and knowledge. *American Journal of Occupational Therapy, 31,* 675-689.

Kielhofner, G., & Burke, J. P. (1980). A model of human occupation, Part 1. Conceptual framework and content. *American Journal of Occupational Therapy, 34,* 572-581.

Kielhofner, G., Burke, J. P., & Igi, C. H. (1980). A model of human occupation, Part 4. Assessment and intervention. *American Journal of Occupational Therapy, 34,* 777-788.

Knox, S. (1974). A play scale. In M. Reilly (Ed.), *Play as exploratory learning* (pp. 247-266). Beverly Hills, CA: Sage Publications.

Kogan, K. L, & Tyler, N. (1973). Mother-child interaction in young physically handicapped children. *American Journal of Mental Deficiency, 77,* 492-497.

Kronenberg, F., Algado, S. S., & Pollard, N. (2005). *Occupational therapy without borders: Learning from the spirit of survivors.* London: Churchill Livingstone.

Largo, R. H., & Howard, J. A. (1979). Developmental progression in play behavior of children between nine and thirty months. I. Spontaneous play and imitation. *Developmental Medicine and Child Neurology, 21,* 299-310.

Lazarus, M. (1883). *Die reize des spiels.* Berlin: Ferd, Dummlers Verlagsbuchhandlung.

Matsutsuyu, J. S. (1969). The interest check list. *American Journal of Occupational Therapy, 23,* 323-328.

Mead, G. H. (1934). *Mind, self, and society.* Chicago: University of Chicago Press.

Melchert-McKearnan, K., Deitz, J., Engel, J. M., & White, O. (2000). Children with burn injuries: Purposeful activity versus rote exercise. *American Journal of Occupational Therapy, 54*(4), 381-390.

Mellou, E. (1994). Play theories: A contemporary review. *Early Child Development and Care, 102,* 91-100.

Merriam-Webster Online. Retrieved Sept. 4, 2007 from http://www.m-w.com/.

Meyer, A. (1922). The philosophy of occupation therapy. *Archives of Occupational Therapy, 1,* 1-10.

Miller, L. J., Wilbarger, J. L., Stackhouse, T. M., Trunnell, S. T., & Hanft, B. E. (2002). Use of clinical reasoning in occupational therapy: The STEP-SI model of intervention of sensory modulation dysfunction. In Bundy, A. C., Lane, S. J., & Murray, E. A. (Eds.), *Sensory integration: Theory and practice* (2nd ed.). Philadelphia: F.A. Davis.

Missiuna, C., & Pollock, N. (1991). Play deprivation in children with physical disabilities: The role of the occupational therapist in preventing secondary disability. *American Journal of Occupational Therapy, 45*(10), 882-888.

Okimoto, A. M., Bundy, A., & Hanzlik, J. (2000). Playfulness in children with and without disability: Measurement and intervention. *American Journal of Occupational Therapy, 54,* 73-82.

Ornstein, R., & Sobel, D. (1989). *Healthy pleasures.* Reading, MA: Addison-Wesley.

Parham, L. D. (1995, April). *The proper domain of occupational therapy research is the study of occupation and its applications to health care.* Paper presented at the Research Colloquium of the American Occupational Therapy Foundation, Denver, CO.

Parham, L. D. (1996). Perspectives on play. In R. Zemke & F. Clark (Eds.), *Occupational science: The evolving discipline.* Philadelphia: F.A. Davis.

Parham, L. D., Cohn, E. S., Spitzer, S., Koomar, J. A., Miller, L. J., Burke, J. P., et al. (2007). Fidelity in sensory integration intervention research. *American Journal of Occupational Therapy, 61*(2), 216-227.

Parham, L. D., & Mailloux, Z. (2005). Sensory integration. In J. Case-Smith (Ed.), *Occupational therapy for children*(5th ed., pp. 356-411). St. Louis: Mosby.

Parten, M. B. (1932). Social participation among preschool children. *Journal of Abnormal Psychology, 27*, 243-269.

Patrick, G. T. (1916). *The psychology of relaxation*. Boston: Houghton-Mifflin.

Pellegrini, A. D. (2002). Perceptions of play-fighting and real fighting: Effects of sex and participant status. In J. L. Roopnarine (Ed.), *Conceptual, social-cognitive, and contextual issues in the fields of play, Vol. 4* (pp. 223-233). Westport, CT: Ablex Publishing.

Pellegrini, A. D. (2005). *Recess: Its role in development and education*. Mahwah, NJ: Lawrence Erlbaum.

Pellegrini, A. D., & Davis, P. D. (1993). Relations between children's playground and classroom behaviour. *British Journal of Educational Psychology 63*(Pt 1), 88-95.

Pellegrini, A. D., & Smith, P. K. (1998). Physical activity play: The nature and function of a neglected aspect of playing. *Child Development, 69*, 577-598.

Piaget, J. (1962). *Play, dreams, and imitation in childhood*. (C. Gattegno & F. M. Hodgson, Trans.). New York: W.W. Norton. (Original work published in 1951.)

Poulsen, A. A., & Ziviani, J. M. (2004). Can I play too? Physical activity engagement of children with developmental coordination disorders. *Canadian Journal of Occupational Therapy 71*(2), 100-107.

Power, T. (1985). Mother and father-infant play: A developmental analysis. *Child Development, 56*, 1514-1524.

Primeau, L.A. (1995). *Orchestration of work and play within families* (Unpublished dissertation, University of Southern California, Los Angeles).

Primeau, L. A., Clark, F., & Pierce, D. (1989). Occupational therapy alone has looked upon occupation: Future applications of occupational science to pediatric occupational therapy. *Occupational Therapy in Health Care, 6*, 19-32.

Reilly, M. (1966). A psychiatric occupational therapy program as a teaching model. *American Journal of Occupational Therapy, 20*, 61-67.

Reilly, M. (1969). The educational process. *American Journal of Occupational Therapy, 23*, 299-307.

Reilly, M. (Ed.). (1974). *Play as exploratory learning*. Beverly Hills, CA: Sage Publications.

Reynolds, P. D. (1971). *A primer in theory construction*. Indianapolis: Bobbs-Merrill Educational Publishing.

Richardson, P. K. (2002). The school as social context: Social interaction patterns of children with physical disabilities. *American Journal of Occupational Therapy, 56*(3), 296-304.

Rigby, P., & Gaik, S. (2007). Stability of playfulness across environmental settings: A pilot study. *Physical and Occupational Therapy in Pediatrics 27*(1), 27-43.

Robinson, A. L. (1977). Play: The arena for acquisition of rules for competent behavior. *American Journal of Occupational Therapy, 31*, 248-253.

Rood, M. S. (1956). Neurophysiological mechanisms utilized in the treatment of neuromuscular dysfunction. *American Journal of Occupational Therapy, 10*, 220-224.

Roopnarine, J. L., & Johnson, J. E. (1994). The need to look at play in diverse cultural settings. In Roopnarine, J. L., Johnson, J. E., & Hooper, F. H. (Eds.), *Children's play in diverse cultures* (pp. 1-8). Albany, NY: State University of New York Press.

Rosenbaum, P. (1998). Physical activity play in children with disabilities: A neglected opportunity for research? *Child Development, 69*, 607-608.

Roth, J., Brooks-Gunn, J., Linver, M., & Hofferth, S. (2002). What happens during the school day? Time diaries from a national sample of elementary school teachers. *Teachers College Record [Online]*. Available: http://www.tcrecord.org, ID Number: 11018.

Rubin, K. H., Fein, G. G., & Vandenberg, B. (1983). Play. In P. H. Mussen (Series Ed.), E. M. Hetherington (Vol. Ed.), *Handbook of child psychology. Vol. 4. Socialization, personality, and social development* (4th ed., pp. 693-774). New York: John Wiley & Sons.

Saunders, E. B. (1922). Psychiatry and occupational therapy. *Archives of Occupational Therapy, 1*, 99-114.

Schaaf, R. C. (1990). Play behavior and occupational therapy. *American Journal of Occupational Therapy, 44*, 68-75.

Schaaf, R. C., Merrill, S. C., & Kinsella, N. (1987). Sensory integration and play behavior: A case study of the effectiveness of occupational therapy using sensory integrative techniques. *Occupational Therapy in Health Care, 4*, 61-75.

Schaaf, R. C., & Mulrooney, L. L. (1989). Occupational therapy in early intervention: A family-centered approach. *American Journal of Occupational Therapy, 43*(11), 745-754.

Schiller, F. (1795/1967). *On the aesthetic education of man*. (E. M. Wilkinson & L. A. Willoughby, trans.). Oxford, UK: Oxford University Press.

Schwartzman, H. B. (1978). *Transformations: The anthropology of children's play*. New York: Plenum Press.

Shannon, P. D. (1974). Occupational choice: Decision making play. In M. Reilly (Ed.), *Play as exploratory learning* (pp. 285-314). Beverly Hills, CA: Sage Publications.

Singer, D. G., & Singer, J. L. (1990). *The house of make-believe*. Cambridge, MA: Harvard University Press.

Siviy, S. M. (1998). Neurobiological substrates of play behavior: Glimpses into the structure and function of mammalian playfulness. In M. Bekoff & J. A. Byers (Eds.), *Animal play: Evolutionary, comparative, and ecological perspectives* (pp. 221-242). Cambridge, UK: Cambridge University Press.

Slagle, E. C. (1922). Training aides for mental patients. *Archives of Occupational Therapy, 1*, 11-17.

Slagle, E. C. (1934). Occupational therapy: Recent methods and advances in the United States. *Occupational Therapy and Rehabilitation, 13*, 289-298.

Slobin, D. (1964). The fruits of the first season: A discussion of the role of play in childhood. *Journal of Humanistic Psychology, 4*, 59-79.

Smith, N. (1958). Occupational therapy in a pediatric section. *American Journal of Occupational Therapy, 12*, 306-313.

Soto, L. D., & Negron, L. (1994). Puerto Rican children. In J. Johnson & J. Roopnarine (Eds.), *Children's play in diverse cultures*. Albany, NY: State University of New York Press.

Spencer, H. (1978). Aesthetic sentiments. In D. Muller-Schwarze (Ed.), *Evolution of play behavior* (pp. 10-15). Stroudsburg, PA: Dowden, Hutchinson, & Ross. (Reprinted from *The principles of psychology*. Vol. 2, pp. 627-632, by H. Spencer, 1878, Appleton & Company.)

State of Connecticut: General Assembly. (2004). *Raised Bill No. 5344: An act concerning childhood nutrition in schools, recess, and lunch breaks.* Retrieved July 31, 2007 from www.cga.state.ct.us/2004/TOB/h/pdf/2004HB05344-R00.HB.pdf.

State of Michigan: State Board of Education. (2000). *Policies for creating effective learning environments.* Retrieved July 31, 2007 from www.michigan.gov/documents/bdpolicy001214 26470 7.pdf.

State of Virginia. (2000). 8VAC20-131-80. Instructional program in elementary schools. *Virginia Register, 15* (25).

Stevenson, G. H. (1932). The healing influence of work and play in a mental hospital. *Archives of Occupational Therapy, 11,* 85-89.

Sutton-Smith, B. (1966). Piaget on play: A critique. *Psychological Review, 73,* 104-110.

Sutton-Smith, B. (1967). The role of play in cognitive development. *Young Children, 22,* 361-370.

Sutton-Smith, B. (1977). Play as adaptive potentiation. In P. Stevens (Ed.), *Studies in the anthropology of play.* Cornwall, NY: Leisure Press.

Sutton-Smith, B. (1980). Children's play: Some sources of play theorizing. In K. H. Rubin (Ed.), *New directions for child development: No. 9. Children's play* (pp. 1-16). San Francisco: Jossey-Bass.

Sutton-Smith, B. (1997). *The ambiguity of play.* Cambridge, MA: Harvard University Press.

Sutton-Smith, B. (2003). Play as a parody of emotional vulnerability. In D. Lytle (Ed.), *Play and culture studies, Vol. 5.* (pp. 3-17). Westport, CT: Praeger.

Takata, N. (1974). Play as a prescription. In M. Reilly (Ed.), *Play as exploratory learning* (pp. 209-246). Beverly Hills, CA: Sage Publications.

Tandy, C. A. (1999). Children's diminishing play space: A study of inter-generational change in children's use of their neighbourhoods. *Australian Geographical Studies, 37,* 154-164.

Tanta, K., Deitz, J., White, O., & Billingsley, F. (2005). The effect of peer-play level on initiations and responses of preschool children with delayed play skills. *American Journal of Occupational Therapy, 59,* 437-445.

Tobin, J. J., Wu, D. Y. H., & Davidson, D. H. (1989). *Preschool in three cultures: Japan, China, and the United States.* New Haven, CT: Yale University Press.

Vandenberg, B. (1978). Play and development from an ethological perspective. *American Psychologist, 33,* 724-738.

Watson, R., & Swartz, L. (2004). *Transformation through occupation.* London: Whurr Publishers.

Weisler, A., & McCall, R. B. (1976). Exploration and play: Resume and redirection. *American Psychologist, 31,* 492-508.

White, R. W. (1959). Motivation reconsidered: The concept of competence. *Psychological Review, 66,* 297-333.

White, R. W. (1971). The urge towards competence. *American Journal of Occupational Therapy, 25,* 271-274.

Whiteford, G. (2000). Occupational deprivation: Global challenge in the new millennium. *British Journal of Occupational Therapy, 65,* 200-205.

Whittier, I. L. (1922). Occupation for children in hospitals. *Occupational Therapy and Rehabilitation, 1,* 41-47.

Wilcock, A., & Townsend, E. (2000). Occupational terminology: Interactive dialogue. *Journal of Occupational Science, 7*(2), 84-86.

Williams, M. S., & Shellenberg, S. (1996). *How does your engine run? Leader's guide to the Alert Program for Self-Regulation* (rev. ed.). Albuquerque: TherapyWorks.

Wittgenstein, L. (1958). *Philosophical investigations* (3rd ed.) (G. E. M. Anscombe, Trans.). New York: Macmillan. (Original work published in 1953.)

Wood, W. (1996). The value of studying occupation: An example with primate play. *American Journal of Occupational Therapy, 50,* 327-337.

Yerxa, E. J., Clark, F. A., Frank, G., Jackson, J., Parham, D., Pierce, D., et al. (1989). An introduction to occupational science, a foundation for occupational therapy in the 21st century. *Occupational Therapy in Health Care, 6,* 1-17.

Ziegler, L. H. (1924). Some observations on recreations. *Archives of Occupational Therapy, 3,* 255-265.

Zuckerman, M. (1994). *Behavioral expressions and biosocial bases of sensation seeking.* Cambridge, UK: Cambridge University Press.

INTERNET RESOURCES

Play Advocacy

American Association for the Child's Right to Play
http://www.ipausa.org

Association for Childhood Education International
http://www.acei.org

International Play Association: Promoting the Child's Right to Play
http://www.ipaworld.org

National Institute for Play
http://nifplay.org

Playing for Keeps
http://www.playingforkeeps.org

Strong National Museum of Play
http://strongmuseum.org

Where Do the Children Play? A National Education & Community Engagement Campaign
http://www.childrenplay.org/matriarch/default.asp

Play Spaces

ADA Accessibility Guidelines for Play Areas
http://www.access-board.gov/play/index.htm

Center for Creative Play
http://www.cfcp.org

Children's Play Areas, Playhouses
http://www.B4UBuild.com

Kaboom
http://www.kaboom.org

National Center for Boundless Play
http://boundlessplaygrounds.org

Playhouse Plans, Playgrounds and Forts
http://www.B4Ubuild.com/links/play_areas.html

Play Research

Active Living Research
http://www.activelivingresearch.org

Association for the Study of Play
http://www.csuchico.edu/kine/tasp

President's Council on Physical Fitness and Sports Research Digest
http://www.presidentschallenge.org/misc/news_research/research_digests.59547a.pdf

Pretend Play & Children's Development
http://www.ericdigests.org/2002-2/play.htm

School-Based Physical Activity Interventions to Prevent or Treat Childhood Overweight
http://www.mcg.edu/institutes/gpi/ResearchPaper.pdf

Recess

American Association for the Child's Right to Play: Recess
http://www.ipausa.org/recess.htm

Elementary Recess Handbook
http://www.ipausa.org/elemrecessbook.html

National Recess Week
http://www.rescuingrecess.com/getinformedaboutprogram

Recess in Elementary School: What Does the Research Say?
http://www.ericdigests.org/2003-2/recess.html

Toys for Children with Disabilities

Able Crew
http://www.theablecrew.org

Able Play
http://www.ableplay.org

Beyond Play
http://www.beyondplay.com

Disability Resource Monthly Guide to Disability Resources on the Internet
http://www.disabilityresources.org

Dr. Toy: The Best Advice on Children's Products
http://www.drtoy.com

Early Intervention Products for Young Children with Special Needs
http://www.whitehutchison.com/children

Lekotek: The Country's Central Source on Toys & Play for Children with Special Needs
http://www.lekotek.org

STEPS: Developmental Adapted Toy and Switch Library
http://www.stepscharity.org

II

Assessment of Play

2

Narrative Contributions to the Play History

Kimberly C. Bryze

The opportunity to assess a child's skills and abilities provides the occupational therapist with a unique glimpse into the child's life in progress. Each child has a past history, is living the present, and is moving toward his or her individual future. The child's past, complete with achievements and struggles, is foundational to who the child is at this present moment. It is the present into which the occupational therapist is invited, to learn, to assess, to influence. Through a narrative process the therapist can begin to understand the child's present in light of his or her past and to imagine the child's future story. The occupational therapist's role is to enter into one episode, or one chapter, in the ongoing story of the child's life. Specifically, the child's life of play is already in process; the occupational therapist is allowed into the child's life because of the unique contributions the therapist can offer to the child's present and future stories.

Most likely the child has been referred to occupational therapy because of concerns about the appropriateness or quality of his or her occupational performance, of which play is one of the most important dimensions in a child's life. Occupational therapists have traditionally assessed the child's play through observation and administration of various play scales. They have then made inferences regarding the impact of delayed skill performance on the child's play, and they have reasoned that by improving the skills that support play, they can improve this overarching occupation of the child. These skill-based methods of assessing play provide therapists with information about the child's current play abilities. However, these tools do not provide a historical perspective of how the child has developed into the player he or she is at present. The Play History (Takata, 1974) has been designed to provide an instrument by which occupational therapists can assess the child's present abilities in light of his or her past play experiences.

This chapter addresses some conceptual and practical concerns about play and the use of the Play History as part of the evaluation process for children. The unique contributions of the narrative approach for collecting information about a child's past and present play are discussed. Guidelines for using a narrative approach to supplement information obtained by more formal means are also offered.

STUDY OF PLAY AND OCCUPATIONAL THERAPY

Occupational therapists have struggled to define clearly what they mean by "play." Although therapists have collected together an extensive body of knowledge about play from such disciplines as education, anthropology, and psychology, relatively little has been done to develop an occupational therapy theory of play. The related bodies of knowledge have contributed to occupational therapists' learning "about play," but this learning has been limited to the interpretations reflective of each discipline. For example, because of their interest in development, researchers in psychology have studied early stages of play as transitions to higher levels of social interaction or pretend play. Occupational therapists have approached the study of play by developing taxonomies for describing play behavior in children. Again, these taxonomies usually reflect other disciplines' knowledge base about play.

Occupational therapists, however, cannot derive from other disciplines' literature all the information they need about play and thus cannot fully understand how play contributes to and supports occupational behavior.

In addition to diverse information from other disciplines, the interpretations of play vary within occupational therapy itself. This variation may result from the influences of theory or frames of reference from which individual therapists practice (Burke, 1993). Therapists with perspectives in practice models such as sensory integration or neurodevelopmental treatment may relate the child's play to an outcome of the ability to process and use sensory input for the production of an adaptive response or as a reflection of neuromotor output. As such, play may be a means to an end (e.g., improved function).

M. Brewster Smith (1974) asserted that the developmental roots of competence lie in the human capacity for play. Play begins the developmental process of occupational behavior and promotes competence, achievement, and acquisition of occupational roles. The child who adequately learns the skills of occupational behavior through play can transform these skills into the habits and roles of daily life. Play is also one way children can learn how they "fit" within an environment. Play is one process by which children learn how they can affect the environment and how they are affected by the environment, and by which they adapt to the environment or adapt the environment to themselves. Moreover, play is a way to derive meaning from environmental interactions; play is a persistent strategy individuals use to apprehend the unknown (Reilly, 1974).

Play can be conceptualized as a transaction between the child and the environment that is intrinsically motivated, internally controlled, and not bound by objective reality (Neumann, 1971). As such, play can be an internal phenomenon or an external event and may be considered to be a continuum of behaviors that are more or less observable, depending on the degree to which the child is internally controlled, intrinsically motivated, and able to suspend reality (Bundy, 1991; Neumann, 1971). Any activity can be playful if the player so wishes; playfulness depends more on process than on the outcome, or product, of play. Play is also a mastery process in which activity is related to capacity; the outcome is skill (Reilly, 1974).

Play may assume various forms of interaction (e.g., sensorimotor, social-emotional, linguistic, or cognitive) and may be realized through various methods of playing, such as qualities of exploration, repetition, replication, or transformation. Play may be directed toward people, objects, or specific functions (e.g., information seeking, social learning, sensorimotor activity, emotional or creative expression). The relationship of the child in dynamic interaction within an environmental context is a continual process that results in the child's learning about herself or himself and the social and physical environment(s). This

relationship is dependent on the cognitive, creative, and interactional abilities of the child. The quality of a child's play is related to the range of these characteristics as they influence action within and on the environment (Takata, 1974).

Each stage of development reflects a stepping stone toward maturity through play and its contribution to the acquisition of occupational behavior. If specific skills do not develop within appropriate developmental stages, a child may be at a disadvantage in progressing toward a subsequent stage. Moreover, if the requisite opportunities for activity and interaction are lacking at a critical period, particular skills may not appear, may be delayed in their appearance, or may be deficient. In this way the processes of development and play parallel each other (Takata, 1974). Moreover, when the physical or human-social environment does not support play, the potential for developing those skills and behaviors may also be reduced. When medical, physical, or cognitive limitations exist, the possibility of learning those skills and behaviors that typically are direct consequences of playful experiences may be affected (Burke, 1993; Reilly, 1974). A child with physical or cognitive disabilities may lack both the abilities and the opportunities for successful play experiences and may be vulnerable to limitations posed by cultural and environmental constraints (Reilly, 1974). Moreover, there is always the risk that the child will not develop the quality of play reflective of his or her stage of maturity. It is most important therefore that inadequate play habits be detected and treated (Behnke & Fetkovich, 1984).

Assessment of Play

An occupational therapist will assess a child's play as an important dimension of understanding the child's ability to participate in one of the most important areas of occupational performance. Assessment in itself is the process of gathering data relevant to a particular child or a particular set of skills or abilities and may include a variety of methods by which to gather these data. An occupational therapist may choose to directly observe the child performing the occupation of play or may choose to gather relevant information by interviewing the child's parent or caregiver. Both types of assessment format are important and provide unique information for use in planning and implementing occupation-based intervention.

Many scholars (Fisher, Bryze, & Hume, 2002; Hinojosa & Kramer, 1998; McLean, Wolery, & Bailey, 2003) have reported the most desirable qualities of assessment processes for use by occupational therapists. In addition to an assessment's reliability and validity, other qualities are especially important in the gathering of information about a child's occupational performance, or play. The *relevance* of the assessment to the reported concerns that prompted the occupational therapy referral is a reminder to therapists to assess that which is most important from the perspective of the parent or caregiver, and this is usually the child's ability to participate in the activity of playing. The assessment should focus on *familiar* play experiences, should include toys and objects to which the child is accustomed, and should be conducted in settings that are *natural* and effortless for the child and family (Pellegrini, 2001). Allowing the child or family to choose the environmental setting or toys and objects increases the level of relevance, familiarity, and authenticity for the assessment process. To provide an effective assessment process, however, the occupational therapist must consider the extent to which the play opportunities present a level of *challenge* that will ensure that exquisite balance between not-enough and too-much difficulty. If one of the operational defining points of play is fun, the challenge of the toys and play opportunities must be "just right" to ensure that the characteristics of internal control and intrinsic motivation are protected.

Although the above-described qualities of occupational therapy assessments are easily considered when a child's performance skills of play are being measured through direct observation, how can these ideals be integrated into an interview- or discussion-based assessment process? The dimensions of relevance, familiarity, naturalness or authenticity, and challenge may all be addressed through an interview assessment process, such as when the Play History is used. The Play History, originally developed by Nancy Takata (1974), provides a structure by which an occupational therapist learns about the child's play interests, skills, and qualities over the timeline of that child's life, whether a short time (e.g., under 2 years) or longer (e.g., more than 7 or 8 years). The Play History is a tool that has been underused by occupational therapists. It will allow them to learn about the child's history of development, the many supports that interweave to facilitate the many forms of play, and the many contributions of play to development.

OVERVIEW OF THE ORIGINAL PLAY HISTORY

The Play History (Takata, 1974) was developed on the premise that play and development are intertwined and that assessment of, and intervention for, play dysfunction is vital to the continued development of the child (Behnke & Fetkovich, 1984; Takata, 1974). Since development is viewed as a process that takes place over time, it is important to look at the past as well as the present play behaviors of the child. Therefore occupational therapists' assessments of play should reflect the premise that play reflects development and thus increases in complexity over time (Behnke & Fetkovich, 1984).

The Play History (Takata, 1974) was developed as a guide to address important concerns regarding the extent to which the past and the present environments support,

guide, and elicit growth and development of competence and skills for competence in life (Behnke & Fetkovich, 1984). The gathering of the child's unique history is believed to be important in the total process of occupational therapy assessment. Development proceeds in an orderly manner with predictability as well as increasing complexity from one step to the next. Therefore a historical perspective can provide important information pertaining to the child's development and competence in play, which may be used in the planning and implementing of intervention.

The instrument consists of an interview schedule designed to identify a child's play experiences, interactions, environments, and opportunities across the time progression of his or her life. The Play History is designed to relate information about the quality and quantity of a child's play to each of five developmental phases or epochs: (1) sensorimotor, (2) symbolic and simple constructive, (3) dramatic and complex constructive, (4) games, and (5) recreational. (See Chapter 1 for a summary of these epochs.) These epochs provide the taxonomy for an analysis of the play phenomenon, and in each of these epochs the following four categories are analyzed: (1) materials (with what does the child play?), (2) action (how does the child play?), (3) people (how does the child play with others?), and (4) setting (where and when does the child play?). These epochs and categories strongly reflect the work of Piaget (1951/1962), Gesell (1945), and other authors in the field of developmental psychology, as well as other occupational therapists working from an occupational behavior perspective (Florey, 1971; Reilly, 1974).

As it was originally designed, the Play History is semistructured, qualitative, and open ended in format (Takata, 1974). It includes a basic set of questions that the interviewer may ask in a meaningful order, depending on the progression of the interview and the content, or depth, of the information provided by the child's parent(s) or primary caregiver(s). Examples of the questions include: With what does the child play? How does the child play? How does the child use tools and materials? What type of play is avoided or liked the least? With whom does the child play? How does the child play with others? The entire Play History is shown in Box 2-1.

Using the original examples of questions (Box 2-1) will often lead the parent to answer in a descriptive manner, rather than by simply saying "yes" or "no." The therapist is required to identify whether the particular criterion under each question has been answered with supporting "evidence," "no evidence," or "no opportunity" in each of the categories within each epoch. The therapist then interprets the results of the interview using a taxonomy of play (Table 2-1). The taxonomy is based on the play epochs outlined by Takata (1974) and has been designed to allow analysis of the child's play in comparison to the typical development of play (Behnke & Fetkovich, 1984; Burke, 1993; Takata, 1974).

Box 2-1 *The Play History*

(1) GENERAL INFORMATION
Name: Birthdate: Sex:
Date: Informant(s):
Presenting Problem:

(2) PREVIOUS PLAY EXPERIENCES
  A. Solitary play
  B. Play with others:
       mother   father   sisters   brothers   playmates   other family members
       pets
  C. Play with toys and materials (earliest preferences)
  D. Gross physical play
  E. Pretend and make-believe play
  F. Sports and games: group collaboration   group competition
  G. Creative interests: arts   crafts
  H. Hobbies, collections, other leisure time activities
  I. Recreation/social activities

(3) ACTUAL PLAY EXAMINATION
  A. *With what* does the child play?
       toys   materials   pets
  B. *How* does the child play with toys and other materials?
  C. What type of play is *avoided* or liked least?
  D. *With whom* does the child play?
       self   parents   brothers   sisters   peers   others
  E. *How* does the child play with others?
  F. *What body postures* does the child use during play?
  G. *How long* does the child play with objects? with people?
  H. *Where* does the child play?
       home: indoors   outdoors
       community: park   school   church   other areas
  I. *When* does the child play?
       daily schedule for weekday and weekend

(4) PLAY DESCRIPTION

(5) PLAY PRESCRIPTION

From Takata, N. (1974). Play as prescription. In M. Reilly (Ed.), *Play as exploratory learning.* Beverly Hills, CA: Sage Publications.

One study (Behnke & Fetkovich, 1984) provided evidence for the reliability and validity of therapists' judgments regarding play development using the Play History. The researchers developed an ordinal scale to quantify information obtained through interviews using the Play History and found high interrater reliability on overall play scores. Test-retest coefficients fell in a moderate range, perhaps reflecting inconsistency in the details recalled by parents from one interview to the next, or increased sensitivity to particular aspects of their children's play as a result of the first interview. Total Play History scores were significantly associated with subscale scores on the Minnesota Child Developmental Inventory. This finding indicates that the Play History yields valid information regarding the child's developmental level.

Behnke and Fetkovich (1984) provided encouraging evidence that the Play History is a reliable and valid measure of general developmental trends in play. The numerical scores they used in their study, however, do not capture the rich qualitative information that an interview produces. In an interview, themes emerge that reflect a child's early and current dominant play behaviors or schemas. Because the emerging themes and specific play patterns paint a unique portrait of the child being assessed, they provide essential information for planning treatment. Therefore the interpretation of interview material is critical in the assessment process. The actual interpretation, or reconstruction, of a child's play history constitutes a difficult yet important step, the basis for which is the depth and quality of the information obtained from the interview.

Although the Play History is designed to be an open-ended interview, its application may be limited by problems inherent in all interviews. The purpose of interviews is to obtain information about certain aspects of behavior or experience. Interviews have a different form and function than more casual or everyday conversations. In casual or friendly conversations each participant takes turns and shares responsibility for keeping the conversation going. In interviews the interviewer and the informant take

Table 2-1
Use of a Play Milieu and Taxonomy

	Sensorimotor Play (0-2 Years)	*Symbolic and Simple Constructive Play (2-4 Years)*	*Dramatic and Complex Constructive Play (4-7 Years)*	*Play Including Games (7-12 Years)*	*Recreation (12-16 Years)*
Emphasis	Independent play with exploration; trial and error	Parallel and beginning to share; symbolic play, and simple constructional use of materials	Cooperative play with purposeful use of materials for constructions, dramatization of reality, and building habits of skill and tool use	Enhancement of constructional and sports skills as expressed in rule-bound behavior, competition, and appreciation of process cooperative play	Team participation and independent action expressed in organized sports, interest groups, and hobbies during leisure time
Materials	Toys, objects for sensory experiences (see, mouth, touch, hear, smell): rattles, ball, nesting blocks, straddle toys, chimes, simple pictures, color cones, large blocks	Toys, objects, raw materials (water, sand, clay, paints, crayons) for fine motor manipulation and simple combining and taking apart Wheeled vehicles and adventure toys to practice gross motor actions	Objects, toys, raw materials for fine motor actions and role playing; large adventure toys for refining gross actions for speed and coordination; pets; nonselective collections	Games played with rules (dominoes, checkers, table card games, Ping-Pong); raw materials and tools for making complex products (weaving, woodwork, carving, needlework) Gross muscle sports—hopscotch, kite flying, skating, basketball Books—puzzles, "things to do," biography, adventure, sports Selective collection or hobby Pet	Team games and sports and special interest groups for music, dancing, singing, discussing Collections and hobbies; parties, books, table games

Continued

Table 2-1
Use of a Play Milieu and Taxonomy—cont'd

	Sensorimotor Play (0-2 Years)	*Symbolic and Simple Constructive Play* (2-4 Years)	*Dramatic and Complex Constructive Play* (4-7 Years)	*Play Including Games* (7-12 Years)	*Recreation* (12-16 Years)
Action	Gross—stand/fall, walk, pull, sit on, climb, open/close Fine—touch, mouth, hold, throw/pick up, bang, shake, carry Motoric imitation of domestic actions	Gross—climb, run, jump, balance, drag, dump, throw Fine—empty/fill; scribble/draw; squeeze/pull; combine/take apart; arrange in spatial dimensions Imagination with storytelling, fantasy; objects represent events/ things	Gross— "daredevil" feats of hopping, skipping, turning somersaults; dance Fine—combining materials and making products to do well, to use tools, to copy reality Dramatic role playing— imitating reality in part/whole costumes, storytelling	Gross—refining and combining skills of jumping, hopping, running Fine—precision in using variety of tools, finer object manipulation and construction Making, following, breaking rules; competition and compromise with peers	Gross—team sports and individual precision sports (tennis, golf) Fine—applying and practicing fine manipulative skills to develop craftsmanship, special talents Organized group work
People	Parents and immediate family	Parents, peers, other adults	Peer group (2 to 5 members); "imaginary friends"; parents, immediate family, other adults	Peer group of same sex; organized groups, e.g., scouts; parents, other adults	Peer group of same and opposite sex; parents and other adults
Setting	Home—crib, play- pen, floor, yard, immediate sur- roundings	Outdoors— playground; play equipment immediate neighborhood Indoors—home, "nursery"	School; neighborhood and extended surroundings (excursions); upper space and off the ground	Neighborhood, playground, school, home	School; neighborhood and extended community; home

Modified from Takata, N. (1974). Play as prescription. In M. Reilly (Ed.), *Play as exploratory learning.* Beverly Hills, CA: Sage Publications.

turns, but a clear differentiation exists between who asks the questions and who provides information regarding his or her individual experience; the interviewer asks most of the questions and the informant offers responses to the questions (Spradley, 1979). Moreover, because the inter- viewer seeks specific types of information, the informant's overriding concern may be to provide the "right" answer; this may interfere with the process of the interview and may affect the quality of the results of the overall assess- ment. Although the questions on the Play History can be arranged and reframed so that the content and order are most meaningful for the informant, the interviewer may be inclined to ask the questions in the same order or in the same phrases in which they have been written and thereby limit the meaningfulness and breadth of the information obtained by the interview process.

The interviewer will be able to use the categories of play and correlating ages as a framework within which the par- ent or caregiver is engaged, but the larger purpose of the interview is in gleaning increasingly deep and expansive explanations of the child's play history, thereby providing rich, descriptive information that the therapist may use in the overall assessment process and design of intervention for enhancing play. One way to facilitate skillful inter- viewing is to use a narrative approach, which contributes greater depth and validity to such an assessment process.

CONCEPTUAL BASES OF THE NARRATIVE APPROACH

Narrative is a natural means of communication between persons regarding daily life situations and events. Narratives are the stories people relate regarding those everyday occurrences that shape people's days and life (Helfrich, Kielhofner, & Mattingly, 1994). For example, the following is a story related by a parent to her child's occupational therapist:

(Mrs. Thompson and 14-month-old Amy arrive at the clinic for their occupational therapy appointment. Nancy, the therapist, greets them at the waiting room door):

Nancy: Good morning Amy, Mrs. Thompson. My, what a bruise you have, Amy! *(to Mrs. Thompson)* How did that happen?

Mrs. Thompson: You wouldn't believe the week we've had. You know, Amy is getting so active, she's quite a handful. Well, two days ago Amy was playing in the living room. I had taken the couch cushions off the couch so Amy could play and crawl on them—you know, from the couch to the cushions on the floor and back up to the couch? That's her "mountain climbing," we call it. Well, Amy was having a great time, crawling around. The phone rang, so I went to get it. It's in the hallway near the kitchen. It was my sister calling to say she was coming for dinner that night. After I hung up the phone, I walked back into the living room just as Amy was toppling off the arm of the couch. She had crawled up to the couch and up to the arm. Well, even though I ran as fast as I could, I couldn't catch her real good. She fell and bumped her head here, see? *(shows Nancy the bruise on her forehead)* I felt so bad. She cried a little bit, but calmed down with some milk and a quiet rock in the rocking chair with me.

Nancy: That must have been scary for you and for Amy! I'm glad she's O.K.

Mrs. Thompson: You wouldn't believe how scared I was. The funny part was after she stopped crying and had her bottle of milk, believe it or not, she went back to climbing her "mountain," as if nothing had happened. Up to the couch and back down to the cushions. She did stay away from the arms of the couch, but, boy, does she like to play that rough stuff! I suppose that's normal, huh? What do you think?

Narrative methodology has been described as being a natural means by which to obtain information about an individual's unique life experiences. Narrative methods are modeled after a normal conversation rather than a formal question and answer exchange. In the hearing and interpretation of the shared narratives, the therapist seeks to understand the other person's frame of reference, to see things from the other person's point of view (Mattingly & Fleming, 1994). The therapist regards what the informant says and does as a product of how the informant defines his or her own world.

Mattingly and Fleming (1994) have written that stories place events within a temporal context and that a historical sense is needed to help link people with the past and with some anticipated future. People organize their knowledge of the past and the future aspects of their lives through narratives. From this perspective, it is important to learn how the child and the family experience life and therefore how they are inclined to experience meaning in their daily lives. Using narrative, people structure their understandings of themselves and their respective lives. Because the parents of children who come to occupational therapy for assessment are the best sources of information concerning their particular child's play, therapists need to listen intently to their stories, to how they experience meaning and view the future (Figure 2-1). Moreover, while listening to and understanding the parents' stories of their child and his or her play, the therapist can begin to comprehend the family's world into which therapy may be inserted. The therapist and the family often begin to see the child's play life as an integrated whole, or as a picture, and not as a composite list of deficits or needs and problems to be changed.

The therapist is able to listen to the shared stories as chapters of the yet unfolding story of the child's play life. This foundation of narratives helps create a more complete picture of the child and his or her play. As these stories are organized in temporal fashion, the therapist will have a sense of development over time, making the views and goals for the future more relevant and meaningful for the child and family. Furthermore, by listening carefully to the kinds of questions and stories the families have about their children, the therapist may learn what kinds of information are important to them as they engage in the assessment process or therapy (Burke, 1993). Their interests will also be reflected in the meaningfulness of their narrative stories. For example:

Mrs. Phillips: Susie is such a good girl. Maybe she is almost too good, though. Does that go along with her heart condition? I mean, maybe because she doesn't move around and explore so much, maybe she really can't get into trouble like the other kids did. I kind of miss that. Actually, last week she did something completely unexpected, and it was great! I was cleaning the kitchen and bathroom areas, and was pretty intent on getting the place spic and span before my husband got home. Susie was playing with her stuffed animals on the kitchen floor. Well, I went into the bathroom to scrub the tub, and I wasn't in there too very long,

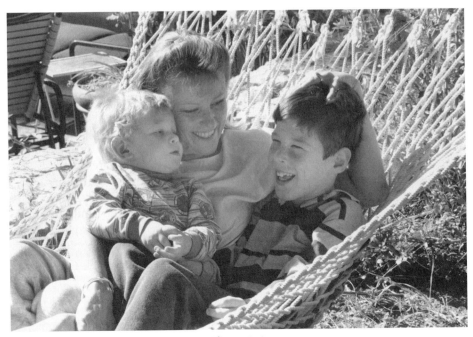

Figure 2-1

Because parents are the best sources of information concerning their child's play, therapists need to listen intently to their stories. (Courtesy Shay McAtee.)

but when I got out of the bathroom was I surprised! Susie had gotten into the pantry cupboard we have— it's a tall cabinet with floor to ceiling shelves. We keep crackers and baking stuff in there. The cupboard door must not have been closed all the way. Guess what happened? Susie got into the crackers and cereal boxes and dumped about five of them over her head! She was sitting in a huge pile of crackers and cereal and was covered. She had tossed it all over, and she had such a big smile on her face. At first I was pretty angry, then I realized she didn't understand why I was frustrated. It's the first kind of naughty thing she ever did, and she looked awfully proud of herself. I even took a picture of her in all this mess. Wanna see it? Here it is.

Narrative is one way in which therapists can incorporate many fragments of past experience into a coherent whole to be understood. Narratives provide powerful experiences of successfully met challenges, where the child has developed increasing confidence and inner drive to take on challenges as development progresses (Mattingly & Fleming, 1994). The exploration of the child's past play, through the parents' stories, is one way to connect a series of early experiences that occur over the child's years; these stories give events and actions meaning and context (Helfrich et al., 1994). In this way a child's play strengths and play needs can be viewed in light of a coherent life story, and the goals for the future may be interpreted and realized with the foundation of a meaningful past.

The goal of learning about a child's play history through narrative is not achieving correctness in its detail, but coming to understand the child within the integrity of his or her life story of play (Helfrich et al., 1994). As the parent relays the child's play history, the story lines may evolve and change as the child's developmental progress is conveyed. The meaning of actions or events across stories may change as the parent tells the story and as the child's play and family worlds come to be understood. Specific to the example of Susie, above, what has once been labeled as being "too good" may now be seen as a paucity of exploratory play; what has once been identified as "naughty" may now be seen within the context of fun, or even typical and "normal." Preliminary interpretations may be modified to adapt to the reality of developmental challenge or progress (Helfrich et al., 1994).

Using narrative can be empowering for the parents as they tell their child's stories, but listening carefully to their narratives is crucial for the therapist because the narratives provide insight into their perceptions of their shared life. Narratives offer a meaningful structure to a child's life across time and illustrate how the child and his or her play change over time (Mattingly & Fleming, 1994).

Clark (1993) has noted that meaningful therapy helps people to create and continue their life stories into the future. Therapists can only help transform a child's life if the people involved see meaning and relevance to their life stories; therapy is viewed as an event or as a chapter in the life of the child and family.

CONSIDERATIONS FOR ELICITING NARRATIVES

Using narrative as a means by which to obtain information about the child's play history may be likened to an art. There are guidelines that can be followed, but there are not strict rules under which these methodological guidelines fall. The methods by which the therapist conducts an interview can influence how narratively rich the parent's responses are. Ideally, the narrative interview is a collaborative process in which the therapist and family work together to find a shared meaning of the child's play. In this process the therapist wants to establish an atmosphere of partnership rather than an expert-patient relationship. The therapist attempts to construct a situation that resembles those in which people naturally talk to each other about important things. The interview should be relaxed and conversational, in the way that people usually interact. The therapist relates to the parents on a more personal level. The therapist is wise to accept whatever hesitant ideas the parent offers without making judgments and to accept the parent as a conversational equal (Taylor & Bogdan, 1984).

During the early parts of an interview the therapist sets the tone of the relationship with the parent. The therapist's initial goal is to establish rapport with the parent. The therapist should convey an attitude of someone who is willing to learn from the informants. In a narrative interview approach there is a danger of appearing to know all there is about how children "should" play. If the therapist maintains the affect and behavior of one who is just searching for meaningful information about the child within the context of his or her particular family, the parent will be much less guarded or fearful of giving the "wrong" answer about this most precious child. The therapist must create an atmosphere in which the parent feels comfortable to talk freely and openly about his or her child's past and present play.

Therapists should remember that interviews are purposeful conversations (Bogdan & Biklen, 1992) and beginning with informal "small talk" may establish the common ground necessary for the rest of the interview process. Early in the process the therapist should explain the purpose of the interview and that the information the parent or caregiver will provide will be important in better understanding the child (his or her development, play, etc.). By setting the frame for the Play History interview in such a way, the therapist puts the parent or caregiver at ease, which contributes to an abundance of rich data about the child's play. Keeping the interview as a conversation or dialogue, rather than a question-then-answer format, ensures elaboration and enhancement of the informants' report. To see the child's play world, a therapist must pay close attention to what is said throughout the interview process. Although this sounds commonplace, a therapist may need to overcome years of selective attention to the "stories" parents tell him or her about their children's lives. Watching, listening, and concentrating involve the hard work that is needed to uncover the meanings embedded in the story lines (Taylor & Bogdan, 1984).

A narrative approach to interviewing is flexible and dynamic. It can be described as being nondirective, unstructured, nonstandardized, and open ended in nature. Narrative approaches may be used in a one-session interview or over the course of several sessions directed toward understanding parents' perspectives on their child's abilities, experiences, or situations as expressed in their own words. An in-depth, narrative-oriented interview is modeled after a conversation between equals, rather than a formal question and answer exchange. The purpose is not merely to obtain answers, but to learn about meaningful contexts in which the child has played throughout development. The narrative approach makes it easier for the therapist to gather information by allowing the informant to guide the direction the interview takes, rather than rigidly sticking to an agenda of particular questions that require answers (Taylor & Bogdan, 1984). The therapist will want to ask questions or seek elaboration of information in a way that expresses interest in the child and the parent or family while following the parent's lead in the line of questioning. The therapist seeks the child's and the parents' perspective, as well as the parents' perceptions of the child's play, and finds ways of encouraging the parents to begin talking about these perspectives and experiences without structuring the conversation and defining what "should" be said.

The therapist may find use of an interview guide helpful to make sure the key topics are explored. This guide is not a structured series of questions or protocol but rather a list of general areas to cover with a parent. For example, consistent with the categories within the Play History, the interview guide may include the following descriptors as cues: (1) previous play experiences; (2) play with others; (3) nature of play with toys and materials in early childhood; (4) nature of gross motor physical play; (5) pretend and make-believe play; (6) participation in sports and games; (7) pursuit of creative interests; (8) pursuit of hobbies, collections, or other leisure-time activities; and (9) participation in recreation and social activities. The interview guide presupposes the therapist's knowledge of the development of play and understanding of various ages and stages through a child's maturation. In the interview situation the therapist decides how to phrase questions and when to ask them; the interview guide serves solely to remind the therapist to ask about certain things.

Early in the interview the therapist asks nondirective and nonjudgmental questions. As the therapist acquires knowledge and understanding of how the parent conveys information about his or her child, questioning may become more focused and directive. As themes and perspectives emerge, the therapist may need to seek clarification of the stories for depth and accuracy of the interpretation (Bogdan & Biklen, 1992). This offers the interview process a rich, natural quality as more complete information is gathered. An example of how a therapist might begin the interview process follows:

Therapist: As an occupational therapist, I am interested in how children perform everyday activities in different environments. One of the areas I am very interested in is how children play. In particular, I would like to get an idea of how Bernardo has played as he has grown and how he plays now. One of the best ways for me to learn about this is by listening to you—the expert on Bernardo—tell me a story about Bernardo playing. Can you tell me of one memorable incident of him playing, either by himself or with other children, that occurred within the past year or so? Tell me about his playing.

One of the best ways to begin an interview is to ask the parent to describe, list, or remember and describe one key event or play experience of the child. Of particular importance is how the therapist asks questions. Questions should be phrased in gentle, caring terms that support the parent's disclosure of personal insights or perceptions of the child and, to some extent, the parent herself or himself. Asking questions as if from the parent's perspective will provide a nonthreatening and open atmosphere in which to explore the child's unique characteristics in play. As the parent begins talking, the therapist can encourage expansion of ideas and detail by using encouraging words, cues, and gestures to indicate interest (Taylor & Bogdan, 1984). If possible, the therapist may encourage the parent to show a personal memento, such as photographs of the child playing or taken during some memorable time of the child's life, which can be used to guide the interview without imposing a structure on the parent (Figure 2-2).

An important principle in asking descriptive questions is that expanding the length of the question tends to encourage an expanded response from the parent (Mattingly & Fleming, 1994). A therapist might ask, "Could you tell me how Bernardo plays with his stuffed monkey?" and a descriptive answer would be obtained. A broader way of asking for such descriptive information might be, "From what you have said, Bernardo has many toys. Could you tell me about what he does when he plays with his monkey, how he plays, and how he may change his play when he plays with his monkey? Could you tell me what it is like when Bernardo plays?"

As the parent mentions specific experiences, the therapist can probe for greater detail, and the therapist may take notes of topics to which to return at a later time. Knowing when and how to probe is important. Throughout the interview, the therapist follows up on topics that have

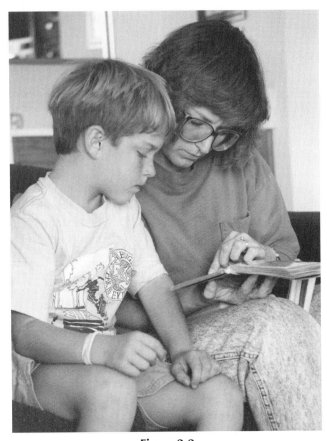

Figure 2-2
The therapist may encourage the parent to share personal mementos, such as photographs, which then can be used to further shape the interview. (Courtesy Shay McAtee.)

been raised by asking specific questions, encourages the parent to describe experiences in detail, and presses for clarification of particular words or phrases (Taylor & Bogdan, 1984). The therapist will want to probe gently for the details of the child's and parent's experiences and the meanings the child and parent attach to them. The therapist is interested in the everyday play events as well as the struggles and successful play experiences in which the child engages. The therapist should be aware that any form of sustained questioning implies evaluation and carries the risk of inadvertently returning to a more formal, distant interview process.

It is important not to interrupt a parent's story, even though the topic may not be interesting to the therapist. A therapist can use subtle gestures, such as not nodding, not taking notes, or gently changing the subject during breaks in the conversation, to redirect the conversation. The therapist must use this subtle control very carefully, however, to avoid directing the conversation in a way that prevents important information regarding the child's play history.

The therapist should ask for clarification of the informants' remarks by restating what was said and requesting confirmation of the restatement. Therapists must conduct interviews with the premise that words and symbols used in their own worlds may have different meanings in the worlds of their clients. They must be attuned to and explore the meanings of words or phrases with which they are not familiar. Therapists should not assume that they have always accurately understood phrases used in the context of a narrative story. If they do not attend to this issue, the essential meaning may be lost. Restating what the parent has said demonstrates a nonjudgmental attitude that contributes to the development of rapport. When the therapist restates what a parent says, a powerful, unstated message is communicated. Consider the following example:

Mrs. Lopez: Bernardo loves to play with his dad, Bernardo, Sr. He loves to be chased. Bernie (we call him Bernie so we won't confuse others with two Bernardos—when I say Bernie I mean little Bernardo) will be on the floor playing with his toys, and Bernardo will lay down close to him. Won't look at him, just lay close. Bernie will look over at his dad every once in a while, and still Bernardo won't look at him—or at least he doesn't let Bernie see him looking! Bernie will eventually ask Bernardo to play. Sometimes it takes a few minutes, but usually it only takes a short time.

Therapist: How does Bernie ask? What does he say?

Mrs. Lopez: Oh, Bernie doesn't talk yet. He asks with his eyes, or he says, "ah, ah, ah." He might even toss a toy at his dad as he lays there ignoring him. Bernie gets his point across!

Therapist: So Bernie asks his dad to play—then what happens?

Mrs. Lopez: Oh it drives me crazy! All of a sudden Bernardo will growl and roll over to his stomach and lunge for Bernie. Bernie usually screams—his scream is so loud, but he is really laughing and excited—and he tries to scoot away, as fast as he can, before Bernardo catches him! It gets really loud in here, and they're moving around on the floor. Sometimes Bernie goes too fast, and he's gonna hurt himself trying to move so fast.

Therapist: You're concerned that Bernie will fall over and bump his head. Has he ever gotten hurt in this game?

Mrs. Lopez: Oh, no. Bernardo always catches him before he hits the floor. They just go so fast. Bernie is scooting and squealing, and Bernardo is commando crawling and growling like a big bear, and it is so rowdy!

Therapist: That is quite a game! Who wins?

Mrs. Lopez: Oh, I think they both do. It usually ends with Bernardo catching little Bernie, of course, and holding him while they roll around on the floor. Lots of hugging and roughhousing. Bernie loves to play with his dad this way. I can't play with him that way, but Bernardo can. I wonder who has the most fun—Bernie or Bernardo?

The vocabulary used in a setting usually provides important clues to how people define situations and classify their world and thus suggests lines of inquiry and questioning. Certain assumptions may be built into a vocabulary. Therapists must learn to examine the words used as a function of the assumptions and purposes of the users, rather than as objective characterizations of the people or objects of reference, even when seemingly common words and phrases are used. The meaning and significance of people's verbal and nonverbal communication can be determined only in the context of what they actually discuss and how they contextualize their child's play experiences over time. The hallmark of narrative interviewing is learning about what is important in the minds of the parents: their meanings, perspectives, and definitions.

Some aspects of the narrative process mandate caution. With this less structured approach to interviewing, there is a danger of imputing meanings that people do not intend. The therapist is advised to pay attention, which implies an openness or an honoring of the person who is being interviewed. The therapist should bring an attitude of sensitivity to the interview situation.

Taylor and Bogdan (1984) suggest that a therapist look for key words in a parent's remarks that will enable the therapist to recall the parent's meaning. It is sometimes helpful to concentrate on the first and last remarks in each conversation. Conversations usually follow an orderly sequence—a certain question elicits a certain response, one remark provokes another, one topic leads to another related topic for discussion. The temporal flow of the interview offers a continuity for greater understanding for the therapist and the parent.

The therapist actively solicits the parent's remembrance and storytelling about the child's play experiences and constructs the child's play history as the final product. The narrative approach to interviewing is directed toward learning about events and activities that cannot be observed directly. In this type of interviewing the parents act as the therapist's eyes and ears with which to perceive the child's play. The parent's role is not simply to reveal his or her own views but to describe the play situations that have occurred. By asking for clarification, restating ideas, and listening attentively, the therapist supports the parent in becoming a good informant, which will further the process of understanding the child's play.

The quality and quantity of the information obtained rest with the therapist's knowledge of play and its developmental nature. Great skill in listening and interviewing is necessary to extract rich and thorough information that enables the therapist to contribute a salient chapter in a child's developing life story.

Review Questions

1. Describe the Play History, with respect to development, format, and purpose.
2. Why is the child's life story of concern to the occupational therapist?
3. Define narrative and narrative methodology.
4. How does the narrative approach affect the administration of the Play History?
5. What are the specific strategies a therapist can use to elicit narratives from parents about their child's play?

REFERENCES

Behnke, C. J., & Fetkovich, M. M. (1984). Examining the reliability and validity of the Play History. *American Journal of Occupational Therapy, 38*(2), 94-100.

Bogdan, R. C., & Biklen, S. K. (1992). *Qualitative research for education: An introduction to theory and methods.* Boston: Allyn & Bacon.

Brewster Smith, M. (1974). Foreword. In M. Reilly (Ed.), *Play as exploratory learning.* Beverly Hills, CA: Sage Publications.

Bundy, A. C. (1991). Play theory and sensory integration. In A. G. Fisher, E. A. Murray, & A. C. Bundy (Eds.), *Sensory integration: Theory and practice.* Philadelphia: F.A. Davis.

Burke, J. P. (1993). Play: The life role of the infant and young child. In J. Case-Smith (Ed.), *Pediatric occupational therapy and early intervention* (2nd ed.). Boston: Andover Medical Publishers.

Clark, F. (1993). Occupation embedded in a real life: Interweaving occupational science and occupational therapy. *American Journal of Occupational Therapy, 47*(12), 1067-1078.

Fisher, A. G., Bryze, K., & Hume, V. (2002). *School AMPS: School version of the Assessment of Motor and Process Skills.* Ft. Collins, CO: Three Star Press.

Florey, L. L. (1971). An approach to play and play development. *American Journal of Occupational Therapy, 25,* 275-280.

Gesell, A. (1945). *The embryology of behavior.* New York: Harper & Bros.

Helfrich, C., Kielhofner, G., & Mattingly, C. (1994). Volition as narrative: Understanding motivation in chronic illness. *American Journal of Occupational Therapy, 48*(4), 311-317.

Hinojosa, J., & Kramer, P. (1998). *Evaluation: Obtaining and interpreting data.* Bethesda, MD: American Occupational Therapy Association.

Mattingly, C., & Fleming, M. H. (1994). *Clinical reasoning: Forms of inquiry in a therapeutic practice.* Philadelphia: F.A. Davis.

McLean, M., Wolery, M., & Bailey, D. B. (2003). *Assessing infants and preschoolers with special needs* (3rd ed.). Upper Saddle River, NJ: Prentice Hall.

Neumann, E. A. (1971). *The elements of play.* New York: MSS Information.

Pellegrini, A. D. (2001). Practitioner review: The role of direct observation in the assessment of young children. *Journal of Child Psychology and Psychiatry, 42*(7), 861-869.

Piaget, J. (1962). Play, dreams, and imitation in childhood. (C. Gattegno & F. M. Hodgson, Trans.). New York: W.W. Norton. (Original work published in 1951).

Reilly, M. (Ed.). (1974). *Play as exploratory learning.* Beverly Hills, CA: Sage Publications.

Spradley, J. P. (1979). *The ethnographic interview.* Fort Worth, TX: Harcourt Brace Jovanovich.

Takata, N. (1974). Play as prescription. In M. Reilly (Ed.), *Play as exploratory learning.* Beverly Hills, CA: Sage Publications.

Taylor, S. J., & Bogdan, R. (1984). *Introduction to qualitative research methods: The search for meanings.* New York: John Wiley & Sons.

3

Development and Current Use of the Revised Knox Preschool Play Scale

Susan Knox

KEY TERMS

Revised Knox Preschool Play Scale
space management
material management
pretense-symbolic
participation

Play is an automatic, integral part of the lives of young children. All children engage in some form of play, and it is through play that they develop an understanding of the world and competence in interacting with it. The way children play reveals physical and cognitive abilities, social participation, imagination, independence, and coping mechanisms (Bergen, 1988; Brown & Gottfried, 1985; Bruner et al., 1976; Garvey, 1977; Hartley & Goldenson, 1963).

From the 1930s through the 1960s, developmental theorists began to describe aspects of play within a normative framework. This work became the precursor to the diagnostic use of play. Assessment of children's abilities through play became popular in the 1950s and 1960s. In the 1970s and 1980s, the growing body of literature on play led to the development of a variety of play assessments, based on normative data, that could be used in clinical settings (Schaefer et al., 1991). Play assessments reflect a variety of professional frameworks and examine different aspects of play, such as neurological functioning, cognitive functioning, organization of behavior, playfulness, and dramatic and social play (Bergen, 1988; Hulme & Lunzer, 1966; Kalverboer, 1977; Lieberman, 1977; Rosenblatt, 1977; Smilansky, 1968). This chapter addresses a widely used assessment instrument, the Revised Knox Preschool Play Scale (Knox, 1968, 1974, 1997b), and discusses its reliability, validity, research applications, and clinical use.

HISTORICAL PERSPECTIVE ON PLAY ASSESSMENT IN OCCUPATIONAL THERAPY

Play has been described as the child's occupation. Play has been characterized as intrinsic, spontaneous, fun, flexible, totally absorbing, vitalizing, challenging, nonliteral, and an end in and of itself. No single characteristic is common to all kinds of play, but a combination of any of the characteristics is usually seen. Play behavior can be analyzed in relation to cultural and societal roles and the effects of the physical and interpersonal environment (Cohen, 1987; Ellis, 1973; Reilly, 1974; Rubin et al., 1983; Takata, 1971) (Figure 3-1).

Assessment of play and of the child's abilities as seen through play is necessary to provide the therapist with tools to analyze play and to plan treatment. Analysis of how children play gives valuable information regarding their cognitive, motor, and social competencies. Occupational therapy focuses on the whole child functioning within the environment; therefore all aspects of development are considered important.

Although occupational therapists have long valued play as a treatment medium and have recognized the value of play as a reflection of child development, formal assessment of play in occupational therapy did not occur until the 1960s. It was during this time that the theory of occupational behavior, having particular relevance to the study of play, was developed by Mary Reilly (1974). Occupational behavior was described as the continuum between play and work, and play was considered one of the child's primary occupations. Reilly (1974) defined play as a multidimensional system for adaptation to the environment. She believed that the exploratory drive of curiosity underlies play behavior. This curiosity drive has three hierarchical stages: exploration, competency, and achievement. Exploratory behavior is seen primarily

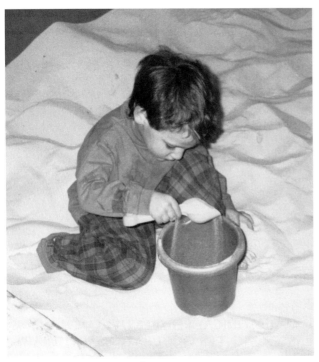

Figure 3-1
In play the child becomes totally absorbed.

in early childhood and is fueled by intrinsic motivation. Competency behavior is fueled by effectance motivation, identified by White (1959), and is characterized by experimentation and practice to achieve mastery. The third stage, achievement, is linked to goal expectancies and is fueled by a desire to achieve excellence (Reilly, 1974) (Figure 3-2).

Students working under Reilly developed clinical tools to assess various aspects of occupational behavior. Interviews examining a person's work or play history were developed (Moorehead, 1969; Takata, 1969, 1974). An interest inventory was designed to assess leisure in adults (Matsutsuyu, 1969). Developmental assessments of play were devised (Florey, 1971, 1981; Knox, 1968, 1974), and specific aspects of play were examined, such as intrinsic motivation (Florey, 1969) and the acquisition of rules (Robinson, 1977).

Despite the availability of play assessments, they were infrequently used until recently. In 1998, Couch and associates conducted a study examining the role of play in pediatric occupational therapy. Of the practitioners surveyed, 91% stated that play was very important and 92% said that they used play "as a modality to elicit motor, sensory, or psychosocial outcomes in their clients " (Couch et al., 1998, p. 113). Only 63% stated that they assessed play behavior, however, and this was primarily through clinical observations. Less than 15% used either criterion- or norm-referenced assessments. Stagnitti (2004) speculated that the low use of play assessments in clinical practice was due to a number of factors: (1) difficulty in assessing

in "natural" environments such as homes or community settings, (2) difficulty in defining play, and (3) unavailability of reliable and valid assessments designed specifically for use in clinical settings.

With the adoption of the Occupational Therapy Practice Framework (American Occupational Therapy Association, 2002), the current emphasis in assessment is on engagement in occupation. Since play is one of the child's primary occupations, the evaluation of play is gaining recognition and use.

REVISED KNOX PRESCHOOL PLAY SCALE

The Play Scale was developed in 1968 (Knox, 1968), and it was later published in *Play as Exploratory Learning* (Reilly, 1974). Play was defined for the purposes of the Preschool Play Scale as "the medium through which the child learns about himself and the world around him. It is that spontaneous activity through which he rehearses, experiences, experiments and orients himself to the actual world" (Knox, 1968, p. 5). The assessment was pilot tested on a population of children with mental retardation and correlated with the children's developmental ages (Knox, 1968). The Play Scale was revised and renamed the Preschool Play Scale (PPS) by Bledsoe and Shepherd (1982), who collected normative data on 90 children and conducted reliability and validity studies. Reliability and validity data were also gathered on a population with disabilities by Harrison and Kielhofner (1986). After its initial development and revision by Bledsoe and Shepherd, the PPS was used to demonstrate differences in the play behavior of different populations (Bundy, 1989; Clifford & Bundy, 1989; Howard, 1986; Kielhofner et al., 1983), to assess pretreatment and posttreatment status (Schaaf & Mulrooney, 1989), and to examine the effects of postural facilitation on free play (Germain & Dwyre, 1988). The PPS has also been used clinically for assessment and as a guide to the developmental nature of play.

The PPS was further revised and renamed the Revised Knox Preschool Play Scale (RKPPS) in 1997 (Knox, 1997b). In the remainder of this chapter the content of the RKPPS is described and studies of its reliability and validity are discussed. Clinical use of the RKPPS is demonstrated through case examples, and its strengths and limitations are critically examined.

Description

The Revised Knox Play Scale (Knox, 1968, 1974, 1997b) is an observational assessment designed to give a developmental description of typical play behavior from birth through the age of 6 years. Play is described in 6-month increments for the first 3 years and in yearly increments for ages 4 through 6. The items are grouped into four dimensions: (1) space management, (2) material management,

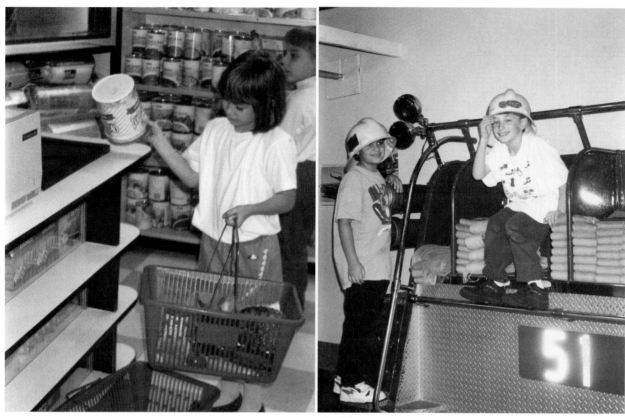

Figure 3-2
Children's play reflects their interest in adult roles.

(3) pretense-symbolic, and (4) participation. Each dimension contains a number of factors, as described in the following:

    Space management: the way children learn to manage their bodies and the space around them. This is achieved through the processes of experimentation and exploration.

      Gross motor activity—play involving the whole body

      Interest—attention to specific types of activity

    Material management: the way in which children handle materials and the purposes for which materials are used. Through material management, children learn control and use of material surroundings.

      Manipulation—fine motor control

      Construction—combining objects and making products

      Purpose—goals of the activity

      Attention—length of time in independent play

    Pretense-symbolic: the way children gain an understanding of the world through imitation and the development of the ability to understand and separate reality from make-believe.

      Imitation—mirroring aspects of the cultural environment

      Dramatization—pretend, introduction of novelty, and role play

    Participation: the amount and manner of interaction with persons in the environment and the degree of independence and cooperation demonstrated in play activities.

      Type—level of social interaction in play

      Cooperation—ability to get along with others in play

      Humor—understanding and expression of humorous or incongruous words or events

      Language—communication with others in play

The behavioral descriptions under each dimension were determined through a review of existing developmental and play scales (Knox, 1968, 1997b) and are written as actions that the child performs. In this way children can be assessed in a variety of settings with available playthings, instead of in standard settings with required playthings. Table 3-1 depicts the RKPPS as it is used today.

Administration

Settings

Children should be observed both indoors and outdoors in as naturalistic or familiar an environment as possible, with peers present. Indoor and outdoor settings are essential so the assessor can see the variety of behaviors necessary to score the dimensions of space and material management adequately. Although a natural setting is

Table 3-1
Revised Knox Preschool Play Scale

0 to 6 Months	*6 to 12 Months*	*12 to 18 Months*
Space Management		
Gross motor: swipes, reaches, plays with hands and feet, moves to continue pleasant sensations	**Gross motor:** reaches in prone, crawls, sits with balance, able to play with toy while sitting, pulls to stand, cruises	**Gross motor:** stands unsupported, sits down, bends and recovers balance, walks with wide stance, broad movements involving large muscle groups, throws ball
Interest: people, gazes at faces, follows movements, attends to voices and sounds, explores self and objects within reach	**Interest:** follows objects as they disappear, anticipates movement, goal-directed movement	**Interest:** practices basic movement patterns, experiments in movement, explores various kinesthetic and proprioceptive sensations, moving objects (i.e., balls, trucks, pull toys)
Material Management		
Manipulation: handles, mouths toys, bangs, strokes, hits	**Manipulation:** pulls, turns, pokes, tears, racks, drops, picks up small object	**Manipulation:** throws, inserts, pushes, pulls, carries, turns, opens, shuts
Construction: brings two objects together	**Construction:** combines related objects, puts object in container	**Construction:** stacks, takes apart, puts together, little attempt to make product, relates two objects appropriately (e.g., lid on pot)
Purpose: sensation—uses materials to see, touch, hear, smell, mouth	**Purpose:** action to produce effect, cause and effect toys	**Purpose:** variety of schemas, process important, trial and error, relational play
Attention: follows moving objects with eyes, 3 to 5 sec attention	**Attention:** 15 sec for detailed object, 30 sec for visual and auditory toy	**Attention:** rapid shifts
Pretense-Symbolic		
Imitation: of observed facial expressions and physical movement (i.e., smiling, pat-a-cake), imitates vocalizations	**Imitation:** imitates observed actions, emotions, sounds and gestures not part of repertoire, patterns of familiar activities	**Imitation:** of simple actions, present events and adults, imitates novel movements, links simple schemas (e.g., puts person in car and pushes it)
Dramatization: not evident	**Dramatization:** not evident	**Dramatization:** beginning pretend using self (e.g., feed self with spoon), pretend on animated and inanimate objects
Participation		
Type: solitary, no effort to interact with other children, enjoys being picked up, swung	**Type:** infant to infant interaction, responds differently to children and adults	**Type:** combination of solitary and onlooker, beginning interaction with peers
Cooperation: demands personal attention, simple give and take interaction with caretaker (tickling, peekaboo)	**Cooperation:** initiates games rather than follows, shows and gives objects	**Cooperation:** seeks attention to self, demands toys, points, shows, offers toys but somewhat possessive, persistent

Continued

Table 3-1
Revised Knox Preschool Play Scale—cont'd

0 to 6 Months	6 to 12 Months	12 to 18 Months
Humor: smiles	**Humor:** smiles, laughs at physical games and in anticipation	**Humor:** laughs at incongruous events
Language: attends to sounds and voices, babbles, uses razzing sounds	**Language:** gestures intention to communicate, responds to familiar words and facial expressions, responds to questions	**Language:** jabbers to self during play, uses gestures and words to communicate wants, labels objects, greets others, responds to simple requests, teases, exclaims, protests, combines words and gestures

18 to 24 Months	24 to 30 Months	30 to 36 Months
Space Management		
Gross motor: runs, squats, climbs on and off chairs, walks up and down stairs (step to gait), kicks ball, rides kiddy car	**Gross motor:** beginning integration of entire body in activities—concentrates on complex movements, jumps off floor, stands on one foot briefly, throws ball in stance without falling	**Gross motor:** runs around obstacles, turns corners, climbs nursery apparatus, walks up and down stairs (alternating feet), catches ball by trapping it, stands on tiptoe
Interest: means—end, multipart tasks	**Interest:** explores new movement patterns (e.g., jumping), makes messes	**Interest:** rough and tumble play
Material Management		
Manipulation: operates mechanical toy, pulls apart pop beads, strings beads	**Manipulation:** feels, pats, dumps, squeezes, fills	**Manipulation:** matches, compares
Construction: uses tools	**Construction:** scribbles, strings beads, puzzles 4 to 5 pieces, builds horizontally and vertically	**Construction:** multischeme combinations
Purpose: foresight before acting	**Purpose:** process important—less interested in finished product (e.g., scribbles, squeezes), plans actions	**Purpose:** toys with moving parts (e.g., dump trucks, jointed dolls)
Attention: quiet play 5 to 10 min; play with single object 5 min	**Attention:** intense interest, quiet play up to 15 min, plays with single object or theme 5 to 10 min	**Attention:** 15 to 30 min
Pretense-Symbolic		
Imitation: representational, recognizes ways to activate toys in imitation, deferred imitation	**Imitation:** of adult routines with toy-related mimicry (e.g., child feeding doll); imitates peers, representational play	**Imitation:** toys as agents (e.g., doll feeds self), more abstract representation of objects, multischeme combinations (e.g., feed doll, pat it, put to bed)
Dramatization: acts on doll (e.g., dresses, brushes hair), pretend actions on more than one object or person, combines two or more actions in pretend, imaginary objects	**Dramatization:** personifies dolls, stuffed animals, imaginary friends, portrays single character, elaborates daily events with details	**Dramatization:** evolving episodic sequences (e.g., mixes cake, bakes it, serves it)

Continued

Table 3-1
Revised Knox Preschool Play Scale—cont'd

18 to 24 Months	24 to 30 Months	30 to 36 Months
Participation		
Type: onlooker, simple actions and contingent responses between peers	**Type:** parallel (plays beside others but play remains independent), enjoys the presence of others, shy with strangers	**Type:** parallel, beginning associative, plays with 2 or 3 children, plays in company 1 to 2 hr
Cooperation: more complex games with a variety of adults (hide and seek, chasing), commands others to carry out actions	**Cooperation:** possessive, much snatch and grab, hoarding, no sharing, resists toys being taken away, independent, initiates own play	**Cooperation:** understands needs of others
Humor: laughs at incongruous labeling of objects or events	**Humor:** laughs at simple combinations of incongruous events and use of words	**Humor:** laughs at complex combinations of incongruous events and words
Language: comprehends action words, requests information, refers to persons and objects not present, combines words together	**Language:** talkative, very little jabber, begins to use words to communicate ideas, information, questions, comments on activity	**Language:** asks wh- questions, relates temporal sequences

36 to 48 Months	48 to 60 Months	60 to 72 Months
Space Management		
Gross motor: more coordinated body movement, smoother walking, jumping, climbing, running, accelerates, decelerates, hops on one foot 3 to 5 times, skips on one foot, catches ball, throws ball using shoulder and elbow, jumps distances	**Gross motor:** increased activity level, can concentrate on goal instead of movement, ease of gross motor ability, stunts, tests of strength, exaggerated movement, clambers, gallops, climbs ladder, catches ball with elbows at side	**Gross motor:** more sedate, good muscle control and balance, hops on one foot 5+ times, hops in a straight line, bounces and catches ball, skips, somersaults, skates, lifts self off ground
Interest: anything new, fine motor manipulation of play materials, challenges self with difficult takes	**Interest:** takes pride in work (e.g., shows and talks about products, compares with friends, likes pictures displayed), complex ideas, rough and tumble play	**Interest:** in reality—manipulation of real-life situations, making something useful, permanence of products, toys that "really work"
Material Management		
Manipulation: small muscle activity—hammers, sorts, inserts small objects, cuts	**Manipulation:** increased fine motor control, quick movements, force, pulling, yanks	**Manipulation:** uses tools to make things, copies, traces, combines materials
Construction: makes simple products, combines play material, takes apart, three-dimensional, design evident	**Construction:** makes products, specific designs evident, builds complex structures, puzzles 10 pieces	**Construction:** makes recognizable products, likes small construction, attends to detail, uses products in play
Purpose: beginning to show interest in finished product	**Purpose:** product very important and used to express self, exaggerates	**Purpose:** replicates reality
Attention: span around 30 min, plays with single object or theme 10 min	**Attention:** amuses self up to 1 hr, plays with single object or theme 10 to 15 min	**Attention:** plays with single object or theme 15+ min

Continued

Table 3-1
Revised Knox Preschool Play Scale—cont'd

36 to 48 Months	48 to 60 Months	60 to 72 Months
Pretense-Symbolic		
Imitation: more complex imitation of real world, emphasis on domestic play and animals, symbolic, past experiences	**Imitation:** pieces together new scripts of adults (e.g., dress-up), reality important	**Imitation:** continues to construct new themes with emphasis on reality—reconstruction of real world
Dramatization: complex scripts for pretend sequences in advance, story sequences, pretend with replica toys, uses one toy to represent another, portrays multiple characters with feelings (mostly anger and crying), little interest in costumes, imaginary characters	**Dramatization:** uses familiar knowledge to construct a novel situation (e.g., explaining on theme of a story or TV show), role playing for or with others, portrays more complex emotions, sequences stories, themes from domestic to magic, enjoys dress-up, shows off	**Dramatization:** sequences stories, costumes important, props, puppets, direct actions of three dolls—making them interact, organizes other children and props for role play
Participation		
Type: associative play, no organization to reach a common goal, more interest in peers than activity, enjoys companions, beginning cooperative play, group play	**Type:** cooperative, groups of 2 or 3 organized to achieve a goal, prefers playing with others to alone, group games with simple rules	**Type:** cooperative groups of 3 to 6, organization of more complex games and dramatic play, competitive games, understands rules of fair play
Cooperation: limited, some turn taking, asks for things rather than grabbing, little attempt to control others, separates easily, joins others in play	**Cooperation:** takes turns, attempts to control activities of others, bossy, strong sense of family and home, quotes parents as authorities	**Cooperation:** compromises to facilitate group play, rivalry in competitive play, games with rules, collaborative play where roles are coordinated and themes are goal directed
Humor: laughs at nonsense words, rhyming	**Humor:** distortions of the familiar	**Humor:** laughs at multiple meanings of words
Language: uses words to communicate with peers, interest in new words, sings simple songs, uses descriptive vocabulary, changes speech depending on listener	**Language:** plays with words, fabricates, long narratives, questions persistently, communicates with peers to organize activities, brags, threatens, clowns, sings whole songs, uses language to express roles, verbal reasoning	**Language:** prominent in sociodramatic play, uses words as part of play as well as to organize play, interest in present, conversation like adults', uses relational terms, sings and dances to reflect meaning of songs

Modified from Knox, S. (1974). A play scale. In M. Reilly (Ed.), *Play as exploratory learning*, Beverly Hills, CA: Sage Publications; and from Bledsoe, N., & Shepherd, J. (1982). A study of reliability and validity of a preschool play scale. *American Journal of Occupational Therapy, 36,* 783-788.

preferable, the scale can be used in a clinic setting if opportunities, equipment, and toys are available for adequate assessment of both gross and fine motor skills. Peers are necessary so that participation can be assessed.

True play behavior is spontaneous, child initiated, and self-directed. The behavior observed should be as free as possible from adult intervention and direction. While this is not always possible (e.g., in a preschool setting), the adults present should take care to avoid directing the activity.

Length of Observation
The child should be observed for a minimum of two 30-minute periods, indoors and outdoors. This is important to observe shifts in play episodes and to see the differences in play that the two settings afford. In a study of play styles of preschool children, Knox (1997a) found that typical preschool children often spent long periods of time in complex play episodes emphasizing primarily one type of play, such as construction or pretend, so observation of the child on

multiple occasions will yield a broader repertoire of play behaviors.

Instructions for Scoring

Within the factors the observer places a mark above each descriptor each time it is observed. Then the factor is ranked at the highest level unless the descriptor is insignificant (i.e., done for less than 1 minute or by chance). Descriptors typical of the child's behavior may be underlined. Each factor is scored at the upper age of the age grouping. For example, the 6- to 12-month level is scored as 12 months; the 30- to 36-month level is scored as 36 months. To score each dimension, the observer takes the mean of the factor scores. To score an overall play age, the observer takes the mean of the dimension scores.

STUDIES USING THE PRESCHOOL PLAY SCALE
Reliability and Validity Studies

The original Play Scale was pilot tested on a population of 12 preschool children with diagnoses of mental retardation. The children were observed indoors and outdoors in a preschool setting and rated on all of the factors in the four dimensions. Scoring consisted of marking each factor with either a + when the behavior was present or a − when the behavior was absent. If there was no opportunity to observe a factor, NA was marked. Items of special interest were underlined. A score on a particular dimension was determined by the age level containing the majority of factor pluses. An overall play age was determined by taking the means of the dimension scores and computing an overall mean. The author found that play ages correlated significantly with developmental ages of the children (Knox, 1968).

Two studies examined the validity and reliability of the PPS as revised by Bledsoe and Shepherd (1982). These authors conducted validity and reliability studies with typically developing children. Each subject was observed and rated for three half-hour sessions over a period of 7 days. Subjects were observed in day-care centers and nursery schools during free play periods. All observations were done indoors in settings that had a wide variety of toys and adequate space. Interrater and test-retest reliability studies were significant at the $p = .0001$ level. Validity studies correlated the PPS with Lunzer's Scale of Organization of Play Behavior, Parten's Social Play Hierarchy, and chronological age. Lunzer's Scale of Organization of Play Behavior (Hulme & Lunzer, 1966) measures cognitive development in play and is correlated in this study with the dimensions of material management and imitation. Parten's Social Play Hierarchy (Parten, 1933) measures social participation in play and is correlated with the participation dimensions of the PPS. All the validity studies were significant at the $p = .0001$ level. The authors concluded that "the scale measured play on a developmental continuum of increasing complexity including physical, cognitive and social components" (Bledsoe & Shepherd, 1982, p. 787).

Harrison and Kielhofner (1986) conducted reliability and validity studies on the PPS with a group of 60 preschool children who had disabilities, including cerebral palsy, mental retardation, and developmental delay. They observed free play in classrooms or medical settings for two 15-minute sessions. They collected data with the PPS, the Parten Social Play Hierarchy, and the Lunzer Scale of Organization of Behavior. Their results also showed statistically significant reliability and validity of the PPS at the $p = .0001$ level for the population with disabilities. Their study had the limitations that all the observations took place indoors and that observations of imitation, imagination, and cooperation were infrequent.

Both studies show that the PPS is a valid and reliable tool with which to assess the developmental aspects of play. Jankovich and associates (2006) examined interrater agreement and construct validity of the RKPPS. They studied 38 typically developing children, ages 36 to 72 months. Interrater agreement within 8 months on the overall play age score was almost 90%. On each dimension, agreement ranged from 91.7% to 100% within 12 months or less. On the 12 categories the two raters agreed within one age level difference between 83% and 100%. The researchers also supported the construct validity of the scale because they found matches between play ages and chronological ages (within one age range) at 92% to 100%.

Fallon (2006) measured interrater reliability among six therapists on five case studies. No therapist received training on the RKPPS. For four of the cases the percent of agreement was 83%, and on the fifth case agreement was 66%. The percent of agreement on the twelve categories ranged from 40% to 76%. Lee (2007) measured interrater reliability and validity on the RKPPS on 61 children with autism. Interrater reliability was r = .94, and the scale correlated significantly with the total score of the Vineland Adaptive Behavior Scales at r = .52.

Studies Using Different Populations

Several studies have examined scores on the PPS and other measures for different diagnostic or socioeconomic groups. These studies contribute to the validity of the PPS by examining how children with identified disabilities, from different social classes, or reared under different circumstances show differing play patterns.

Kielhofner and co-workers (1983) studied playfulness and level of play development of three 2-year-old children who had been hospitalized most of their lives and three 2-year-old children living at home. Playfulness was measured by a modified version of Lieberman's Playfulness Scale (Lieberman, 1977). Level of play development was measured by a modified version of the PPS. The children were observed in three different environments: (1) the child's familiar environment with the caretaker present and participating, (2) a standardized play environment with the caretaker present but passive, and (3) a standard play environment with the caretaker present and participating. The study authors found statistically significant differences in the developmental level of play and in playfulness between the two groups. They also analyzed differences based on the environments and found the play ages were lower for both groups in the second environment (standard environment, passive caretaker). Playfulness was not statistically significant across environmental groups. Limitations of this study included a very small sample size and medical complications affecting certain areas of play, such as tracheotomies that limited speech and social interaction. An important addition in this study was the use of a measure of playfulness, since this aspect of play is not covered by the PPS. Also important was the finding of the differences in play between a familiar environment and a standard environment. The study underlines the importance of observing play naturalistically.

Howard (1986) used the PPS to compare developmental play ages of two groups of children, of whom 12 were physically abused and 12 were not abused. Children were from 1 to 5 years of age and were paired by age and family income. Children were observed for 40 minutes, independent of the mother, but with at least one other child present. Mothers were also given a questionnaire asking three questions related to the amount of time spent with the child in play and the amount of time the child spent watching television. Statistically significant deficits in the overall developmental play age and in the play imitation category, as well as a trend toward lower participation, were found in the abused group. These children interacted less imaginatively and were less socially interactive. The abused group also showed a statistically significant difference in the amount of television watched, averaging 1 hour more per day than the unabused group. This study used a more prolonged observation period and also ensured that peers were available, helping to create a more natural environment conducive to play.

Bundy (1989) compared play behavior between two groups of 4- to 6-year-old boys. One group comprised 31 boys with sensory integrative dysfunction, and the other included 30 boys without sensory integration problems. She found significant differences between the mean scores of the two groups on the PPS and its four dimensions. On discriminative analysis of the four play dimensions, space management was the best single predictor of group membership. As individuals, however, many of the boys with sensory integrative dysfunction had age-appropriate

skills in one or more areas of play. Bundy recommended that, with this population, observations of playfulness and quality of movement should accompany use of the PPS.

Clifford and Bundy (1989), as part of the same study, studied 31 preschool boys with sensory integrative dysfunction and 35 without dysfunction. They examined play preference, as measured by the Preschool Play Materials Preference Inventory (Wolfgang & Phelps, 1983); play performance, as measured by the PPS; and verbal receptive language, as measured on the Revised Peabody Picture Vocabulary Test (Dunn & Dunn, 1981). The boys were observed both indoors and outdoors. Clifford and Bundy found no significant difference in the means on the play materials preference scores between the groups because both groups preferred toys representing sensorimotor play over construction and symbolic toys. They did find a difference, however, in how the two groups used toys and how well the boys played with the toys as measured on the PPS. The mean scores on this scale and three of its dimensions (space management, material management, and participation) were significantly lower for the boys with sensory integrative dysfunction. Two types of play deficits were defined. The first type was seen in boys who were unsuccessful at engaging in preferred activities. The second type was seen in boys who showed poor skills but altered their play preferences to compensate. This study is important in that it evaluated play preferences as well as performance.

Von Zuben, Crist, and Mayberry (1991) explored play behavior and its relation to socioeconomic status. They modified the PPS into a rating scale that teachers used for 4- and 5-year-old children attending the same school; 41 children were of middle socioeconomic status and 43 of low socioeconomic status. No significant differences between the socioeconomic groups were found for play age, dimensions, or categories. The authors discussed a number of study limitations. The schools were socioeconomically integrated, contained a variety of educational play resources, and were staffed by trained teachers. These factors may have affected the children's experience level and peer interaction. Modification of the PPS into a checklist may have additionally altered findings. The teachers were not blind to the socioeconomic status, and no interrater reliability studies were conducted. On the other hand, the teachers had opportunities to observe the children in a variety of play settings and over time. These are important limitations that may have significantly altered the findings. It would have been interesting to have observed the children both at school and in their homes or neighborhoods to determine whether the school environment fostered different levels of play.

Morrison, Bundy, and Fisher (1991) examined the contribution of playfulness and motor skills to play performance in children without disabilities and in those with juvenile rheumatoid arthritis (JRA). They defined playfulness in terms of the child's feelings of internal control over the environment, as measured on the Preschool and Primary Internal-External Locus of Control Scale (Norwicki & Duke, 1974), and ability to be creative or imaginative, as measured by tests of associative fluency from the Walloch and Koogan Scale, revised by Ward (Ward, 1968). Motor proficiency was measured by the Bruininks-Oseretsky Test of Motor Proficiency (Bruininks, 1978). Play was measured by the PPS.

Two groups of children, 15 without disabilities and 14 with JRA, ranging in age from 4 years, 6 months to 6 years, 6 months, were tested. The authors set a significance level of $p < .10$. They found no significant differences in the two groups on the PPS, the internal locus of control test, the tests of associative fluency, total Bruininks, or fine motor Bruininks. There were significant differences, however, on the gross motor section of the Bruininks. The authors correlated the dimensions of the PPS with the other scales for both groups. For the group without disabilities, associative fluency correlated with material management and space management, internal locus of control correlated with material management, and the gross motor and fine motor Bruininks correlated with participation. For the group with JRA, the fine motor Bruininks correlated with the total PPS, and the gross motor Bruininks correlated with the dimension of space management.

The authors concluded that minor dysfunction did not always result in play deficits and that some children with disabilities could compensate for areas of dysfunction and play normally. A limitation of this study was that the authors were not able to observe the children in their usual play environments with familiar peers. The children with JRA were tested during clinic visits and the nondisabled children in preschools. This would affect overall play and specifically participation.

Restall and Magill-Evans (1994) studied the play of preschool children with autism. The purposes of their study were to "compare the play of children with autism with the play of children without dysfunction in their homes" and to "examine the relationship between children's play preferences and their communication, social, and motor abilities" (p. 113). Nine children with a diagnosis of autism and nine children with typical development were studied. Children were between the ages of 3 and 6 years and were matched for gender, age (chronological age for those without dysfunction and mental age for those with autism), and socioeconomic status. The children were observed under two conditions: unstructured play and a structured setting with specific toys and the parents available to the child. Children were rated on the PPS, the Vineland Adaptive Behavior Scales (Sparrow et al., 1984), and types of play materials chosen.

The results showed a statistically significant difference between the two groups on the total PPS score and on the participation dimension. There was no difference between groups on the play materials chosen. The group with autism showed significantly lower Vineland scores. The PPS was significantly correlated with the Vineland for both groups, and the total PPS score was correlated with the communication variable of the Vineland for the autistic group and on the socialization variable for the nonautistic group. This study lends support to naturalistic observations in familiar settings. Limitations included limited opportunities for peer social interaction and limited opportunities to observe a variety of play within the time periods designated.

Shepherd and associates (1994) compared the play skills of preschool children who had speech and language delays with those of children having typical language development. They tested 20 children with speech-language delays but no identified physical or cognitive disability and 21 children with typical language. A teacher checklist was also used to supplement the free play observation. The authors found significant differences of $p = .0001$ in overall play age and for the dimensions of imitation, material management, and participation. In space management the p level was .01.

Misale and Murphy (1997) studied the effects of expressive language and motor delays on play skills and playfulness in children. They tested 10 children, 5 with delays in both language and motor skills and 5 with just language delays, using the RKPPS and the Test of Playfulness (ToP). They found no significant differences in the play skills between the two groups, but there were differences in playfulness. The lowest score on the RKPPS, however, was in the pretense-symbolic dimension. This was supported by the results on the ToP and suggests that these children had difficulty in imaginative play.

Rüdlinger (1998) compared the play behavior of two Swedish children with low vision and their best friends. The play skills of all four children were within normal limits for their chronological age. Rüdlinger observed qualitative differences, however, in some of the adaptations the children with low vision made to play with preferred materials, such as coming closer to the object with which they were playing. She also found that the children with low vision usually directed the play so that they could participate. When other children were present and the games became difficult, they would leave and start their own game. This study raised the question of when low vision stops a child from participating versus when the child's own will does. The study also demonstrated the importance of the type of environment on children's play.

Using the RKPPS, O'Sullivan (2000) assessed 20 deaf and 20 typically hearing children. She found differences between the two groups in overall play age and in each of the dimensions.

In summary, the studies using the PPS with different categories of children showed varied results. Groups of children who were autistic, physically abused, deaf, or language delayed or who had prolonged hospitalization showed statistically significant differences in total play ages from their normally developing counterparts. The children with autism had the most difficulty in social participation, the children with physical abuse showed problems in imitation, and those with sensory integrative dysfunction had problems with space management. The studies of children with juvenile rheumatoid arthritis (JRA), comparing children with motor and language delays and those with just language delay, and of children from different socioeconomic groups found no significant differences. These studies show the usefulness of the PPS in differentiating developmental play abilities in a variety of populations but also point out the individual nature of play and the children's ability to overcome some disabilities and develop typical play skills. The studies also demonstrate the need for additional measures of play, such as play style or playfulness and play material preference, to tap into some of the more qualitative aspects of play.

Studies of Treatment Effects

Studies have used the PPS as a measure of treatment effects. Schaaf and Mulrooney (1989) used the PPS along with an unpublished Parent/Teacher Play Questionnaire and the Peabody Developmental Motor Scales (Folio & Fewell, 1984) to assess the effectiveness of specific occupational therapy intervention on five subjects enrolled in an early intervention program. All subjects had developmental delay and were scheduled to receive occupational therapy. The study authors collected data during a 4-week baseline period and a 10-week intervention period. The PPS was administered twice during the baseline period and four to five times during intervention. Teachers filled out the questionnaire weekly, and the Peabody was administered before and after intervention. Intervention consisted of direct and consultative occupational therapy with an emphasis on the facilitation of play behaviors. The authors found the PPS helpful in determining change, but because of their small sample size and other limitations, they recommended more extensive exploration.

Germain and Dwyre (1988) used the PPS to determine effectiveness of occupational therapy intervention on play behavior. Six physically handicapped children were observed under each of two conditions: (1) handled, in which the therapist facilitated postural responses while the child was playing, and (2) unhandled, in which the child engaged in free play. They found that the children displayed greater play skills, as demonstrated on the PPS, in the unhandled condition, which was contrary to their expectations. The study raised the question as to the effects of therapist's handling on child performance. As the authors pointed out, there is a delicate balance between giving a child enough support or assistance to facilitate play and giving too much, so that the child becomes

dependent on the therapist, thus decreasing self-initiated behaviors.

Over (2006, in press) used the RKPPS to assess the effects of therapeutic listening on the occupation of play in three children diagnosed with autism. The children were receiving occupational therapy services that used a sensory integration approach. They were assessed on the RKPPS before and after receiving a 10-week course of therapeutic listening. Because the study time was too short to see differences in the dimension and overall play ages, Over analyzed the new play skills that emerged after treatment based on the descriptors. All children showed significant increases in the number of behavioral descriptors. The author concluded that "active involvement of the auditory system in combination with proprioceptive, tactile, and vestibular systems can positively impact the occupational performance of play" (Over, in press).

Other Studies

The RKPPS has been and is currently being used in other ways. Tanta (2002) used the PPS to determine eligibility and peer pairings in her study of the effect of peer-play level on the behavior of preschool children with delayed play skills. Fallon (2006) used the RKPPS and focus groups with parents to study the play of children with intellectual disabilities All of the children showed play ages significantly below their chronological ages. A study being conducted in Israel (Weintraub, 2006, personal correspondence) is examining an intervention focused on improving mother-child interest and play skills of the children in a shelter for women who have been abused. Another study (Keilson & English, 2006, personal correspondence) is examining whether parents are reliable raters of their child's play.

The scale has been used by numerous academic occupational therapy programs to structure the students' observations of children. It has been translated into Spanish, German, Japanese, Korean, Norwegian, French, and Portuguese.

Summary of Study Use

The studies using the PPS have shown good reliability and validity with populations of normal children, as well as those with disabilities. The PPS has also proved useful in differentiating developmental play abilities in a variety of populations with handicaps. In addition, it has been helpful for assessing the effectiveness of various treatment techniques, for screening children for research projects, and for a variety of other uses.

CLINICAL USE

In the clinical setting the PPS has been useful in assessment and in denoting progress, as illustrated by the two case studies below. In clinical assessment, observing overall play level is usually not as important as looking at the profile of play skills, recognizing strengths and weaknesses, and determining interest areas.

The PPS has been especially helpful when a child is not testable on standardized tests. For example, young children with autism often do not respond to direction and refuse standard test items. Because the PPS correlates significantly with developmental age, it is often possible to estimate developmental levels by observing free play.

The PPS is useful with children who, because of their disability, may need adult intervention, such as in a testing situation, but in free play settings do not show the same skills. An illustration of this is the case example of Jane. This case also illustrates the use of the PPS to assess progress.

Another clinical use of the PPS is as a guide to the developmental aspects of play. Here, therapists can use the descriptions to help parents understand typically developing play and encourage appropriate play skills (Figure 3-3).

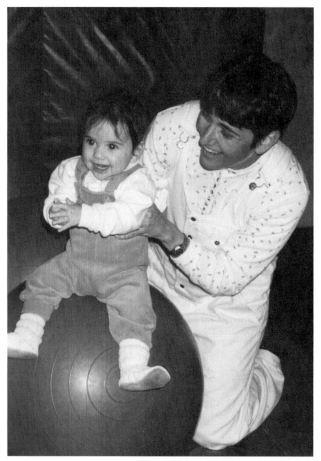

Figure 3-3

Suggestions can be given to parents for appropriate and fun play activities.

Case Examples

CASE EXAMPLE 1
Andrew

Andrew was a 3-year-old boy with a diagnosis of autism. When standardized testing was attempted, he refused to sit in the chair, threw or pushed aside all test items, and tried to leave the room, so the therapist decided to assess him with the PPS during free play. She took him into a large clinic room equipped with swings, trampoline, bolsters and other climbing equipment, sandbox, toys for manipulation, and toys that provided sensory input. Andrew was allowed to choose his activities, and the therapist provided assistance if necessary. At times, the therapist offered various types of toys to observe his response.

On the RKPPS, Andrew was observed to be most interested in gross motor activity, choosing swings, trampoline, and climbing apparatus. Gross motor activity was characterized by the use of his entire body, throwing, jumping, and climbing. He was very curious about the unfamiliar objects in the room and explored them. Movements were coordinated, and he was able to accelerate, decelerate, and change course. On the space management dimension, he showed play skills at the 36-month level (Figure 3-4).

In material management, Andrew's play was at the 12- to 18-month level. Manipulation consisted of throwing, pounding, squeezing, and mouthing objects with unusual textures. Primary interest was in sensation and movement. Andrew showed no aversive response to textures, except to shaving cream. His mother reported that he did not play with toys at home.

On the dimension of pretense-symbolic, skills were at the 12-month level. No imitation was observed in the clinic; however, Andrew's mother reported that he had learned most of his activities of daily living by observation and imitation.

Participation skills were also at the 12-month level. Play was generally solitary in nature. Andrew occasionally watched others in the room but did not imitate them or enter into their play. In language he hummed to himself and primarily used gestures to communicate his desires.

The most striking findings with Andrew were the discrepancies between space management and the other dimensions. Although he showed coordinated gross motor movements, he avoided manipulative activity or played with toys and objects for their sensory qualities alone. Imitation was severely limited, and participation with peers was nonexistent. Analysis of these discrepancies assisted in treatment planning. Goals in therapy included improving purposeful play with toys and imitation of and interaction with adults and peers in play.

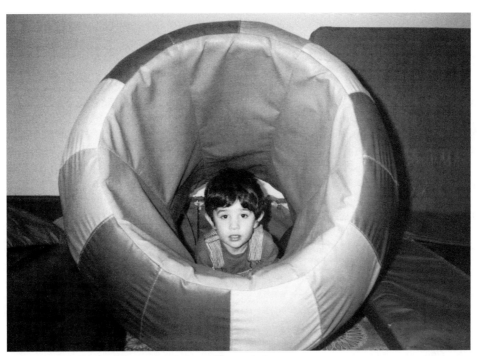

Figure 3-4
Andrew's play preferences were for gross motor activity.

CASE EXAMPLE 2

Jane

Jane was a twin born at 26 weeks of gestational age. She had an atrial septal defect repaired at 15 months of age, as well as severe visual problems caused by retrolental fibroplasia. She also had a history of seizures and was receiving medication. Jane experienced feeding difficulties that interfered with the transition from the bottle to the cup and from liquid to solid foods. Her twin was developing typically. Jane was referred to occupational therapy at 20 months of chronological age (corrected age of 16 months) after she had stabilized from surgery to repair the heart defect. Jane's parents stated that before the surgery they had been told she was "too fragile" to be handled much, so most of the time she was in her crib or propped in a corner of the couch with pillows around her.

When Jane was seen initially, a complete developmental and feeding evaluation and observations of free play were conducted. Results of the full evaluation are not presented at this time except for findings that relate to the results on the PPS. Jane showed a strong aversive response to touch stimulation on her hands and face. As a result, she avoided holding, handling, or mouthing toys. She enjoyed being swung, bounced, and moved. She responded to auditory input, but her only visual response was slight turning toward strong light.

On the RKPPS, all dimensions were scored at the lowest level. In space management, Jane played with her hands and feet in the supine position, and she moved to continue pleasant sensations, such as shaking her head from side to side. She made no attempt to explore her environment with hands or body and stayed in the position in which she was placed.

In material management, manipulation could not even be scored because Jane avoided holding or handling any toys or objects. When given a toy, she would hold it for only a few seconds, then drop it. She made no attempt to find toys with her hands once they were dropped. She attended to voices and sounds but could not see persons or objects in her environment. In imitation, she attended to sounds and made some imitative noises. After adult intervention she imitated pat-a-cake.

In participation, Jane demanded personal attention by crying, fussing, or smiling when she heard familiar voices. She babbled to herself when alone in the crib. She attended to sounds and turned toward them. She did not initiate any social games with caretakers but seemed to enjoy them when engaged. She made no effort to interact with her twin sister. Evident throughout the PPS was Jane's extreme dependence on adult intervention for almost all sensory and social input because of her visual impairment and extreme tactile defensiveness. Self-initiated play was virtually nonexistent. Again, the results on the PPS helped define goals for occupational therapy intervention.

Jane was treated by the occupational therapist twice weekly in the home until she was 2½, when treatment changed to a center-based program. At the time of the change, she was again assessed on the PPS. Although she was still primarily dependent on adults to facilitate her play, she actively manipulated toys with a variety of textures. She was beginning to reach for dropped toys and for those that made noise. She also could operate a push pad to activate a fan or sound toy. She transferred toys at midline and actively manipulated or explored them. She banged a piano and drum with her hands and was interested in cause and effect toys that made noise. In space management, she could transition from prone to sitting and back and was beginning to crawl toward sounds. In imitation, she really enjoyed songs and simple hand play initiated by adults. Participation was still primarily with adults, but she was more aware of her siblings and smiled and vocalized when they played with her.

In Jane's case, significant changes were seen on the RKPPS during the 10 months of treatment, primarily in terms of factor descriptors but also in a higher age level in the material management dimension

STRENGTHS AND LIMITATIONS OF THE REVISED KNOX PRESCHOOL PLAY SCALE

It has been rewarding to me, as the original creator of the RKPPS, to see how much the scale has been used and to see its value clinically. However, the studies discussed here and my clinical experience have revealed both strengths and limitations in the RKPPS. One of the advantages is that it covers all areas of development and reflects developmental status, as demonstrated in the validity studies. Thus, if a child cannot be evaluated on a standardized developmental assessment, that child can be observed during free play and assessed on the RKPPS, and the therapist can feel fairly confident that play levels approximate developmental level.

A big advantage of the RKPPS is that it does not require specialized toys or equipment and can be used to assess the child in natural settings. In addition, it assesses natural behaviors rather than requested ones. This is particularly important to occupational therapists, who are concerned with children's occupational role behaviors within their everyday environments. Although the scale was designed to be used in natural settings, it has been used successfully in clinical settings as long as the setting has equipment for both gross and fine motor skills and the availability of peers to assess participation.

One limitation of the PPS is that the measurement is in fairly large increments (6 months for ages up to 3 years and yearly from 4 to 6 years of age). This can be a problem, particularly for assessment of progress, because the child may make significant changes but may not change levels, as demonstrated in the case of Jane. However, there may be changes within the item descriptors that may denote progress, so the PPS is still helpful in the clinical setting. Studies that have taken place over limited time periods have adjusted the scoring to look at how the behavioral descriptions have changed or increased (Over, 2006).

The RKPPS looks only at developmental aspects of play and does not consider affect, emotions, or other qualities of play that might be considered under play style or playfulness. At the time of testing, additional information should be gathered from parental interview. The scale should be used in conjunction with other measures of play such as play histories, play style, playfulness, or toy preference and with other measures of development (Knox, 1997).

It is important to note that the RKPPS still needs additional standardization, reliability, and validity studies.

SUMMARY

The Preschool Play Scale is reviewed from its initial development in 1968. Standardization, reliability, and validity studies with children developing normally and those with disabilities have shown that the PPS is a valid and reliable test of the developmental nature of play. Further validity has been demonstrated through a number of studies using different populations.

Studies have used the PPS to assess effects of treatment and for a variety of other uses. Case studies are presented in the chapter to further illustrate clinical use. Strengths and limitations of the RKPPS are also addressed.

Review Questions

1. Describe the Revised Knox Preschool Play Scale. Discuss its history, intention, and methodology.
2. Discuss reliability and validity studies of the Preschool Play Scale. What might be the strengths and limitations of the scale? What are the clinical implications of these strengths and weaknesses?
3. The Revised Knox Preschool Play Scale includes the dimensions of space management, material management, pretense-symbolic, and participation. Describe what is addressed in each of these dimensions.
4. Discuss the developmental changes (from birth to age 5 years) that are outlined within each of the four dimensions of the Revised Knox Preschool Play Scale.
5. Describe how the Revised Knox Preschool Play Scale may be administered and scored, as suggested in the chapter.

REFERENCES

American Occupational Therapy Association (2002). Occupational therapy practice framework: Domain and process. *American Journal of Occupational Therapy, 56*, 609-639.

Bergen, D. (1988). *Play as a medium for learning and development.* Portsmouth, NH: Heinemann Educational Books.

Bledsoe, N., & Shepherd, J. (1982). A study of reliability and validity of a pre-school play scale. *American Journal of Occupational Therapy, 36*(12), 783-788.

Brown, C., & Gottfried, A. (Eds.). (1985). *Play interactions*, Skillman, NJ: Johnson & Johnson Baby Products.

Bruininks, R. (1978). *Bruininks-Oseretsky Test of Motor Proficiency.* Circle Pines, MN: American Guidance Service.

Bruner, J. S., Jolly, A., & Sylva, K. (Eds.). (1976). *Play—its role in development and evolution.* New York: Basic Books.

Bundy, A. (1989). A comparison of the play skills of normal boys with sensory integrative dysfunction. *Occupational Therapy Journal of Research, 9*(2), 84-100.

Clifford, J., & Bundy, A. (1989). Play preference and play performance in normal boys and boys with sensory integrative dysfunction. *Occupational Therapy Journal of Research, 9*(4), 202-217.

Cohen, D. (1987). *The development of play.* New York: New York University Press.

Couch, K., Dietz, J., & Kanny, E. (1998). The role of play in pediatric occupational therapy. *American Journal of Occupational Therapy, 52*(2), 111-117.

Dunn, L., & Dunn, L. (1981). *Peabody Picture Vocabulary Test—Revised.* Circle Pines, MN: American Guidance Service.

Ellis, M. (1973). *Why people play.* Englewood Cliffs, NJ: Prentice Hall.

Fallon, J. (2006). *An exploratory study of the free play of children with intellectual disabilities* (Unpublished master's thesis, Trinity College, Dublin, Ireland).

Florey, L. (1969). Intrinsic motivation: The dynamics of occupational therapy theory. *American Journal of Occupational Therapy, 23*, 319-322.

Florey, L. (1971). An approach to play and play development. *American Journal of Occupational Therapy, 25*, 275-280.

Florey, L. (1981). Studies of play: Implications for growth, development and for clinical practice. *American Journal of Occupational Therapy, 35*(8), 519-524.

Folio, R., & Fewell, R. (1984). *Peabody Developmental Motor Scales.* Allen, TX: Developmental Learning Materials.

Garvey, C. (1977). *Play.* London: Fontana/Open Books Publishing.

Germain, A., & Dwyre, M. (1988). Unpublished paper presented at the annual conference of the American Occupational Therapy Association, Phoenix, AZ, 1988.

Harrison, H., & Kielhofner, G. (1986). Examining reliability and validity of the Preschool Play Scale with handicapped children. *American Journal of Occupational Therapy, 40*(3), 167-173.

Hartley, R., & Goldenson, R. (1963). *The complete book of children's play.* New York: The Cornwall Press.

Howard, A. (1986). Developmental play ages of physically abused and non-abused children. *American Journal of Occupational Therapy, 40*(10), 691-695.

Hulme, I., & Lunzer, E. A. (1966). Play, language and reasoning in subnormal children. *Journal of Child Psychology and Psychiatry, 7*, 107.

Jankovich, M., Mullen, J., Rinear, E., Tanta, K., & Deitz, J. (2006). *Inter-rater agreement and construct validity of the Revised Knox Preschool Play Scale.* Unpublished manuscript.

Kalverboer, A. (1977). Measurement of play: Clinical applications. In B. Tizard & D. Harvey (Eds.), *Biology of play* (pp. 100-122). Philadelphia: J.B. Lippincott.

Keilson, M. & English, L., (2006). Personal correspondence.

Kielhofner, G., Barris, R., Bauer, D., Shoestock, B., & Walker, L. (1983). A comparison of play behavior in non-hospitalized and hospitalized children. *American Journal of Occupational Therapy, 37*(5), 305-312.

Knox, S. (1968). *Observation and assessment of the everyday play behavior of the mentally retarded child* (Unpublished master's thesis, University of Southern California).

Knox, S. A play scale. In M. Reilly (Ed.), *Play as exploratory learning* (pp. 247-266). Beverly Hills, CA: Sage Publications.

Knox, S. (1997a). *Play and play styles of preschool children* (Unpublished doctoral dissertation, University of Southern California).

Knox, S. (1997b). Development and current use of the Knox Preschool Play Scale. In L. D. Parham & L. Fazio (Eds.), *Play in occupational therapy for children* (pp. 35-51). St. Louis: Mosby.

Lee, S. (2007). *Reliability and validity of the Preschool Play Scale (revised) of Preschool Children With Autism.* Unpublished paper presented at the annual conference of the American Occupational Therapy Association, St. Louis, MO, April 23, 2007.

Lieberman, J. (1977). *Playfulness: Its relationship to imagination and creativity.* New York: Academic Press.

Matsutsuyu, J. (1969). The interest check list. *American Journal of Occupational Therapy, 23*, 323-328.

Misale, J., & Murphy, C. (1997). *The effects of expressive language and motor delays on play skills and playfulness in children* (Unpublished master's thesis, McMaster University, Ontario, Canada).

Moorehead, L. (1969). The occupational history. *American Journal of Occupational Therapy, 23*, 329-334.

Morrison, C., Bundy, A., & Fisher, A. (1991). The contribution of motor skills and playfulness to the play performance of preschoolers. *American Journal of Occupational Therapy, 45*(8), 687-694.

Norwicki, S., & Duke, M. (1974). A preschool and primary internal-external control scale. *Developmental Psychology, 10*, 874-880.

O'Sullivan, K. (2000). *Deaf and typical hearing children, ages 3-6*, Poster Session, American Occupational Therapy Association Annual Conference, Seattle, WA, 2000.

Over, K. (2006). *The effect of Therapeutic Listening on the occupation of play.* Presentation at the American Occupational Therapy Association Annual Conference, Charlotte, NC, 2006.

Over, K. (in press). The effect of therapeutic listening on the development of play, *American Journal of Occupational Therapy*.

Parten, M. (1933). Social play among pre-school children. *Journal of Abnormal and Social Psychology, 28*, 136-147.

Reilly, M. (1974). *Play as exploratory learning.* Beverly Hills, CA: Sage Publications.

Restall, G., & Magill-Evans, J. (1994). Play and preschool children with autism. *American Journal of Occupational Therapy, 48*(2), 113-120.

Robinson, A. (1977). Play: The arena for acquisition of rules of competent behavior. *American Journal of Occupational Therapy, 31*, 248-253.

Rosenblatt, D. (1977). Developmental trends in infant play. In B. Tizard & D. Harvey (Eds.), *Biology of play* (pp. 33-44). Philadelphia: J.B. Lippincott.

Rubin, K., Fein, G., & Vandenberg, B. Play. In P. Mussen (Ed.), *Handbook of child psychology* (Vol. 4, 4th ed., pp. 693-774). New York: John Wiley & Sons.

Rüdlinger, M. (1998). *The use of the Knox Preschool Play Scale in assessing children with low vision* (Unpublished master's thesis, Göteborg University, Göteborg, Sweden).

Schaaf, R., & Mulrooney, L. (1989). Occupational therapy in early intervention: A family centered approach. *American Journal of Occupational Therapy, 43*(11), 745-754.

Schaefer, C., Gitlin, K., & Sandgrund, A. (1991). Introduction. In C. Schaefer, K. Gitlin, & A. Sandgrun (Eds.), *Play diagnosis and assessment.* New York: John Wiley & Sons.

Shepherd, J., Broillier, C., & Dandow, R. (1994). Play skills of preschool children with speech and language delays. *Physical and Occupational Therapy in Pediatrics, 14*, 1-20.

Smilansky, S. (1968). *The effects of sociodramatic play on disadvantaged preschool children.* New York: John Wiley & Sons.

Sparrow, S., Balla, D., & Cicchetti, D. (1984). *Vineland Adaptive Behavior Scales.* Circle Pines, MN: American Guidance Service.

Stagnitti, K. (2004). Understanding play: The implications for play assessment. *Australian Occupational Therapy Journal 14*(2), 1-20.

Takata, N. (1969). The play history. *American Journal of Occupational Therapy, 23*(4), 314-318.

Takata, N. (1971). The play milieu—A preliminary appraisal. *American Journal of Occupational Therapy, 25*, 281-284.

Takata, N. Play as a prescription. In M. Reilly (Ed.), *Play as exploratory learning* (pp. 209-246). Beverly Hills, CA: Sage Publications.

Tanta, K. (2002). *The effect of peer-play level on the behavior of preschool children with delayed play skills* (Unpublished doctoral dissertation, University of Washington).

Von Zuben, M., Crist, P., & Mayberry, W. (1991). A pilot study of differences in play behavior between children of low and middle socioeconomic status. *American Journal of Occupational Therapy, 45*(2), 113-118.

Ward, W. C. (1968). Creativity in young children. *Child Development, 39*, 737-754.

Weintraub, N. (2006). Personal correspondence.

White, R. (1959). Motivation reconsidered: The concept of competence. *Psychological Review, 66*, 297-333.

Wolfgang, C., & Phelps, P. (1983). Preschool play materials preference inventory. *Early Child Development and Care, 12*, 127-141.

4

Test of Playfulness

GEVA SKARD AND ANITA C. BUNDY

KEY TERMS

playfulness
intrinsic motivation
internal control
suspension of reality
framing
environment
environmental supportiveness
Test of Environmental Supportiveness (TOES)
Test of Playfulness (ToP)

Occupational therapists are responsible for assessing and promoting play because it is the primary occupation of young children. While much has been written about play, and studies have found that people recognize it when they see it (Smith, Takhvar, Gore, & Vollstedt, 1985), play remains an elusive concept that has defied universal definition for decades (cf. Berlyne, 1966; Rubin, Fein, & Vandenberg, 1983). This chapter presents a model for observing and assessing playfulness. Playfulness has been defined simply as the disposition to play (Barnett, 1991). It might also be thought of as the way that a child approaches play (and other tasks). Playfulness is only one aspect of play. The totality of play also includes play activities and the skills children use in play, to name just two other aspects. However, the high correlation of playfulness with adaptability and coping (Hess & Bundy, 2003; Saunders, Sayle, & Goodall, 1999) suggests that playfulness may be one of the most important aspects of play.

In this chapter we outline a model for the systematic evaluation of playfulness and the supportiveness of the environment in which play takes place. This model has been operationalized in two observational assessments: the Test of Playfulness (ToP) (Bundy, Nelson, Metzger, & Bingaman, 2001) and the Test of Environmental Supportiveness (TOES) (Bronson & Bundy, 2001). To illustrate the model, we present two case examples.

A MODEL OF PLAYFULNESS

The model we will put forward draws from agreement in the literature that playfulness can be determined by evaluation for the presence of three elements: intrinsic motivation, internal control, and the freedom to suspend reality (Bundy, 1991, 1993; Kooij, 1989; Kooij & Vrijhof, 1987; Morrison, Bundy, & Fisher, 1991; Neumann, 1971).

Play is intrinsically motivated. Players engage in a play activity simply because they want to, not for any other reason. The doing (process) is more important than the outcome (product) (Rubin, Fein, & Vandenberg, 1983) (Figure 4-1). For example, although winning a game may be fun, winning is not the primary reason for playing. In fact, not knowing who will win increases the motivation to play, whereas knowing in advance who will win decreases the fun. For this reason very skilled players may

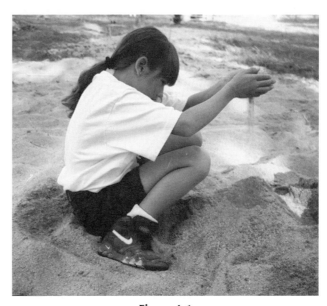

Figure 4-1

Play involves more attention to process than product. (Courtesy Becca Austin.)

be given a "handicap" in games like tennis or golf. When chance plays a big part in a game (e.g., cards), players usually begin again once a clear winner is identified (Caillois, 1979). The source of the motivation or the reasons why a particular activity is intrinsically motivating vary widely; we refer to these as personal motivations. Some children are motivated by activities that provide social interaction, and others seek sensation or mastery.

Internal control means that players are largely in charge of their actions and at least some aspects of the activity's outcome (Figures 4-2 and 4-3). Players decide such things as who to play with, what to play, and how and when the play should end. When attempting a new activity, a person may be heard to say, "I was playing with it to see what would happen" (Figure 4-4). Games with rules, a common form of play, may seem to be outside the definition of play; rules suggest that there is indeed a particular way to play. Nonetheless, rules can be modified to suit the style and needs of players. For example, Scrabble players may decide to look up words in a dictionary. And, while play cannot be bound by too may rules, neither can it have no rules. Otherwise players would not know how

to act and would not feel in control. Even pretend play, which seems to be a flight of pure fantasy, actually has rules of a kind. For example, two 9-year-old girls planning prom night for Barbie dolls must negotiate the "rules" of the evening—often multiple times.

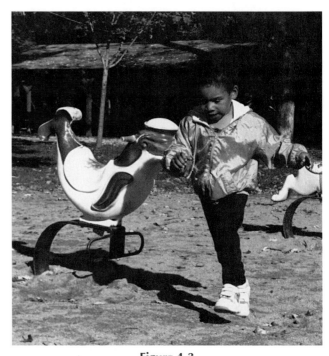

Figure 4-3

All players must retain enough control to say (verbally or nonverbally), "I'm finished. I want to do something else now." (Courtesy Becca Austin.)

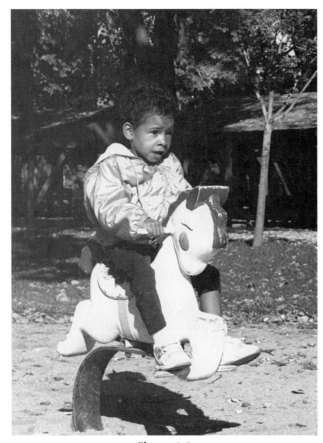

Figure 4-2

A horse is a horse, but that horse can be transportation or imply a source of sensation—the choice is the player's. (Courtesy Becca Austin.)

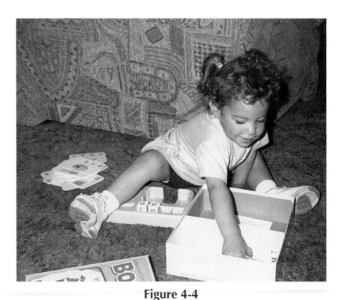

Figure 4-4

There is no "right way" to play with a game or toy. (Courtesy Becca Austin.)

Freedom to suspend reality means that the individual chooses how close to objective reality the play will be (Figure 4-5). Players may pretend that they are someone else or that an object is something other than what it really is. They may pretend to do something they are not actually doing. For example, they may pretend to be fighting but the verbal and physical cues they give say, "This is not for real." Players may also suspend reality by stretching the rules slightly, teasing, or telling jokes. For example, a 4-year-old pretending to be the teacher can assume a bossy persona that would not be allowed except in play.

Each of the three elements (intrinsic motivation, internal control, and freedom to suspend reality) can be represented by a continuum reflecting the relative presence of the trait in a particular transaction. The summative contribution of all three continua tips the balance and determines the relative presence of playfulness. Playfulness and nonplayfulness also represent a continuum (Bundy, 1991, 1993; Neumann, 1971) (Figure 4-6).

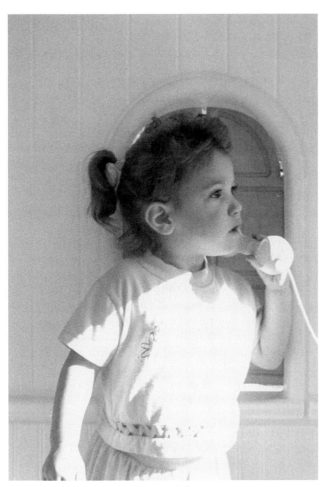

Figure 4-5
"As if" serves the same function as rules. (Courtesy Becca Austin.)

It is unlikely—and perhaps not even desirable—for any transaction to be totally intrinsically motivated, internally controlled, or free of the constraints of reality. Thus this model should be viewed with the knowledge that the continua are not scales in any strict sense. Nonetheless, the concept is useful in presenting an impression of the relative absence or presence of traits, particularly when therapists are in need of a quick, informal means for evaluating a particular transaction in an intervention session.

In addition to the three primary elements of play, Bateson (1971, 1972) described a fourth concept, framing, that seems critical to play and playfulness. Bateson likened the play frame to a picture frame that separates the wallpaper from the picture. He described play as a frame in which players give cues to others about how they want to be treated. To be a good player, a person must be able to both give and read cues. Of course, the ability to give and read social cues is also a part of many nonplay transactions. Bateson, however, argued that, in play, cues are exaggerated and thus easier to learn. Furthermore, people do not need language to learn about play cues, making infant-adult play an excellent early medium for learning to give and read social cues.

Framing seems somewhat more difficult to explain than the other elements of playfulness, perhaps because giving and reading cues are so much a part of culture that knowledge of them is tacit: only their impairment or absence is obvious. Furthermore, social cues may involve affective processing as much as cognitive (Stern, 1985).

The four elements of playfulness reflect the player's contributions to a play transaction. Their expression, however, will be affected by the supportiveness of the environment. The environment is addressed in depth later in the chapter.

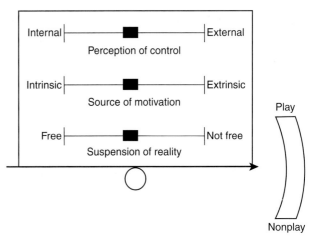

Figure 4-6
Schematic representation of the elements of playfulness.

Operationalizing the Elements of Playfulness

If the concept of playfulness as a reflection of the combined presence of intrinsic motivation, internal control, freedom to suspend reality, and framing is to be used in a more formal manner to evaluate playfulness, each trait must be defined in a more readily usable or operational manner. How will children act if they are intrinsically motivated, internally controlled (Figure 4-7), free of unnecessary constraints of reality, or entering or maintaining the frame? This operationalization of the elements is a vital step in the development of a valid assessment of playfulness—one that may allow therapists to capture the important aspects of play and thus include it routinely in their evaluations of young children. The operationalization of these concepts leads to the creation of the actual test items (Bundy, 1993).

Many of the traits of play that are most commonly listed in play literature can be viewed as an aspect of intrinsic motivation, internal control, or the suspension of reality. They can be considered a part of one or more of the more encompassing elements of play. They answer one or more questions about how intrinsic motivation,

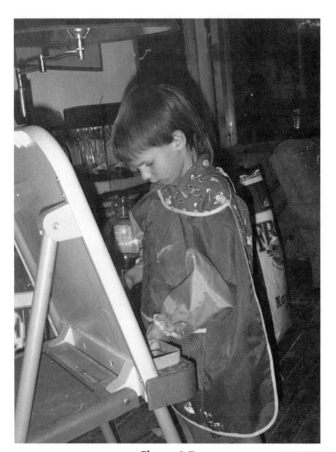

Figure 4-7

A player who experiences internal control can make material things do whatever his competence allows. (Courtesy Becca Austin.)

internal control, or the suspension of reality is recognized when they are seen.

Intrinsic motivation, internal control, and freedom from some constraints of reality are not mutually exclusive. Certain behaviors may reflect more than one of these elements. For example, maintaining a play theme for a significant period of time suggests that a player is skilled at framing but also may reflect the player's social skills or skills for interacting with objects, both aspects of internal control.

The relationship between the elements of play has been explored in the development of the Test of Playfulness (ToP), which has made use of a statistical procedure called Rasch analysis (Wright & Masters, 1982; Wright & Stone, 1979) to compare performance of children on different items and thus find out which features of play are "easier" or "harder" for children to master. Although the elements of play are not mutually exclusive, the items from the ToP seem to be somewhat more strongly associated with one element than the others. These associations are represented in Box 4-1. The items are defined in Table 4-1.

Administering the Test of Playfulness

The ToP is designed for assessing the play of children and adolescents who are between the ages of 6 months and 18 years and whose playfulness is a concern. The ToP is scored after free play is observed, preferably in both indoor and outdoor play situations. Tyler (1996) found that boys and girls did not differ in their scores on the ToP. The ToP appears to be valid across a number of cultural groups: Porter and Bundy (2000) found evidence for its validity with African American children, and Griffith (2000) and Phillips (1998) found that it was valid for Hispanic children in the United States and in Central America, respectively.

Although there is evidence that the ToP is valid and reliable with adolescents (Hess & Bundy 2003), use of the assessment has not, so far, been studied with adults. The greatest threat to the reliability and validity of the ToP in relation to adults may be the tendency for adults to become self-conscious when being observed rather than the possibility that playfulness, which many consider to be a trait, will change with age (Guitard, Ferland, & Dutil, 2005; Lieberman, 1977). In response to this problem, one of us (ACB) has developed a self-report version of the ToP for use with adults, The Experience of Leisure Scale (TELS) (Meakins, Bundy, & Gliner, 2005). Since self-consciousness is a factor for many adolescents, TELS may prove to be a better measure than the ToP for them also.

Box 4-1	*How ToP Items Associate with the Elements in the Play Model of Playfulness*		
Motivation	**Freedom from**	**Control**	Intensity
Engaged	**constraints of reality**	*Self*	Skill
Extent	Mischief	Decides	Supports
Intensity	Teases	Safe	Enters
Process	Pretends	Modifies	Initiates
Persists	Extent	Interacts with objects	Shares
Affect	Skill	Transitions	
	Clowns and jokes		**Frame**
	Extent	*Shared*	Gives cues
	Intensity	Negotiates	Reads cues
	Creative	Social play	Engaged (skill)
		Extent	

Table 4-1
Definitions of ToP Items

Item	Description
Is actively engaged.	Extent—Proportion of time player is involved in activities rather than aimless wandering or other nonfocused activity or temper tantrums. Intensity—Degree to which the child is concentrating on the activity or playmates. Skill—Players' ability to stay focused or carry a play theme from activity to activity.
Decides what to do and how to do it.	Extent—Proportion of time when players actively choose what they are doing. Players may decide to do what another is doing, but no one is forcing them or rewarding them for doing the activity.
Maintains level of safety sufficient to play.	Extent—Proportion of time when players feel safe enough to play. If necessary, players may alter the environment.
Tries to overcome barriers or obstacles to persist with an activity.	Intensity—Degree to which the child perseveres in order to overcome obstacles to continuing the activity.
Modifies activity to maintain challenge or make it more fun.	Skill—Ease with which the child actively changes the requirements or complexity of the task in order to vary the challenge or degree of novelty.
Engages in playful mischief or teasing.	Extent—Proportion of time when players are involved in playful teasing or minor infractions of the rules designed to make the play more fun. Skill—The ease, cleverness, or adeptness with which players create and carry out mischief or teasing.
Engages in activity for the sheer pleasure of it (process) rather than primarily for the end product.	Extent—Proportion of time when players seem to want to do the activity simply because they enjoy it rather than to attain a particular outcome or for some extrinsic reward.
Pretends (to be someone else; to do something else; that an object is something else; that something else is happening).	Extent—Proportion of time when there are overt indicators players are assuming different character roles, pretending to be doing something, pretending something is happening, or pretending an object or person is something else. Skill—The degree to which the "performance" convinces the examiner.

Continued

Table 4-1
Definitions of ToP Items—cont'd

Item	Description
Incorporates objects or other people into play in unconventional or variable ways.	Extent—Proportion of time when players (1) use objects commonly thought of as toys in ways other than those the manufacturer clearly intended, (2) incorporate objects not classically thought of as toys into the play (e.g., bugs, table legs), or (3) use one toy or object in a number of different ways. Creativity is a key. Skill—The ease or cleverness with which players incorporate objects or other people in creative ways.
Negotiates with others to have needs/desires met.	Skill—Ease and finesse with which players verbally or nonverbally ask for what they need.
Engages in social play.	Extent—Proportion of time during which player interacts with others involved in the same or similar activity. Intensity—The depth of the player's interactions with other people during play. Skill—The level of social play. Ranges from playing alone to being the leader.
Supports play of others.	Skill—Ease with which players support play of others (e.g., encouragement, ideas).
Enters a group already engaged in an activity.	Skill—Ease with which player does something to become part of a group (two or more) already engaged in an activity; the action is not disruptive to what is going on.
Initiates play with others.	Skill—Ease with which player initiates a new activity with another.
Clowns or jokes.	Extent—Proportion of time when players tell jokes or funny stories or engage in exaggerated, swaggering behavior, usually for the purpose of gaining others' attention. Skill—The ease or cleverness with which a player clowns or jokes. Ranges from not gaining others' attention to gaining positive reactions from others to being overtly funny.
Shares (toys, equipment, friends, ideas).	Skill—The ease with which players allow others to use toys, personal belongings, or equipment they are using or share playmates (friends) or ideas.
Gives readily understandable cues (facial, verbal, body) that say, "This is how you should act toward me."	Extent—Proportion of time during which players act in a way to give out clear messages about how others should interact with them.
Responds to others' cues.	Extent—Proportion of time during which the child acts in accord with others' play cues.
Demonstrates positive affect during play.	Intensity—Degree to which player's affect is positive; ranges from mild enjoyment to real exuberance.
Interacts with objects.	Intensity—The degree to which players get involved with objects. Skill—The ease with which players interact with objects.
Transitions from one play activity to another with ease.	Skill—The ease with which players move from activity to activity when one has ended or is not evolving and another is available.

Scoring the Test of Playfulness

The ToP Keyform may be used to score a child's playfulness. The ToP Keyform (Figure 4-8) shows the relative difficulty of each item plotted against the means and standard deviations for the items, called the measure score. To score the ToP Keyform, the examiner circles all the scores awarded on ToP items on the ToP Protocol Sheet (Figure 4-9) and then draws a line through the points so that half are above it and half below. That line passes through a measure score on the right. The measure score is an interval level score that can be entered into statistical calculations (e.g., for research purposes). An idea of how this particular score compares with that of the approximately 2000 children who are a part of the ToP data set can be obtained by using Figure 4-10.

Development of the Test of Playfulness and Evidence for Validity and Reliability

Initially the ToP was a 60-item assessment scored from videotaped segments of free play. The ToP has undergone three notable revisions. Retaining its observational format, the current version (Version 4) comprises 29 items that can be scored directly, without videotaping, because we have found that the scores are equivalent (Nichols, 1997).

In the revision process some items (e.g., is physically active in play) were eliminated because statistical analysis suggested that they did not contribute to the construct of playfulness. Other items (e.g., using unconventional objects in play) were revised to reflect improved operational definitions that were easier to score in a consistent fashion. New items were generated to make the ToP more sensitive to small changes that come from intervention (Bundy, Nelson, Metzger, & Bingaman, 2001; Muneto, 2002).

In addition to item revision and generation, the scoring procedure for the ToP was changed. Initially all scoring was based on the proportion of time an item could be observed (extent). This, however, did not always seem to be the most relevant criterion. For example, with some items (e.g., persists in overcoming obstacles to play) the more relevant feature seemed to be the intensity with which the child engaged in the behavior. Thus an "intensity" scale was created to capture the degree to which some items were present. For other items (e.g., enters a group already engaged in an activity), a relevant feature seemed to be the skill or the ease with which a child was able to accomplish a task. Thus a third scale, "skillfulness," was created. In the current version none of the scales pertains to all the descriptors but more than one scale is applied to many descriptors. Scales that do not apply are shaded out in the sample scoring sheet (Figure 4-9).

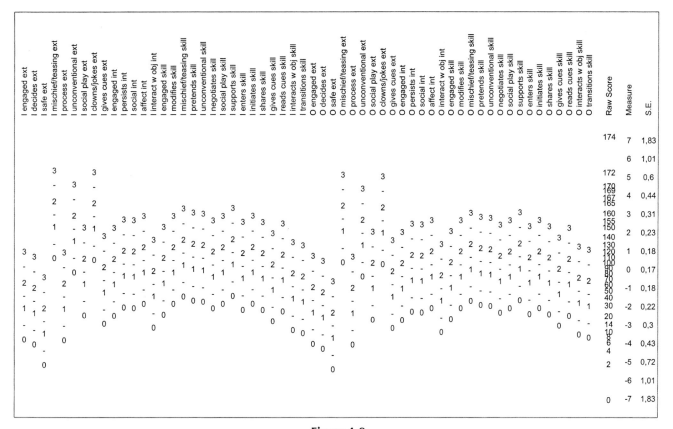

Figure 4-8

ToP Keyform indicating the relative difficulty of each item plotted against the means and standard deviations for the items.

TEST OF PLAYFULNESS (ToP) (Version 4.0–5/05)

Child (#): _____ Age: _____ Rater: _____ In Out Video Live (Circle)	**EXTENT** 3 = Almost always 2 = Much of the time 1 = Some of the time 0 = Rarely or never NA = Not Applicable	**INTENSITY** 3 = Highly 2 = Moderately 1 = Mildly 0 = Not NA = Not Applicable	**SKILLFULNESS** 3 = Highly skilled 2 = Moderately skilled 1 = Slightly skilled 0 = Unskilled NA = Not Applicable

ITEM	EXT	INT	SKILL	COMMENTS
Is actively <u>engaged</u>.				
<u>Decides</u> what to do.				
Maintains level of <u>safety</u> sufficient to play.				
Tries to overcome barriers or obstacles to <u>persist</u> with an activity.				
<u>Modifies</u> activity to maintain challenge or make it more fun.				
Engages in playful mischief or <u>teasing</u>				
Engages in activity for the sheer pleasure of it (<u>process</u>) rather than primarily for the end product.				
<u>Pretends</u> (to be someone else; to do something else; that an object is something else; that something else is happening).				
Incorporates objects or other people into play in unconventional or variable **and** <u>creative</u> ways.				
<u>Negotiates</u> with others to have needs/ desires met.				
Engages in <u>social play</u>.				
<u>Supports</u> play of others.				
<u>Enters</u> a group already engaged in an activity.				
<u>Initiates</u> play with others.				
<u>Clowns</u> or <u>jokes</u>.				
<u>Shares</u> (toys, equipment, friends, ideas).				
<u>Gives</u> readily understandable <u>cues</u> (facial, verbal, body) that say, "This is how you should act toward me."				
Responds to others' cues.				
Demonstrates positive <u>affect</u> during play.				
Interacts <u>with objects</u>.				
<u>Transitions</u> from one play activity to another with ease.				

Figure 4-9

ToP protocol sheet.

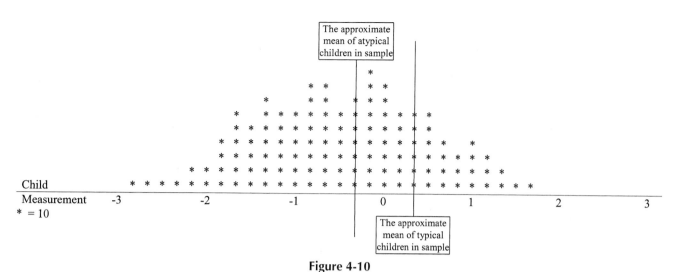

Figure 4-10
Graphic representation of the entire ToP data set, including the approximate means of typical and atypical children in the sample.

In the course of development of ToP, raw ToP data from nearly 2000 children have been subjected to Rasch analysis, a statistical modeling technique that measures how well performance on the items meets two basic assumptions: (1) easy items are easy for everybody, and (2) more capable (or in this case more playful) people have higher scores. By use of Rasch analysis it is also possible to determine whether items define a single unidimensional construct, the relative difficulty of each item, the relative playfulness of each child, and the degree of severity of each rater.

Over time, data from approximately 96% of items, 93% of participants, and 95% of raters have met the assumptions of the Rasch model consistently. Thus we can say that items of the ToP define a unidimensional construct reflecting playfulness. Since 95% fit to the model is desired, the data from the participants fall somewhat short of the standard. On further reflection we have learned that the construct of playfulness seems to differ slightly for some groups of children.

Although there are no large samples of children with any one diagnosis, it seems possible that some of the data that failed to conform to the expectations of the Rasch model reflect diagnostic information. In other words, children with particular disabilities may tend to attain ToP scores that reflect characteristics of their disability. Data collected by Leipold and Bundy (2000) and Harkness and Bundy (2001) are consistent with this hypothesis. These studies found that children with attention deficit hyperactivity disorder tended to have unexpectedly low scores on remaining engaged and unexpectedly high scores on mischief and teasing (Leipold & Bundy, 2000). Similarly, children with physical difficulties but no known cognitive limitations tended to have unexpectedly low scores on remaining engaged and deciding but unexpectedly high scores on clowning and joking (Harkness & Bundy, 2001). Clearly, more research is needed to investigate playfulness in children with disabilities.

The ToP has been examined for test-retest reliability in three studies (Brentnall, 2005; O'Brien & Shirley, 2001; Scott, 2003). Using a very small sample, O'Brien and Shirley found that ToP scores remained stable over several years. Both Brentnall and Scott, using data from the same videotaped play sessions at a day-care center, found only moderate test-retest coefficients. They suggested that in situations with many choices of playmates and activities, it is relatively easy to change the nature of the test and thus decrease the reliability of the scores. In particular, they found that whether a child was playing alone or with others was an important factor that affected scoring. This suggests that children tested twice to evaluate for changes occurring as a result of intervention should be seen either alone or with a playmate (not necessarily the same playmate) in both tests to ensure that any change in scores is the result of the intervention.

Brentnall also found differences in scoring that resulted from length of observation. She concluded that ToP scores were most reliable when based on 15-minute observations.

ENVIRONMENTAL INFLUENCE ON PLAYFULNESS

So far in this chapter, playfulness, defined as a disposition to play, has been assumed to be a characteristic of the individual (Lieberman, 1977). Yet even the most playful child may behave in a less playful way when the environment is unsupportive. By the same token, a child's actions may become more playful in a very supportive environment (Bronson & Bundy, 2001). Many researchers have examined how individuals interact with their environments and how this interaction affects behavior and performance (Barker, 1968; Gibson, 1979; Lewin, 1955; Pervin, 1968; Stern, 1970). For some years now, theorists have been advocating a dynamic person-environment system, in which personal and environmental factors are seen to have a reciprocal influence on one another (e.g., Kielhofner, 1995; Magnussen, 1981; Wicker, 1987).

It follows then that, just as we examine factors in the individual related to playfulness, so too should we assess features of the environment for their influence on play. Both the physical and social environments can influence play through affording opportunities and "pulling for" certain behaviors (Gibson, 1979; Kielhofner, 1995). For example, playground climbing equipment pulls for active group play, whereas books and craft materials suggest quiet solitary play. The sociocultural ambience (e.g., accepted norms, expectations, and rules) influences the freedom and confidence with which an individual interacts with elements of the environment (Rowles, 1991). Overly strict or inconsistent rules reduce play, whereas carefully considered rules promote it. Other situational properties include complexity and clarity (Magnussen, 1981). To promote play, environments must enable children to move from "what does this do?" (exploration) to "what can I do with this?" (play).

A positive fit between the player and the environment occurs when opportunities meet the needs of the individual and when the ability of the individual matches the demands of the environment (Pervin, 1968). Congruence between the choices offered in the setting and the player's motivation, self-determination, and desire for autonomy contributes to fit (Eccles et al., 1993; O'Conner & Vallerand, 1994).

An environment that pulls for behavior below the player's capacity (e.g., baby toys for an older child) may result in boredom. Environments that pull for behaviors beyond the individual's abilities can cause anxiety. Settings pulling for behaviors at the upper levels of an individual's capacity promote involvement, attentiveness, maximum performance, and adaptation (Csikszentmihalyi, 1990). Other environmental properties that promote a positive fit include choice and the presence of playthings that match the individual's motivations (Holland, 1966; Jordan et al., 1991). Players' motivations are discussed in more detail in the next section.

Assessment of an environment's capacity to support playfulness may be especially important in the case of players with physical, cognitive, or sensory impairments, who may receive less feedback from, and be less able to access and affect, playmates and the environment than typically developing players (Holaday et al., 1997). The cues given by players with disabilities may be more difficult for caregivers and playmates to read; thus they may miss the player's cues and, thinking the player is passive and unresponsive, decrease their interactions (Jennings & MacTurk, 1995). They may also fail to understand cues and therefore respond inappropriately. Both of these situations may result in negative consequences for the play and the player's sense of efficacy.

Test of Environmental Supportiveness (TOES)

The TOES was developed to assess the extent to which elements of a particular environment support a player's motivations for play (Bronson & Bundy, 2001). The TOES is meant to be administered in conjunction with the ToP. Understanding the effects that different elements of the child-environment interaction have in facilitating or restricting play allows therapists to develop and monitor appropriate modifications for established contexts. Specifically, the TOES examines fit between the players' motivations and caregivers, playmates, objects, play spaces, and the sensory environment (Bundy, 1997). The TOES scoring sheet is presented in Figure 4-11; a description of the items is presented in Table 4-2.

Researchers in education and health care now recommend evaluation of clients within naturalistic contexts. Consideration of people in their everyday environment promotes a positive, adaptive relationship between a functioning person and a supportive environment (Letts et al., 1994). This approach informs services supporting the activities of people in everyday environments as opposed to the remediation of underlying impairments (Pacheo & Lucca-Irizarry, 1995). Changing the environment may be far easier and more appropriate than changing the person (Healthy Toronto 2000 Subcommittee, 1988). Conjunctive use of the ToP and TOES addresses the need for a person-in-environment assessment of play and playfulness.

The first step in administering the TOES is to attempt to determine the source of the player's motivations. That is, what benefit(s) do players seem to be seeking from the activities in which they are engaging? Since the TOES is set within a context of the player's personal motivations, the therapist may need to discuss these with caregivers. Once personal motivations are established, the therapist can assess the degree to which each element (e.g., playmates, space) contributes to these motivations' being met.

Scoring the TOES
At present the items of the TOES can be scored but there is no means for summing them into a meaningful score. Since the primary purpose of the TOES is as a tool for consultation with caregivers, however, it is appropriate that the information the instrument yields relative to each item should be descriptive.

Evidence for TOES Validity and Reliability
TOES items were selected after an extensive review of relevant literature and input from a panel of expert occupational therapists (from the United States, Canada, and Sweden) who had focused their work on the environment. Two studies (Harding, 1997; Bronson & Bundy, 2001) have provided preliminary evidence of the construct validity and reliability of the TOES.

TEST OF ENVIRONMENTAL SUPPORTIVENESS (TOES)–7/03

Child's Name:	Apparent Source(s) of Motivation:
Date of Observation:	
Child's Birth Date:	Location of Observation:
Age at Observation:	Examiner:

CONTINUA OF ITEMS

2 = strongly favors description on right
1 = slightly favors description on right
−1 = slightly favors description on left
−2 = strongly favors description on left
NA = not applicable

Comments

Caregivers interfere with player's activities and opportunities	−2 −1 1 2 NA	Caregivers promote player's activities and opportunities	
Caregivers change the rules	−2 −1 1 2 NA	Caregivers adhere to consistent boundaries/rules	
Caregivers enforce unreasonably strict boundaries or fail to set boundaries	−2 −1 1 2 NA	Caregivers adhere to reasonable boundaries/rules	
Peer playmate's response to player's cues interferes with transaction	−2 −1 1 2 NA	Peer playmate's response to player's cues supports transaction	
Peer playmates do not give clear cues or give cues that interfere with the transaction	−2 −1 1 2 NA	Peer playmates give clear cues that support the transaction	
Peer playmates are dominated by player or dominate players	−2 −1 1 2 NA	Peer playmates participate as equals with player	
Older playmate's response to player's cues interferes with transaction	−2 −1 1 2 NA	Older playmate's response to player's cues supports transaction	
Older playmates fail to give clear cues or give cues that interfere with transaction	−2 −1 1 2 NA	Older playmates give clear cues that support the transaction	
Older playmates are dominated by or dominate player	−2 −1 1 2 NA	Older playmates participate as equals with player	
Younger playmate's response to player's cues interferes with transaction	−2 −1 1 2 NA	Younger playmate's response to player's cues supports transaction	
Younger playmates fail to give clear cues or give cues that interfere with transaction	−2 −1 1 2 NA	Younger playmates give clear cues that support the transaction	
Younger playmates are dominated by or dominate player	−2 −1 1 2 NA	Younger playmates participate as equals with player	
Natural/fabricated objects do not support activity of player	−2 −1 1 2 NA	Natural/fabricated objects support activity of player	
Amount and configuration of space do not support type of play	−2 −1 1 2 NA	Amount and configuration of space support activity of player	
Sensory environment does not offer adequate invitation to play	−2 −1 1 2 NA	Sensory environment offers adequate invitation to play	
Space is not physically safe	−2 −1 1 2 NA	Space is physically safe	
Space is not accessible	−2 −1 1 2 NA	Space is accessible	

Additional comments:

Figure 4-11
TOES scoring sheet.

Table 4-2
Elements for Evaluation of Human and Nonhuman Environment

Item	Description
Caregiver promotes player's activities and opportunities.	Gives player access to possibilities if needed (e.g., ideas, props, or playthings). Facilitates interactions of entire group (including player). Acts in a way that says play and player's motivations are important (e.g., does not interrupt player or stop play unnecessarily). Responds to player's cues in a way that sanctions play. Available for help if needed. Shows respect for players. Is unobtrusive when appropriate. Gives only amount of direction necessary to facilitate play.
Caregiver adheres to consistent boundaries and rules.	Rules can be flexible but do not change unexpectedly or irrationally.
Caregiver adheres to reasonable boundaries and rules.	Enough to make player safe and comfortable. Not derived from power struggle. Not excessively strict; flexible when appropriate. Tacit or explicit permission to choose objects, activities, type of play, play locations.
Playmate(s) response to player's cues supports transaction.	Behaves toward player in logical, supportive way. Waits for responses (timing). Contributes to maintaining the flow of the play.
Playmate(s) gives clear cues that support transaction.	Gives clear messages about how player should interact with him or her. Messages reflect a continuation of the frame or a logical change.
Playmate(s) participates as equal with player.	Gets involved in activity. Adapts activity so it is play for self and player. Contributes good ideas. Does not get suppressed by player. Has skills to engage in the play. Plays with (rather than directs) player. Not bossy, manipulative. Shares common interests. Seems happy with status and roles in the situation.
Natural and fabricated object(s) support activity and apparent motivations of player.	Support player in his or her efforts to fulfill motivations. Allow modification of challenges. Sufficient number exists to support play. Engender feeling to do something with them.
Amount and configuration of space support activity.	Allow modification of challenges. Boundaries of play space evident when necessary.
Sensory environment offers adequate invitation to play.	Meets player's needs (this is the most important element). Colors—neither overstimulating nor drab. Level and type of noise are conducive to play (anger, crying versus laughing, chatting). Neither sterile nor overly cluttered. Temperature well controlled.
Space is physically safe.	No objects or surfaces pose an imminent threat to player's safety.
Space is accessible.	Objects are placed where player can get them readily. Readily permits movement. Provides physical support as needed for player.

Evidence of Reliability

Bronson and Bundy (2001) examined interrater reliability and estimated item model error. Goodness of fit statistics revealed that data from 100% of raters (n = 10) conformed to the expectations of the Rasch model. Furthermore, estimated item model errors were low (<.25) for all but one item ("younger playmates read player's cues"; error = .26).

Evidence of Validity

Bronson and Bundy (2001) also examined fit of items and participants (n = 160) to the Rasch model, as well as logic of item order. Data from 94% of items (all except "space is physically safe"), 95% of environments, and 96% of ratings conformed to the expectations of the Rasch model. Bronson and Bundy concluded that the scoring criteria for "space is physically safe" should be more clearly defined; Bundy has attempted to do this in the version presented in this chapter.

Bronson and Bundy suggested that the ordering of the items is logical. For example, "space is physically safe" was found to be the easiest item, which accords with the commonsense assumption that, unless children feel physically safe, they will be unlikely to play (Vandenberg, 1981). Items that refer to younger playmates were the most difficult. This is also logical, since younger playmates lack the skills that peer or older playmates have for enhancing play (Bailey et al., 1993).

CASE EXAMPLES

Whether or not therapists assign scores to the ToP and TOES, they can easily use the ToP to undertake systematic examination of playfulness in their young clients using an approach illustrated by the following two case studies.

CASE EXAMPLE 1
Daniel

Daniel is a 4-year-old boy who experiences delays across all domains of development. The greatest concern is that he does not play well with other children. There are also concerns about his social interaction with adults. He speaks a little with his parents, but at kindergarten (which he attends every day) he rarely speaks at all. Daniel is observed by the occupational therapist for 15 minutes indoors in the kindergarten. He is part of a group of children ranging in age from 3 to 6 years. When the observation starts, Daniel is wandering around the room in an apparently aimless fashion. After a couple of minutes, he sits down by a toy castle where there are animal and human figures. He manipulates the figures somewhat awkwardly.

He places one "man" up in the tower of the castle, but there are no signs he is engaging in pretend play and the activity does not seem to develop. After a while, a girl of the same age comes to play with him. She picks up a toy lion. She makes the lion walk up the wall of the castle while she makes a threatening roaring sound. Daniel repeats her actions, moving his lion and making a roaring sound. The girl moves her lion toward Daniel's and shakes it slightly it as if it were trying to communicate; Daniel simply repeats the roaring sounds. After failing to get a response following several repetitions of the same movement and sounds, the girl gives up and leaves to play elsewhere. Daniel stays where he is and repeats the lion's movements up the wall, but he does not make any sound or develop the play further. Instead, Daniel sits quietly by the castle, doing nothing.

After a while, Daniel leaves the castle and goes into one of the other rooms. There are mattresses and pillows on the floor, and some older boys are jumping, and, by the sound of it, having a lot of fun. Cautiously, Daniel joins in with the jumping. He starts jumping on the edge of the mattress, perhaps waiting to see if the others will protest, then jumps nearer. The older boys are looking at him welcomingly and giving him space to jump with them. For 5 minutes, Daniel jumps and smiles and seems to enjoy himself, but there is no laughter or any other obvious signs of joy. Then the older boys stop jumping and start to negotiate a new game to play. Daniel watches but does not take part in the planning process. When the older boys start playing, he watches for a while and then leaves the room.

On his way out, Daniel passes some children who are playing with a toy railway. Daniel stops to watch for a while. When he picks up part of a train that is lying idle on the floor, a younger boy cries out, "No! That's mine. Go away!" Daniel hesitates for a few seconds, but then drops the train on the floor. He sits down, picks up a rail part, and keeps it in his hands, watching the others play. At this point the observation ends.

Daniel's Playfulness Profile

Daniel's scores on the ToP are shown in Figure 4-12. Through examination of scores on the items associated with each of the elements (see Figure 4-8), a playfulness profile has been created for Daniel (Figure 4-13). Daniel's ToP Keyform is shown in Figure 4-14. Each of the elements of playfulness is discussed separately before Daniel's playfulness profile is summarized.

Source of Motivation

The mark on the continuum representing motivation is rather far toward the "extrinsic" side. Toys and other children's play seemed to influence Daniel's choices of

TEST OF PLAYFULNESS (ToP) (Version 4.0–5/05)

	EXTENT	INTENSITY	SKILLFULNESS
Child (#): Daniel Age: 4 years Rater: G. Skard [In] Out Video [Live] (Circle)	3 = Almost always 2 = Much of the time 1 = Some of the time 0 = Rarely or never NA = Not Applicable	3 = Highly 2 = Moderately 1 = Mildly 0 = Not NA = Not Applicable	3 = Highly skilled 2 = Moderately skilled 1 = Slightly skilled 0 = Unskilled NA = Not Applicable

ITEM	EXT	INT	SKILL	COMMENTS
Is actively <u>engaged</u>.	2	0	1	Engages in several disconnected play themes, and sometimes whether he is playing is in question.
<u>Decides</u> what to do.	3			
Maintains level of <u>safety</u> sufficient to play.	3			
Tries to overcome barriers or obstacles to <u>persist</u> with an activity.		1		
<u>Modifies</u> activity to maintain challenge or make it more fun.			0	
Engages in playful <u>mischief</u> or <u>teasing</u>.	0		NA	
Engages in activity for the sheer pleasure of it (<u>process</u>) rather than primarily for the end product.	2			
<u>Pretends</u> (to be someone else; to do something else; that an object is something else; that something else is happening).	0		1	He makes lion sound and moves the lion. Plastic lions do not make sounds or move, but uncertain whether he is really pretending or just copying his playmate.
Incorporates objects or other people into play in unconventional or variable **and** <u>creative</u> ways.	0		NA	
<u>Negotiates</u> with others to have needs/desires met.			1	
Engages in <u>social play</u>.	1	0	1	
<u>Supports</u> play of others.			0	
<u>Enters</u> a group already engaged in an activity.			2	
<u>Initiates</u> play with others.			0	
<u>Clowns</u> or <u>jokes</u>.	0		NA	
<u>Shares</u> (toys, equipment, friends, ideas).			0	Shares a little too readily.
<u>Gives</u> readily understandable <u>cues</u> (facial, verbal, body) that say, "This is how you should act toward me."	1		1	
Responds to others' cues.			1	
Demonstrates positive <u>affect</u> during play.		0		
Interacts <u>with objects</u>.		1	1	
<u>Transitions</u> from one play activity to another with ease.			1	

Figure 4-12

Daniel's scores on the ToP.

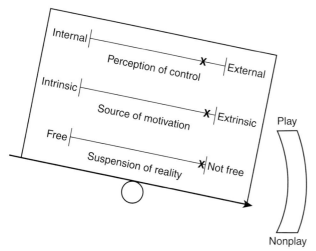

Figure 4-13
Daniel's playfulness profile.

play was the only activity in the observation where the activity actually matched his play skills.

Suspension of Reality
The marker on the continuum representing suspension of reality is also placed very far to the "not free" end. Daniel did show brief behavior consistent with pretending (i.e., roaring like a lion at the castle); however, it was not clear whether he was actually pretending or simply imitating his playmate without really understanding what she was doing.

Framing
Although Daniel did give out a few relatively subtle cues as to how others should interact with him, they were so difficult to notice that only a very skilled player would be able to read them. By the same token, Daniel seemed aware of other children's cues (as evidenced by his response to the younger boy's retaliation), but did not seem able to read them unless they were very blatant (e.g., missing the girl's cues to engage in pretend play).

Environmental Supportiveness
The TOES scores for Daniel are shown in Figure 4-15. In use of the TOES to assess Daniel's play environment, the first step would have been to determine what motivated him during the play episode observed. However, the fact that he showed so little intrinsic motivation makes this somewhat difficult. The only period when there was a clear indication of interest and enjoyment was when he was jumping on the mattress, an activity seemingly motivated by a desire for sensation.

In establishing the degree to which the environment supported Daniel's play, both human and nonhuman environments must be considered. In the observed play transaction the relevant human environmental factors to consider were peer, older, and younger playmates. Daniel's peer playmate behaved toward him in a logical and supportive way. She involved herself in his play activity, giving him clear cues as to how she wanted to play. She contributed good ideas and waited for his response before finally giving up and leaving when no response was forthcoming. Daniel seemed unable to respond to her initiatives.

The older playmates' response to Daniel's cues seemed to support the transaction. They behaved toward him in a logical and supportive way, although they did not actively include him as an equal. And as they planned the new activity, Daniel seemed not to find a role for himself and chose to leave. The younger playmate did not behave toward Daniel in a logical and supportive way, being unable to share his friends,

what he wanted to do. He did not, however, seem interested enough or able to overcome any barrier (e.g., the girl leaving or the older boys changing the game) to continue playing. Most of the time, he did not show significant levels of interest, engagement, or affect. (The reason for this could be that the accessible activities and toys were too difficult for his skills.) The only clear indication of interest and enjoyment was when he was jumping on the mattress. In this 5-minute period, Daniel seemed to be motivated by mastery of the environment (he is able to jump and do the same thing as the older boys) (White, 1959) and by the sheer sensation associated with the gross motor activity (Caillois, 1979). This indicates that Daniel might be more motivated if the environment presents him with possibilities to engage in appropriate gross motor activities.

Perception of Control
The marker on the continuum representing control is placed relatively far toward the "external" side. Daniel seemed to feel safe. He also decided the activities in which he wanted to take part. He is the decision maker as long as he has the real option to do something else; active choice is the main issue. "Decides" is a very easy item. The overall impression, however, was that Daniel did not feel much in control; especially with regard to items that reflect shared control, he received very low scores.

The score on "enters a group already engaged in an activity," a shared control item, is a surprisingly high score among a long row of 1 and 0 scores. This social skill constitutes an important resource in developing play skills and social interaction, so it is worth pondering why Daniel scored so well here; perhaps his performance resulted from active training in social skills. One other possible explanation is that the gross motor

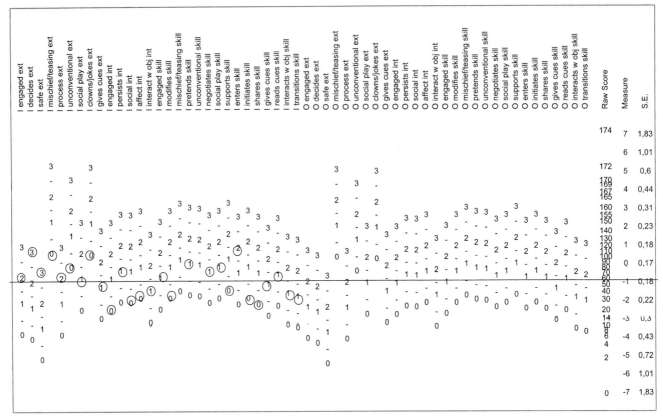

Figure 4-14
Daniel's ToP Keyform.

the space, or even the toys he was not playing with at the time that Daniel approached.

With regard to the nonhuman environment, the space available and the objects available for play should be considered. The space was physically safe and offered adequate invitation to play for many of the children. Daniel seemed motivated by gross motor activity, however, and the only space available for this kind of activity was occupied by a group of older children. Moreover, objects other than the mattress (i.e., the castle and figures) did not seem to support Daniel's motivations. Daniel would probably have played better with toys designed for younger children, but in a kindergarten for 3- to 6-year-olds, toys of this kind were not available.

Summary

When viewed overall, Daniel's profile describes a child who is not very playful. He has a raw score of about 65 and a scaled score (measure) slightly above −1 (see Figure 4-14). Daniel's score in reference to the whole sample can be determined by consulting Figure 4-10. Although this profile may in part reflect factors internal to Daniel, any tendencies toward playfulness were not adequately supported by the environment.

Derja

Derja is a 4½-year-old girl who has spastic hemiplegic cerebral palsy. Her right side is affected, and she needs a walker to move around in the kindergarten she attends every day. She has relatively good control of movement in her spastic arm but has some problems with tactile discrimination in her hand. She displays no sign of learning disabilities. She has some limitations in the field of vision on her right side. She also has some minor problems with articulation but otherwise does not seem to have any language problems.

Derja is observed for 15 minutes playing indoors at the kindergarten, where she is the only disabled child. The observation begins when Derja is approaching a group of peers who are sitting in a corner, on the floor, playing with Barbie dolls. Derja tries to sit down next to them, but her walker gets in the way, threatening to knock over some of the toys. The girls protest a little, reaching out to save the toys from being knocked over, but when Derja is seated, they immediately return to their play. Derja starts playing with a doll that has not been taken by the other children. She finds a dress and

TEST OF ENVIRONMENTAL SUPPORTIVENESS (TOES)–7/03

Child's Name: **Daniel**	Apparent Source(s) of Motivation:
Date of Observation: **xx-2005**	**Toys and gross motor activity**
Child's Birth Date: **xxxx**	Location of Observation: **Kindergarten, Indoors**
Age at Observation: **4 years**	Examiner: **G. Skard**

CONTINUA OF ITEMS 2 = strongly favors description on right 1 = slightly favors description on right −1 = slightly favors description on left −2 = strongly favors description on left NA = not applicable			Comments
Peer playmate's response to player's cues interferes with transaction	−2 −1 1 **2** NA	Peer playmate's response to player's cues supports transaction	
Peer playmates do not give clear cues or give cues that interfere with the transaction	−2 −1 1 **2** NA	Peer playmates give clear cues that support the transaction	
Peer playmates are dominated by player or dominate players	−2 −1 1 **2** NA	Peer playmates participate as equals with player	
Older playmate's response to player's cues interferes with transaction	−2 −1 1 **2** NA	Older playmate's response to players cues supports transaction	
Older playmates fail to give clear cues or give cues that interfere with transaction	−2 −1 1 **2** NA	Older playmates give clear cues that support the transaction	
Older playmates are dominated by or dominate player	−2 −1 **1** 2 NA	Older playmates participate as equals with player	
Younger playmate's response to player's cues interferes with transaction	**−2** −1 1 2 NA	Younger playmate's response to player's cues supports transaction	
Younger playmates fail to give clear cues or give cues that interfere with transaction	**−2** −1 1 2 NA	Younger playmates give clear cues that support the transaction	
Younger playmates are dominated by or dominate player	**−2** −1 1 2 NA	Younger playmates participate as equals with player	
Natural/fabricated objects do not support activity of player	−2 **−1** 1 2 NA	Natural/fabricated objects support activity of player	
Amount and configuration of space do not support type of play	−2 **−1** 1 2 NA	Amount and configuration of space support activity of player	
Sensory environment does not offer adequate invitation to play	−2 −1 1 **2** NA	Sensory environment offers adequate invitation to play	
Space is not physically safe	−2 −1 1 **2** NA	Space is physically safe	
Space is not accessible	−2 **−1** 1 2 NA	Space is accessible	
Additional comments:			

Figure 4-15

TOES scoring sheet for Daniel (only relevant items are shown).

TEST OF PLAYFULNESS (ToP) (Version 4.0–5/05)

	EXTENT	INTENSITY	SKILLFULNESS
Child (#): ____Derja____ Age: __4½ years__ Rater: ____G. Skard____ [In] Out Video [Live] (Circle)	3 = Almost always 2 = Much of the time 1 = Some of the time 0 = Rarely or never NA = Not Applicable	3 = Highly 2 = Moderately 1 = Mildly 0 = Not NA = Not Applicable	3 = Highly skilled 2 = Moderately skilled 1 = Slightly skilled 0 = Unskilled NA = Not Applicable

ITEM	EXT	INT	SKILL	COMMENTS
Is actively <u>engaged</u>.	3	3	3	
<u>Decides</u> what to do.	3			
Maintains level of <u>safety</u> sufficient to play.	3			
Tries to overcome barriers or obstacles to <u>persist</u> with an activity.		3		Her lack of movement control and tactile discrimination in her hand are major obstacles
<u>Modifies</u> activity to maintain challenge or make it more fun.			2	
Engages in playful <u>mischief</u> or <u>teasing</u>.	0		NA	
Engages in activity for the sheer pleasure of it (<u>process</u>) rather than primarily for the end product.	3			
<u>Pretends</u> (to be someone else; to do something else; that an object is something else; that something else is happening).	2		3	
Incorporates objects or other people into play in unconventional or variable **and** <u>creative</u> ways.	0		NA	
<u>Negotiates</u> with others to have needs/ desires met.			3	
Engages in <u>social play</u>.	2	2	1	
<u>Supports</u> play of others.			2	
<u>Enters</u> a group already engaged in an activity.			3	She enters effortlessly even in a situation where she due to movement problems threatens to knock down toys.
<u>Initiates</u> play with others.			NA	
<u>Clowns</u> or <u>jokes</u>.	1		3	Turns a potential problem into a something positive by pretending to fall in a funny way.
<u>Shares</u> (toys, equipment, friends, ideas).			3	
<u>Gives</u> readily understandable <u>cues</u> (facial, verbal, body) that say, "This is how you should act toward me."	3		3	
<u>Responds</u> to others' cues.			3	
Demonstrates positive <u>affect</u> during play.		1		
Interacts <u>with objects</u>.		3	3	
Transitions from one play activity to another with ease.			NA	

Figure 4-16

Derja's scores on the ToP.

a jacket she can reach from where she is sitting. She points and asks in a polite way if one of the girls would pass her a pair of shoes and a hat that are out of her reach. For about 5 minutes, Derja dresses the doll with great difficulty. She seems to be concentrating hard and struggles to close the Velcro of the dress and the jacket. During this period Derja does not pay the other girls any attention, nor they her. The girls constantly change the dolls' clothes and pretend that their dolls are taking care of babies. They pretend that the dolls are talking, drinking coffee, and having lunch, but after a while the play does not seem to have developed very much. When finally Derja's doll is dressed with shoes and hat, Derja can focus her attention on the play interaction. She moves her doll toward them and says, "Now I am coming." Then she tries to seat her doll on a chair at the toy table but knocks it over. She pretends that the doll is afraid of falling by crying out, "I am falling down. Help me! Help me!" All the girls laugh. One of them helps Derja's doll to sit down and offers her a cup of coffee. Derja pretends that her doll is drinking and moves her own mouth to make the appropriate noises. Derja's participation seems to have given new life to the play for a few minutes, but then the other girls leave to do something else. Derja stays behind and keeps on playing with the dolls. She lays the table with plates and cups. She makes the dolls talk to each other. She moves them around and makes one of them pick up a baby and put it in a pram. She makes the doll rock the pram while she sings a lullaby in a very low voice. Derja is still playing alone when the 15-minute observation finishes.

Derja's Playfulness Profile
Derja's scores on the ToP are shown in Figure 4-16. By examinations of the scores on the items associated with each of the elements (see Figure 4-8), a playfulness profile has been created for Derja (Figure 4-17). Derja's ToP Keyform is shown in Figure 4-18.

Source of Motivation
The placement of the marker along the continuum representing motivation is relatively far toward the "intrinsic" end, since Derja received high scores on all the items reflecting that element. Despite her obvious difficulties with movement, she remained actively and intensely engaged in playing with the dolls for most of the 15 minutes. Throughout this time Derja seemed to be enjoying herself but was without much enthusiasm. Most of the time she seemed so focused on the challenges presented by the activities she was undertaking that she did not demonstrate joy. This is commonly observed in players of all ages; in fact, manifest joy seems to be observed only in certain kinds of activities

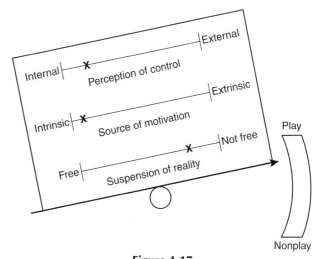

Figure 4-17
Derja's playfulness profile.

such as gross motor play or play including performance (e.g., playing clowns or comedians, or even acting as children playing).

In addition to the social interaction with her peers, it seems likely that the mastery and experience of playing house with the dolls were Derja's main sources of motivation. This impression is based on her persistence in dressing the doll, which was very difficult for her, and the fact that she stayed behind to continue playing with the dolls alone after all the others left to do something else.

Perception of Control
The placement of the marker along the continuum representing control is also on the "internal" side, but more toward the middle than that for motivation. Derja received higher scores on items that reflect self-control than on those that reflect shared control (e.g. "social play" and "supporting play of others"). This is to be expected, given her problems with tactile discrimination in the hand and subsequent movement control and because sharing control is more difficult than self-control. The dressing of the dolls is very difficult to perform, and this makes it difficult to be attentive to shared control as well. Derja appeared to feel safe and to be the decision maker with regard to the activity on which she focused. Dressing and role play were important parts of the activity, which the other girls performed simultaneously. Derja, on the other hand, seemed to modify the challenge by splitting these activities and performing them one at a time. When she performed the difficult task of dressing the doll, she had to focus all her attention on controlling her movements. In this period she did not take part in any other interactive play. Later, when the doll was dressed, she focused her attention on the pretend play

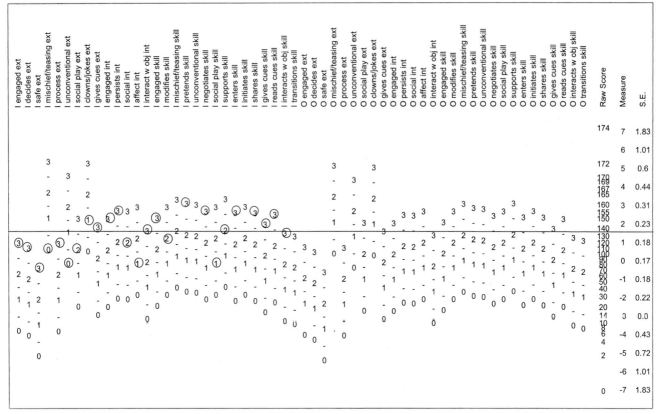

Figure 4-18
Derja's ToP Keyform.

and the social interaction and did not change the doll's clothes again.

Derja's social play score is relatively low not because of a lack of social skills, but rather because of her disability. The short clowning incident showed how skillful she was in getting the positive attention of others and encouraging other children to follow her lead.

Suspension of Reality

The placement of the marker on the continuum representing suspension of reality is toward the "not free" end. That is, aside from pretending and the short incident of clowning, the overall transaction appeared quite bound by objective reality. Derja's performance in this area seemed once again to be a reflection of her disability. In addition, one item relating to suspension of reality, the use of objects in variable or unconventional ways, never occurred, with all the toys being used in their prescribed ways.

Framing

Derja seemed very good at all the items related to framing. There were no obvious points at which she failed to interact with others in expected ways, and it would have been easy to know how to interact with her. Furthermore, the play session seemed quite cohesive.

Environmental Supportiveness

The TOES scores for Derja are shown in Figure 4-19. When the TOES is used to assess Derja's play environment, the first step is to determine what motivated her during the play observed. Of course, the observer can never be certain of the sources of a player's motivations, but a good place to start is often to consider what benefits a player might be seeking from the activities in which he or she is engaging. As suggested previously, and in addition to social interaction with her peers, it seems likely that the mastery and experience of playing house with the dolls were Derja's main sources of motivation.

In this play transaction the only relevant human environmental factor to consider is that relating to peer playmates. Although the period of interaction between Derja and her playmates was very short, their response to Derja's cues seemed to support the transaction. The playmates' play cues were quite clear and made it easy for Derja to enter the group and

TEST OF ENVIRONMENTAL SUPPORTIVENESS (TOES)–7/03

Child's Name: **Derja**	Apparent Source(s) of Motivation:
Date of Observation: **xx-2005**	**Social interaction with her peers, and the mastery and sensation of playing with dolls**
Child's Birth Date: **xxxx**	Location of Observation: **Kindergarten, Indoors**
Age at Observation: **4¹/₂**	Examiner: **G. Skard**

CONTINUA OF ITEMS

  2 = strongly favors description on right
  1 = slightly favors description on right
 −1 = slightly favors description on left
 −2 = strongly favors description on left
 NA = not applicable

			Comments
Peer playmate's response to player's cues interferes with transaction	−2 −1 1 **2** NA	Peer playmate's response to player's cues supports transaction	
Peer playmates do not give clear cues or give cues that interfere with the transaction	−2 −1 1 **2** NA	Peer playmates give clear cues that support the transaction	
Peer playmates are dominated by player or dominate players	−2 −1 1 **2** NA	Peer playmates participate as equals with player	
Natural/fabricated objects do not support activity of player	−2 −1 **1** 2 NA	Natural/fabricated objects support activity of player	
Amount and configuration of space do not support type of play	−2 **−1** 1 2 NA	Amount and configuration of space support activity of player	
Sensory environment does not offer adequate invitation to play	−2 −1 1 **2** NA	Sensory environment offers adequate invitation to play	
Space is not physically safe	−2 −1 1 **2** NA	Space is physically safe	
Space is not accessible	−2 **−1** 1 2 NA	Space is accessible	
Additional comments:			

Figure 4-19

TOES scoring sheet for Derja (only relevant items are shown).

take part in the transaction when she was able to do so. Another important feature is that all the players seemed to participate as equals.

With regard to the nonhuman environment, the objects seemed to support Derja's activity relatively well. Although the small details of Barbie dolls' clothes presented a significant problem for Derja, her motivation to play with these particular dolls helped her to rise to meet the challenge. Adjusting the difficulty by offering alternative dolls with fewer accessories but potentially less attraction would probably not have increased the supportiveness. Amount and configuration of space, by comparison, were not very supportive of Derja's participation. In the corner dedicated to playing with dolls there was not enough room for Derja to move her walker around without knocking things over. It would

probably have been better for Derja if there had been a table and chairs to play at instead of just the floor to sit on. Sitting at a table might also have made it easier for Derja to get up and follow her playmates when they left to do something else, supposing she had wanted to. At the same time, however, the sensory environment of the kindergarten offered adequate invitation to play and the space was certainly physically safe.

Summary

When viewed overall, Derja's profile describes a relatively playful child who was playing in a fairly supportive environment. She has a raw score of about 135 and a scaled score (measure) between 1 and 2 (Figure 4-18). Derja's score in reference to the whole sample can be seen by looking at Figure 4-10.

SUMMARY

In this chapter we have argued that assessing an individual's playfulness is very important. Playfulness can be assessed in the context of any activity (play or nonplay). The chances of seeing playfulness, however, may be greatest during free play. We have provided a model for the evaluation of playfulness and introduced an assessment based on that model. We have also introduced an assessment for the evaluation of environmental supportiveness of play. We have illustrated the use of the model and the assessments in two case studies.

Review Questions

1. What is meant by the phrase "operationalizing the elements of playfulness"?
2. Discuss the concept of framing and how it is operationalized in the Test of Playfulness (ToP).
3. What are the four dimensions measured by the ToP? Define each one, and describe the behaviors and behavioral qualities that each one addresses.
4. How can the ToP be used in clinical practice to generate a playfulness profile for a child? Sketch an example to show a colleague what a playfulness profile might look like.
5. Explain how to administer and score the ToP.
6. What is the TOES, and why was it developed?
7. Explain how to administer and score the TOES.

REFERENCES

Bailey, D. B., Jr., McWilliam, R. A., Ware, W. B., & Burchinal, M. A. (1993). Social interactions of toddlers and preschoolers in same- age and mixed age play groups. *Journal of Applied Developmental Psychology, 14,* 261-267.

Barker, R. G. (1968). *Ecological psychology: Concepts and methods for studying the environment of human behavior.* Stanford, CA: Stanford University.

Barnett, L. (1991). The playful child: Measurement of a disposition to play. *Play and Culture, 4,* 51-74.

Bateson, G. (1971). The message, "this is play." In R. E. Herron & B. Sutton-Smith (Eds.), *Child's play* (pp. 261-269). New York: John Wiley & Sons.

Bateson, G. (1972). Toward a theory of play and phantasy. In G. Bateson (Ed.), *Steps to an ecology of the mind* (pp. 14-20). New York: Bantam.

Berlyne, D. (1966). Notes on intrinsic motivation and intrinsic reward in relation to instruction. In J. Bruner (Ed.), *Learning about learning* (Cooperative Research Monograph No. 15). Washington, DC: U.S. Department of Health, Education, and Welfare, Office of Education.

Brentnall, J. (2005). *The effect of the length of observation on the test-retest reliability of the Test of Playfulness* (Unpublished honours thesis, University of Sydney, Sydney, Australia).

Bronson, M., & Bundy, A. C. (2001). A correlational study of the Test of Playfulness and the Test of Environmental Supportiveness. *Occupational Therapy Journal of Research, 21,* 223-240.

Bundy, A. C. (1991). Play theory and sensory integration. In A. G. Fisher, E. A. Murray, & A. C. Bundy (Eds.), *Sensory integration: Theory and practice* (pp. 48-68). Philadelphia: F.A. Davis.

Bundy, A. C. (1993). Assessment of play and leisure: Delineation of the problem. *American Journal of Occupational Therapy, 47,* 217-222.

Bundy, A. C. (1997). Play and playfulness: What to look for. In L. D. Parham & L. S. Fazio (Eds.), *Play in occupational therapy for children* (pp. 56-62). St. Louis: Mosby.

Bundy, A., Nelson, L., Metzger, M., & Bingaman, K. (2001). Validity and reliability of a test of playfulness. *Occupational Therapy Journal of Research, 21*(4), 276-292.

Caillois, R. (1979). *Man, play and games.* New York: Schocken.

Csikszentmihalyi, M. (1990). *Flow: The psychology of optimal experience.* New York: Harper Perennial.

Eccles, J. S., Midgley, C., Wigfield, A., Buchanan, C. M., Reuman, D., Flanagan, C., et al. (1993). Development during adolescence: The impact of stage-environment fit on young adolescents' experiences in schools and families. *American Psychologist, 48,* 90-101.

Gibson, J. J. (1979). *The ecological approach to visual perception.* Boston: Houghton Mifflin.

Griffith, L. R. (2000). *Hispanic American children and the Test of Playfulness* (Unpublished master's thesis, Colorado State University, Ft. Collins, CO).

Guitard, P., Ferland, F., & Dutil, E. (2005.) Toward a better understanding of playfulness in adults. *Occupational Therapy Journal of Research, 25,* 9-22.

Harding, P. S. (1997). *Validity and reliability of a Test of Environmental Supportiveness* (Master's thesis, Colorado State University, Ft. Collins, CO).

Harkness, L., & Bundy, A. C. (2001). Playfulness and children with physical disabilities. *Occupational Therapy Journal of Research, 21,* 73-89.

Healthy Toronto 2000 Subcommittee. (1988). *Healthy Toronto 2000.* Toronto, Ontario, Canada: Board of Health, City of Toronto.

Hess, L., & Bundy, A. C. (2003). The association between playfulness and coping in adolescents. *Physical and Occupational Therapy in Pediatrics. 23*(2), 5-17.

Holaday, B., Swan, J. H., & Turner-Henson, A. (1997). Images of the neighborhood and activity patterns of chronically ill school age children. *Environment and Behavior, 29,* 348-373.

Holland, J. L. (1966). *The psychology of vocational choice: A theory of personality types and model environments.* Waltham, MA: Blaisdell.

Jennings, K. D., & MacTurk, R. H. (1995). The motivational characteristics of infants and children with physical and sensory impairments. In R. H. MacTurk & G. A. Morgan (Eds.), *Mastery motivation: Origins, conceptualizations and applications* (pp. 201-219). Norwood, NJ: Ablex Publishing.

Jordan, S. A., Wellborn, W. R. III, Kovnick, J., & Saltzstein, R. (1991). Understanding and treating motivation difficulties in ventilator-dependent SCI patients. *Paraplegia, 29,* 431-442.

Kielhofner, G. W. (1995). *A model of human occupation: Theory and application* (2nd ed.). Baltimore: Williams & Wilkins.

Kooij, R. V. (1989). Research on children's play. *Play & Culture, 2*, 20-34.

Kooij, R. V., & Vrijhof, H. J. (1987). Play and development. *Topics in Learning Disabilities, 1*, 57-67.

Leipold, E., & Bundy, A. C. (2000). A comparison of playfulness of children with attention deficit hyperactive disorder and children with no known disorder. *Occupational Therapy Journal of Research, 20*, 61-82.

Letts, L., Lew, M., Rigby, P., Cooper, B., Stewart, D., & Strong, S. (1994). Person-environment assessments in occupational therapy. *American Journal of Occupational Therapy, 48*, 608-618.

Lewin, K. (1955). *Dynamic theory of personality*. New York: McGraw-Hill.

Lieberman, J. N. (1977). *Playfulness: Its relationship to imagination and creativity*. New York: Academic Press.

Magnussen, D. (1981). Wanted: A psychology of situations. In D. Magnussen (Ed.), *Toward a psychology of situations: An interactional perspective* (pp. 9-32). Hillsdale, NJ: Lawrence Erlbaum.

Meakins, C., Bundy, A. C., & Gliner, J. (2005). Reliability and validity of The Experience of Leisure Scale (TELS). In F. McMahon, D. E. Lytle, & B. Sutton-Smith (Eds.), *Play: An interdisciplinary synthesis* (pp. 255-267). Play & Culture Studies, Vol. 6. Lanham, MD: University Press of America.

Morrison, C. D., Bundy, A. C., & Fisher, A. G. (1991). The contribution of motor skills and playfulness to the play performance of preschoolers. *American Journal of Occupational Therapy, 45*, 687-694.

Muneto, P. K. (2002). *The development of additional items for the Test of Playfulness* (Unpublished master's thesis, Colorado State University, Ft. Collins, CO).

Neumann, E. A. (1971). *The elements of play*. New York: MSS Information.

Nichols, K. (1997). *Relationship between live and videotape scores on the Test of Playfulness* (Unpublished master's thesis, Colorado State University, Ft. Collins, CO).

O'Brien, J. C., & Shirley, R. J. (2001). Does playfulness change over time? A preliminary look using the Test of Playfulness. *Occupational Therapy Journal of Research, 21*, 132-139.

O'Connor, B. P., & Vallerand, R. J. (1994). Motivation, self-determination, and person-environment fit as predictors of psychological adjustment among nursing home residents. *Psychology and Aging, 9*, 189-194.

Pacheo, A. M., & Lucca-Irizarry, N. (1995). Relations between environmental psychology and allied fields: Research implications. *Environment and Behavior, 27*, 100-108.

Pervin, L. A. (1968). Performance and satisfaction as a function of individual-environment fit. *Psychological Bulletin, 69*, 56-68.

Phillips, H. A. (1998). *Guatemalan and Nicaraguan children and the Test of Playfulness* (Unpublished master's thesis, Colorado State University, Ft. Collins, CO).

Porter, C. A., & Bundy, A. C. (2000). Validity and reliability of three tests of playfulness with African American children and their parents. In S. Reifel (Ed.), *Play and culture studies (Vol. 3): Theory in context and out* (pp. 315-334). Westport, CT: Ablex Publishing.

Rowles, G. D. (1991). Beyond performance: Being in place as a component of occupational therapy. *American Journal of Occupational Therapy, 45*, 265-271.

Rubin, K., Fein, G. G., & Vandenberg, B. (1983). Play. In P. H. Mussen (Ed.), *Handbook of child psychology: Vol. 4, Socialization, personality and social development* (4th ed., pp. 693-774). New York: John Wiley & Sons.

Saunders, I., Sayer, M., & Goodale, A. (1999). The relationship between playfulness and coping in preschool children: A pilot study. *American Journal of Occupational Therapy, 53*, 221-226.

Scott, F. C. (2003). *The test-retest reliability of the Test of Playfulness* (Unpublished master's thesis, University of Toronto, Toronto, Ontario, Canada).

Smith, P. K., Takhvar, M., Gore, N., & Vollstedt, P. (1985). Play in young children: Problems of definition, categorization, and measurement. *Early Child Development and Care, 19*, 25-41.

Stern, D. N. (1985). *The interpersonal world of the infant: a view from psychoanalysis and developmental psychology*. New York: Basic Books.

Stern, G. G. (1970) *People in context: Measuring person-environment congruence in education and industry*. New York: John Wiley & Sons.

Tyler, R. G. (1996). *Influence of gender and environment on the Test of Playfulness* (master's thesis, Colorado State University, Ft. Collins, CO).

Vandenberg, B. (1981). Environmental and cognitive factors in social play. *Journal of Experimental Child Psychology, 31*, 169-175.

White, R. (1959). Motivation reconsidered: The concept of competence. *Psychological Review, 66*, 297-323.

Wicker, A. W. (1987). Behavior settings reconsidered: Temporal stages, resources, internal dynamics, context. In D. Stokols & I. Altman (Eds.), *Handbook of environmental psychology* (pp. 613-653). New York: John Wiley & Sons.

Wright, B. D., & Masters, G. N. (1982). *Rating scale analysis*. Chicago: MESA.

Wright, B. D., & Stone, M. H. (1979). *Best test design*. Chicago: MESA.

SUGGESTED READING

Bond, T. G., & Fox, C. M. (2001). *Applying the Rasch Model: Fundamental measurement in the human sciences*. Mahwah, NJ: Lawrence Erlbaum.

5

Assessment of Play and Leisure in Children and Adolescents

ALEXIS HENRY

KEY TERMS

observation-based assessments
self-report measures
Pediatric Interest Profiles

IMPORTANCE OF PLAY AND LEISURE

Along with work and self-care, play is considered to be a principal occupation of human beings across the lifespan (Neistadt & Crepeau, 1998). People of all ages play. Generally, play activities are those that are freely chosen, intrinsically motivated, and done for personal enjoyment or a sense of challenge. Play can promote a sense of physical and mental well-being. It affords the individual chances to learn, socialize, or be physically fit. Play allows a respite from more obligatory life activities such as school, work, and caregiving.

For children, play is a particularly important occupation. It provides essential opportunities for the development of sensorimotor, cognitive, and social-emotional capacities (Hinojosa & Kramer, 1997; Piaget, 1962). From earliest infancy, play is the medium through which children learn to move their bodies, solve problems, relate to others, and cope with their own feelings. Although engaging in play activities facilitates development across many areas, play is important for its own sake. As a truly child-directed activity, play is done for its intrinsic pleasure and enjoyment. Ask any child why he or she is playing and the answer is likely to be, "Because it's fun!"

Play has been described as the primary occupation of young children (Parham & Fazio, 1997; Reilly, 1969). Drawing a picture, building a block tower, playing house, playing hide-and-seek with friends, and riding a bike are only a few examples of the activities that encompass childhood play. It is through such experimental, manipulative, physical, interactive, and imitative play activities that young children learn about themselves and their

world. In a review of the research on the developmental benefits of play, Barnett (1990) suggested that empirical evidence supports play as a facilitator for the development of problem-solving skills, abstract reasoning skills, social-communication skills, and anxiety management skills. Participation in physical activities enhances the development of sensorimotor skills, physical fitness, and a healthy lifestyle (DeMarco & Sidney, 1989). Throughout childhood, play serves as an important vehicle for the development of skills needed for successful engagement in student, family, and social roles (Christiansen, 1991; Coleman & Iso-Ahola, 1993).

The benefits of play continue into adolescence. Research has shown that adolescents spend considerable time in play and leisure activities (Csikszentmihalyi & Larson, 1984; Fine, Mortimer, & Roberts, 1990). A study of typically developing, middle-class adolescents, conducted by Kleiber, Larson, and Csikszentmihalyi (1986), found that study participants spent 40% of their waking hours engaged in leisure activities, including socializing, playing sports, watching TV, and working on hobbies. Shared leisure interests can provide the foundation for the development of peer relationships in adolescence. Moreover, leisure activities often give adolescents their first opportunity to structure their own time and thus develop a sense of independence (Larson & Kleiber, 1993).

In a review of the role of schools in promoting adolescent health, Kane and Duryea (1991) maintained that physical education, fitness, and sports participation can have physiological, cognitive, emotional, social, and intrapersonal benefits for adolescents. Larson and Kleiber (1993) suggested that participation in leisure activities promotes self-direction, self-expression, and motivated involvement among adolescents. Because leisure activities are freely chosen, they provide an important opportunity for the development of self-identity. Moreover, typical adolescent leisure activities, such as socializing, playing an instrument, and participating in sports, can provide an "important transitional link between the spontaneous play of childhood and the more disciplined activities of adulthood" (Larson & Kleiber, 1993, p. 125).

Adolescents who are actively involved in leisure activities tend to report higher life satisfaction, a greater sense of competence, and more self-esteem than adolescents with low involvement in leisure activities (Brennan, 1985; Feldman & Gaier, 1980; Williams & McGee, 1991). Furthermore, adolescents who participate in positive leisure activities are less likely to engage in negative activities such as drug and alcohol abuse (Scafidi, Field, Prodromidis, & Rahdert, 1997; Vicary, Smith, Caldwell, & Swisher, 1998). Leisure activities also help individuals cope with stress by providing direct relief and by facilitating the development of friendships (Coleman & Iso-Ahola, 1993). For both children and adolescents, an understanding of a youngster's play or leisure provides insight into his or her current quality of life.

Undoubtedly, engagement in play and leisure has many varied benefits for children and adolescents. Because of beliefs about the benefits of play and the importance of play in its own right, many service providers—including occupational therapists, recreational therapists, early childhood educators, special educators, physical therapists, and school psychologists—use play-based interventions to promote development, teach skills, and help youngsters become more competent and satisfied players. A first step in the use of play-based interventions is to gain an understanding of the young person's involvement in play and leisure activities.

Assessing Play and Use of Leisure Time

Most scholars agree that play is a highly complex behavior that can be assessed from many vantage points (Barnett, 1990; Bundy, 1993; Parham & Fazio, 1997). Various strategies have been developed to assess play and leisure in children and adolescents. Measures of play and leisure may have clinical and research applications. Although the goal of research measures is to describe the phenomenon of interest as it is manifested in a particular group of individuals, the purpose of clinical measures is to identify potential problems or areas for intervention for a single individual. Many measures serve both purposes.

In general, information for assessments of childhood play has been obtained through evaluator observations of a child's play behavior or a parent interview. Behavioral observations are typically done while the child engages in a natural play setting (e.g., a playground). These observations may describe the types of play activities in which a child engages (e.g., construction play, imitation play), the manner in which the child engages in play (e.g., the child's level of spontaneity, joyfulness, overall playfulness), or the level of cognitive, social, or physical development the child exhibits during play (i.e., whether the child demonstrates age-appropriate skills). Examples of such

observation-based assessments include the Children's Playfulness Scale (Barnett, 1991), the Play Intensity Scale (Van der Kooij, 1989), the Playground Skills Test (Butcher, 1991), the Preschool Play Scale (Knox, 1997), and the Test of Playfulness (Bundy, 1997). The Preschool Play Scale and the Test of Playfulness are both clinical measures designed to help service providers identify play-related difficulties and plan play-based interventions.

In addition to observations of the child at play, parent interviews are often excellent sources of information about a young child's play involvement and experiences. Several parent interviews have been developed. The Play Activity Questionnaire is a parent interview regarding a child's play preferences (Finegan, Niccols, Zacher, & Hood, 1991). The Play History (Behnke & Fetkovich, 1984; Bryze, 1997; Takata, 1969) is a parent interview that examines a child's play experiences, environments, and behavior from a developmental and historical perspective.

Because play is such a complex behavior, it is unlikely that any single assessment method can fully describe a child's play. Although behavioral observations and parent interviews provide important information that contributes to an understanding of a child's involvement in play, they fail to include the *child's own perspective* regarding his or her play. When the goal of an assessment is to better understand the individual's perspective on the domain being assessed, a self-report approach can be very useful. However, few child self-report measures of play preferences or play perceptions have been developed. One exception is the Play Skills Self Report Questionnaire (PSSRQ) (Sturgess, 2007; Sturgess & Ziviani, 1995). Designed for use with 5- to 10-year-old children, the PSSRQ is a self-report measure of a child's perceptions of his or her play competencies across different types of play experiences (e.g., playing alone versus playing with others, or engaging in pretend versus creative versus sensorimotor play). A need exists for a self-report measure of a child's involvement in and preference for specific play activities.

Self-report measures, in the form of checklists and questionnaires, are the most common strategy for assessing play or leisure among adolescents. Such self-report measures may be used to assess the individual's level of interest in leisure activities, past or anticipated future involvement in leisure activities, or motivations for use of leisure time (Beard & Ragheb, 1983; Gregory, 1983; Matsutsuyu, 1969; McKechnie, 1975).

Unfortunately, because few adolescent-specific measures have been developed, measures developed for adults are used most often. Adult measures are clearly inappropriate, since they rarely include items of interest to adolescents (Chang et al., 1993). For example, the Interest Checklist (Matsutsuyu, 1969), one of the measures most commonly used by occupational therapists to assess leisure interests (Hemphill, 1980), includes such nonleisure items as dusting and ironing but does not include such common adolescent activities as talking on the phone or "hanging out" with friends. An exception is the Leisure Interest Checklist for Teenagers (LIC-T) (Rosenthal, Muram, Arheart, & Bryant, 1994). While the items of the LIC-T are appropriate for adolescents, the LIC-T can be used only to assess level of interest in leisure activities. It does not examine other aspects of activity involvement (e.g., frequency of participation or level of enjoyment).

Although multiple measures are available to assess play and use of leisure time among children and adolescents, and each can contribute to the understanding of a child's or adolescent's involvement in the occupation of play, age-appropriate measures that capture youngsters' perspectives on their play and leisure preferences, involvement, and enjoyment have been lacking. The Pediatric Interest Profiles were developed to fill this gap in the measures available for service providers and researchers.

PEDIATRIC INTEREST PROFILES

The Pediatric Interest Profiles (see the appendixes at the end of this chapter) are three age-appropriate profiles of play and leisure interests and participation that can be used both with children and adolescents who have disabilities and with those who do not. The decision about which profile to administer to any particular child should be based on the child's life experience, maturity, and disability, if any. The Kid Play Profile is designed for use with children from about ages 6 to 9 (Appendix 5-A), the Preteen Play Profile is appropriate for children from about ages 9 to 12 (Appendix 5-B), and the Adolescent Leisure Interest Profile can be used with adolescents from about ages 12 to 21 (Appendix 5-C).

Conceptual Foundation

The conceptual underpinnings of the Pediatric Interest Profiles are drawn from occupational behavior perspectives (Reilly, 1962), particularly the Model of Human Occupation (Kielhofner, 2002a). The Model of Human Occupation is an occupational therapy practice model that addresses people's "motivations for occupations, the routine patterning of occupational behavior, nature of skilled performance and the influence of the environment on occupation" (Kielhofner & Barrett, 1998, p. 527). The Model of Human Occupation has informed the development of the Pediatric Interest Profiles in two important ways. First, the Model of Human Occupation theorists have emphasized that play is a fundamental human occupation that engages individuals across the lifespan (Kielhofner, 2002b). While the content and form of play evolve as the individual develops and changes, the need for the occupation of play is always present. Second, in considering the self-knowledge and inner dispositions that motivate engagement in occupations (the so-called

volition subsystem), Model of Human Occupation theorists have emphasized the importance of understanding the individual's unique preferences (i.e., interests) for occupations and how these preferences influence the choices the individual makes for engaging in occupations on a daily basis (Kielhofner, 2002c).

In addition to the conceptual influences of the Model of Human Occupation, the development of the Pediatric Interest Profiles has been informed by the "top-down" approach to occupation-centered assessment of children advocated by Coster (1998). In describing an approach to the assessment process and the development of assessment instruments for occupational therapists, Coster contended that the first level at which children with dysfunction need to be assessed is social participation. The critical question is whether the child is fully participating in the occupations typically expected of, or available to, a child of this age and culture (Coster, 1998). Once the extent of the child's participation is determined, more discrete assessment may be needed to identify factors that are restricting participation. Coster also noted the importance of understanding the child's perspective regarding his or her participation and suggested that a self-assessment may be a useful strategy for gathering such information. A complete assessment of a child's or adolescent's participation in play or leisure requires the incorporation of a self-assessment approach because play and leisure are, by definition, determined by the individual.

An emphasis on participation is also consistent with current international models of enablement and disablement, such as the World Health Organization's (2001) International Classification of Functioning, Disability and Health (ICF). The ICF proposes that participation, which is defined as an individual's involvement in life situations (including participation in recreation and leisure), is influenced by the person's health condition, which may impose body level functional or structural impairments and activity limitations, as well as various environmental and personal factors. The Pediatric Interest Profiles are designed to help providers understand a child's or adolescent's participation in play and leisure.

Rationale for Development

The initial motivation for developing the Pediatric Interest Profiles stemmed from findings during my doctoral dissertation research. I conducted a short-term follow-up study of adolescents and young adults hospitalized for a first episode of psychosis. In that study I found variables derived from the Interest Checklist (Matsutsuyu, 1969) that reflected the participants' interest in leisure activities, particularly social-recreational activities, to be good predictors of the participants' functioning at 6 months after discharge (Henry, 1994). Although I had always believed that active involvement in social recreational activities was important, these findings were somewhat surprising. As a result, I became more interested in the role of leisure interests and involvement in the health and well-being of young persons, particularly those with psychiatric disorders. It was also clear that the existing measures were insufficient to adequately assess leisure interests and involvement in adolescents. A more appropriately age-targeted measure of leisure was needed for this age group.

The first efforts toward developing a new measure of leisure interests for adolescents were undertaken in collaboration with students in the research methods course of the occupational therapy program at Worcester State College in Massachusetts. These initial student projects focused on item development and reliability testing of a pilot version of the adolescent measure (Brophy et al., 1995; Hann, Regele, Walsh, Fontana, & Bentley, 1994). After further refinement, an additional reliability study of the Adolescent Leisure Interest Profile was undertaken (Henry, 1998b).

Discussions with pediatric occupational therapy colleagues led me to realize that a similar age-targeted measure was needed for younger children, since interest in play and leisure activities and the level of involvement in activities change as children mature (i.e., the play interests and involvement of a 6-year-old are not likely to be the same as the leisure interests and involvement of a 15-year-old). Again, in collaboration with occupational therapy students taking the research methods course at Worcester State College, studies were undertaken that focused on item development and pilot testing of preliminary versions of the child measures (Andrews et al., 1995; Beck et al., 1996; Budd et al., 1997). The results of these initial efforts are the Kid Play Profile and the Preteen Play Profile.

Need for Self-Report Measures

In recent years, service providers have come under increasing demand to develop collaborative models of service delivery in which the provider works in partnership with the client (child, parent, and other family members) to identify problems and possible solutions to the client's problems (Brown & Bowen, 1998; Hanft, 1988; Law et al., 1994). The emphasis on the collaborative nature of intervention requires that service providers understand the perspective of the persons with whom they work (Mattingly, 1991). Principally because play and leisure are determined by the player (Bundy, 1993), it is important that play and leisure be assessed from the player's viewpoint.

Paper-and-pencil self-report measures are an easy method for beginning the collaborative process because they provide a vehicle for further discussion and exploration of the domain being assessed. Thus a play and leisure profile can be a starting point from which a clinician and client collaboratively identify play-related problems and plan for play-related interventions.

In many service settings it may be difficult to observe a child or adolescent in a natural play environment (e.g., playground, home) or it may be too time consuming when the service provider needs to assess many domains in a brief time. A self-report measure provides a quick way to gather information. Moreover, information provided directly by a child or adolescent is unique and cannot be obtained with other methods. Parent reports cannot replace child reports, especially when the goal is to obtain information about the child's feelings (Flanery, 1990). A metaanalytical study by Achenbach and colleagues (1987) found low correlations between data provided by parent informants and the child's own report. A self-report tool allows for a direct measure of the child's or adolescent's perceptions.

Considerations in Development of Self-Report Measures for Young Children

Is a paper-and-pencil self-report measure an appropriate tool to use with young children? Can a young child respond appropriately and reliably to paper and-pencil self-report measures? Several researchers have successfully developed self-report measures for young children. For example, the Pictorial Scale of Perceived Competence for Young Children (Harter, 1990; Harter & Pike, 1984) is a measure of perceived competence that has been shown to be reliable with 4- to 7-year-old children.

In the development of measures for young children, consideration should be given to basic intellectual capacities (i.e., comprehension and information processing) and social-cognitive processes involving perceptions of the self and others that are typical for the targeted age group. It is important to ensure that the task of taking the test is within the child's capabilities (Flanery, 1990). The wording of questions must be age appropriate, the questions and stimuli must be meaningful to the child, and the complexities of the test must match the child's abilities (Flanery, 1990). Harter (1990) and Royeen (1985) have recommended that stimuli in child self-report measures be concrete and, preferably, behaviorally represented. Pictorial representations of stimuli have been used successfully in child measures.

As children change over time, the phenomenon of interest (in this case, play and leisure interests) also undergoes developmental transition. These issues have been taken into consideration in the development of the content and format for each of the Pediatric Interest Profiles.

Purpose of the Pediatric Interest Profiles

The Pediatric Interest Profiles are intended to provide a quick and easy method of gathering information about play interests directly from the child or adolescent. The activity items, the questions about the activities, and the response formats of each version of the Pediatric Interest Profiles have been designed to be appropriate for and easily understood by children within the targeted age range. Each version lists or depicts via drawings a variety of play and leisure activities and asks the child or adolescent to respond to multiple questions about the activities. The questions address the child's participation in the activities, feelings of enjoyment and competence in the activities, and whether the activities are done alone or with others.

Service providers can use the information gathered with the Pediatric Interest Profiles to identify children or adolescents who may be at risk for play-related problems. The Pediatric Interest Profiles can also be used to identify specific play activities of interest to an individual child or adolescent so that those activities can be used to engage the child in therapeutic or educational interventions.

Self-report instruments such as the Pediatric Interest Profiles are often most valuable when they are used to facilitate a conversation between the provider and the child. The Pediatric Interest Profiles can provide a means to engage the child or adolescent in a more detailed interview about his or her play experiences. Children, in particular, seem to enjoy telling stories about their play. Such interviews can enhance rapport between the child and provider and can give a more detailed picture of any play-related problems the child has. Both providers and researchers can use the Pediatric Interest Profiles to better understand child and adolescent involvement in play and leisure.

Using a paper-and-pencil checklist format, the child or adolescent answers questions about his or her interest or participation in a variety of different play and leisure activities. The format and the specific activity items vary across the three profiles that make up the Pediatric Interest Profiles, so that each is appropriate for the intended age group. Each profile asks the respondent multiple questions about the play or leisure activities.

In the Kid Play Profile the child answers up to three questions about each of 50 activity items. For each activity item, the child is asked, "Do you do this activity?" If the answer is yes, the child is also asked, "Do you like this activity?" and "Who do you do this activity with?" The child answers the questions by circling or coloring in a response. Simple stick-figure drawings and words are used to depict each activity. In addition, simple drawings and words are used to represent each possible response. The Kid Play Profile activity items are grouped into eight categories: sports activities, outside activities, summer activities, winter activities, indoor activities, creative activities, lessons and classes, and socializing.

In the Preteen Play Profile the child answers up to five questions about each of 59 activity items. For each activity item, the child is asked, "Do you do this activity?" If the answer is yes, the child is also asked, "How often do you do this activity?", "How much do you like this activity?", "How good are you at this activity?", and "Who do you do this activity with?" The child answers the questions by circling a response. As with the Kid Play Profile,

stick figure drawings are used to depict each activity. The Preteen Play Profile activity items are grouped into eight categories: sports activities, outside activities, summer activities, winter activities, indoor activities, creative activities, lessons and classes, and socializing.

In the Adolescent Leisure Interest Profile the adolescent answers up to five questions about each of 83 activity items. For each activity item the adolescent is asked, "How interested are you in this activity?" and "How often do you do this activity?" If the adolescent does the activity, he or she also is asked, "How well do you do this activity?", "How much do you enjoy this activity?", and "Who do you do this activity with?" The adolescent is instructed to place a checkmark beside one of the responses to each question. No drawings are used in the adolescent profile. The Adolescent Leisure Interest Profile activity items are grouped into eight categories: sports activities, outside activities, exercise activities, relaxation activities, intellectual activities, creative activities, socializing, and club and community organizations.

User Qualifications

The Pediatric Interest Profiles can be used by all service providers, including occupational therapists, recreational therapists, physical therapists, social workers, educators, child life workers, and school psychologists, who are concerned with the play and leisure experiences of children and adolescents.

Administration and Scoring

Before administering the Pediatric Interest Profiles, the service provider should take time to become familiar with the material in this chapter and with each of the three profiles. Familiarity with normal child and adolescent development, particularly cognitive and social development, is also needed. The following administration and scoring procedures will help in gathering information about children's and adolescents' play interests.

Determination of Which Profile to Administer

Although the format and activity items in each profile are appropriate for a specific age range, the age ranges on the three profiles do overlap. The decision about which profile to administer to any particular child should be based on the child's life experience, maturity, and disability, if any. Providers should use their best judgment in determining whether the activity items are appropriate for the child and whether the child understands and can respond to the questions being asked on the profile. For example, the Kid Play Profile might be the appropriate choice for an immature 9-year-old child with a cognitive disability, but the Preteen Play Profile might be a better choice for a mature, typically developing 9-year-old child. Generally, only one version of the Pediatric Interest Profiles should be administered to a child. Table 5-1 provides a quick overview of each profile.

Administration of the Pediatric Interest Profiles
Kid Play Profile

The Kid Play Profile is designed for young school-aged children. It is composed of pictures and simple words that represent 50 play and leisure activities. The format of the Kid Play Profile and the activity items make it appropriate for children from about ages 6 to 9, or children in first to third grades. A combination of pictures and simple words is used so that children who are just beginning to read can complete the Kid Play Profile. The activities are those commonly done by school-aged children. Some 5-year-old children who are not yet reading may be able to complete the Kid Play Profile if they understand the purpose of the profile and are given assistance with reading. The Kid Play Profile is probably not appropriate for children younger than 5.

The Kid Play Profile can be administered either individually or with groups of three to five children. Written instructions for completing the profile are provided on its cover sheet. The instructions can be read to children who are unable to read. In addition, the person administering the Kid Play Profile should ensure that the child understands the words or the pictures that represent the activities and the available responses to each question regarding the activities. Several colored markers or pencils should be available when the Kid Play Profile is administered. Although some children circle their responses, others prefer to color in the pictures representing their responses.

When completing the Kid Play Profile, the child first answers question 1 (Do You Do This Activity?). If the child does the activity, he or she then answers question 2 (Do You Like This Activity?) and question 3 (Who Do You Do This Activity With?). If the child does not do the activity, questions 2 and 3 are not answered. In answering question 2, the child should circle or color only one response. If

Table 5-1
Overview of Pediatric Interest

Profile	Categories	Questions
Kid Play Profile		
6 to 9 Years	Sports Activities	Do You Do This Activity?
15 Minutes for Child to Complete 50 Activities	Outdoor Activities	Do You Like This Activity?
	Summer Activities	Who Do You Do This Activity With?
	Winter Activities	
	Indoor Activities	
	Creative Activities	
	Lessons And Classes	
	Socializing Activities	
Preteen Play Profile		
9 to 12 Years	Sports Activities	Do You Do This Activity?
20 Minutes for Child to Complete 59 Activities	Outdoor Activities	How Often Do You Do This Activity?
	Summer Activities	How Much Do You Like This Activity?
	Winter Activities	How Good Are You At This Activity?
	Indoor Activities	Who Do You Do This Activity With?
	Creative Activities	
	Lessons and Classes	
	Socializing Activities	
Adolescent Leisure Interest Profile		
12 to 21 Years	Sports Activities	How Interested Are You In This Activity?
30 Minutes for Adolescent to Complete 83 Activities	Outdoor Activities	How Often Do You Do This Activity?
	Exercise Activities	How Well Do You Do This Activity?
	Relaxation Activities	How Much Do You Enjoy This Activity?
	Intellectual Activities	Who Do You Do This Activity With?
	Creative Activities	
	Socializing Activities	
	Club/Community Activities	

unsure how to answer, the child can be encouraged to circle how he or she feels "most of the time." In answering question 3, the child may circle more than one response, indicating, for example, that he or she does the activity both "With Friends" and "With a Grown-Up." At the end of the profile are five blank spaces for the child to add "other" activities if he or she desires. The child may be given reading or physical assistance to complete the Kid Play Profile; however, the responses must be the child's own. Assuring the child that there are no right or wrong answers will encourage honesty. Children without disabilities should be able to complete the Kid Play Profile in approximately 15 minutes.

Preteen Play Profile

The Preteen Play Profile is designed for older children, generally between the ages of 9 and 12, or children in fourth to sixth grades. The Preteen Play Profile uses pictures to represent 59 play and leisure activities that are commonly done by children of this age. The child circles his or her responses to the questions asked about each activity. The administration of the Preteen Play Profile is virtually the same as that of the Kid Play Profile.

The Preteen Play Profile can be administered either individually or with small groups (three to five children). Written instructions for completing the Preteen Play Profile are provided on its cover sheet. The instructions can be read to children who are unable to read. It is important to ensure that the child understands either the words or pictures that represent the activities, as well as the responses to each question asked regarding the activities.

When completing the Preteen Play Profile, the child first answers question 1 (Do You Do This Activity?). If the response is "yes," the child then answers questions 2 through 5. If the response to question 1 is "no," questions 2 through 5 are not answered. In answering questions 2 through 4, the child should circle only one response. If unsure how to answer, the child should be encouraged to circle how he or she feels "most of the time." The child may circle more than one response to question 5 (Who Do You Do This Activity With?). Again, there are five blank spaces at the end of the profile so that the child can add "other" activities he or she does. As with the Kid Play Profile, assistance with reading or physical assistance may be given, but the person administering the profile should make sure that the responses are the child's own. Assuring the child that there are no right or wrong answers encourages honesty. Children without disabilities should be able to complete the Preteen Play Profile in approximately 20 minutes.

Adolescent Leisure Interest Profile

The Adolescent Leisure Interest Profile is designed to be used with adolescents aged 12 to 21. It consists of 83 leisure activities in which adolescents commonly engage. The Adolescent Leisure Interest Profile can be administered either individually or in groups of three to five adolescents. When administering the Adolescent Leisure Interest Profile, the service provider should ensure that the young person understands how to complete the profile. The adolescent should answer the first two questions for every activity item. The next three questions should be answered only if he or she does the activity. If the adolescent does not do the activity, those columns should be left blank. The adolescent can add "other" activities in the five blank spaces at the end of the profile.

The young person completing the Adolescent Leisure Interest Profile should be encouraged to be honest and assured that there are no right or wrong answers. If the Adolescent Leisure Interest Profile is administered in a group, group members should not be permitted to share responses or ask one another how to respond. Physical or reading assistance can be given, if needed, but the adolescent should not be coached on how to respond. If he or she asks for the service provider's opinion on how to respond, a neutral answer such as "Just say how you feel" is appropriate. The Adolescent Leisure Interest Profile can be administered in more that one session, if necessary, but the sessions should take place within a day or two of each other. Adolescents without disabilities can generally complete the Adolescent Leisure Interest Profile in approximately 30 minutes.

Review of the Pediatric Interest Profiles

The first thing to do after administering one of the Pediatric Interest Profiles is to review the profile with the child or adolescent. The profile administrator should note any patterns in the child's responses, such as the following:

- What individual activities or types of activities does the child seem to like best?
- Does the child seem to have a variety of interests?
- Does the child have at least some activities that he or she does with others?
- Does the child seem to be interested only in passive activities such as watching TV?
- Does the child enjoy the activities he or she does?
- Does the child feel competent in doing activities?

The review provides an opportunity to ask the child or adolescent to tell more about his or her participation in play and leisure. Using the Pediatric Interest Profiles to conduct a play-related interview is discussed further on pp. 105 to 106.

Scoring of the Pediatric Interest Profiles and Use of Summary Score Sheets

Methods for scoring each of the Pediatric Interest Profiles, with numerical values assigned to the child's or adolescent's responses, are described here. Service providers who wish to report findings from the Pediatric Interest Profiles in a child's or adolescent's clinic, school, or hospital record may elect to use the Summary Score Sheets that accompany each of the profiles for documentation purposes. The

Summary Score Sheets are provided on pp. 149 to 154, 171 to 177, and 184 to 193. The Summary Score Sheets are designed so that a provider can do the following:

- Summarize a child's or adolescent's scores on one of the versions of the Pediatric Interest Profile
- Summarize information from a play-related interview conducted after the profile is administered (see p. 105)
- Record play observations
- Make recommendations for interventions

If there is no need to document findings from the Pediatric Interest Profiles, the provider may elect not to score the profile or use the Summary Score Sheet. In such cases, reviewing the profile with the child or adolescent in the manner described above and on p. 105 will probably be sufficient.

The scoring method described in the following paragraphs will also be useful to those who wish to use the Pediatric Interest Profiles as a research tool. These scoring methods are parallel to the ones used in the reliability studies of the Pediatric Interest Profiles (discussed on p. 114).

Scoring of the Kid Play Profile

Directions for scoring the Kid Play Profile are also included in its accompanying Summary Score Sheet (Appendix 5-A). Scores can be assigned to the child's responses in the following manner (Figure 5-1):

Question 1. Do You Do This Activity? Yes = 1, No = 0

Question 2. Do You Like This Activity? A lot = 3, A little = 2, Not at all = 1

Question 3. Who Do You Do This Activity With? By myself = 1, With friends = 1, With a grown-up = 1

For questions 1 and 2, mean scores for each category (e.g., sports, indoor activities, summer activities) can be calculated. A category score for question 1 is calculated by adding the number of "yes" responses to the question Do You Do This Activity?, then dividing the sum by the number of activities within that category. The result is multiplied by 100 to calculate the percentage of activities in which the child participates. A total percentage for question 1 can be calculated by summing the total number of activities the child does, dividing this sum by 50, and then multiplying by 100 (any "other" activities are excluded).

In the case of question 1, a higher score indicates that the child does a greater percentage of the activities within the category.

For question 2, the scorer should sum the child's responses for the activities that he or she does (3 = a lot, 2 = a little, 1 = not at all) in the category. The sum is then divided by the total number of activities that the child does within that category (the sum of question 1). The category score is intended to reflect how much the child enjoys the activities of that particular type that he or she actually does. In the case of question 2, the nearer the score is to 3, the more the child enjoys the activities within the category.

A total score for question 2 is calculated by summing the scores for the 8 categories and dividing by 8 (any "other" activities are excluded). As with the category

Indoor Activities	Yes	A lot	A little	Not at all	By myself	With friends	With a grown-up
25. Play cards		3	2	1			
26. Play board games	✔	3 ✔	2	1		✔	✔
27. Read	✔	3	2 ✔	1	✔		
28. Use computer	✔	3 ✔	2	1	✔		
29. Watch TV	✔	3 ✔	2	1	✔		
30. Listen to music		3	2	1			
31. Collect things	✔	3	2 ✔	1	✔		
32. Take care of pet		3	2	1			
Total	5	9	4	0	4	1	1

Number of indoor activities child participates in ___5___

Percent of indoor activities child participates in ___63%___

How much the child likes indoor activities ___2.6___

Percent of activities the child does
By myself ___80%___
With friends ___20%___
With a grown-up ___20%___

Play interview

Figure 5-1
Category scores calculated for the indoor activities category of the Kid Play Profile.

scores for question 2, the nearer the score is to 3, the more the child enjoys all of the activities that he or she does.

For question 3, the most useful summary score to calculate is the percentage of the total activities that a child does alone, with friends, or with an adult. These percentages are calculated by summing the *By Myself* responses, summing the *With Friends* responses, summing the *With a Grown-Up* responses, and dividing each total by the number of activities the child does. Multiplying the decimal by 100 gives the percentage. Because children may give more than one answer for this question (e.g., a child may do an activity both *By Myself* and *With Friends),* the total for the three responses may exceed 100%.

For question 3, the total percentage of activities done *By Myself, With Friends,* and *With a Grown-Up* is calculated by summing the percentage across the 8 activity categories and dividing by 8.

For both category and total scores on the Kid Play Profile, higher scores mean that the child:
- Does more of the activities (question 1)
- Enjoys the activities more (question 2, scores range from 1 to 3)
- Does more of the activities alone, with friends, or with an adult (question 3, scores range from zero to 100% for each of the three responses)

Scoring of the Preteen Play Profile

The scoring of the Preteen Play Profile is similar to the scoring of the Kid Play Profile. Again, directions for scoring the Preteen Play Profile are included in its accompanying Summary Score Sheet (Appendix 5-B). Scores can be assigned to the child's responses in the following manner (Figure 5-2):

Question 1. Do You Do This Activity? Yes = 1, No = 0
Question 2. How Often Do You Do This Activity? Once a week or more = 3, Once a month or more = 2, Once a year or more = 1
Question 3. How Much Do You Like This Activity? A lot = 3, A little = 2, Not at all = 1
Question 4. How Good Are You At This Activity? Very good = 3, So-so = 2, Not so good = 1
Question 5. Who Do You Do This Activity With? By myself = 1, With friends = 1, With a grown-up = 1

As with the Kid Play Profile, mean scores can be calculated for the activity categories and for the total scores for these questions. A category score for question 1 is calculated by summing the child's "yes" responses to the question Do You Do This Activity? Then the sum is divided by the number of activities within that category, and the result is multiplied by 100 to calculate the percentage of activities in which the child participates.

In the case of question 1, a higher score indicates that the child does more of the activities within the category. A total percentage for question 1 is calculated by adding the total number of activities the child does, dividing by 59, and then multiplying by 100 (any "other" activities are excluded).

For questions 2 through 4, in each category the child's responses for the activities the child does in that category are added up. Each sum is divided by the total number of activities the child does within that category (the sum

Sports Activities	Yes	Once a week or more	Once a month or more	Once a year or more	A lot	A little	Not at all	Very good	So-so	Not so good	By myself	With friends	With a grown-up
1. Play baseball or softball	✔	3	2	1 ✔	3	2 ✔	1	3	2 ✔	1		✔	
2. Play basketball	✔	3	2	1 ✔	3	2 ✔	1	3	2 ✔	1		✔	
3. Play soccer	✔	3 ✔	2	1	3 ✔	2	1	3 ✔	2	1		✔	
4. Play football	✔	3	2	1 ✔	3	2 ✔	1	3	2	1 ✔		✔	
5. Play ice or field hockey		3	2	1	3	2	1	3	2	1			
Total	*4*	*3*	*0*	*3*	*3*	*6*	*0*	*3*	*4*	*1*	*0*	*4*	*0*

Number of sports activities child participates in _*4*_ Percent of sports activities child participates in _*80%*_	How often the child does sports activities _*1.5*_	How much the child likes sports activities _*2.25*_	How good the child perceives him- or herself to be at the activities _*2*_	Percent of activities the child does By myself _*0*_ With friends _*100%*_ With a grown-up _*0*_

Play interview

Figure 5-2

Category scores calculated for the indoor activities category of the Preteen Play Profile.

of question 1). A total score for questions 2 through 4 is calculated by summing the scores of the 8 categories and dividing by 8 (excluding any "other" activities). It should be remembered that total scores for questions 2 through 4 are calculated using only the number of activities that the child does across all the activity categories.

For question 5, the most useful summary score to calculate is the percentage of the total activities that a child does alone, with friends, or with an adult. These percentages are calculated by summing the *By Myself* responses, summing the *With Friends* responses, summing the *With a Grown-Up* responses, and dividing each total by the number of activities the child does. The decimal is multiplied by 100 to achieve the percentage. As with the Kid Play Profile, because children may give more than one answer for this question, the total for the three responses may exceed 100%.

For question 5, the total percentage of activities done *By Myself, With Friends,* and *With a Grown-Up* is calculated by summing the percentage across the 8 activity categories and dividing by 8 ("other" activities are excluded).

For both category and total scores on the Preteen Play Profile, higher scores mean that the child:
* Does more of the activities (question 1)
* Does the activities more often (question 2, scores range from 1 to 3)
* Enjoys the activities more (question 3, scores range from 1 to 3)
* Feels that he or she does the activities well (question 4, scores range from 1 to 3)
* Does more of the activities alone, with friends, or with an adult (question 5, scores range from zero to 100% for each of the three responses)

Scoring of the Adolescent Leisure Interest Profile

As with the other profiles, directions for scoring the Adolescent Leisure Interest Profile are included in its accompanying Summary Score Sheet (Appendix 5-C). Scores can be assigned to the adolescent's responses in the following manner (Figure 5-3):

Question 1. How Interested Are You in This Activity?
Very = 3, Somewhat = 2, Not at all = 1

Exercise Activities	How interested are you in this activity?			How often do you do this activity?						How well do you do this activity?			How much do you enjoy this activity?			Who do you do this activity with?		
	Very	Some-what	Not at all	3 to 7 times a week	Less than 3 times a week	Once or twice a month	Less than once a month	Never		Very well	Well	Not very well	Very much	Some-what	Not at all	By myself	With friends	With family
20. Bicycling	3✔	2	1	5	4✔	3	2	1		3✔	2	1	3✔	2	1		✔	
21. Skating/ skateboarding	3	2✔	1	5	4	3	2✔	1		3	2✔	1	3✔	2	1		✔	✔
22. Swimming	3	2	1✔	5	4	3	2✔	1		3	2✔	1	3	2	1✔		✔	✔
23. Jogging	3	2✔	1	5✔	4	3	2	1		3✔	2	1	3✔	2	1	✔		
24. Tennis	3	2	1✔	5	4	3	2	1✔		3	2	1	3	2	1			
25. Aerobics	3	2✔	1	5	4	3	2✔	1		3✔	2	1	3	2✔	1	✔		
26. Gymnastics	3	2	1✔	5	4	3	2	1✔		3	2	1	3	2	1			
27. Martial arts	3	2	1✔	5	4	3	2	1✔		3	2	1	3	2	1			
28. Power walking	3	2✔	1	5	4	3	2✔	1		3	2✔	1	3	2✔	1	✔	✔	
29. Weight lifting	3✔	2	1	5	4✔	3	2	1		3	2✔	1	3✔	2	1	✔		
Total	6	8	4	5	8	0	8	3		9	8	0	12	4	1	4	4	2
	How interested the adolescent is in exercise activities *1.8*			How often the adolescent participates in exercise activities *2.4*						How good the adolescent perceives him- or herself to be at exercise activities *2.43*			How much the adolescent enjoys exercise activities *2.43*			Percent of exercise activities the adolescent does By myself *57%* With friends *57%* With family *29%*		
Leisure interview																		

Figure 5-3

Category scores calculated for the exercise activities category of the Adolescent Leisure Interest Profile.

Question 2. How Often Do You Do This Activity? 3 to 7 times a week = 5, Less than 3 times a week = 4, 1 to 2 times a month = 3, Less than 1 time a month = 2, Never = 1

Question 3. How Well Do You Do This Activity? Very well = 3, Well = 2, Not very well = 1

Question 4. How Much Do You Enjoy This Activity? Very much = 3, Somewhat = 2, Not at all = 1

Question 5. Who Do You Do This Activity With? By myself = 1, With friends = 1, With family = 1

A mean score can be calculated for each activity category and for the total score for each question. Category scores for question 1 (How Interested Are You in This Activity?) are calculated by summing the responses within an activity category (e.g., exercise activities) and then dividing by the total number of activities within that category. Category scores for question 2 are calculated in the same manner. Total scores for questions 1 and 2 are calculated by summing the totals of the 8 categories on the Adolescent Leisure Interest Profile and then dividing by 8 (any "other" activities are excluded). Category and total scores for questions 3 and 4 are calculated using only the items where the adolescent has indicated participation in the activity. The category scores for questions 3 and 4 reflect how the adolescent feels about the activities he or she actually does. For each activity category the number of items used in the calculation is the number of activities the adolescent does within the category. This number will vary for each adolescent.

In a similar manner, separate total scores for questions 3 and 4 are calculated by summing the scores for the 8 categories on the Adolescent Leisure Interest Profile and then dividing by 8 (excluding any "other" activities).

For question 5, the most useful summary score to calculate is the percentage of the total activities that the adolescent does alone, with friends, or with family members. These percentages are calculated by summing the *By Myself* responses, summing the *With Friends* responses, summing the *With Family* responses, and dividing each total by the number of activities the adolescent does. The decimal is multiplied by 100 to achieve the percentage. As with the other two profiles, because adolescents may give more than one answer for this question, the total for the three responses may exceed 100%.

For question 5, the total percentage of activities done *By Myself, With Friends,* and *With Family* is calculated by summing the percentage across the 8 activity categories and dividing by 8 (excluding any "other" activities).

For both category scores and total scores, higher scores mean the adolescent:
- Is more interested in the activities (question 1, scores range from 1 to 3)
- Does the activities more often (question 2, scores range from 1 to 5)
- Feels that he or she does the activities well (question 3, scores range from 1 to 3)
- Enjoys the activities (question 4, scores range from 1 to 3)
- Does more of the activities alone, with friends, or with a family member (question 5, scores range from zero to 100% for each of the three responses)

Interpretation and Use of Results of the Pediatric Interest Profiles in Practice

Once the appropriate version of the Pediatric Interest Profiles has been administered to a child or adolescent, how can the provider make the best use of the information gathered? Although there might be several approaches to using the information from the Pediatric Interest Profiles, this chapter focuses on three specific ways:
- To conduct a play interview (i.e., engage the child or adolescent in a more detailed discussion about his or her play or leisure participation)
- To identify children or adolescents who may be at risk for play-related problems
- To set play-related goals and identify play or leisure activities to use in intervention

Use of the Pediatric Interest Profiles as a Basis for a Play Interview

Self-report measures such as the Pediatric Interest Profiles are probably most useful when they serve as a starting point for a conversation. After the child or adolescent has completed one of the Pediatric Interest Profiles, he or she can review the profile with the provider. The child's or adolescent's responses to the Pediatric Interest Profile can help focus and guide the discussion. Because play and leisure are so individually determined, the goal of the discussion is to achieve a better understanding of the meaning of the child's or adolescent's responses. In reviewing an individual child's or adolescent's profile, the provider will, of course, be looking for patterns in the responses. Does Shawna seem to prefer specific types of activities to others? How often does Matthew seem to do the things he enjoys? Does Jose feel that he does activities well or not? How much does Andrea tend to do activities with others versus alone? It is important, too, to understand the child's or adolescent's perception of his or her play and leisure. How does Kelly feel about her participation in play? Is it a source of pleasure, satisfaction, and self-esteem for her? How does her participation in play affect her relationships with peers and family members?

A discussion with the child or adolescent might begin by focusing on an activity the child does often or really enjoys, for example, "Robin, I see that you really like ice-skating. Tell me more about that. What is it about ice-skating that you really like? How did you get interested in it? Who do you like to go skating with?" Questions such as these encourage a child to tell a more detailed story than would be obtained with the Pediatric Interest Profiles alone.

Because play participation intersects with so many other areas of life, a play-related interview will help to provide insights into how the child makes friends, engages with peers, perceives himself or herself, relates to family members, and so on. Many clinicians have recommended this storytelling or narrative approach to interviewing as an effective means of understanding the client's perspective (Henry, 1998a; Kielhofner & Mallinson, 1995; Mattingly, 1991).

The following questions can be used to interview a child or adolescent about his or her participation in play or leisure activities. Although the intention is not to provide a complete structured play interview, these questions may help in planning the approach to such an interview.

What are your favorite activities?

Why are these your favorites?

What do you really like about _____?

How did you get interested in _____?

What things do you do particularly well?

What are you most proud of?

Tell me about something you can do that is a real challenge for you.

What things would you like to do better?

What are your favorite activities to do with friends? With family? By yourself?

What do you spend the most time doing?

Is this how you would like to spend your time?

Tell me about a time when you really had fun.

How good are you at _____ in comparison to classmates/friends/peers?

Are there things you would like to do but don't or can't?

What do you think makes it hard for you to do _____ _____?

What most gets in the way?

What would help you do better?

What would help you do _____ better?

Clearly, not all of the preceding questions are appropriate for younger children. To describe their feelings and experiences, young children need to acquire the requisite cognitive and linguistic capacities. Before the age of 7 or 8, children tend to describe themselves in terms of observable characteristics and behavior (Stone & Lemanek, 1990). Thus in interviews with younger children questions should be direct, focus on behavior, and involve simple vocabulary and short sentences (Cohn, 1994). As children mature, their capacity for self-reflection increases. By adolescence, children have generally developed a greater sense of self-awareness and are capable of more sophisticated responses in an interview situation (Stone & Lemanek, 1990).

Use of Other Sources of Information

In addition to interviews with the child or adolescent, discussion with the child's parents and teachers and direct observation of the child in play situations will enhance understanding of the child's play and leisure participation. If the child's play and leisure participation is clearly hampered in some way, a more discrete assessment will probably be needed to identify the factors interfering with his or her participation. The "top-down" approach advocated by Coster (1998) suggests that assessment should proceed by an identification of the critical tasks the child must accomplish to participate and the specific aspects of task performance that most limit the child's participation. For example, a child may not be participating successfully in playground activities at recess. Further assessment may reveal that the child is not able to engage in a critical task (e.g., playing kickball) because of gross motor coordination problems (e.g., he can't run and kick the ball simultaneously) (Coster, 1998). These more discrete assessments may be accomplished with such tools as the School Function Assessment (Coster, Deeney, Haltiwanger, & Haley, 1998), the Sensory Integration and Praxis Tests (Ayres, 1989), or the Bruininks-Osteretsky Test of Motor Proficiency (Bruininks, 1978).

Other factors in addition to the child's or adolescent's characteristics influence his or her participation in play or leisure. Among these factors are parental interests and expectations for the child, peer influences, family financial resources, and availability of opportunities in the child's community. Considering the child in the context of his or her family, culture, peer group, and community can enhance understanding of the child's play and leisure participation.

Use of the Pediatric Interest Profiles to Identify Children or Adolescents with Play-Related Problems

The research done thus far with the Pediatric Interest Profiles, as well as other research on play and leisure, has not provided clear data to indicate that a specific "pattern" of play and leisure participation can identify a child or adolescent with a problem. Exceptions, of course, are children or adolescents who engage in antisocial, self-destructive, or highly risky activities (Raphael, 1996). It is probably best to take a commonsense approach when thinking about how the Pediatric Interest Profiles can help identify children at risk for play-related problems. One of the following patterns on the Pediatric Interest Profiles might be considered a "red flag" that would call for further assessment. The child or adolescent:

- Has very few interests
- Has play interests that vary significantly from typical interests of peers
- Experiences little enjoyment in play activities
- Feels little sense of competence in play activities
- Tends to engage only in solitary activities

None of the activity items on the Pediatric Interest Profiles are generally considered risky, deviant, or harmful. Certainly many adolescents, and even some younger children, do engage in risky or deviant behaviors. These may include sexual activity, smoking, alcohol and drug use or abuse, truancy, fighting, theft, and gang activity, just to name a few. Although the Pediatric Interest Profiles do not include any of these activities, the provider can, and probably should, ask about such activities during an interview, especially if the child or adolescent is known or suspected to have engaged in risky or harmful behaviors.

To explore harmful activities and behaviors with an adolescent or younger child, the interviewer might begin by asking such questions as:

Are there other activities that you do that we haven't talked about?

Are there things you do that your parents don't know about?

Do you do things that could get you into trouble?

Research Conducted with the Pediatric Interest Profiles: What Activities Do Kids Do?

The research conducted thus far with the Pediatric Interest Profiles has yielded some very preliminary data showing the item activities most often done and most preferred by the study participants. These initial data are presented as a starting point for thinking about how children typically respond to the Pediatric Interest Profiles and whether an individual child or adolescent may be responding atypically. The data should be viewed cautiously, however, for several important reasons. First, the sample sizes are very small. These samples were drawn for the purpose of examining reliability of the Pediatric Interest Profiles and not for establishing norms. Second, all of the item development and reliability studies involving the Pediatric Interest Profiles were conducted in New England. Thus both the items and the children's responses to the items probably represent a geographical bias. Third, the activities and questions on the research versions of the Pediatric Interest Profiles have been modified during different phases of research. Fourth, it is not clear whether a child or adolescent with an "atypical" response is, in fact, at risk for play or leisure difficulties. Data from much larger samples are needed to begin to explore this question.

Kid Play Profile: What Activities Kids Do and What They Like.

Thirty-eight first- through third-grade children without disabilities participated in the test-retest reliability study of a 30-item research version of the Kid Play Profile. (The study is discussed in more detail on p. 114.) Using data from the first administration of the Kid Play Profile, Table 5-2 shows the activities most commonly done and most liked by children participating in the study.

Not surprisingly, watching television was both the most commonly done and most preferred activity. Other highly favored indoor activities included using computers, drawing or painting, listening to music, playing cards, and playing board games. Highly favored outside activities included riding bikes, swimming, going to the beach,

Table 5-2

Play Activities Most Commonly Done and Most Preferred by Children Using the 30-Item Version of the Kid Play Profile

What Children Do (n = 38)	%	What Children Like	
Watch Television	97.40	Watch Television (37)	2.89
Use Computers	97.40	Use Computers (37)	2.73
Ride Bikes	97.40	Ride Bikes (36)	2.72
Draw or Paint	97.40	Draw or Paint (36)	2.72
Go Swimming	92.10	Go Swimming (35)	2.66
Go to the Beach	92.10	Go to the Beach (35)	2.63
Listen to Music	92.10	Listen to Music (34)	2.68
Go Sledding	89.50	Go Sledding (34)	2.68
Play Board Games	89.50	Play Board Games (34)	2.55
Play Tag	89.50	Play Tag (34)	2.51
Read	86.80	Read (33)	2.46
Play Cards	84.20	Play Cards (32)	2.66
Go to Playground	84.20	Go to Playground (32)	2.56

Numbers in () indicate the number of children who reported doing the activity. Ratings range from 3 to 1: 3 = like it a lot, 2 = like it a little, 1 = don't like it at all.

sledding, going to the playground, and playing tag. Some of the favored outdoor activities probably reflect the geographical bias of some of the activity items. Going to the beach and sledding are activities that are readily available in New England.

Tables 5-3 and 5-4 show the most commonly done and most liked activities for boys and girls from the same group of children. Although boys and girls show many similarities (and although these sample sizes are very small), the data do reflect some gender differences. Boys reported playing with Lego blocks more often than girls did (95% of boys versus 66% of girls), while girls reported reading more often than boys did (100% of girls versus 75% of boys). It should be noted that these data are from the 30-item version of the Kid Play Profile. There would likely be differences on the most commonly done and preferred activities with the expanded, 50-item version of the Kid Play Profile. Data on the 50-item version have not yet been collected.

Preteen Play Profile: What Activities Preteens Do and What They Like.
Thirty-two fourth- and fifth-grade students without disabilities participated in the test-retest reliability study of the Preteen Play Profile (discussed in more detail on p. 115). Data from the first administration of the Preteen Play Profile are presented in Tables 5-5 to 5-7. The tables show the most commonly done and most liked activities among the students (and separately for boys and girls) completing the Preteen Play Profile for

this study. As Table 5-5 shows, hanging out with friends, going to the movies, playing in the snow, and watching television were the most common and some of the most highly preferred activities among students in the study. Although there were many similarities between boys and girls in terms of the activities they reported doing and enjoying, boys were more likely than girls to play sports, to play video games, and to go to arcades. Girls were more likely to draw or paint and to go out to eat. Again, some of the preferred activities (e.g., playing in the snow) probably reflect a regional bias.

Adolescent Leisure Interest Profile: What Activities Adolescents Do and What They Like.
Twenty-eight adolescents without disabilities and 88 adolescents with psychiatric disorders, learning disabilities, and physical disabilities participated in two separate test-retest reliability studies of the Adolescent Leisure Interest Profile (Henry, 1998b). (These studies are discussed in more detail on p. 116.) Data from the first administration of the Adolescent Leisure Interest Profile in both studies were combined in order to describe the leisure interests and participation of the four groups of adolescents (three with disabilities, one without).

Questions on the Adolescent Leisure Interest Profile are slightly different from those on the Kid Play Profile and Preteen Play Profile. With the Adolescent Leisure Interest Profile, adolescents are asked to respond to the

Table 5-3

Play Activities Most Commonly Done and Most Preferred by Boys Using the 30-ltem Version of the Kid Play Profile

What Boys Do (n = 20)	%	What Boys Like	
Watch Television	100	Watch Television (20)	2.90
Use Computers	100	Use Computers (20)	2.75
Ride Bikes	95	Ride Bikes (19)	2.68
Listen to Music	95	Listen to Music (19)	2.68
Go to the Beach	95	Go to the Beach (19)	2.63
Go Swimming	95	Go Swimming (19)	2.63
Play with Legos	95	Play with Legos (19)	2.63
Go Sledding	95	Go Sledding (19)	2.58
Play Cards	90	Play Cards (18)	2.77
Play Board Games	90	Play Board Games (18)	2.61
Draw or Paint	85	Draw or Paint (17)	2.71
Play Dodgeball	85	Play Dodgeball (17)	2.47
Play Tag	85	Play Tag (17)	2.34

Note: Numbers in () indicate the number of boys who reported doing the activity. Ratings range from 3 to 1: 3 = like it a lot, 2 = like it a little, 1 = don't like it at all.

Table 5-4
Play Activities Most Commonly Done and Most Preferred by Girls Using the 30-Item Version of the Kid Play Profile

What Girls Do (n = 18)	%	What Girls Like	
Draw or Paint	100.00	Draw or Paint (18)	2.83
Read	100.00	Read (18)	2.61
Watch Television	94.40	Watch Television (17)	2.68
Ride Bikes	94.40	Ride Bikes (17)	2.76
Use Computers	94.40	Use Computers (17)	2.71
Go Swimming	88.90	Go Swimming (16)	2.69
Play Tag	88.90	Play Tag (16)	2.69
Play Hide and Seek	88.90	Play Hide and Seek (16)	2.63
Go to the Beach	88.90	Go to the Beach (16)	2.63
Play Board Games	88.90	Play Board Games (16)	2.56
Go to Playground	88.90	Go to Playground (16)	2.56
Go Sledding	83.30	Go Sledding (15)	2.80
Listen to Music	83.30	Listen to Music (15)	2.67

Numbers in () indicate the number of girls who reported doing the activity. Ratings range from 3 to 1: 3 = like it a lot, 2 = like it a little, 1 = don't like it at all.

Table 5-5
Play Activities Most Commonly Done and Most Preferred by Preteens Using the Preteen Play Profile

What Preteens Do (n = 32)	%	What Preteens Like	
Hang Out With Friends	96.90	Hang Out with Friends (31)	2.94
Go to Movies	96.90	Go to Movies (31)	2.94
Play in Snow	96.90	Play in Snow (31)	2.87
Watch Television	96.90	Watch Television (31)	2.77
Go Swimming	93.80	Go Swimming (30)	2.83
Ride a Bike	93.80	Ride a Bike (30)	2.65
Use Computers	90.60	Use Computers (29)	2.90
Listen to Music	90.60	Listen to Music (29)	2.83
Go Sledding	90.60	Go Sledding (29)	2.83
Read	90.60	Read (29)	2.62
Play Cards	84.00	Play Cards (27)	2.74
Go Out to Eat	84.00	Go Out to Eat (27)	2.69
Draw or Paint	81.00	Draw or Paint (26)	2.77
Play Basketball	81.00	Play Basketball (26)	2.65
Roller Blade	81.00	Roller Blade (26)	2.61
Play Board Games	81.00	Play Board Games (26)	2.61

Numbers in () indicate the number of preteens who reported doing the activity. Ratings range from 3 to 1: 3 = like it a lot, 2 = like it a little, 1 = don't like it at all.

Table 5-6
Play Activities Most Commonly Done and Most Preferred by Boys Using the Preteen Play Profile

What Boys Do (n = 13)	%	What Boys Like	
Hang Out with Friends	100.00	Hang Out with Friends (13)	3.00
Go to the Movies	100.00	Go to the Movies (13)	2.92
Play Baseball	100.00	Play Baseball (13)	2.62
Play on Computer	92.30	Play on Computer (12)	2.92
Play in the Snow	92.30	Play in the Snow (12)	2.83
Listen to Music	92.30	Listen to Music (12)	2.83
Watch Television	92.30	Watch Television (12)	2.83
Go to the Beach	92.30	Go to the Beach (12)	2.67
Swim	92.30	Swim (12)	2.58
Ride a Bike	92.30	Ride a Bike (12)	2.58
Play Basketball	92.30	Play Basketball (12)	2.58
Play Video Games	84.60	Play Video Games (11)	3.00
Read	84.60	Read (11)	2.91
Go to Arcade	84.60	Go to Arcade (11)	2.82
Go Sledding	84.60	Go Sledding (.11)	2.73

Numbers in () indicate the number of boys who reported doing the activity. Ratings range from 3 to 1: 3 = like it a lot, 2 = like it a little, 1 = don't like it at all.

Table 5-7
Play Activities Most Commonly Done and Most Preferred by Girls Using the Preteen Play Profile

What Girls Do (n = 19)	%	What Girls Like	
Watch Television	100.00	Watch Television (19)	2.72
Go to the Movies	94.70	Go to the Movies (18)	2.94
Hang Out with Friends	94.70	Hang Out with Friends (18)	2.89
Play in the Snow	94.70	Play in the Snow (18)	2.89
Go Sledding	94.70	Go Sledding (18)	2.89
Play Cards	94.70	Play Cards (18)	2.83
Swim	94.70	Swim (18)	2.72
Draw or Paint	94.70	Draw or Paint (18)	2.72
Ride a Bike	94.70	Ride a Bike (18)	2.72
Read	94.70	Read (18)	2.44
Play on Computer	89.50	Play on Computer (17)	2.89
Listen to Music	89.50	Listen to Music (17)	2.89
Go Out to Eat	89.50	Go Out to Eat (17)	2.69
Play Board Games	89.50	Play Board Games (17)	2.58

Numbers in () indicate the number of girls who reported doing the activity. Ratings range from 3 to 1: 3 = like it a lot, 2 = like it a little, 1 = don't like it at all.

first question by specifying their level of interest in the activity. They respond to the second question by indicating the frequency of their participation.

Tables 5-8 and 5-9 show the 10 activities most preferred and most often done by the four groups of adolescents participating in the studies. There was great similarity among the activities in which all four groups were interested and in which they participated. The four activities most often done were the same for all four groups (adolescents with and without disabilities): listening to music, hanging out with friends, watching television, and talking on the phone. There were some differences across the groups. The adolescents with learning disabilities indicated more frequent participation in physical activities. The adolescents without disabilities reported going to parties more often. There were no other meaningful differences in activity preferences among the four groups.

Use of the Pediatric Interest Profiles to Set Goals and Plan Play-Related Interventions

Once the service provider has administered a version of the Pediatric Interest Profiles and has reviewed the profile and discussed the child's or adolescent's participation in play and leisure, the final step, if appropriate, is to set goals and plan interventions. The Pediatric Interest Profile, discussions with the child, comments by parents and teachers, and the provider's observations all contribute to the formulation of goals for the interventions. At the forefront, however, should be the child's own goals and the family's goals (Cohn & Cermak, 1998; Coster,

1998). What do the child or adolescent and the family want in terms of expanding his or her participation in play and leisure? How might engaging in play and leisure activities help the child meet goals for participation in other domains such as the classroom and family life?

By using the Pediatric Interest Profiles in the manner described in this chapter, the provider can develop a sense of what the child's needs are in terms of participation in play and leisure. In addition, the Pediatric Interest Profiles and other sources of information will help the provider determine factors that might be impeding participation. The Pediatric Interest Profiles can be used to identify specific activities that could be pursued to enhance participation or that could engage the child in interventions for specific performance problems (e.g., difficulties with fine or gross motor coordination, problem solving, memory, or social skills). For example, if an adolescent girl identified jewelry making as an interest on the Adolescent Leisure Interest Profile, that activity could be used to help her develop a new hobby, thus increasing her participation in a meaningful leisure activity and helping enhance her fine motor coordination. As another example, the provider's discussion with an 8-year-old boy based on his Kid Play Profile reveals that he wants to play baseball with the other children. From observations and discussions with the boy's teacher, however, the provider knows that he lacks the social skills needed to interact with his peers appropriately. In this case role-playing exercises might be used to help the boy learn how to ask to be included in a game at recess or how to deal better with frustration.

Table 5-8

The 10 Activities from the Adolescent Leisure Interest Profile Most Preferred by Adolescents with and Without Disabilities

Adolescents with Psychiatric Disabilities (n=27)	Adolescents with Learning Disabilities (n=33)	Adolescents with Physical Disabilities (n=28)	Adolescents Without Disabilities (n=29)
1. Listening to Music	Hanging Out With Friends	Watching TV	Listening to Music
2. Sleeping Late	Watching TV	Visiting Relatives	Hanging Out With Friends
3. Hanging Out With Friends	Listening to Music	Talking on the Phone	Going to Parties
4. Going to Parties	Celebrating Holidays	Taking Vacations	Going to Movies
5. Taking Vacations	Going to Movies	Sleeping Late	Taking Vacations
6. Swimming Going to Amusement Parks Going to Movies Dating	Taking Vacations	Shopping	Celebrating Holidays
7. Celebrating Holidays	Going Out to Eat Talking on the Phone Playing Basketball	Listening to Music	Watching TV
8.	Going to Parties	Hanging Out With Friends	Going to the Beach
9.		Going to Parties	Talking on the Phone
10.		Going to Movies	Dating

From Henry, A. D. (1998). Development of a measure of adolescent leisure interests. *American Journal of Occupational Therapy, 52,* 531-539.

Table 5-9

The 10 Activities From the Adolescent Leisure Interest Profile Most Often Done by Adolescents with and Without Disabilities

Adolescents with Psychiatric Disabilities (n=27)	Adolescents with Learning Disabilities (n=33)	Adolescents with Physical Disabilities (n=28)	Adolescents Without Disabilities (n=29)
1. Listening to Music	Hanging Out With Friends	Listening to Music	Listening to Music
2. Hanging Out With Friends	Watching TV	Hanging Out With Friends	Hanging Out With Friends
3. Watching TV	Listening to Music	Watching TV	Watching TV
4. Talking on the Phone	Talking on the Phone	Talking on the Phone	Talking on the Phone
5. Sleeping Late	Playing Basketball	Reading	Riding in a Car
6. Reading	Bicycling	Sleeping Late	Reading
7. Cooking	Riding in a Car	Using Computer	Going to Parties
8. Drawing or Painting Using Computer	Going Out to Eat	Studying Math	Swimming
9. Riding in a Car	Roller Skating	Going to Movies	Sleeping Late
10.	Swimming	Shopping	Lying in the Sun
	Shopping	Playing Video Games	

From Henry, A. D. (1998). Development of a measure of adolescent leisure interests. *American Journal of Occupational Therapy, 52,* 531-539.

In addition to providing direct service to the child or adolescent, the provider can enhance a child's participation in play and leisure activities by working with school personnel or the family to develop opportunities for that child to engage in play and leisure in the classroom (e.g., gym class); at home with siblings, parents, and grandparents; or in the community. The provider might give parents information about community services and opportunities such as a soccer league, YMCA programs, arts-and-crafts classes, and swimming lessons. The provider might need to advocate for access for children with disabilities or for financial support for children with limited resources. Information from the Pediatric Interest Profiles and other sources can make it possible to provide enhanced direct and indirect play- and leisure-related services to children and adolescents who need them. In Chapter 6 some specific case examples are presented to illustrate the use of the Pediatric Interest Profiles.

Development of and Research on the Pediatric Interest Profiles

Item Development for the Kid Play Profile and the Preteen Play Profile

Development of the Kid Play Profile and Preteen Play Profile began in 1995 (Andrews et al., 1995). To compile the initial pool of leisure activity items for the Kid Play Profile and the Preteen Play Profile, the test developers conducted several small group interviews with a total of 18 children between the ages of 6 and 12. During the interviews, the children were asked such open-ended questions as:

What do you do for fun or to relax?

What do you do when you get together with friends?

What types of activities do you do with your family?

Based on these interviews, a checklist-format interest inventory of 75 activity items was developed. The items were organized into 12 preliminary categories based on similarity of type (e.g., sports, outdoor activities, music activities). The respondent was asked to indicate whether he or she did each activity with a "yes" or "no" response and to list any "other" activities he or she did that were not included in the inventory. This inventory was administered to 481 New England schoolchildren between the ages of 8 and 12 (mean age=10). Boys constituted 49.3% (n=237) of the respondents and girls 46.5% (n=224); 4.1% (n=20) of the children did not identify their gender on the inventory form.

The percentage of children who responded "yes" to each activity item was calculated. Activities with a participation rate above 5% were retained. Only one item had a participation rate below 5%, providing evidence of the items' content validity. A review of the 481 response forms yielded an additional 9 "other" activities that were consistently identified by the children, resulting in an initial pool of 84 potential items. These items were reviewed for redundancies and, in several instances, multiple activity items were collapsed into a somewhat broader item. For example, the items naming the games Monopoly, Sorry, and Trouble were collapsed into a single item called "board games." Five expert occupational therapy pediatric clinicians reviewed the items. They were asked to consider the clarity, age appropriateness, and overall appeal of the set of items for both boys and girls. They were also asked to suggest any additional activity items that might be appropriate for younger children, since 6- and 7-year-olds were not represented in the item development sample. These efforts resulted in a final pool of 63 items. These items were used in the development of both the Kid Play Profile and the Preteen Play Profile.

Development of the Pilot Kid Play Profile Format

Because the usefulness of a self-report instrument depends on the ability of the respondent to comprehend what is being asked, the development of the Kid Play Profile posed a special challenge. The goal was to develop a checklist format with questions and stimuli that preliterate children could understand with only minimal assistance from the person administering the measure. A review of the literature on the development of self-report measures for young children suggested that presenting concrete, pictorially represented stimuli was an appropriate approach for this age group (Harter, 1990; Royeen, 1985). Thus the pilot Kid Play Profile used simple pictures and words to represent activity items. The responses to each of the three pilot questions asked in the Kid Play Profile were also represented with simple pictures and words. To respond to the first question, "Do you do this?", the child indicated "yes" or "no" by circling the appropriate word or picture. If the child indicated "yes," he or she was to answer two additional questions: (1) "Do you like this?" and (2) "Who do you do it with?"

Pilot Study of the Kid Play Profile

A pilot study was conducted to examine how young children (ages 6 through 9) responded to the Kid Play Profile content and format (Beck et al., 1996). Data from the item development phase described previously were used to develop a pilot version of the Kid Play Profile. This version included 19 items that the data (along with the expert reviewers) suggested were often done by younger children. This pilot version was administered once to 29 first- to third-grade school children (mean age = 7.26 years) in Rhode Island. The children completed the pilot Kid Play Profile in regular classroom settings, with their teacher and a trained undergraduate research student present. The research student gave the group verbal instructions on how to complete the profile, but children were given individual instructions only if necessary.

The appropriateness of the children's responses was determined by calculation of a "consistent response" score for each item for each child (1 = consistent, 0 = not consistent). A response was considered to be "consistent" under either one of two conditions: (1) if the child indicated that he or she did the activity (i.e., answered "yes" to question one), and the child also answered questions two and three, or (2) if the child answered "no" to question one, and the child did not answer questions two and three. The percentage of consistent responses could then be calculated for each item and child. In addition to consistency of responses, gender differences in the actual responses to the three questions and the time required to complete the pilot version were examined.

The consistent response score for the total group of children averaged across all items was 81%. The mean consistent response scores were 73% for first-grade students (n = 7), 78% for second-grade students (n = 10), and 88% for third-grade students (n = 12). These scores were not significantly different across the three grades. As well, no significant gender differences in the consistent response scores were found. The relatively high consistent response scores suggest that young children, even first graders, can generally comprehend and respond appropriately to the format of the Kid Play Profile.

The mean time to complete the profile was 7.76 minutes. Although the activity items appeared to appeal to both boys and girls, the total scores for questions one and two suggested that, overall, the activity items were both done and liked more by boys than girls.

The results of the pilot showed that young children could complete the 19-item version quickly and relatively accurately. Based on these results, and drawing from the item pool described previously, a 30-item version of the Kid Play Profile was developed. It seemed that a number of items could be added without creating a profile that was too lengthy. The added items included more activities that would either appeal to girls or be gender neutral. In addition, a cover sheet with simple written directions for completing the Kid Play Profile was created. The 30-item version was subjected to a test-retest reliability study with typically developing children.

Development of the Pilot Preteen Play Profile Format

In keeping with the goal of developing age-appropriate measures of leisure activity, the Preteen Play Profile has a more complex format, includes more items, and asks more questions than the Kid Play Profile, although it also uses pictures to represent the activity items. The Preteen Play Profile was designed to appeal to children 9 through 12 years of age.

Drawn from the item pool described previously, 53 items were chosen that the data and the expert reviewers suggested were often done by older children. Stick-figure drawings were created to represent each activity. These activity items were grouped into eight activity categories based on similarity of type. In addition, the relatively simple question format developed for the Kid Play Profile was elaborated to include additional questions about frequency of participation in the activities and the child's feeling of competence in doing the activities. A cover sheet with written directions on how to complete the profile was developed. The pilot Preteen Play Profile had five pilot questions about each activity item. The first question was "Do you do this?" The child indicated his or her response by circling "yes" or "no." If the child did the activity, he or she then answered four additional questions: (1) "How often do you do it?" (2) "How much do you like it?" (3) "How good are you at it?" (4) "Who do you do it with?"

Pilot Study of the Preteen Play Profile

As with the Kid Play Profile, a pilot study was conducted to examine whether 9- through 11-year-old children could respond to the Preteen Play Profile format in a consistent manner. Thirty-five fourth- and fifth-grade students from a public elementary school in eastern Massachusetts took part in the pilot study. The participants included 16 boys and 19 girls, ages 9 through 11. These students were administered the Preteen Play Profile as a group in a regular classroom setting. The students were expected to read the directions for completing the profile independently, but a pediatric occupational therapist and a teacher were present to answer questions as needed.

The consistency of the students' responses to the Preteen Play Profile was examined in exactly the same manner as described for the Kid Play Profile. Students' responses were considered to be consistent under either one of two conditions: (1) if the child indicated that he or she did the activity (i.e., answered "yes" to question one), then the child also answered questions two through five, or (2) if the child answered "no" to question one, then did not answer questions two through five. The percentage of "consistent responses" was calculated for each item and child. The mean percentage of consistent responses for the total group of children was 90%, indicating that most students understood and accurately completed the Preteen Play Profile.

Although the time required to complete the Preteen Play Profile was not formally recorded, the occupational therapist present during the administration reported that all children had completed the form within 20 minutes. This same group of children participated in the test-retest reliability study of the Preteen Play Profile.

Item Development for the Adolescent Leisure Interest Profile

As with the Kid Play Profile and Preteen Play Profile, the item development process for the Adolescent Leisure Interest Profile began with preliminary, open-ended interviews. Ten adolescents, ages 11 through 15, participated in the interviews in the fall of 1994. They were asked such questions as "What do you do for fun or to relax?" "What do you do when you get together with friends?" "What types of activities do you do with your family?" Based on the interview data, an 80-item checklist-format leisure interest inventory was generated.

This initial inventory was administered to 856 public junior high and high school students (425 girls, 431 boys), ages 12 through 20, in central Massachusetts and central Connecticut (Hann, Regele, Walsh, Fontana, & Bentley, 1994). As with the initial inventory for the Kid Play Profile and Preteen Play Profile, the respondents were asked to indicate their participation in the activities with a "yes" or "no" response and to list any "other" activities they did that were not included in the inventory. Participation rates were calculated for each of the items. None had a rate below 7%, which provided evidence of the content validity of the items.

Development of the Pilot Adolescent Leisure Interest Profile Format

The 856 data forms from the item development study were reviewed and six "other" activities that were consistently identified by the respondents were added to the original 80 items. These 86 items were grouped into 10 activity categories based on similarity of type (e.g., socializing activities, sports activities, and intellectual activities). Gregory's (1983) Activity Index and Meaningfulness of Activity Scale was adapted to ask specific questions about each leisure activity item. Using a checklist format, the adolescent was asked to answer two questions for each item: (1) "How interested are you in this?" and (2) "How often do you do this?" For those activities in which he or she participated, the adolescent was asked an additional four questions: (3) "Why do you do this activity?" (4) "How well do you do this?" (5) "How much do you enjoy doing this?" and (6) "Do you do this with others?" A cover sheet providing written instruction on completing the Adolescent Leisure Interest Profile was also developed.

Test-retest and internal consistency reliability studies with typically developing adolescents and adolescents with disabilities were then conducted.

Reliability Studies of the Pediatric Interest Profiles

Test-retest and internal consistency reliability studies of the three pilot versions of the Pediatric Interest Profiles have been conducted with typically developing children and adolescents (i.e., those without identified disabilities). In addition, test-retest and internal consistency reliability studies of the pilot version of the Adolescent Leisure Interest Profile have been conducted with adolescents with psychiatric, physical, and learning disabilities (Henry, 1998b).

Kid Play Profile

Thirty-one first- to third-grade children, ages 6 through 9 (mean age = 7.29), participated in a test-retest reliability study of the 30-item pilot version of the Kid Play Profile (Budd et al., 1997). The children were recruited from after-school programs, Sunday school programs, and day-care centers in central Massachusetts. During both administrations the children were administered the Kid Play Profile in either small groups or individual sessions, with a trained undergraduate research student present. The research student reviewed the written instructions with the children and was available to provide clarification if needed. During the first administration the research student also recorded the number of minutes required for each child to complete the Kid Play Profile form. The second administration of the Kid Play Profile took place 7 to 14 days after the first.

The mean time required to complete the 30-item Kid Play Profile was 11.32 minutes. Pearson correlations were used to examine reliability of the category scores and total score for all three questions (responses on the third question were recoded to reflect whether the child did the activity alone or with others; 0 = alone, 1 = with others). Reliability coefficients for the category and total scores are presented in Table 5-10. Coefficients for the total scores were .91 for the first question ("Do you do this?"), .70 for the second question ("Do you like this?"), and .45 for the third question ("Who do you do it with?"). The coefficients for the first two questions exceed a standard for acceptable test-retest reliability of .60 (Benson & Clark, 1982; Crocker & Algina, 1986). The test-retest reliability coefficients for the category and total scores for the third question were generally lower than desirable. Low variability in responses to the third question probably contributed to the low reliability coefficients.

Data from the first administration of the Kid Play Profile were used to calculate internal consistency reliability coefficients (Cronbach's alpha) for the category and total scores for the first question ("Do you do this?").

Coefficients for the category scores ranged from .31 to .58; the coefficient for the total score was .80. After this reliability study was completed, the Kid Play Profile was expanded again to a 50-item version.

Preteen Play Profile

Thirty-two fourth- and fifth-grade students, aged 9 and 10, participated in a test-retest reliability study of the 53-item pilot version of the Preteen Play Profile. During both administrations of the Preteen Play Profile, the children completed the profile as a group in a regular classroom setting with their teacher and a pediatric occupational therapist present. The occupational therapist reviewed the instructions on completing the Preteen Play Profile with the children and was available to answer questions if necessary, but did not provide any individualized assistance. The second administration of the Preteen Play Profile took place within 2 to 3 weeks after the first.

Table 5-10

Test-Retest Reliability Coefficients for Category and Total Scores on the Kid Play Profile Among Children Without Disabilities (n = 31)

	Do You Do It?	*Do You Like It?*	*Who Do You Do It with?*
Sports	.84‡	.42* (28)	.80‡ (28)
Ball Activities	.72‡	.42* (26)	.20ns (26)
Outside Activities	.56†	.69‡ (31)	.39* (31)
Summer Activities	.70‡	.38* (31)	.05ns (31)
Winter Activities	.83‡	.47† (29)	.60‡ (29)
Indoor Activities	.83‡	.46† (29)	.45* (29)
Creative Activities	.56†	.43* (29)	.56† (29)
Music Activities	.77‡	.46† (30)	.21ns (30)
Relaxation Activities	.74‡	.64* (30)	.28ns (30)
Total	.91‡	.70‡ (31)	.45† (31)

Numbers in parentheses indicate the number of children who participated in at least one activity within the category.
*$p < .05$.
†$p < .01$.
‡$p < .001$.
ns, Not significant.

Pearson correlations were used to examine the test-retest reliability for the category and total scores of the Preteen Play Profile; coefficients are presented in Table 5-11. The coefficients for the category scores across all five questions ranged from .05 to .94. The coefficients for the total scores for question 1 ("Do you do this?"), question 2 ("How often do you do it?"), and question 4 ("How good are you at it?") were high (.91, .73, and .70, respectively). The reliability coefficients for questions 3 ("How much do you like it?") and 5 ("Who do you do it with?") were lower than desirable. As with the Kid Play Profile, low variability in responses among the participants may have contributed to the lowered coefficients for these questions.

As with the Kid Play Profile, internal consistency reliability coefficients (Cronbach's alpha) were calculated for the category and total scores for the first question ("Do you do this?") using data from the first administration of the Preteen Play Profile. Coefficients for the category scores ranged from .16 to .71; the coefficient for the total score was .72. After this reliability study was completed, the Preteen Play Profile was expanded to 59 items.

Adolescent Leisure Interest Profile

Twenty-eight typically developing adolescents, ages 14 through 19, participated in a test-retest reliability study of an initial pilot version of the Adolescent Leisure Interest Profile (Brophy et al., 1995). The participants included 24 high school and 4 college students in central Massachusetts. The high school students completed both administrations of the Adolescent Leisure Interest Profile during a study hall session, and the college students completed the Adolescent Leisure Interest Profile in a college dormitory room. During both administrations a trained undergraduate research student was present to answer questions. For all participants the second administration took place 1 week after the first.

Pearson correlations were used to examine reliability of the category scores and total scores for all six questions (presented in Table 5-12). Coefficients for the six total scores ranged from .61 to .85. These correlations all exceed a standard for acceptable test-retest reliability of .60 (Benson & Clark, 1982; Crocker & Algina, 1986). In addition, by use of data from the first administration

Table 5-11

Test-Retest Reliability Coefficients for Category and Total Scores on the Preteen Play Profile Among Preteens Without Disabilities (n = 32)

	Do You Do It?	How Often Do You Do It?	How Much Do You Like It?	Are You Good at It?	Do You Do It with Others or Alone?
Sports	0.95‡	0.36* (28)	0.61‡ (28)	0.74‡ (28)	
Outdoor Activities	0.40*	0.71‡ (32)	0.66‡ (32)	0.47† (32)	0.62‡ (32)
Summer Activities	0.86‡	0.84‡ (31)	0.35* (31)	0.51† (31)	0.72‡ (31)
Winter Activities	0.77‡	0.69‡ (31)	0.51* (31)	0.38† (31)	0.05‡ (31)
Music Activities	0.82‡	0.70‡ (30)	0.41* (30)	0.57† (30)	0.43‡ (30)
Making Things	0.79‡	0.61‡ (28)	0.53* (28)	0.30ns (28)	0.42* (28)
Socializing	0.67‡	0.75‡ (31)	0.38* (31)	0.66† (31)	0.12ns (31)
Indoor Activities	0.57‡	0.71‡ (32)	0.48* (32)	0.62† (32)	0.57‡ (32)
Total	0.92‡	0.75‡ (32)	0.51* (32)	0.72† (32)	0.57† (32)

Numbers in parentheses indicate the number of preteens who participated in at least one activity within the category.

*$p < .05$.
†$p < .01$.
‡$p < .001$.
ns, Not significant.

Table 5-12

Test-Retest Reliability Coefficients for Category and Total Scores of the Adolescent Leisure Interest Profile Among Adolescents Without Disabilities (n = 28)

	How Interested? *(n = 28)*	*How Often?* *(n = 28)*	*Why?*	*How Well?*	*How Much* *Enjoy?*	*Others or* *Alone?*
Exercise Activities	.89‡	.90‡	.83‡ (26)	.75‡ (26)	.34ns (26)	.49* (26)
Sports	.87‡	.46*	.37ns (22)	.52† (22)	.69‡ (22)	.61† (22)
Creative Activities	.76‡	.83‡	.87‡ (23)	.76‡ (24)	.26ns (24)	.21ns (24)
Intellectual Activities	.54‡	.53†	.44ns (19)	−.33ns (18)	−.06ns (19)	.60† (18)
Clubs/Organizations	.89‡	.77‡	.45ns (18)	.24ns (17)	.66‡ (18)	.28ns (18)
Family Activities	.76‡	.66‡	.07ns (24)	.35ns (24)	.38ns (24)	.26ns (24)
Social Activities	.83‡	.83‡	.80‡ (26)	.52† (25)	.64‡ (26)	.15ns (27)
Relaxation Activities	.63‡	.64‡	.24ns (25)	.27ns (25)	.25ns (25)	.30ns (24)
Outdoor Activities	.85‡	.89‡	.98‡ *(20)*	.48* (19)	.63† (19)	.25ns (19)
Miscellaneous Activities	.53†	.64‡	.10ns (17)	.62† (17)	.47* (17)	.83‡ (17)
Total	.85‡	.83‡	.61‡	.61‡	.73‡	.53†

From Henry, A. D. (1998). Development of a measure of adolescent leisure interests. *American Journal of Occupational Therapy, 52,* 531-539.

Numbers in parentheses indicate the number of adolescents who participated in at least one activity within the category.

*p < .05.

†p < .01.

‡p < .001.

ns, Not significant.

of the Adolescent Leisure Interest Profile, internal consistency estimates were calculated for the category scores (i.e., the activity categories) and total score on the first question ("How interested are you?") using Cronbach's alpha. Coefficients ranged from .58 to .80 for the category scores. The coefficient for the total score was .92. The coefficient for the total score exceeds a standard for acceptable internal consistency reliability of .80 (Benson & Clark, 1982; Crocker & Algina, 1986).

After this first reliability study was completed, the Adolescent Leisure Interest Profile was reviewed by a small group of occupational therapists experienced in working with adolescents. Based on their feedback

and on findings of the first reliability study, revisions to the Adolescent Leisure Interest Profile were made. These included rewording some activity items and questions and developing more detailed directions for completing the Adolescent Leisure Interest Profile. A second reliability study of this revised pilot version of the Adolescent Leisure Interest Profile was then undertaken.

The participants in the second reliability study of the Adolescent Leisure Interest Profile (revised pilot version) included 88 adolescents (ages 12 to 21) with psychiatric (n = 27), physical (n = 28), and learning (n = 33) disabilities (Henry, 1998b). These adolescents were recruited from five different school and hospital settings in Massachusetts and Rhode Island. For the most part, the adolescents completed the Adolescent Leisure Interest Profile in individual or small group (three to five persons) sessions, except for those with learning disabilities, who completed the Adolescent Leisure Interest Profile in a larger classroom setting. In all instances an experienced occupational therapist administered the Adolescent Leisure Interest Profile. The therapist provided reading or physical assistance or clarification to those who needed it. The second administration was completed within 7 to 14 days after the first.

Pearson correlations were used to examine reliability of the category score and total scores for the six questions (presented in Table 5-13). The results of the reliability study with adolescents with disabilities were similar to the study with adolescents without disabilities. Based on data from the first administration of the Adolescent Leisure Interest Profile to adolescents with disabilities, internal consistency estimates were calculated for the category scores and total score on the first question ("How interested?") using Cronbach's alpha. Coefficients ranged from .59 to .80 for the category scores. The coefficient for the total score was .93, which exceeds the standard for acceptable reliability of .80 (Benson & Clark, 1982; Crocker & Algina, 1986). Test-retest reliability coefficients for the six total scores for the total group all exceeded .60, ranging from .62 to .78. Reliability of the total scores for the three groups of adolescents with disabilities was also examined. Scores were most stable among the adolescents

Table 5-13

Test-Retest Reliability Coefficients for Category and Total Scores on the Adolescent Leisure Interest Profile Among Adolescents with Disabilities (n = 88)

	How Interested? (n = 88)	How Often? (n = 88)	Why?	How Well?	How Much Enjoy?	Others or Alone?
Exercise Activities	.76‡	.75‡	.36† (81)	.60‡ (81)	.54‡ (81)	.72‡ (81)
Sports	.78‡	.80‡	.45‡ (65)	.62‡ (65)	.56‡ (65)	.51‡ (65)
Creative Activities	.76‡	.75‡	.63‡ (83)	.48‡ (82)	.63‡ (82)	.61‡ (82)
Intellectual Activities	.71‡	.64‡	.59‡ (66)	.56‡ (64)	.64‡ (65)	.70‡ (65)
Clubs/ Organizations	.73‡	.71‡	.48† (43)	.73‡ (43)	.57‡ (43)	.26ns (43)
Family Activities	.58‡	.54‡	.62‡ (85)	.61‡ (83)	.65‡ (84)	.71‡ (85)
Social Activities	.73‡		.50‡ (87)	.58‡ (85)	.52‡ (87)	.58‡ (87)
Relaxation Activities	.48‡	.38‡	.04ns (81)	.67‡ (80)	.55‡ (81)	.62‡ (81)
Outdoor Activities	.70‡	.79‡	.21ns (60)	.50‡ (59)	.33* (59)	.47‡ (58)
Miscellaneous Activities	.63‡	.53‡†	.10 ns (69)	.40‡ (68)	.43‡ (68)	.59‡ (69)
Total	.78‡	.77‡	.62‡	.74‡	.68‡	.78‡

From Henry, A. D. (1998). Development of a measure of adolescent leisure interests. *American Journal of Occupational Therapy, 52,* 531-539.

Numbers in parentheses indicate the number of adolescents who participated in at least one activity within the category.

*$p < .05$.

†$p < .01$.

‡$p < .001$.

ns, Not significant

with psychiatric disorders (from .62 to .89), followed by those with physical disabilities (from .56 to .88). The adolescents with learning disabilities showed the lowest reliability (from .50 to .75); only two of the six reliability coefficients exceeded .60 among these adolescents (presented in Table 5-14).

To examine whether the Adolescent Leisure Interest Profile discriminates between adolescents with and without disabilities, study administrators combined data from the first administrations of the Adolescent Leisure Interest Profile in both reliability studies. Although the data showed considerable similarity among the four groups of adolescents (three with disabilities and one without) in terms of leisure activity interest and participation (see Tables 5-8 and 5-9, discussed on p. 111), there was evidence that certain questions on the Adolescent Leisure Interest Profile (e.g., feelings of enjoyment) could point out some differences among the groups of adolescents. In particular, the adolescents with psychiatric disorders reported significantly lower levels of enjoyment in leisure activities than the other three groups, as shown in Table 5-15 (Henry, 1998b).

After these studies were completed, additional revisions were made to the Adolescent Leisure Interest Profile.

Conclusions and Future Research with the Pediatric Interest Profiles

For the most part the studies conducted with the Pediatric Interest Profiles indicate that the three pilot versions had acceptable test-retest reliability. In particular, across the three pilot versions of the Pediatric Interest Profiles, the questions regarding play and leisure activity participation and interest level were shown to be the most stable. Questions regarding feelings of competence or enjoyment in activities had generally lower reliability. It is possible that children's and adolescents' feelings about enjoyment or competence in play and leisure activities may be naturally somewhat unstable. When using the Pediatric Interest Profiles, providers should be aware that children's responses to some of the questions could change.

Providers should also be aware that the three pilot versions of the Pediatric Interest Profiles used in the reliability

Table 5-14

Test-Retest Reliability for Total Scores on the Adolescent Leisure Interest Profile for Three Subgroups of Adolescents with Disabilities

	Adolescents with Psychiatric Disabilities (n=27)	Adolescents with Learning Disabilities (n=33)	Adolescents with Physical Disabilities (n=28)
How Interested?	.87†	.53*	.88†
How Often?	.89†	.50*	.80†
Why?	.62†	.69†	.56*
How Well?	.87†	.55†	.74†
How Much Enjoy?	.75†	.53*	.71†
With Others or Alone?	.86†	.75†	.72†

From Henry, A. D. (1998). Development of a measure of adolescent leisure interests. *American Journal of Occupational Therapy, 52,* 531-539.
*$p<.01$.
†$p<.001$.

Table 5-15

Mean Total Scores on the Adolescent Leisure Interest Profile for Adolescents with and Without Disabilities

	Adolescents with Psychiatric Disabilities (n=27)	Adolescents with Learning Disabilities (n=33)	Adolescents with Physical Disabilities (n=28)	Adolescents Without Disabilities (n=29)
Total Scores:				
How Interested?	1.85	1.67	1.75	1.66
How Often?	2.31	2.07	2.07	2.08
Why?	1.86	1.88	1.88	1.88
How Well?	2.27	2.48	2.33	2.41
How Much Enjoy?	2.39	2.56	2.50	2.50
With Others or Alone?	1.74	1.77	1.80	1.71

From Henry, A. D. (1998). Development of a measure of adolescent leisure interests. *American Journal of Occupational Therapy, 52,* 531-539.

studies just described underwent additional revisions before their publication in this text. The revisions included reformatting each of the three versions, improving the clarity of the questions asked about the activities, reorganizing and retitling some activity categories, and adding activity items for a broader geographical representation of play and leisure interests. In addition, one question that was included in the pilot version of the Adolescent Leisure Interest Profile ("Why do you do this?" with responses "have to" or "want to") was dropped from the version shown in Appendix 5-C. Because the person doing the leisure activity chooses the activity, it was felt that this question was unnecessary. In addition, dropping this question reduced the administration time for the adolescent version.

It is unlikely that these revisions will negatively affect the reliability of the Pediatric Interest Profiles. However, additional research with the Pediatric Interest Profiles is warranted. For example, because the children and adolescents who participated in the item development studies were overwhelmingly middle-class and Caucasian, the activity items may reflect cultural, ethnic, or socioeconomic bias. Testing of the Pediatric Interest Profiles with varying groups of children and adolescents is needed.

The current data on the Pediatric Interest Profiles are insufficient to describe patterns of play and leisure interest and participation for children and adolescents in any meaningful way, or to determine if certain patterns of participation put children at risk. With larger samples of children and adolescents, both with and without disabilities, responding to all three versions of the Pediatric Interest Profiles, factor analytical and other studies could be conducted to begin to address questions regarding the meaning of patterns of play and leisure participation.

Case Examples Using the Pediatric Interest Profiles

Each of the following three case examples describes the use of one of the Pediatric Interest Profiles with a child or adolescent. These cases are presented to offer ideas on how a service provider can use information gathered with the Pediatric Interest Profiles (and other sources) to guide interventions.

CASE EXAMPLE 1

Using the Kid Play Profile: Jerome

Jerome is 6 years old and attends first grade at an urban, public elementary school in Maryland. He lives with his mother, maternal grandmother, and 8-year-old brother, Joe. Jerome's mother works full time in a manufacturing plant and attends school one evening a week to earn a BS in education. Jerome's parents are divorced. Jerome and his brother visit their father in Pennsylvania one weekend each month and for three week-long vacations each year. Jerome's grandmother provides child care for Jerome and his brother when their mother is working or at school.

His mother reports that Jerome has always been more "difficult" than her other son. As a baby he was not easily soothed, was a "picky" eater, and rarely slept through the night. She felt that she had to carry him all the time. As a toddler, he was very physically active and frequently got "bumps and bruises." His high level of physical activity continues to the present. Jerome's mother describes him as "literally bouncing off the walls" at the end of the day. In addition, since toddlerhood he has been very particular about his clothing, disliking most types of underwear, socks, turtleneck shirts, and jeans. His mother reports, "Sometimes we go through five shirts in the morning before he is ready for school."

Jerome enjoyed kindergarten, but his progress in developing preacademic skills such as letter recognition and writing was slower than most of his classmates. First grade has been more difficult. Jerome has trouble paying attention in class, is often disruptive because he cannot sit still, and is falling further behind in developing reading-readiness skills. He is having difficulty with handwriting and other fine motor tasks. While his teacher is very supportive and patient, she is beginning to feel frustrated with her ability to manage his behavior in the classroom and worries about his ability to keep up with the pace of classroom activities. He interacts only minimally with classmates and on the playground spends most of his time on the swings or "running in circles." Since the middle of the school year, Jerome has been receiving resource room help for language arts and classroom-based occupational therapy for fine motor activities and handwriting.

At a recent parent meeting, Jerome's mother expressed concern about his increasing social isolation. She is concerned because Jerome tells her that he eats lunch alone, usually plays by himself during recess, and does not get included in most social activities. Jerome's classroom teacher confirms this. The school psychologist and the occupational therapist were identified as the service providers responsible for addressing these issues. The occupational therapist administered the Kid Play Profile to gain Jerome's perspective on his play participation and interviewed Jerome's mother and teacher about his behavior at home and school.

Findings Using the Kid Play Profile
Jerome was able to complete the Kid Play Profile with considerable assistance from the occupational therapist. His responses on the Kid Play Profile indicate that he primarily enjoys outdoor, gross motor activities

such as biking, roller-blading, swimming, sledding, going to the playground, and playing "superheroes." He seems to enjoy few indoor or fine motor activities but did indicate that he likes to build things. He told the occupational therapist that his favorite play activities are riding his bike and climbing on the jungle gym at the playground. He reports that he most often plays by himself or sometimes with his older brother but says that his brother "doesn't always like to do stuff with me." He says he has "a few" friends at school but could name only one boy in his class (Andrew) with whom he plays during recess. When asked if he has any other friends, he stated, "Well, they don't really like me." He reports that there are "no kids in the neighborhood" that he can play with. His mother confirms that Jerome and his older brother don't always play together. She says that Jerome is actually more skilled at gross motor activities such as biking and roller-blading than his older brother and that the older brother prefers more creative or indoor activities such as drawing, listening to music, reading, or watching TV. She says, "They are like night and day." Her biggest concern about Jerome is his academic performance and the fact that he doesn't seem to know how to make friends.

The classroom teacher confirms that Jerome doesn't seem to be making friends in school. She is concerned that his disruptive behavior is causing him to be marginalized by other classmates. On the playground, she has observed that he has difficulty following the rules of organized games such as soccer and kickball and is not often invited to play by other children.

Interventions

The interventions recommended by the occupational therapist primarily addressed Jerome's social skills and his behavior in the classroom. She referred Jerome to the Friendship Group, jointly run by herself and the school psychologist. The goal of this group is to help referred children develop appropriate social-interaction skills in the context of structured dyadic play with one other child. Jerome was encouraged to invite one classmate to participate in the Friendship Group with him. The play activities used in the group require cooperation, turn-taking, and negotiation. The group teaches skills in communication and self-regulation.

The occupational therapist also encouraged Jerome's mother to foster more play between Jerome and his brother. She suggested that Joe might be encouraged to share with Jerome his interest in drawing or building things with construction toys such as Lego or K-Nex. Such activities would also help the development of Jerome's fine motor skills. Because Jerome enjoys and is good at a variety of gross motor activities, the occupational therapist encouraged his mom to help him

develop friendships building on these interests. The occupational therapist suggested that participating in recreational programs at the local community center might help Jerome find friends with similar interests and that his mom could help Jerome arrange occasional "play dates" with one other child.

The occupational therapist also indicated that Jerome should continue receiving classroom-based occupational therapy for handwriting and other fine motor skill development and should continue receiving resource room assistance with language arts.

CASE EXAMPLE 2

Using the Preteen Play Profile: Consuela

Consuela is 10 years old and attends fifth grade at a public middle school in a relatively affluent, suburban community in southern Texas. She lives with her parents and two siblings, a 13-year-old brother and an 11-year-old sister. Both parents are well educated and have earned graduate degrees, and the family is financially well off. Consuela's father is employed in the computer industry, and her mother works part time for a biotechnology firm.

When Consuela was 8, she began complaining of stiffness and pain in her back and hips. When these symptoms had persisted for a few weeks, her mother took her to the pediatrician. After a thorough medical workup and a series of laboratory tests, it was determined that Consuela has juvenile rheumatoid arthritis. In the past year, she has had two flare-ups of the disease, and at this time she has involvement in her hips, knees, back, and fingers. Her pediatric rheumatologist recently referred her to outpatient occupational and physical therapy for help with daily activities (including self-care, school, and play activities) and for help in maintaining her strength, mobility, and endurance.

As part of the initial assessment, the occupational therapist administered the Preteen Play Profile and interviewed Consuela to learn more about her interests and involvement in play. She also interviewed Consuela's parents during an outpatient therapy session and consulted with Consuela's teacher about her functioning in school.

Findings Using the Preteen Play Profile

Consuela appears to be a bright and generally happy child. She reports that she has friends both at school and in her neighborhood, and her teacher and parents confirm this. Her teacher reports that Consuela is doing well academically and has been able to keep up with schoolwork even when she was absent during recent flare-ups. Consuela is able to engage in most classroom activities without difficulty, although her pace is sometimes slowed due to joint stiffness. Her teacher has noticed that her ability to complete written assignments within the time allotted in class has slowed because of stiffness in her hands. Consuela also requires more time to travel from one classroom to another than she has in the past. Her parents report similar experiences at home; Consuela needs more time to complete activities of daily living (e.g., dressing herself in the morning). They express concern that Consuela often "overdoes it" and clearly want to protect her from another flare-up of the disease.

The Preteen Play Profile showed that Consuela has a wide range of interests. She reports enjoying biking, roller-blading, and swimming but generally does these activities only in the summer. She told the occupational therapist that, in the past, she had enjoyed camping and hiking with her family but that this has become more difficult for her during the past year. She also used to play soccer in a city league but no longer has the endurance for this.

Consuela has an interest in creative activities. She enjoys painting and likes to bake with her mom and sister. Two years ago, she and her sister began a garden with their mother, but bending over or kneeling in the garden has gotten more difficult for her. She also told the occupational therapist that the stiffness in her hands is making it harder for her to paint or to write during class. Consuela reports that she has "about three or four" close friends in school and two friends in her neighborhood. She enjoys "hanging out" with friends, going to the movies, or shopping at the local mall but is often tired before her friends are ready to leave.

Consuela reports that her favorite subjects in school are art, science, and social studies. She sometimes gets stiff if she has to sit too long in school or if she is watching TV or working on the computer. She is beginning to have difficulty carrying her tray at lunchtime, and it is getting more difficult for her to carry her books back and forth from home to school. Despite the friends she has at school, she says that some kids tease her because she walks so slowly, and she is beginning to feel self-conscious. She expressed some concern about her future, saying, "If things are hard now, what will it be like in a few years?"

Interventions

The outpatient occupational therapist made several recommendations to help Consuela maintain joint mobility and endurance and continue participation in activities that are important to her. For their individual therapy sessions, which focus on maintaining hand function, Consuela chose jewelry making (e.g., beading). As they made jewelry, the occupational therapist taught Consuela joint protection and therapeutic exercise activities for her hands. The occupational therapist also taught Consuela to evaluate her pain level and to adjust her activity level in response to the pain she is experiencing.

Together, the outpatient occupational therapist and physical therapist made recommendations for home, school, and community-based activities to help Consuela maintain mobility of both large and small joints and to help maintain her endurance. Consuela's parents were encouraged to allow her to begin to take responsibility for monitoring her own pain level and to adjust her activity level accordingly. The occupational therapist and physical therapist both encouraged Consuela's continued participation in low-impact, gross motor activities, such as swimming or bike riding. They suggested roller-blading at an indoor rink (with appropriate protective equipment) rather than on the street to decrease joint stress. The therapists also suggested that Consuela's parents request (or purchase) a second set of schoolbooks to keep at home so that Consuela does not need to carry books back and forth. Consuela and her mother made a plan to walk their dog together in the morning to help with Consuela's stiffness before she dressed for school.

The occupational therapist and physical therapist also consulted with Consuela's teacher and the school-based occupational therapist regarding classroom accommodations. Consuela's teacher helped her arrange for a "lunchtime buddy" to help her with her lunch tray. The school-based occupational therapist and the teacher also made minor changes within the classroom. For example, the occupational therapist provided Consuela with rubber "pencil grips" to decrease joint stress during handwriting, and the teacher allowed Consuela to take stretch breaks and to stand during some classroom activities.

Consuela's parents were referred to the American Juvenile Arthritis Organization for support and information. Consuela was referred to a support group for children with persistent conditions that is offered at a local hospital.

CASE EXAMPLE 3

Using the Adolescent Leisure Interest Profile: Michael

Michael is an 18-year-old who dropped out of high school at 16. He has been hospitalized for the past 4 months at an intermediate-care adolescent psychiatric unit at a state-funded hospital in California. After leaving high school, Michael had three short-term psychiatric hospitalizations, once with symptoms of mania and twice with symptoms of depression with psychotic features. In the past 2 years he has been unable to maintain a job for more than 2 weeks and has spent much of the day in his room listening to music.

Michael currently has a diagnosis of bipolar (manic-depressive) disorder.

Before this hospitalization Michael lived with his father, 16-year-old sister, and 14-year-old brother. He also has an older sister, age 23, who is currently attending college. Michael's father is a salesman who has struggled financially in recent years. Michael's mother died in an automobile accident 4 years ago. His father describes Michael before his mother's death as a "happy and bright kid" who did well in school and had many friends and leisure interests. After his mother's death, Michael began using alcohol and marijuana heavily and became increasingly irritable and isolated. Eventually he dropped out of school. His current hospitalization followed a serious suicide attempt.

During this hospitalization Michael has received medication that has been effective in controlling his symptoms. He has begun working on earning a GED and has been actively involved in vocational readiness groups. He will soon be discharged to live at home with his father and two younger siblings and plans to find a job. He expresses concern about his ability to make friends, saying, "I don't know what to do with people." He has few leisure interests, although in the hospital he has begun to learn to play the guitar. While working with Michael to develop aftercare plans, the occupational therapist administered the Adolescent Leisure Interest Profile.

Findings Using the Adolescent Leisure Interest Profile

Michael's responses on the Adolescent Leisure Interest Profile show that he has few leisure interests. He has indicated strong interest only in listening to music, going to concerts, doing creative writing, and attending worship. His responses on the Adolescent Leisure Interest Profile show that he doesn't feel he does any activities well and does most things alone. Unlike most adolescents, Michael indicated no interest in hanging out with friends. He told the occupational therapist, "Any friends I had, I lost a long time ago."

Before his mother's death Michael had attended church regularly with her and the rest of his family, but he stopped going after her death.

During an interview the occupational therapist talked more with Michael about his past leisure interests. He reported that he used to enjoy hiking and that he and his family went camping often, but that no one in his family has gone since his mother's death. He said, "She was the one who would organize a trip and get everyone excited about it." He told the occupational therapist that he misses camping and hiking and that he would like to get more involved in outdoor activities after discharge, but said he was unsure how to start. "Maybe I'd like a job where I could work outside."

Interventions

Before discharge, Michael and the occupational therapist explored opportunities in the community for Michael to complete GED classes, take guitar lessons, and find a job. They found that guitar lessons and a GED class were available at a local community center, and Michael registered for both. In addition, he has made plans to join a youth group at the church he had attended before his mother's death.

The occupational therapist worked with Michael to develop a resume and to practice job-interviewing skills. Michael made a list of the types of jobs he thought he might like, and together they looked at job ads in the local papers. He found advertisements for four jobs that interested him; two jobs were for landscaping assistants and two were messenger jobs. By the time he was ready for discharge, Michael had two interviews scheduled. In addition, his aftercare plans include a weekly work support group for young adults held at the local community mental health center, psychotherapy sessions, and AA meetings.

Review Questions

1. Briefly describe the three specific ways to use the Pediatric Interest Profiles.
2. Young children (before age 7) and adolescents tend to describe their feelings and experiences differently. These differences call for different methods in facilitating responses to assessments. Briefly summarize these different ways of describing feelings and experiences for the young child and for the adolescent.
3. A child or adolescent's participation in play or leisure may be influenced by several contextual factors. Briefly describe some of these.
4. Several sampling factors are cause for cautious use of the data thus far collected. What are these sampling factors?

REFERENCES

Achenbach, T. M., McConaughy, S. H., & Howell, C. T. (1987). Child/adolescent behavioral and emotional problems: Implications of cross-informant correlations for situational specificity. *Psychological Bulletin, 101*, 213-232.
Andrews, P. M., Bleecher, R., Genoa, A. M., Molloy, P., Monahan, K., & Sargent, J. (1995). *Leisure interests of children.* (Unpublished manuscript, Worcester State College, Worcester, MA).
Ayres, A. J. (1989). *Sensory integration and praxis tests.* Los Angeles: Western Psychological Services.
Barnett, L. A. (1990). Developmental benefits of play. *Journal of Leisure Research, 22*, 138-153.

Barnett, L. A. (1991). The playful child: Measurement of a disposition to play. *Play and Culture, 4,* 51-74.

Beard, J. G., & Ragheb, M. G. (1983). Measuring leisure motivation. *Journal of Leisure Research, 15,* 219-228.

Beck, D., Benson, S., Curet, J., Froehlich, D., McCrary, L., Rasmussen, L., et al. (1996). *Pilot study of a child's play interest profile* (Unpublished manuscript, Worcester State College, Worcester, MA).

Behnke, C., & Fetkovich, M. (1984). Examining the reliability and validity of the Play History. *American Journal of Occupational Therapy, 23,* 314-318.

Benson, J., & Clark, E. (1982). A guide for instrument development and validation. *American Journal of Occupational Therapy, 36,* 789-800.

Brennan, A. (1985). Participation and self-esteem: A test of six alternative patterns. *Adolescence, 4,* 385-400.

Brophy, P., Caizzi, D., Crete, B., Jachym, T., Kobus, M., & Sainz, C. (1995). *Preliminary reliability study of the Adolescent Leisure Interest Profile* (Unpublished manuscript, Worcester State College, Worcester, MA).

Brown, C., & Bowen, R. E. (1998). Including the consumer and environment in occupational therapy treatment planning. *Occupational Therapy Journal of Research, 18*(1), 44-62.

Bruininks, R. (1978). *Bruininks-Osteretsky Test of Motor Proficiency.* Circle Pines, MN: DLM Teaching Resources.

Bryze, K. (1997). Narrative contribution to the play history. In L. D. Parham & L. S. Fazio (Eds.), *Play in occupational therapy for children* (pp. 23-34). St. Louis: Mosby.

Budd, P., Ferraro, D., Lovely, A., McNeil, T., Owanisian, L., Parker, J., et al. (1997). *Pilot study of the revised child's play interest profile* (Unpublished manuscript, Worcester State College, Worcester, MA).

Bundy, A. C. (1993). Assessment of play and leisure: Delineation of the problem. *American Journal of Occupational Therapy, 47,* 217-222.

Bundy, A. C. (1997). Play and playfulness: What to look for. In L. D. Parham & L. S. Fazio (Eds.), *Play in occupational therapy for children* (pp. 52-65). St. Louis: Mosby.

Butcher, J. (1991). Development of a playground skills test. *Perceptual and Motor Skills, 72,* 259-266.

Chang, A. F, Rosenthal, T. L., Bryant, E. S., Rosenthal, R. H. Heidlage, R. M., & Fritzler, B. K. (1993). Comparing high school and college students' leisure interests and stress ratings. *Behavioral Research and Therapy, 31,* 179-184.

Christiansen, C. (1991). Occupational performance assessment. In C. Christiansen & C. Baum (Eds.), *Occupational therapy: Overcoming human performance deficits* (pp. 375-424). Thorofare, NJ: Slack.

Cohn, E. S. (1994). *Interviewing children* (Unpublished manuscript, Boston University, Boston).

Cohn, E. S., & Cermak, S. A. (1998). Including the family perspective in sensory integration outcomes research. *American Journal of Occupational Therapy, 52,* 540-546.

Coleman, D., & Iso-Ahola, S. E. (1993). Leisure and health: The role of social support and self-determination. *Journal of Leisure Research, 25,* 111-128.

Coster, W. (1998). Occupation-centered assessment of children. *American Journal of Occupational Therapy, 52,* 337-344.

Coster, W. J., Deeney, T., Haltiwanger, J., & Haley, S. M. (1998). *The School Function Assessment: Standardization version.* Boston: Boston University.

Crocker, L., & Algina, J. (1986). *Introduction to classical and modern test theory* (pp. 133-134). San Antonio: Harcourt, Brace, Jovanovich.

Csikszentmihalyi, M., & Larson, R. (1984). *Being adolescent.* New York: Basic Books.

DeMarco, T., & Sidney, K. (1989). Enhancing children's participation in physical activity. *Journal of School Health, 59,* 337-340.

Feldman, M. J., & Gaier, E. L. (1980). Correlates of adolescent life satisfaction. *Youth and Society, 12,* 131-144.

Fine, G. A., Mortimer, J. T., & Roberts, D. F. (1990). Leisure work, and the mass media. In S. S. Feldman & G. R. Elliott (Eds.), *At the threshold: The developing adolescent* (pp. 225-252). Cambridge, MA: Harvard University Press.

Finegan, J. K., Niccols, G. A., Zacher, M. A., & Hood, J. E. (1991). The play activity questionnaire: A parent report measure of children's play preferences. *Archives of Sexual Behavior, 20,* 393-409.

Flanery, R. C. (1990). Methodological and psychometric considerations in child reports. In A. M. La Greca (Ed.), *Through the eyes of the child: Obtaining self-reports from children and adolescents* (pp. 57-79). Needham Heights, MA: Allyn & Bacon.

Gregory, M. D. (1983). Occupational behavior and life satisfaction among retirees. *American Journal of Occupational Therapy, 37,* 548-553.

Hanft, B. (1988). The changing environment of early intervention services: Implications for practice. *American Journal of Occupational Therapy, 42,* 724-731.

Hann, J., Regele, K., Walsh, C., Fontana, L., & Bentley, R. (1994). *Item development for a new measure of adolescent leisure interests* (Unpublished manuscript, Worcester State College, Worcester, MA).

Harter, S. (1990). Issues in the assessment of the self-concept in children and adolescents. In A. M. La Greca (Ed.), *Through the eyes of the child: Obtaining self-reports from children and adolescents* (pp. 292-325). Needham Heights, MA: Allyn & Bacon.

Harter, S., & Pike, R. (1984). The pictorial perceived competence scale for young children. *Child Development, 55,* 1969-1982.

Hemphill, B. J. (1980). Mental health evaluations used in occupational therapy. *American Journal of Occupational Therapy, 34,* 721-726.

Henry, A.D. (1994). *Predicting psychosocial functioning and symptomatic recovery among adolescents and young adults with a first psychotic episode: A six-month follow-up study* (Unpublished doctoral dissertation, Boston University, Boston).

Henry, A. D. (1998a). Interview process in occupational therapy. In M. E. Neistadt & E. B. Crepeau (Eds.), *Willard and Spackman's occupational therapy* (9th ed., pp. 155-168). Philadelphia: Lippincott.

Henry, A. D. (1998b). Development of a measure of adolescent leisure interests. *American Journal of Occupational Therapy, 52,* 531-539.

Hinojosa, J., & Kramer, P. (1997). Integrating children with disabilities into family play. In L. D. Parham & L. S. Fazio

(Eds.), *Play in occupational therapy for children,* (pp. 159-170). St. Louis: Mosby.

Kane, W. M., & Duryea, F. J. (1991). The role of education and extracurricular activities. In W. R. Hendee (Ed.), *The health of adolescents: Understanding and facilitating biological, behavioral and social development* (pp. 139-161). San Francisco: Jossey-Bass.

Kielhofner, G. (2002a). *Model of human occupation: Theory and application* (3rd ed.). Baltimore: Lippincott Williams & Wilkins.

Kielhofner, G. (2002b). Doing and becoming: Occupational change and development. In G. Kielhofner (Ed.), *Model of human occupation: Theory and application* (3nd ed., pp. 145-161). Baltimore: Lippincott Williams & Wilkins.

Kielhofner, G. (2002c). Volition. In G. Kielhofner (Ed.), *Model of human occupation: Theory and application* (3nd ed., pp. 44-62). Baltimore: Lippincott Williams & Wilkins.

Kielhofner, G., & Barrett, J. (1998). The model of human occupation. In M. Neistadt & E. B. Crepeau (Eds.), *Occupational therapy* (9th ed., pp. 527-542). Philadelphia: Lippincott.

Kielhofner, G., & Mallinson, F. (1995). Gathering narrative data through interviews: Empirical observations and suggested guidelines. *Scandinavian Journal of Occupational Therapy, 2,* 63-68.

Kleiber, D., Larson, R., & Csikszentmihalyi, M. (1986). The experience of leisure in adolescence. *Journal of Leisure Research, 18*(3), 169-176.

Knox, S. (1997). Development and current use of the Knox Preschool Play Scale. In L. D. Parham & L. S. Fazio (Eds.), *Play in occupational therapy for children* (pp. 35-51). St. Louis: Mosby.

Larson, R., & Kleiber, D. (1993). Daily experiences of adolescents. In P. H. Tolan & B. J. Cohler (Eds.), *Handbook of clinical research and practice with adolescents. Wiley series on personality process* (pp. 125-145). New York: John Wiley & Sons.

Law, M., Baptiste, S., Carswell, A., McColl, M. A., Polatajko, H., & Pollock, N. (1994). *Canadian Occupational Performance Measure.* Toronto: Canadian Association of Occupational Therapists.

Matsutsuyu, J. S. (1969). The interest check list. *American Journal of Occupational Therapy, 23,* 323-328.

Mattingly, C. (1991). The narrative nature of clinical reasoning. *American Journal of Occupational Therapy, 45,* 998-1005.

McKechnie, G. (1975). *Leisure activities blank.* Palo Alto, CA: Consulting Psychologists Press.

Neistadt, M. E., & Crepeau, E. B. (1998). Introduction to occupational therapy. In M. Neistadt & E. B. Crepeau (Eds.), *Occupational therapy* (9th ed., pp. 5-12). Philadelphia: Lippincott.

Parham, L. D., & Fazio, L. S. (Eds.). (1997). *Play in occupational therapy for children.* St. Louis: Mosby.

Piaget, J. (1962). *Play, dreams, and imitation in childhood.* (C. Gattegno & F. M. Hodgson, Trans.) New York: W.W. Norton. (Original work published in 1951.)

Raphael, D. (1996). Determinants of health of North American adolescents: Evolving definitions, recent findings, and proposed research agenda. *Journal of Adolescent Health, 19,* 6-16.

Reilly, M. (1962). Occupational therapy can be one of the great ideas of 20th century medicine. *American Journal of Occupational Therapy, 6,* 1-9.

Reilly, M. (1969). A psychiatric occupational therapy program as a teaching model. *American Journal of Occupational Therapy 23,* 299-307.

Rosenthal, T. L., Muram, D., Arheart, K. L., & Bryant, E. S. (1994). A brief leisure interests checklist for teenagers: Initial response. *Journal of Sex Education and Therapy, 20,* 30-40.

Royeen, C. B. (1985). Adaptation of Likert scaling for use with children. *Occupational Therapy Journal of Research, 5,* 59-69.

Scafidi, F. A., Field, T., Prodromidis, M., & Rahdert, E. (1997). Psychosocial stressors of drug abusing disadvantaged adolescent mothers. *Adolescence, 32,* 93-100.

Stone, W. L., & Lemanek, K. L. (1990). Developmental issues in children's self-reports. In A. M. LaCreca (Ed.), *Through the eyes of the child: Obtaining self-reports from children and adolescents* (pp. 18-55). Boston: Allyn & Bacon.

Sturgess, J. (2007). *The development of a play skills self-report questionnaire (PSSRQ) for 5-10 year old children and their parents/carers* (Unpublished doctoral dissertation, University of Queensland, Queensland, Australia).

Sturgess, J., & Ziviani, J. (1995). Development of a self-report play questionnaire for children aged 5 to 7 years: A preliminary report, *Australian Occupational Journal, 42,* 107-117.

Takata, N. (1969). The play history. *American Journal of Occupational Therapy, 2,* 314-318.

Van der Kooij, R. (1989). Research on children's play. *Play and Culture, 2,* 20-34.

Vicary, J. R., Smith, E., Caldwell, L., & Swisher, J. D. (1998). Relationship of changes in adolescents' leisure activities to alcohol use. *American Journal of Health Behavior, 22,* 276-282.

Williams, S., & McGee, R. (1991). Adolescents' self-perceptions of their strengths. *Journal of Youth and Adolescence, 20,* 325-337.

World Health Organization (2001). *ICF: International classification of functioning, disability and health.* Geneva: World Health Organization.

Appendix 5-A

Kid Play Profile

Kid Play Profile
Alexis D. Henry, ScD, OTR/L

Directions

There are 50 activities in this booklet. For each activity, there are three questions.

1. Do You Do This Activity?

2. Do You Like This Activity?

3. Who Do You Do This Activity With?

If you answer "No" to question 1, you do not need to answer questions 2 or 3. Just go on to the next activity.

You can color or circle your answers.

At the end, you may add other activities that you do and that you weren't asked about.

Name _____ Date _____

Age _____ Birthday _____ Grade _____ Check ☐ Boy ☐ Girl

Kid Play Profile

Sports Activities	Do You Do This Activity?	Do You Like This Activity?	Who Do You Do This Activity With?
1. Play Baseball	Yes No	A Lot A Little Not at All	By Myself With Friends With a Grown-Up
2. Play Basketball	Yes No	A Lot A Little Not at All	By Myself With Friends With a Grown-Up
3. Play Soccer	Yes No	A Lot A Little Not at All	By Myself With Friends With a Grown-Up

Kid Play Profile

Outdoor Activities	Do You Do This Activity?	Do You Like This Activity?	Who Do You Do This Activity With?
4. Play Catch	Yes No	A Lot A Little Not at All	By Myself With Friends With a Grown-Up
5. Ride a Bike	Yes No	A Lot A Little Not at All	By Myself With Friends With a Grown-Up
6. Play Dodgeball	Yes No	A Lot A Little Not at All	By Myself With Friends With a Grown-Up

Kid Play Profile

Outdoor Activities	Do You Do This Activity?	Do You Like This Activity?	Who Do You Do This Activity With?
 7. Play Frisbee®	 Yes No	 A Lot A Little Not at All	 By Myself With Friends With a Grown-Up
 8. Play Hide-and-Seek	 Yes No	 A Lot A Little Not at All	 By Myself With Friends With a Grown-Up
 9. Jump Rope	 Yes No	 A Lot A Little Not at All	 By Myself With Friends With a Grown-Up

Kid Play Profile

Outdoor Activities	Do You Do This Activity?	Do You Like This Activity?	Who Do You Do This Activity With?
10. Play Kickball	Yes / No	A Lot / A Little / Not at All	By Myself / With Friends / With a Grown-Up
11. Play on Playground	Yes / No	A Lot / A Little / Not at All	By Myself / With Friends / With a Grown-Up
12. Roller-Skate or In-Line Skate	Yes / No	A Lot / A Little / Not at All	By Myself / With Friends / With a Grown-Up

Kid Play Profile

Outdoor Activities	Do You Do This Activity?	Do You Like This Activity?	Who Do You Do This Activity With?
13. Play Tag	Yes No	A Lot A Little Not at All	By Myself With Friends With a Grown-Up

Kid Play Profile

Summer Activities	Do You Do This Activity?	Do You Like This Activity?	Who Do You Do This Activity With?
14. Play at Beach, Lake, or River	Yes No	A Lot A Little Not at All	By Myself With Friends With a Grown-Up
15. Go on Picnic	Yes No	A Lot A Little Not at All	By Myself With Friends With a Grown-Up
16. Swim	Yes No	A Lot A Little Not at All	By Myself With Friends With a Grown-Up

Kid Play Profile

Summer Activities	Do You Do This Activity?	Do You Like This Activity?	Who Do You Do This Activity With?
17. Camp	Yes No	A Lot A Little Not at All	By Myself With Friends With a Grown-Up
18. Hike	Yes No	A Lot A Little Not at All	By Myself With Friends With a Grown-Up
19. Go Fishing	Yes No	A Lot A Little Not at All	By Myself With Friends With a Grown-Up

Kid Play Profile

Summer Activities	Do you do this activity?	Do you like this activity?	Who do you do this activity with?

Kid Play Profile

Winter Activities	Do You Do This Activity?	Do You Like This Activity?	Who Do You Do This Activity With?
21. Go Sledding	Yes No	A Lot A Little Not at All	By Myself With Friends With a Grown-Up
22. Play in Snow	Yes No	A Lot A Little Not at All	By Myself With Friends With a Grown-Up
23. Ice-Skate	Yes No	A Lot A Little Not at All	By Myself With Friends With a Grown-Up

Kid Play Profile

Winter Activities	Do You Do This Activity?	Do You Like This Activity?	Who Do You Do This Activity With?

24. Ski or Snowboard

Do You Do This Activity?
Yes   No

Do You Like This Activity?
A Lot   A Little   Not at All

Who Do You Do This Activity With?
By Myself   With Friends   With a Grown-Up

Kid Play Profile

Indoor Activities	Do You Do This Activity?	Do You Like This Activity?	Who Do You Do This Activity With?
25. Play Cards	Yes No	A Lot A Little Not at All	By Myself With Friends With a Grown-Up
26. Play Board Games	Yes No	A Lot A Little Not at All	By Myself With Friends With a Grown-Up
27. Read	Yes No	A Lot A Little Not at All	By Myself With Friends With a Grown-Up

Kid Play Profile

Indoor Activities	Do You Do This Activity?	Do You Like This Activity?	Who Do You Do This Activity With?
28. Use Computer	Yes / No	A Lot / A Little / Not at All	By Myself / With Friends / With a Grown-Up
29. Watch TV	Yes / No	A Lot / A Little / Not at All	By Myself / With Friends / With a Grown-Up
30. Listen to Music	Yes / No	A Lot / A Little / Not at All	By Myself / With Friends / With a Grown-Up

Kid Play Profile

Indoor Activities	Do You Do This Activity?	Do You Like This Activity?	Who Do You Do This Activity With?
31. Collect Things	Yes / No	A Lot / A Little / Not at All	By Myself / With Friends / With a Grown-Up
32. Take Care of Pet	Yes / No	A Lot / A Little / Not at All	By Myself / With Friends / With a Grown-Up

Kid Play Profile

Creative Activities	Do You Do This Activity?	Do You Like This Activity?	Who Do You Do This Activity With?
33. Do Puzzles	Yes / No	A Lot · A Little · Not at All	By Myself · With Friends · With a Grown-Up
34. Sing	Yes / No	A Lot · A Little · Not at All	By Myself · With Friends · With a Grown-Up
35. Dance	Yes / No	A Lot · A Little · Not at All	By Myself · With Friends · With a Grown-Up

Kid Play Profile

Creative Activities	Do You Do This Activity?	Do You Like This Activity?	Who Do You Do This Activity With?
36. Build Things	Yes No	A Lot A Little Not at All	By Myself With Friends With a Grown-Up
37. Draw or Paint	Yes No	A Lot A Little Not at All	By Myself With Friends With a Grown-Up
38. Cook or Bake	Yes No	A Lot A Little Not at All	By Myself With Friends With a Grown-Up

Kid Play Profile

Lessons/Classes	Do You Do This Activity?	Do You Like This Activity?	Who Do You Do This Activity With?
39. Music Lessons	Yes / No	A Lot / A Little / Not at All	By Myself / With Friends / With a Grown-Up
40. Swimming Lessons	Yes / No	A Lot / A Little / Not at All	By Myself / With Friends / With a Grown-Up
41. Dance Lessons	Yes / No	A Lot / A Little / Not at All	By Myself / With Friends / With a Grown-Up

Kid Play Profile

Lessons/Classes	Do You Do This Activity?	Do You Like This Activity?	Who Do You Do This Activity With?
42. Gymnastics Lessons	Yes / No	A Lot / A Little / Not at All	By Myself / With Friends / With a Grown-Up
43. Arts and Carfts Lessons	Yes / No	A Lot / A Little / Not at All	By Myself / With Friends / With a Grown-Up
44. Martial Arts Lessons	Yes / No	A Lot / A Little / Not at All	By Myself / With Friends / With a Grown-Up

Kid Play Profile

Socializing Activities	Do You Do This Activity?	Do You Like This Activity?	Who Do You Do This Activity With?
45. Hang Out With Friends	Yes / No	A Lot / A Little / Not at All	By Myself / With Friends / With a Grown-Up
46. Go to Scouts	Yes / No	A Lot / A Little / Not at All	By Myself / With Friends / With a Grown-Up
47. Play Superheroes	Yes / No	A Lot / A Little / Not at All	By Myself / With Friends / With a Grown-Up

Kid Play Profile

Socializing Activities	Do You Do This Activity?	Do You Like This Activity?	Who Do You Do This Activity With?
48. Play School	Yes No	A Lot A Little Not at All	By Myself With Friends With a Grown-Up
49. Play House	Yes No	A Lot A Little Not at All	By Myself With Friends With a Grown-Up
50. Play Dress-Up or Make-Up	Yes No	A Lot A Little Not at All	By Myself With Friends With a Grown-Up

Kid Play Profile

Socializing Activities	Do You Do This Activity?	Do You Like This Activity?	Who Do You Do This Activity With?
51. Fill in Your Own	Yes No	A Lot A Little Not at All	By Myself With Friends With a Grown-Up
52. Fill in Your Own	Yes No	A Lot A Little Not at All	By Myself With Friends With a Grown-Up
53. Fill in Your Own	Yes No	A Lot A Little Not at All	By Myself With Friends With a Grown-Up

Kid Play Profile

Socializing Activities	Do You Do This Activity?	Do You Like This Activity?	Who Do You Do This Activity With?
54. Fill in Your Own	Yes No	A Lot A Little Not at All	By Myself With Friends With a Grown-Up
55. Fill in Your Own	Yes No	A Lot A Little Not at All	By Myself With Friends With a Grown-Up

Kid Play Profile
Alexis D. Henry, ScD, OTR/L
Summary Score Sheet

Child's Name _____

School _____

Service Provider's Name _____

Discipline _____

Gender ☐ Male ☐ Female

Grade _____

	Year	Month	Day
Date Tested			
Date of Birth			
Chronological Age			

The child receives the following service(s) _____

Conditions that may affect the child's play _____

Category Scores
Instructions

Transfer the following information from the child's *Kid Play Profile* to each corresponding category table.

Place a checkmark in the "Yes" column of each activity in which the child has participated.

In the next three columns, circle the score that indicates how the child likes the activity (3 = a lot; 2 = a little; 1 = not at all).

Place a checkmark in one or more of the last three columns to indicate with whom the child does the activity.

Scoring

Add the checkmarks in the *Yes* column and place this number in the box labeled *Number of (Sports, Outside, etc.) Activities Child Participates in.*

Divide the number of activities the child participates in by the total number of activities in the category. Then multiply by 100 to calculate the percent of activities the child participates in. Place the percent in the box labeled *Percent of Activities the Child Participates in.*

To calculate how much the child likes the category activities, add the scores of the three columns. Divide the total by the number of activities the child participates in. Place this number in the box labeled *How Much the Child Likes Activities.* Scores will range from 1 to 3. The closer the number is to 3, the more the child likes the activities.

To calculate the percent of activities that the child does alone, with friends, or with an adult, add the checkmarks in each column. Divide the total for each column by the number of activities the child participates in. Multiply each total by 100 and place the percent in the appropriate place in the box labeled *Percent of Activities the Child Does By Myself, With Friends,* or *With a Grown-Up.* Because children may give more than one answer for this question (for example, children may do an activity both "by myself" and "with friends"), the total for the 3 responses may exceed 100%.

Sports Activities	Yes	A Lot	A Little	Not at All	By Myself	With Friends	With a Grown-Up
1. Play Baseball		3	2	1			
2. Play Basketball		3	2	1			
3. Play Soccer		3	2	1			
Total							

Number of Sports Activities Child Participates in _____ Percent of Sports Activities Child Participates in _____	How Much the Child Likes Sports Activities _____	Percent of Activities the Child Does By Myself _____ With Friends _____ With a Grown-Up _____

Play Interview

Outside Activities	Yes	A Lot	A Little	Not at All	By Myself	With Friends	With a Grown-Up
4. Play Catch		3	2	1			
5. Ride a Bike		3	2	1			
6. Play Dodgeball		3	2	1			
7. Play Frisbee®		3	2	1			
8. Play Hide-and-Seek		3	2	1			
9. Jump Rope		3	2	1			
10. Play Kickball		3	2	1			
11. Play on Playground		3	2	1			
12. Roller-Skate or In-Line Skate		3	2	1			
13. Play Tag		3	2	1			
Total							

Number of Outside Activities Child Participates in _____ Percent of Outside Activities Child Participates in _____	How Much the Child Likes Outside Activities _____	Percent of Activities the Child Does By Myself _____ With Friends _____ With a Grown-Up _____

Play Interview

Summer Activities	Yes	A Lot	A Little	Not at All	By Myself	With Friends	With a Grown-Up
14. Play at Beach, Lake, or River		3	2	1			
15. Go on Picnic		3	2	1			
16. Swim		3	2	1			
17. Camp		3	2	1			
18. Hike		3	2	1			
19. Go Fishing		3	2	1			
20. Garden		3	2	1			
Total							

Number of Summer Activities Child Participates in _____

Percent of Summer Activities Child Participates in _____

How Much the Child Likes Summer Activities _____

Percent of Activities the Child Does
By Myself _____
With Friends _____
With a Grown-Up _____

Play Interview

Winter Activities	Yes	A Lot	A Little	Not at All	By Myself	With Friends	With a Grown-Up
21. Go Sledding		3	2	1			
22. Play in Snow		3	2	1			
23. Ice-Skate		3	2	1			
24. Ski or Snowboard		3	2	1			
Total							

Number of Winter Activities Child Participates in _____

Percent of Winter Activities Child Participates in _____

How Much the Child Likes Winter Activities _____

Percent of Activities the Child Does
By Myself _____
With Friends _____
With a Grown-Up _____

Play Interview

Indoor Activities	Yes	A Lot	A Little	Not at All	By Myself	With Friends	With a Grown-Up
25. Play Cards		3	2	1			
26. Play Board Games		3	2	1			
27. Read		3	2	1			
28. Use Computer		3	2	1			
29. Watch TV		3	2	1			
30. Listen to Music		3	2	1			
31. Collect Things		3	2	1			
32. Take Care of Pet		3	2	1			
Total							

Number of Indoor Activities Child Participates in _____

Percent of Indoor Activities Child Participates in _____

How Much the Child Likes Indoor Activities _____

Percent of Activities the Child Does
  By Myself _____
  With Friends _____
  With a Grown-Up _____

Play Interview

Creative Activities	Yes	A Lot	A Little	Not at All	By Myself	With Friends	With a Grown-Up
33. Do Puzzles		3	2	1			
34. Sing		3	2	1			
35. Dance		3	2	1			
36. Build Things		3	2	1			
37. Draw or Paint		3	2	1			
38. Cook or Bake		3	2	1			
Total							

Number of Creative Activities Child Participates in _____

Percent of Creative Activities Child Participates in _____

How Much the Child Likes Creative Activities _____

Percent of Activities the Child Does
  By Myself _____
  With Friends _____
  With a Grown-Up _____

Play Interview

Lessons/Classes	Yes	A Lot	A Little	Not at All	By Myself	With Friends	With a Grown-Up
39. Music Lessons		3	2	1			
40. Swimming Lessons		3	2	1			
41. Dance Lessons		3	2	1			
42. Gymnastics Lessons		3	2	1			
43. Arts and Crafts Lessons		3	2	1			
44. Martial Arts Lessons		3	2	1			
Total							

Number of Lessons Child Participates in _____

Percent of Lessons Child Participates in _____

How Much the Child Likes Lessons _____

Percent of Lessons the Child Does
    By Myself _____
    With Friends _____
    With a Grown-Up _____

Play Interview

Socializing Activities	Yes	A Lot	A Little	Not at All	By Myself	With Friends	With a Grown-Up
45. Hang Out With Friends		3	2	1			
46. Go to Scouts		3	2	1			
47. Play Superheroes		3	2	1			
48. Play School		3	2	1			
49. Play House		3	2	1			
50. Play Dress-Up or Make-Up		3	2	1			
Total							

Number of Socializing Activities Child Participates in _____

Percent of Socializing Activities Child Participates in _____

How Much the Child Likes Socializing Activities _____

Percent of Activities the Child Does
    By Myself _____
    With Friends _____
    With a Grown-Up _____

Play Interview

Other Activities	Yes	A Lot	A Little	Not at All	By Myself	With Friends	With a Grown-Up
51.		3	2	1			
52.		3	2	1			
53.		3	2	1			
54.		3	2	1			
55.		3	2	1			
Total							

Number of Other Activities Child Participates in _____
 	
Percent of Other Activities Child Participates in _____
	How Much the Child Likes Other Activities _____	Percent of Activities the Child Does
		   By Myself _____
		   With Friends _____
		   With a Grown-Up _____

Play Interview

Total (Exclude "other" activities when calculating totals)

Number of Activities Child Participates in (sum the totals of the 8 categories) _____
Percent of Activities Child Participates in (divide the above number by 50)_____
	How Much the Child Likes All Activities He or She Participates in (sum the scores for the 8 categories and divide the number by 8) _____	Percent of All Activities the Child Does
		   By Myself _____
		   With Friends _____
		   With a Grown-Up _____
		(add final percentages from each column and divide by 8)

Play Interview Summary

_____
_____
_____
_____

Play Observations

_____
_____
_____
_____

Interpretations/Recommendations

_____
_____
_____
_____

Appendix 5-B

Preteen Play Profile

Preteen Play Profile
Alexis D. Henry, ScD, OTR/L

Directions

There are 59 activities in this booklet. For each activity, there are five questions.

1. Do you do this activity?
2. How often do you do this activity?
3. How much do you like this activity?
4. How good are you at this activity?
5. Who do you do this activity with?

If you answer "No" to question 1, you do *not* need to answer questions 2 through 5. Just go on to the next activity.

Circle only one answer for questions 1 through 4. You can circle more than one answer for question 5.

There are no right or wrong answers. Your answers should show how you really feel.

At the end, you may add other activities that you do and that you weren't asked about.

Name _____ Date _____

Age _____ Birthday _____ Grade _____ Check ☐ Boy ☐ Girl

Preteen Play Profile

Sports Activities	Do You Do This Activity?	How Often Do You Do This Activity?			How Much Do You Like This Activity?			How Good Are You At This Activity?			Who Do You Do This Activity With?		
1. Play Baseball or Softball	Yes No	Once a Week or More	Once a Month or More	Once a Year or More	A Lot	A Little	Not at All	Very Good	So-So	Not So Good	By Myself	With Friends	With a Grown-Up
2. Play Basketball	Yes No	Once a Week or More	Once a Month or More	Once a Year or More	A Lot	A Little	Not at All	Very Good	So-So	Not So Good	By Myself	With Friends	With a Grown-Up
3. Play Soccer	Yes No	Once a Week or More	Once a Month or More	Once a Year or More	A Lot	A Little	Not at All	Very Good	So-So	Not So Good	By Myself	With Friends	With a Grown-Up
4. Play Football	Yes No	Once a Week or More	Once a Month or More	Once a Year or More	A Lot	A Little	Not at All	Very Good	So-So	Not So Good	By Myself	With Friends	With a Grown-Up
5. Play Ice Hockey or Field Hockey	Yes No	Once a Week or More	Once a Month or More	Once a Year or More	A Lot	A Little	Not at All	Very Good	So-So	Not So Good	By Myself	With Friends	With a Grown-Up

Preteen Play Profile

Outdoor Activities	Do You Do This Activity?	How Often Do You Do This Activity?			How Much Do You Like This Activity?			How Good Are You At This Activity?			Who Do You Do This Activity With?		
6. Play Catch	Yes No	Once a Week or More	Once a Month or More	Once a Year or More	A Lot	A Little	Not at All	Very Good	So-So	Not So Good	By Myself	With Friends	With a Grown-Up
7. Ride Bike	Yes No	Once a Week or More	Once a Month or More	Once a Year or More	A Lot	A Little	Not at All	Very Good	So-So	Not So Good	By Myself	With Friends	With a Grown-Up
8. Play Dodgeball	Yes No	Once a Week or More	Once a Month or More	Once a Year or More	A Lot	A Little	Not at All	Very Good	So-So	Not So Good	By Myself	With Friends	With a Grown-Up
9. Play Frisbee®	Yes No	Once a Week or More	Once a Month or More	Once a Year or More	A Lot	A Little	Not at All	Very Good	So-So	Not So Good	By Myself	With Friends	With a Grown-Up
10. Jump Rope	Yes No	Once a Week or More	Once a Month or More	Once a Year or More	A Lot	A Little	Not at All	Very Good	So-So	Not So Good	By Myself	With Friends	With a Grown-Up

Preteen Play Profile

Outdoor Activities	Do You Do This Activity?	How Often Do You Do This Activity?			How Much Do You Like This Activity?			How Good Are You At This Activity?			Who Do You Do This Activity With?		
11. Play Kickball	Yes No	Once a Week or More	Once a Month or More	Once a Year or More	A Lot	A Little	Not at All	Very Good	So-So	Not So Good	By Myself	With Friends	With a Grown-Up
12. Play on Playground	Yes No	Once a Week or More	Once a Month or More	Once a Year or More	A Lot	A Little	Not at All	Very Good	So-So	Not So Good	By Myself	With Friends	With a Grown-Up
13. Roller-Skate or In-Line Skate	Yes No	Once a Week or More	Once a Month or More	Once a Year or More	A Lot	A Little	Not at All	Very Good	So-So	Not So Good	By Myself	With Friends	With a Grown-Up
14. Skateboard	Yes No	Once a Week or More	Once a Month or More	Once a Year or More	A Lot	A Little	Not at All	Very Good	So-So	Not So Good	By Myself	With Friends	With a Grown-Up

Preteen Play Profile

Summer Activities	Do You Do This Activity?	How Often Do You Do This Activity?	How Much Do You Like This Activity?	How Good Are You At This Activity?	Who Do You Do This Activity With?
15. Play at Beach, Lake, or River	Yes No	Once a Week or More / Once a Month or More / Once a Year or More	A Lot / A Little / Not at All	Very Good / So-So / Not So Good	By Myself / With Friends / With a Grown-Up
16. Go on Picnic	Yes No	Once a Week or More / Once a Month or More / Once a Year or More	A Lot / A Little / Not at All	Very Good / So-So / Not So Good	By Myself / With Friends / With a Grown-Up
17. Swim	Yes No	Once a Week or More / Once a Month or More / Once a Year or More	A Lot / A Little / Not at All	Very Good / So-So / Not So Good	By Myself / With Friends / With a Grown-Up
18. Camp	Yes No	Once a Week or More / Once a Month or More / Once a Year or More	A Lot / A Little / Not at All	Very Good / So-So / Not So Good	By Myself / With Friends / With a Grown-Up
19. Hike	Yes No	Once a Week or More / Once a Month or More / Once a Year or More	A Lot / A Little / Not at All	Very Good / So-So / Not So Good	By Myself / With Friends / With a Grown-Up

Preteen Play Profile

Summer Activities	Do You Do This Activity?	How Often Do You Do This Activity?	How Much Do You Like This Activity?	How Good Are You At This Activity?	Who Do You Do This Activity With?
20. Go Fishing	Yes No	Once a Week or More Once a Month or More Once a Year or More	A Lot A Little Not at All	Very Good So-So Not So Good	By Myself With Friends With a Grown-Up
21. Garden	Yes No	Once a Week or More Once a Month or More Once a Year or More	A Lot A Little Not at All	Very Good So-So Not So Good	By Myself With Friends With a Grown-Up
22. Sail or Canoe	Yes No	Once a Week or More Once a Month or More Once a Year or More	A Lot A Little Not at All	Very Good So-So Not So Good	By Myself With Friends With a Grown-Up

Preteen Play Profile

Winter Activities	Do You Do This Activity?	How Often Do You Do This Activity?			How Much Do You Like This Activity?			How Good Are You At This Activity?			Who Do You Do This Activity With?		
23. Go Sledding	Yes No	Once a Week or More	Once a Month or More	Once a Year or More	A Lot	A Little	Not at All	Very Good	So-So	Not So Good	By Myself	With Friends	With a Grown-Up
24. Play in Snow	Yes No	Once a Week or More	Once a Month or More	Once a Year or More	A Lot	A Little	Not at All	Very Good	So-So	Not So Good	By Myself	With Friends	With a Grown-Up
25. Ice-Skate	Yes No	Once a Week or More	Once a Month or More	Once a Year or More	A Lot	A Little	Not at All	Very Good	So-So	Not So Good	By Myself	With Friends	With a Grown-Up
26. Ski or Snowboard	Yes No	Once a Week or More	Once a Month or More	Once a Year or More	A Lot	A Little	Not at All	Very Good	So-So	Not So Good	By Myself	With Friends	With a Grown-Up

Preteen Play Profile

Indoor Activities	Do You Do This Activity?		How Often Do You Do This Activity?			How Much Do You Like This Activity?			How Good Are You At This Activity?			Who Do You Do This Activity With?		
27. Play Cards	Yes	No	Once a Week or More	Once a Month or More	Once a Year or More	A Lot	A Little	Not at All	Very Good	So-So	Not So Good	By Myself	With Friends	With a Grown-Up
28. Play Board Games	Yes	No	Once a Week or More	Once a Month or More	Once a Year or More	A Lot	A Little	Not at All	Very Good	So-So	Not So Good	By Myself	With Friends	With a Grown-Up
29. Read	Yes	No	Once a Week or More	Once a Month or More	Once a Year or More	A Lot	A Little	Not at All	Very Good	So-So	Not So Good	By Myself	With Friends	With a Grown-Up
30. Use Computer	Yes	No	Once a Week or More	Once a Month or More	Once a Year or More	A Lot	A Little	Not at All	Very Good	So-So	Not So Good	By Myself	With Friends	With a Grown-Up
31. Watch TV	Yes	No	Once a Week or More	Once a Month or More	Once a Year or More	A Lot	A Little	Not at All	Very Good	So-So	Not So Good	By Myself	With Friends	With a Grown-Up

Preteen Play Profile

Indoor Activities	Do You Do This Activity?	How Often Do You Do This Activity?			How Much Do You Like This Activity?			How Good Are You At This Activity?			Who Do You Do This Activity With?		
32. Listen to Music	Yes No	Once a Week or More	Once a Month or More	Once a Year or More	A Lot	A Little	Not at All	Very Good	So-So	Not So Good	By Myself	With Friends	With a Grown-Up
33. Collect Things	Yes No	Once a Week or More	Once a Month or More	Once a Year or More	A Lot	A Little	Not at All	Very Good	So-So	Not So Good	By Myself	With Friends	With a Grown-Up
34. Take Care of Pet	Yes No	Once a Week or More	Once a Month or More	Once a Year or More	A Lot	A Little	Not at All	Very Good	So-So	Not So Good	By Myself	With Friends	With a Grown-Up
35. Play Video Games	Yes No	Once a Week or More	Once a Month or More	Once a Year or More	A Lot	A Little	Not at All	Very Good	So-So	Not So Good	By Myself	With Friends	With a Grown-Up

Preteen Play Profile

Creative Activities	Do You Do This Activity?	How Often Do You Do This Activity?			How Much Do You Like This Activity?			How Good Are You At This Activity?			Who Do You Do This Activity With?		
36. Do Puzzles	Yes No	Once a Week or More	Once a Month or More	Once a Year or More	A Lot	A Little	Not at All	Very Good	So-So	Not So Good	By Myself	With Friends	With a Grown-Up
37. Sing	Yes No	Once a Week or More	Once a Month or More	Once a Year or More	A Lot	A Little	Not at All	Very Good	So-So	Not So Good	By Myself	With Friends	With a Grown-Up
38. Dance	Yes No	Once a Week or More	Once a Month or More	Once a Year or More	A Lot	A Little	Not at All	Very Good	So-So	Not So Good	By Myself	With Friends	With a Grown-Up
39. Build Things	Yes No	Once a Week or More	Once a Month or More	Once a Year or More	A Lot	A Little	Not at All	Very Good	So-So	Not So Good	By Myself	With Friends	With a Grown-Up
40. Draw or Paint	Yes No	Once a Week or More	Once a Month or More	Once a Year or More	A Lot	A Little	Not at All	Very Good	So-So	Not So Good	By Myself	With Friends	With a Grown-Up

Preteen Play Profile

Creative Activities	Do You Do This Activity?	How Often Do You Do This Activity?			How Much Do You Like This Activity?			How Good Are You At This Activity?				Who Do You Do This Activity With?		
41. Cook or Bake	Yes No	Once a Week or More	Once a Month or More	Once a Year or More	A Lot	A Little	Not at All	Very Good	So-So	Not So Good		By Myself	With Friends	With a Grown-Up
42. Make Jewelry	Yes No	Once a Week or More	Once a Month or More	Once a Year or More	A Lot	A Little	Not at All	Very Good	So-So	Not So Good		By Myself	With Friends	With a Grown-Up

Preteen Play Profile

Lessons/Classes	Do You Do This Activity?		How Often Do You Do This Activity?			How Much Do You Like This Activity?			How Good Are You At This Activity?			Who Do You Do This Activity With?		
	Yes	No	Once a Week or More	Once a Month or More	Once a Year or More	A Lot	A Little	Not at All	Very Good	So-So	Not So Good	By Myself	With Friends	With a Grown-Up
43. Music Lessons	Yes	No	Once a Week or More	Once a Month or More	Once a Year or More	A Lot	A Little	Not at All	Very Good	So-So	Not So Good	By Myself	With Friends	With a Grown-Up
44. Swimming Lessons	Yes	No	Once a Week or More	Once a Month or More	Once a Year or More	A Lot	A Little	Not at All	Very Good	So-So	Not So Good	By Myself	With Friends	With a Grown-Up
45. Dance Lessons	Yes	No	Once a Week or More	Once a Month or More	Once a Year or More	A Lot	A Little	Not at All	Very Good	So-So	Not So Good	By Myself	With Friends	With a Grown-Up
46. Gymnastics Lessons	Yes	No	Once a Week or More	Once a Month or More	Once a Year or More	A Lot	A Little	Not at All	Very Good	So-So	Not So Good	By Myself	With Friends	With a Grown-Up
47. Arts & Crafts Lessons	Yes	No	Once a Week or More	Once a Month or More	Once a Year or More	A Lot	A Little	Not at All	Very Good	So-So	Not So Good	By Myself	With Friends	With a Grown-Up

Preteen Play Profile

Lessons/Classes	Do You Do This Activity?	How Often Do You Do This Activity?			How Much Do You Like This Activity?			How Good Are You At This Activity?			Who Do You Do This Activity With?		
48. Martial Arts Lessons	Yes No	Once a Week or More	Once a Month or More	Once a Year or More	A Lot	A Little	Not at All	Very Good	So-So	Not So Good	By Myself	With Friends	With a Grown-Up
49. Horseback Riding Lessons	Yes No	Once a Week or More	Once a Month or More	Once a Year or More	A Lot	A Little	Not at All	Very Good	So-So	Not So Good	By Myself	With Friends	With a Grown-Up

Preteen Play Profile

Socializing Activities	Do You Do This Activity?	How Often Do You Do This Activity?			How Much Do You Like This Activity?			How Good Are You At This Activity?			Who Do You Do This Activity With?		
50. Hang Out With Friends	Yes No	Once a Week or More	Once a Month or More	Once a Year or More	A Lot	A Little	Not at All	Very Good	So-So	Not So Good	By Myself	With Friends	With a Grown-Up
51. Go to Scouts, 4-H, or Campfire	Yes No	Once a Week or More	Once a Month or More	Once a Year or More	A Lot	A Little	Not at All	Very Good	So-So	Not So Good	By Myself	With Friends	With a Grown-Up
52. Play Superheroes	Yes No	Once a Week or More	Once a Month or More	Once a Year or More	A Lot	A Little	Not at All	Very Good	So-So	Not So Good	By Myself	With Friends	With a Grown-Up
53. Play School	Yes No	Once a Week or More	Once a Month or More	Once a Year or More	A Lot	A Little	Not at All	Very Good	So-So	Not So Good	By Myself	With Friends	With a Grown-Up
54. Play Dress-Up or Make-Up	Yes No	Once a Week or More	Once a Month or More	Once a Year or More	A Lot	A Little	Not at All	Very Good	So-So	Not So Good	By Myself	With Friends	With a Grown-Up

Preteen Play Profile

Socializing Activities	Do You Do This Activity?	How Often Do You Do This Activity?	How Much Do You Like This Activity?	How Good Are You At This Activity?	Who Do You Do This Activity With?
55. Go to Movies	Yes No	Once a Week or More Once a Month or More Once a Year or More	A Lot A Little Not at All	Very Good So-So Not So Good	By Myself With Friends With a Grown-Up
56. Go Out to Eat	Yes No	Once a Week or More Once a Month or More Once a Year or More	A Lot A Little Not at All	Very Good So-So Not So Good	By Myself With Friends With a Grown-Up
57. Go Shopping	Yes No	Once a Week or More Once a Month or More Once a Year or More	A Lot A Little Not at All	Very Good So-So Not So Good	By Myself With Friends With a Grown-Up
58. Talk on Phone	Yes No	Once a Week or More Once a Month or More Once a Year or More	A Lot A Little Not at All	Very Good So-So Not So Good	By Myself With Friends With a Grown-Up
59. Go to Arcade	Yes No	Once a Week or More Once a Month or More Once a Year or More	A Lot A Little Not at All	Very Good So-So Not So Good	By Myself With Friends With a Grown-Up

Preteen Play Profile

Other Activities	Do You Do This Activity?		How Often Do You Do This Activity?			How Much Do You Like This Activity?			How Good Are You At This Activity?			Who Do You Do This Activity With?		
	Yes	No	Once a Week or More	Once a Month or More	Once a Year or More	A Lot	A Little	Not at All	Very Good	So-So	Not So Good	By Myself	With Friends	With a Grown-Up
60. Fill in Your Own	Yes	No	Once a Week or More	Once a Month or More	Once a Year or More	A Lot	A Little	Not at All	Very Good	So-So	Not So Good	By Myself	With Friends	With a Grown-Up
61. Fill in Your Own	Yes	No	Once a Week or More	Once a Month or More	Once a Year or More	A Lot	A Little	Not at All	Very Good	So-So	Not So Good	By Myself	With Friends	With a Grown-Up
62. Fill in Your Own	Yes	No	Once a Week or More	Once a Month or More	Once a Year or More	A Lot	A Little	Not at All	Very Good	So-So	Not So Good	By Myself	With Friends	With a Grown-Up
63. Fill in Your Own	Yes	No	Once a Week or More	Once a Month or More	Once a Year or More	A Lot	A Little	Not at All	Very Good	So-So	Not So Good	By Myself	With Friends	With a Grown-Up
64. Fill in Your Own	Yes	No	Once a Week or More	Once a Month or More	Once a Year or More	A Lot	A Little	Not at All	Very Good	So-So	Not So Good	By Myself	With Friends	With a Grown-Up

Preteen Play Profile
Alexis D. Henry, ScD, OTR/L
Summary Score Sheet

Child's Name _____

School _____

Service Provider's Name _____

Discipline _____

Gender ☐ Male ☐ Female

Grade _____

	Year	Month	Day
Date Tested			
Date of Birth			
Chronological Age			

The child receives the following service(s) _____

_____

Conditions that may affect the child's play _____

_____

Category Scores
Instructions

Transfer the following information from the child's *Preteen Play Profile* to each corresponding category table.

Place a checkmark in the "Yes" column of each activity in which the child has participated.

In the next three sets of columns, transfer the child's scores that indicate how the child likes the activity, how often the child does the activity, and how good the child perceives him- or herself at the activity.

Finally, place a checkmark in one or more of the last three columns to indicate with whom the child does the activity.

Scoring

Add the checkmarks in the "Yes" column and place this number in the box labeled *Number of (Sports, Outside, etc.) Activities Child Participates in.*

Divide the number of activities the child participates in by the total number of activities in the category. Then multiply by 100 to calculate the percent of activities the child participates in. Place the percent in the box labeled *Percent of Activities the Child Participates in.*

To calculate how often the child does the category activities, add the scores of the three columns labeled *Once a Week or More, Once a Month or More,* and *Once a Year or More.* Divide the total by the number of activities the child participates in. Place this sum in the box labeled *How Often the Child Does (Sports, Outside, etc.) Activities.* The closer the number is to 3, the more frequently the child participates in the activities.

To calculate how much the child likes the category activities, add the scores of the three columns labeled *A Lot, A Little, Not at All.* Divide the total by the number of activities the child participates in. Place this sum in the box labeled *How Much the Child Likes Activities.* The closer the number is to 3, the more the child likes the activities.

To calcualte how good the child is at doing the category activities, add the scores of the three columns labeled *Very Good, So-So, Not So Good.* Divide the total by the number of activities the child participates in. Place this sum in the box labeled *How Good the Child Perceives Him- or Herself to be at the Activities.* The closer the number is to 3, the more the child perceives him- or herself to be good at the activities

To calculate the percent of activities that the child does alone, with friends, and with an adult, add the checkmarks in each column. Divide the total for each column by the number of activities the child participates in. Multiply each total by 100 and place the percent in the appropriate place in the box labeled *Percent of Activities the Child Does By Myself, With Friends, or With a Grown-Up.* Because children may give more than one answer for this question (for example, children may do an activity both "by myself" and "with friends"), the total for the 3 responses may exceed 100%.

Sports Activities	Yes	Once a Week or More	Once a Month or More	Once a Year or More	A Lot	A Little	Not at All	Very Good	So-So	Not So Good	By Myself	With Friends	With a Grown-Up
1. Play Baseball or Softball		3	2	1	3	2	1	3	2	1			
2. Play Basketball		3	2	1	3	2	1	3	2	1			
3. Play Soccer		3	2	1	3	2	1	3	2	1			
4. Play Football		3	2	1	3	2	1	3	2	1			
5. Play Ice or Field Hockey		3	2	1	3	2	1	3	2	1			
Total													

Number of Sports Activities Child Participates in _____

Percent of Sports Activities Child Participates in _____

How Often the Child Does Sports Activities

_____

How Much the Child Likes Sports Activities

_____

How Good the Child Perceives Him- or Herself to be at the Activities

_____

Percent of Activities the Child Does
By Myself _____
With Friends _____
With a Grown-Up _____

Play Interview

Outdoor Activities	Yes	Once a Week or More	Once a Month or More	Once a Year or More	A Lot	A Little	Not at All	Very Good	So-So	Not So Good	By Myself	With Friends	With a Grown-Up
6. Play Catch		3	2	1	3	2	1	3	2	1			
7. Ride Bike		3	2	1	3	2	1	3	2	1			
8. Play Dodgeball		3	2	1	3	2	1	3	2	1			
9. Play Frisbee®		3	2	1	3	2	1	3	2	1			
10. Jump Rope		3	2	1	3	2	1	3	2	1			
11. Play Kickball		3	2	1	3	2	1	3	2	1			
12. Play on Playground		3	2	1	3	2	1	3	2	1			
13. Roller-Skate or In-Line Skate		3	2	1	3	2	1	3	2	1			
14. Skateboard		3	2	1	3	2	1	3	2	1			
Total													

Number of Outdoor Activities Child Participates in _____

Percent of Outdoor Activities Child Participates in _____

How Often the Child Does the Activities

_____

How Much the Child Likes Outdoor Activities

_____

How Good the Child Perceives Him- or Herself to be at the Activities

_____

Percent of Activities the Child Does
By Myself _____
With Friends _____
With a Grown-Up _____

Play Interview

Summer Activities	Yes	Once a Week or More	Once a Month or More	Once a Year or More	A Lot	A Little	Not at All	Very Good	So-So	Not So Good	By Myself	With Friends	With a Grown-Up
15. Play at Beach, Lake, or River		3	2	1	3	2	1	3	2	1			
16. Go on Picnic		3	2	1	3	2	1	3	2	1			
17. Swim		3	2	1	3	2	1	3	2	1			
18. Camp		3	2	1	3	2	1	3	2	1			
19. Hike		3	2	1	3	2	1	3	2	1			
20. Go Fishing		3	2	1	3	2	1	3	2	1			
21. Garden		3	2	1	3	2	1	3	2	1			
22. Sail or Canoe		3	2	1	3	2	1	3	2	1			
Total													

Number of Summer Activities Child Participates in _____

Percent of Summer Activities Child Participates in _____

How Often the Child Does the Activities

_____

How Much the Child Likes Summer Activities

_____

How Good the Child Perceives Him- or Herself to be at the Activities

_____

Percent of Activities the Child Does
By Myself _____
With Friends _____
With a Grown-Up _____

Play Interview

Winter Activities	Yes	Once a Week or More	Once a Month or More	Once a Year or More	A Lot	A Little	Not at All	Very Good	So-So	Not So Good	By Myself	With Friends	With a Grown-Up
23. Go Sledding		3	2	1	3	2	1	3	2	1			
24. Play in Snow		3	2	1	3	2	1	3	2	1			
25. Ice-Skate		3	2	1	3	2	1	3	2	1			
26. Ski or Snowboard		3	2	1	3	2	1	3	2	1			
Total													

Number of Winter Activities Child Participates in _____

Percent of Winter Activities Child Participates in _____

How Often the Child Does the Activities

_____

How Much the Child Likes Winter Activities

_____

How Good the Child Perceives Him- or Herself to be at the Activities

_____

Percent of Activities the Child Does
By Myself _____
With Friends _____
With a Grown-Up _____

Play Interview

Indoor Activities	Yes	Once a Week or More	Once a Month or More	Once a Year or More	A Lot	A Little	Not at All	Very Good	So-So	Not So Good	By Myself	With Friends	With a Grown-Up
27. Play Cards		3	2	1	3	2	1	3	2	1			
28. Play Board Games		3	2	1	3	2	1	3	2	1			
29. Read		3	2	1	3	2	1	3	2	1			
30. Use Computer		3	2	1	3	2	1	3	2	1			
31. Watch TV		3	2	1	3	2	1	3	2	1			
32. Listen to Music		3	2	1	3	2	1	3	2	1			
33. Collect Things		3	2	1	3	2	1	3	2	1			
34. Take Care of Pet		3	2	1	3	2	1	3	2	1			
35. Play Video Games		3	2	1	3	2	1	3	2	1			
Total													

Number of Indoor Activities Child Participates in _____ Percent of Indoor Activities Child Participates in _____	How Often the Child Does the Activities _____	How Much the Child Likes Indoor Activities _____	How Good the Child Perceives Him- or Herself to be at the Activities _____	Percent of Activities the Child Does By Myself _____ With Friends _____ With a Grown-Up ____

Play Interview

Creative Activities	Yes	Once a Week or More	Once a Month or More	Once a Year or More	A Lot	A Little	Not at All	Very Good	So-So	Not So Good	By Myself	With Friends	With a Grown-Up
36. Do Puzzles		3	2	1	3	2	1	3	2	1			
37. Sing		3	2	1	3	2	1	3	2	1			
38. Dance		3	2	1	3	2	1	3	2	1			
39. Build Things		3	2	1	3	2	1	3	2	1			
40. Draw or Paint		3	2	1	3	2	1	3	2	1			
41. Cook or Bake		3	2	1	3	2	1	3	2	1			
42. Make Jewelry		3	2	1	3	2	1	3	2	1			
Total													

Number of Creative Activities Child Participates in _____ Percent of Creative Activities Child Participates in _____	How Often the Child Does the Activities _____	How Much the Child Likes Creative Activities _____	How Good the Child Perceives Him- or Herself to be at the Activities _____	Percent of Activities the Child Does By Myself _____ With Friends _____ With a Grown-Up ____

Play Interview

Lessons/ Classes	Yes	Once a Week or More	Once a Month or More	Once a Year or More	A Lot	A Little	Not at All	Very Good	So-So	Not So Good	By Myself	With Friends	With a Grown-Up
43. Music Lessons		3	2	1	3	2	1	3	2	1			
44. Swimming Lessons		3	2	1	3	2	1	3	2	1			
45. Dance Lessons		3	2	1	3	2	1	3	2	1			
46. Gymnastics Lessons		3	2	1	3	2	1	3	2	1			
47. Arts & Crafts Lessons		3	2	1	3	2	1	3	2	1			
48. Martial Arts Lessons		3	2	1	3	2	1	3	2	1			
49. Horseback Riding Lessons		3	2	1	3	2	1	3	2	1			
Total													

Number of Lessons/ Classes Child Participates in _____ Percent of Lessons/ Classes Child Participates in _____	How Often the Child Attends the Lessons/ Classes _____	How Much the Child Likes Lessons/ Classes _____	How Good the Child Perceives Him- or Herself to be at the Lesson/Classes _____	Percent of Lessons/ Classes the Child Does By Myself _____ With Friends _____ With a Grown-Up ____

Play Interview

Socializing Activities	Yes	Once a Week or More	Once a Month or More	Once a Year or More	A Lot	A Little	Not at All	Very Good	So-So	Not So Good	By Myself	With Friends	With a Grown-Up
50. Hang Out With Friends		3	2	1	3	2	1	3	2	1			
51. Scouts/4H/ Campfire		3	2	1	3	2	1	3	2	1			
52. Play Superheroes		3	2	1	3	2	1	3	2	1			
53. Play School		3	2	1	3	2	1	3	2	1			
54. Play Dress-Up or Make-Up		3	2	1	3	2	1	3	2	1			
55. Go to Movies		3	2	1	3	2	1	3	2	1			
56. Go Out to Eat		3	2	1	3	2	1	3	2	1			
57. Go Shopping		3	2	1	3	2	1	3	2	1			
58. Talk on Phone		3	2	1	3	2	1	3	2	1			
59. Go to Arcade		3	2	1	3	2	1	3	2	1			
Total													

Number of Social Activities Child Participates in _____

Percent of Social Activities Child Participates in _____

How Often the Child Does the Social Activities

_____

How Much the Child Likes Activities

_____

How Good the Child Perceives Him- or Herself to be at the Activities

_____

Percent of Activities the Child Does
By Myself _____
With Friends _____
With a Grown-Up _____

Play Interview

Other Activities	Yes	Once a Week or More	Once a Month or More	Once a Year or More	A Lot	A Little	Not at All	Very Good	So-So	Not So Good	By Myself	With Friends	With a Grown-Up
60.		3	2	1	3	2	1	3	2	1			
61.		3	2	1	3	2	1	3	2	1			
62.		3	2	1	3	2	1	3	2	1			
63.		3	2	1	3	2	1	3	2	1			
64.		3	2	1	3	2	1	3	2	1			
Total													

Number of Other Activities Child Participates in _____

Percent of Other Activities Child Participates in _____

How Often the Child Does the Other Activities

_____

How Much the Child Likes Activities

_____

How Good the Child Perceives Him- or Herself to be at the Activities

_____

Percent of Activities the Child Does
By Myself _____
With Friends _____
With a Grown-Up _____

Play Interview

Total (exclude "other" activities when calculating totals)

Number of Activities Child Participates in (sum the totals of the 8 categories) _____ Percent of Activities Child Participates in (divide the above number by 59) _____	How Often the Child Does the Activities (sum the scores of the 8 categories and divide the number by 8) _____	How Much the Child Likes the Activities (sum the scores of the 8 categories and divide the number by 8) _____	How Good the Child Perceives Him- or Herself to be at the Activities (sum the scores of the 8 categories and divide the number by 8) ____	Percent of Activities the Child Does (add final percentages from each column and divide by 8) By Myself _____ With Friends _____ With a Grown-Up ____

Play Interview Summary

_____
_____
_____
_____

Play Observations

_____
_____
_____
_____

Interpretations/Recommendations

_____
_____
_____
_____

Appendix 5-C

Adolescent Leisure Interest Profile

Adolescent Leisure Interest Profile
Alexis D. Henry, ScD, OTR/L

Directions

There are 83 leisure activities in this booklet. There are five questions for each activity. The first two questions are

1. How interested are you in this activity?

2. How often do you do this activity?

If you do the activity, please answer the last three questions. If you do not do the activity, leave the last three questions blank and go on to the next activity.

Please check only one answer for each question. However, you may check more than one answer for question 5.

There are no right or wrong answers. Your answers should show how you really feel.

At the end, you may add other activities that you do and that you weren't asked about.

Name _____ Date _____

Age _____ Birthday _____ Grade _____ Gender ☐ Male ☐ Female

Adolescent Leisure Interest Profile

Sports Activities	How Interested Are You In This Activity?			How Often Do You Do This Activity?					How Well Do You Do This Activity?			How Much Do You Enjoy This Activity?			Who Do You Do This Activity With?		
	Very	Some-what	Not at All	3 To 7 Times a Week	Less Than 3 Times a Week	Once or Twice a Month	Less Than Once a Month	Never	Very Well	Well	Not Very Well	Very Much	Some-what	Not at All	By Myself	With Friends	With Family
1. Baseball/Softball																	
2. Basketball																	
3. Soccer																	
4. Football																	
5. Ice or Field Hockey																	
6. Track and Field																	
7. Cheerleading																	
8. Volleyball																	
Outdoor Activities																	
9. BMX/Mountain Biking																	
10. ATV/Dirt Biking																	
11. Camping																	
12. Hiking/Mountain Climbing																	
13. Fishing																	
14. Gardening																	
15. Canoeing/Rowing/Sailing																	
16. Sledding																	
17. Skiing/Snowboarding																	
18. Horseback Riding																	
19. Golfing																	
Exercise Activities																	
20. Bicycling																	
21. Skating/Skateboarding																	
22. Swimming																	
23. Jogging																	
24. Tennis																	
25. Aerobics																	
26. Gymnastics																	
27. Martial Arts																	
28. Power Walking																	
29. Weight Lifting																	

continued

Adolescent Leisure Interest Profile (continued)

Relaxation Activities	How Interested Are You In This Activity?			How Often Do You Do This Activity?					How Well Do You Do This Activity?			How Much Do You Enjoy This Activity?			Who Do You Do This Activity With?		
	Very	Some-what	Not at All	3 To 7 Times a Week	Less Than 3 Times a Week	Once or Twice a Month	Less Than Once a Month	Never	Very Well	Well	Not Very Well	Very Much	Some-what	Not at All	By Myself	With Friends	With Family
30. Watching TV																	
31. Listening to Music																	
32. Talking on the Phone																	
33. Playing Video Games																	
34. Sleeping Late																	
35. Riding in a Car																	
36. Lying in the Sun																	
37. Yoga																	
Intellectual Activities																	
38. Reading																	
39. Computers																	
40. Math																	
41. Science																	
42. History																	
43. Literature																	
44. Politics																	
45. Debates																	
46. Science/ Art Museums																	
Creative Activities																	
47. Drawing or Painting																	
48. Cooking or Baking																	
49. Making Jewelry																	
50. Woodworking																	
51. Playing an Instrument																	
52. Making Models																	
53. Creative Writing/Poetry																	
54. Sewing/Knitting																	
55. Photography																	

continued

Adolescent Leisure Interest Profile (continued)

Socializing Activities	How Interested Are You In This Activity?			How Often Do You Do This Activity?					How Well Do You Do This Activity?			How Much Do You Enjoy This Activity?			Who Do You Do This Activity With?		
	Very	Some-what	Not at All	3 To 7 Times a Week	Less Than 3 Times a Week	Once or Twice a Month	Less Than Once a Month	Never	Very Well	Well	Not Very Well	Very Much	Some-what	Not at All	By Myself	With Friends	With Family
56. Hanging Out With Friends																	
57. Going to the Movies/Theater/Concerts																	
58. Going out to Eat																	
59. Going to the Mall/Shopping																	
60. Going to the Beach/River/Lake																	
61. Amusement Parks																	
62. Going to Dances																	
63. Dating																	
64. Sporting Events																	
65. Playing Pool																	
66. Bowling																	
67. Playing Board/Card Games																	
68. Celebrating Holidays																	
69. Taking Vacations																	
70. Going to Parties																	
71. Visiting Relatives																	
72. Cookouts/Barbecues																	
73. Going to Worship																	
Club/Community Activities																	
74. Scouting																	
75. School Plays/Musicals																	
76. Youth Groups/CYOs																	
77. Honor Societies																	
78. Chorus/Choir																	
79. Drama Club																	
80. Language Club																	

continued

Adolescent Leisure Interest Profile (continued)

Club/Community Activity (continued)	How Interested Are You In This Activity?			How Often Do You Do This Activity?					How Well Do You Do This Activity?			How Much Do You Enjoy This Activity?			Who Do You Do This Activity With?		
	Very	Some-what	Not at All	3 To 7 Times a Week	Less Than 3 Times a Week	Once or Twice a Month	Less Than Once a Month	Never	Very Well	Well	Not Very Well	Very Much	Some-what	Not at All	By Myself	With Friends	With Family
81. Volunteering																	
82. Student Government																	
83. Hiking Club																	

Other Activities

Adolescent Leisure Interest Profile
Alexis D. Henry, ScD, OTR/L
Summary Score Sheet

Adolescent's Name _____   Gender ☐ Male ☐ Female

School _____   Grade _____

Service Provider's Name _____

	Year	Month	Day
Date Tested			
Date of Birth			
Chronological Age			

Discipline _____

The adolescent receives the following service(s) _____

_____

Conditions that may affect the adolescent's leisure activities _____

_____

Category Scores
Instructions

Transfer the following information from the *Adolescent Leisure Interest Profile* to each corresponding category table.

Circle each number that reflects the adolescent's response under the heading *How Interested Are You in This Activity?* Also circle each number that reflects the adolescent's response under the headings *How Often Do You Do This Activity? How Well Do You Do This Activity?* and *How Much Do You Enjoy This Activity?*

Finally, place a checkmark in one or more of the last three columns to indicate with whom the adolescent does the activity.

Scoring

To calculate how interested the adolescent is in the category activities, add the scores of the three columns labeled *Very, Somewhat,* and *Not at All.* Divide the total by the number of activities in the category. Place this sum in the box labeled *How Interested the Adolescent is in (Sports, Outdoor, etc.) Activities.* The closer the number is to 3, the more interesting the adolescent finds the activities.

To calculate how often the adolescent participates in the category activities, add the scores of the five columns labeled *3 to 7 Times a Week, Less Than 3 Times a Week, Once or Twice a Month, Less Than Once a Month,* and *Never.* Divide the total by the number of activities in the category. Place this sum in the box labeled *How Often the Adolescent Participates*

in *(Sports, Outdoor, etc.) Activities.* The closer the number is to 5, the more frequently the adolescent participates in the activities.

To calculate how well the adolescent perceives that he/she does the category activities, add the scores of the three columns labeled *Very Well, Well, Not Very Well.* Divide the total by the number of category activities the adolescent participates in. Place this sum in the box labeled *How Good the Adolescent Perceives Him- or Herself to be at (Sports, Outdoor, etc.) Activities.* The closer the number is to 3, the better the adolescent perceives him- or herself to be at the activities he or she does.

To calculate how much the adolescent enjoys the category activities, add the scores of the three columns labeled *Very much, Somewhat,* and *Not at All.* Divide the total by the number of activities the adolescent participates in. Place this sum in the box labeled *How Much the Adolescent Enjoys (Sports, Outdoor, etc.) Activities.* The closer the number is to 3, the more the adolescent enjoys the activities.

To calculate the percent of activities that the adolescent does alone, with friends, and with family, add the checkmarks in each column. Divide the total for each column by the number of activities the adolescent participates in. Multiply each total by 100 and place the percent in the appropriate place in the box labeled *Percent of Activities the Adolescent Does By Myself, With Friends, or With Family.* Because respondents may give more than one answer for this questions (for example, an adolescent may do an activity both "by myself" and "with friends"), the total for the 3 responses may exceed 100%.

Sports Activities	How Interested Are You In This Activity?			How Often Do You Do This Activity?					How Well Do You Do This Activity?			How Much Do You Enjoy This Activity?			Who Do You Do This Activity With?		
	Very	Some-what	Not at All	3 To 7 Times a Week	Less Than 3 Times a Week	Once or Twice a Month	Less Than Once a Month	Never	Very Well	Well	Not Very Well	Very Much	Some-what	Not at All	By Myself	With Friends	With Family
1. Baseball/Softball	3	2	1	5	4	3	2	1	3	2	1	3	2	1			
2. Basketball	3	2	1	5	4	3	2	1	3	2	1	3	2	1			
3. Soccer	3	2	1	5	4	3	2	1	3	2	1	3	2	1			
4. Football	3	2	1	5	4	3	2	1	3	2	1	3	2	1			
5. Ice or Field Hockey	3	2	1	5	4	3	2	1	3	2	1	3	2	1			
6. Track and Field	3	2	1	5	4	3	2	1	3	2	1	3	2	1			
7. Cheerleading	3	2	1	5	4	3	2	1	3	2	1	3	2	1			
8. Volleyball	3	2	1	5	4	3	2	1	3	2	1	3	2	1			
Total																	
	How Interested the Adolescent is in Sports Activities _____			How Often the Adolescent Participates in Sports Activities _____					How Good the Adolescent Perceives Him- or Herself to be at Sports Activities _____			How Much the Adolescent Enjoys Sports Activities _____			Percent of Sports Activities the Adolescent Does By Myself ____ With Friends __ With Family ___		

Leisure Interview

Outdoor Activities	How Interested Are You In This Activity?			How Often Do You Do This Activity?					How Well Do You Do This Activity?			How Much Do You Enjoy This Activity?			Who Do You Do This Activity With?		
	Very	Some-what	Not at All	3 To 7 Times a Week	Less Than 3 Times a Week	Once or Twice a Month	Less Than Once a Month	Never	Very Well	Well	Not Very Well	Very Much	Some-what	Not at All	By Myself	With Friends	With Family
9. BMX/Mountain Biking	3	2	1	5	4	3	2	1	3	2	1	3	2	1			
10. ATV/Dirt Biking	3	2	1	5	4	3	2	1	3	2	1	3	2	1			
11. Camping	3	2	1	5	4	3	2	1	3	2	1	3	2	1			
12. Hiking/Mountain Climbing	3	2	1	5	4	3	2	1	3	2	1	3	2	1			
13. Fishing	3	2	1	5	4	3	2	1	3	2	1	3	2	1			
14. Gardening	3	2	1	5	4	3	2	1	3	2	1	3	2	1			
15. Canoeing/ Rowing/Sailing	3	2	1	5	4	3	2	1	3	2	1	3	2	1			
16. Sledding	3	2	1	5	4	3	2	1	3	2	1	3	2	1			
17. Skiing/ Snowboarding	3	2	1	5	4	3	2	1	3	2	1	3	2	1			
18. Horseback Riding	3	2	1	5	4	3	2	1	3	2	1	3	2	1			
19. Golfing	3	2	1	5	4	3	2	1	3	2	1	3	2	1			
Total																	
	How Interested the Adolescent is in Outdoor Activities _____			How Often the Adolescent Participates in Outdoor Activities _____					How Good the Adolescent Perceives Him- or Herself to be at Outdoor Activities _____			How Much the Adolescent Enjoys Outdoor Activities _____			Percent of Sports Activities the Adolescent Does By Myself ____ With Friends ___ With Family ___		

Leisure Interview

Exercise Activities	How Interested Are You In This Activity?			How Often Do You Do This Activity?					How Well Do You Do This Activity?			How Much Do You Enjoy This Activity?			Who Do You Do This Activity With?		
	Very	Some-what	Not at All	3 To 7 Times a Week	Less Than 3 Times a Week	Once or Twice a Month	Less Than Once a Month	Never	Very Well	Well	Not Very Well	Very Much	Some-what	Not at All	By Myself	With Friends	With Family
20. Bicycling	3	2	1	5	4	3	2	1	3	2	1	3	2	1			
21. Skating/ Skateboarding	3	2	1	5	4	3	2	1	3	2	1	3	2	1			
22. Swimming	3	2	1	5	4	3	2	1	3	2	1	3	2	1			
23. Jogging	3	2	1	5	4	3	2	1	3	2	1	3	2	1			
24. Tennis	3	2	1	5	4	3	2	1	3	2	1	3	2	1			
25. Aerobics	3	2	1	5	4	3	2	1	3	2	1	3	2	1			
26. Gymnastics	3	2	1	5	4	3	2	1	3	2	1	3	2	1			
27. Martial Arts	3	2	1	5	4	3	2	1	3	2	1	3	2	1			
28. Power Walking	3	2	1	5	4	3	2	1	3	2	1	3	2	1			
29. Weight Lifting	3	2	1	5	4	3	2	1	3	2	1	3	2	1			
Total																	
	How Interested the Adolescent is in Exercise Activities _____			How Often the Adolescent Participates in Exercise Activities _____					How Good the Adolescent Perceives Him- or Herself to be at Exercise Activities _____			How Much the Adolescent Enjoys Exercise Activities _____			Percent of Exercise Activities the Adolescent Does By Myself _____ With Friends __ With Family ___		

Leisure Interview

Relaxation Activities	How Interested Are You In This Activity?			How Often Do You Do This Activity?					How Well Do You Do This Activity?			How Much Do You Enjoy This Activity?			Who Do You Do This Activity With?		
	Very	Some-what	Not at All	3 To 7 Times a Week	Less Than 3 Times a Week	Once or Twice a Month	Less Than Once a Month	Never	Very Well	Well	Not Very Well	Very Much	Some-what	Not at All	By Myself	With Friends	With Family
30. Watching TV	3	2	1	5	4	3	2	1	3	2	1	3	2	1			
31. Listening to Music	3	2	1	5	4	3	2	1	3	2	1	3	2	1			
32. Talking on the Phone	3	2	1	5	4	3	2	1	3	2	1	3	2	1			
33. Playing Video Games	3	2	1	5	4	3	2	1	3	2	1	3	2	1			
34. Sleeping Late	3	2	1	5	4	3	2	1	3	2	1	3	2	1			
35. Riding in a Car	3	2	1	5	4	3	2	1	3	2	1	3	2	1			
36. Lying in the Sun	3	2	1	5	4	3	2	1	3	2	1	3	2	1			
37. Yoga	3	2	1	5	4	3	2	1	3	2	1	3	2	1			
Total																	
	How Interested the Adolescent is in Relaxation Activities _____			How Often the Adolescent Participates in Relaxation Activities _____					How Good the Adolescent Perceives Him- or Herself to be at Relaxation Activities _____			How Much the Adolescent Enjoys Relaxation Activities _____			Percent of Relaxation Activities the Adolescent Does By Myself ____ With Friends __ With Family __		

Leisure Interview

Intellectual Activities	How Interested Are You In This Activity?			How Often Do You Do This Activity?					How Well Do You Do This Activity?			How Much Do You Enjoy This Activity?			Who Do You Do This Activity With?		
	Very	Some-what	Not at All	3 To 7 Times a Week	Less Than 3 Times a Week	Once or Twice a Month	Less Than Once a Month	Never	Very Well	Well	Not Very Well	Very Much	Some-what	Not at All	By Myself	With Friends	With Family
38. Reading	3	2	1	5	4	3	2	1	3	2	1	3	2	1			
39. Computers	3	2	1	5	4	3	2	1	3	2	1	3	2	1			
40. Studying Math	3	2	1	5	4	3	2	1	3	2	1	3	2	1			
41. Studying Science	3	2	1	5	4	3	2	1	3	2	1	3	2	1			
42. Studying History	2	1	5	4	3	2	1	3	2	1	3	2	1				
43. Literature	3	2	1	5	4	3	2	1	3	2	1	3	2	1			
44. Politics	3	2	1	5	4	3	2	1	3	2	1	3	2	1			
45. Debates	3	2	1	5	4	3	2	1	3	2	1	3	2	1			
46. Science/ Art Museums	3	2	1	5	4	3	2	1	3	2	1	3	2	1			
Total																	

How Interested the Adolescent is in Intellectual Activities _____	How Often the Adolescent Participates in Intellectual Activities _____	How Good the Adolescent Perceives Him- or Herself to be at Intellectual Activities _____	How Much the Adolescent Enjoys Intellectual Activities _____	Percent of Intellectual Activities the Adolescent Does By Myself ____ With Friends __ With Family ___

Leisure Interview

Creative Activities	How Interested Are You In This Activity?			How Often Do You Do This Activity?					How Well Do You Do This Activity?			How Much Do You Enjoy This Activity?			Who Do You Do This Activity With?		
	Very	Some-what	Not at All	3 To 7 Times a Week	Less Than 3 Times a Week	Once or Twice a Month	Less Than Once a Month	Never	Very Well	Well	Not Very Well	Very Much	Some-what	Not at All	By Myself	With Friends	With Family
47. Drawing or Painting	3	2	1	5	4	3	2	1	3	2	1	3	2	1			
48. Cooking or Baking	3	2	1	5	4	3	2	1	3	2	1	3	2	1			
49. Making Jewelry	3	2	1	5	4	3	2	1	3	2	1	3	2	1			
50. Woodworking	3	2	1	5	4	3	2	1	3	2	1	3	2	1			
51. Playing an Instrument	3	2	1	5	4	3	2	1	3	2	1	3	2	1			
52. Making Models	3	2	1	5	4	3	2	1	3	2	1	3	2	1			
53. Creative Writing/Poetry	3	2	1	5	4	3	2	1	3	2	1	3	2	1			
54. Sewing/Knitting	3	2	1	5	4	3	2	1	3	2	1	3	2	1			
55. Photography	3	2	1	5	4	3	2	1	3	2	1	3	2	1			
Total																	
	How Interested the Adolescent is in Creative Activities _____			How Often the Adolescent Participates in Creative Activities _____					How Good the Adolescent Perceives Him- or Herself to be at Creative Activities _____			How Much the Adolescent Enjoys Creative Activities _____			Percent of Creative Activities the Adolescent Does By Myself _____ With Friends __ With Family ___		

Leisure Interview

Socializing Activities	How Interested Are You In This Activity?			How Often Do You Do This Activity?					How Well Do You Do This Activity?			How Much Do You Enjoy This Activity?			Who Do You Do This Activity With?		
	Very	Some-what	Not at All	3 To 7 Times a Week	Less Than 3 Times a Week	Once or Twice a Month	Less Than Once a Month	Never	Very Well	Well	Not Very Well	Very Much	Some-what	Not at All	By Myself	With Friends	With Family
56. Hanging Out with Friends	3	2	1	5	4	3	2	1	3	2	1	3	2	1			
57. Going to the Movies/Theater/ Concerts	3	2	1	5	4	3	2	1	3	2	1	3	2	1			
58. Going out to Eat	3	2	1	5	4	3	2	1	3	2	1	3	2	1			
59. Going to the Mall/Shopping	3	2	1	5	4	3	2	1	3	2	1	3	2	1			
60. Going to the Beach/River/Lake	3	2	1	5	4	3	2	1	3	2	1	3	2	1			
61. Amusement Parks	3	2	1	5	4	3	2	1	3	2	1	3	2	1			
62. Going to Dances	3	2	1	5	4	3	2	1	3	2	1	3	2	1			
63. Dating	3	2	1	5	4	3	2	1	3	2	1	3	2	1			
64. Sporting Events	3	2	1	5	4	3	2	1	3	2	1	3	2	1			
65. Playing Pool	3	2	1	5	4	3	2	1	3	2	1	3	2	1			
66. Bowling	3	2	1	5	4	3	2	1	3	2	1	3	2	1			
67. Playing Board/ Card Games	3	2	1	5	4	3	2	1	3	2	1	3	2	1			
68. Celebrating Holidays	3	2	1	5	4	3	2	1	3	2	1	3	2	1			
69. Taking Vacations	2	1	5	4	3	2	1	3	2	1	3	2	1				
70. Going to Parties	3	2	1	5	4	3	2	1	3	2	1	3	2	1			
71. Visiting Relatives	3	2	1	5	4	3	2	1	3	2	1	3	2	1			
72. Cookouts/ Barbecues	3	2	1	5	4	3	2	1	3	2	1	3	2	1			
73. Going to Worship	3	2	1	5	4	3	2	1	3	2	1	3	2	1			
Total																	
	How Interested the Adolescent is in Social Activities _____			How Often the Adolescent Participates in Social Activities _____					How Good the Adolescent Perceives Him- or Herself to be at Social Activities _____			How Much the Adolescent Enjoys Social Activities _____			Percent of Social Activities the Adolescent Does By Myself ____ With Friends __ With Family __		

Leisure Interview

Club/Community Activities	How Interested Are You In This Activity?			How Often Do You Do This Activity?					How Well Do You Do This Activity?			How Much Do You Enjoy This Activity?			Who Do You Do This Activity With?		
	Very	Some-what	Not at All	3 To 7 Times a Week	Less Than 3 Times a Week	Once or Twice a Month	Less Than Once a Month	Never	Very Well	Well	Not Very Well	Very Much	Some-what	Not at All	By Myself	With Friends	With Family
74. Scouting	3	2	1	5	4	3	2	1	3	2	1	3	2	1			
75. School Plays/ Musicals	3	2	1	5	4	3	2	1	3	2	1	3	2	1			
76. Youth Groups/CYOs	3	2	1	5	4	3	2	1	3	2	1	3	2	1			
77. Honor Societies	3	2	1	5	4	3	2	1	3	2	1	3	2	1			
78. Chorus/Choir	3	2	1	5	4	3	2	1	3	2	1	3	2	1			
79. Drama Club	3	2	1	5	4	3	2	1	3	2	1	3	2	1			
80. Language Club	3	2	1	5	4	3	2	1	3	2	1	3	2	1			
81. Volunteering	3	2	1	5	4	3	2	1	3	2	1	3	2	1			
82. Student Government	3	2	1	5	4	3	2	1	3	2	1	3	2	1			
83. Hiking Club	3	2	1	5	4	3	2	1	3	2	1	3	2	1			
Total																	
	How Interested the Adolescent is in Club/ Community Activities _____			How Often the Adolescent Participates in Club/ Community Activities _____					How Good the Adolescent Perceives Him-or Herself to be at Club/ Community Activities _____			How Much the Adolescent Enjoys Club/ Community Activities _____			Percent of Club/ Community Activities the Adolescent Activities Does By Myself ____ With Friends __ With Family __		

Leisure Interview

Other Activities	How Interested Are You In This Activity?			How Often Do You Do This Activity?					How Well Do You Do This Activity?			How Much Do You Enjoy This Activity?			Who Do You Do This Activity With?		
	Very	Some-what	Not at All	3 To 7 Times a Week	Less Than 3 Times a Week	Once or Twice a Month	Less Than Once a Month	Never	Very Well	Well	Not Very Well	Very Much	Some-what	Not at All	By Myself	With Friends	With Family
84.	3	2	1	5	4	3	2	1	3	2	1	3	2	1			
85.	3	2	1	5	4	3	2	1	3	2	1	3	2	1			
86.	3	2	1	5	4	3	2	1	3	2	1	3	2	1			
87.	3	2	1	5	4	3	2	1	3	2	1	3	2	1			
88.	3	2	1	5	4	3	2	1	3	2	1	3	2	1			
Total																	
	How Interested the Adolescent is in Other Activities _____			How Often the Adolescent Participates in Other Activities _____					How Good the Adolescent Perceives Him- or Herself to be at Other Activities _____			How Much the Adolescent Enjoys Other Activities _____			Percent of Other Activities the Adolescent Does By Myself _____ With Friends __ With Family ___		

Leisure Interview

Total (exclude "other" activities when calculating totals)

	How Interested the Adolescent is in all Activities (sum the scores of the 8 categories and divide by 8) _____	How Often the Adolescent Participates in all Activities (sum the scores of the 8 categories and divide by 8) _____	How Good the Adolescent Perceives Him- or Herself to be at Activities He or She Does (sum the scores of the 8 categories and divide by 8) _____	How Much the Adolescent Enjoys Activities He or She Does (sum the scores of the 8 categories and divide by 8) _____	Percent of Activities the Adolescent Does (add percentages from each column for the 8 categories and divide by 8) By Myself _____ With Friends __ With Family ___

Leisure Interview Summary

_____

_____

Leisure Observations

_____

_____

Interpretations/Recommendations

_____

_____

6

Family Narratives and Play Assessment

Janice Posatery Burke, Roseann C. Schaaf,
and T. Brianna Lomba Hall

KEY TERMS

centering the family in care
narrative
making meaning
connected knowing
family story
therapist's story
storytelling
play

A life lived is what actually happened. A life experienced consists of the images, feelings, sentiments, desires, thoughts, and meanings known to the person whose life it is…A life as told, a life history, is a narrative, influenced by the cultural conventions of telling, by the audience, and by the social context.
E. M. Bruner in *Text, Play, and Story*, **1984**

Occupational therapy services continue to evolve and expand to meet the ever-changing demands in health care. Therapists find themselves surrounded by myriad social, cultural, economic, political, and pragmatic issues that affect the children they serve and the service they deliver. Integrating these modern-day demands with therapists' professional commitment to the occupational needs of children and their families continues to be one of the major challenges to the profession.

During these volatile days of health care reform, therapists must constantly weigh children's needs against service delivery parameters. Among the most pressing demands is the reconfiguration of practices to provide effective and efficient service. Such restructuring must be carefully considered in relation to the therapist's focus on the occupational roles of children: player, family member, student, and friend. This chapter seeks to identify a strategy for maintaining an occupational therapy focus on the occupational roles of children and families as the primary forces setting the context for a child's growth and development. With this dual focus on the child as a player and a family member, the chapter presents an occupational therapy approach to play assessment using narrative techniques and methods.

Play is a primary occupation of childhood, as has been recognized and appreciated within the occupational therapy literature (Florey, 1971, 1981; Knox, 1996; Reilly, 1974; Takata, 1969, 1974). A consideration of play within the context of the family life story allows the therapist to see the child as part of a family unit, where certain behaviors and activities are more highly valued than others. This chapter endorses interventions that are aimed at the child's major occupational role, that of the player, interwoven into a particular family pattern gleaned through the family story, as obtained with narrative techniques.

EXTERNAL FORCES SHAPING OCCUPATIONAL THERAPY

The multidimensional quality of occupational therapy practice calls for understanding the whole person and the everyday demands placed on the individual so as to create opportunities for growth and change. In addition to thinking about children and their environments, occupational therapists must now consider shrinking health care dollars, demands for more effective and efficient use of their time (e.g., seeing more clients for shorter lengths of time), administrative directives that ask them to move toward consultative models and managed care models, and pressure from third-party payers. This complicated picture of health care delivery requires a shift in treatment priorities, patterns of practice, and strategies for solving client needs.

Legislative mandates such as those found originally in P.L. 102-119 (The Individuals with Disabilities Education Act Amendments [IDEA], 1991) and more recently in P.L. 108-446 (The Individuals with Disabilities Education Improvement Act, 2004), with their focus on early intervention, exemplify the external forces that have reshaped pediatric occupational therapy practice. No longer satisfied with a traditional model of treatment, wherein the therapists as the experts provide one-to-one intervention based on goals they have designed and developed, the new public law directs therapists to provide family-centered care for infants and toddlers. For instance, the reauthorization of IDEA 2004 includes specific guidelines that call for a "family-directed identification of the needs of each family of such an infant or toddler, to assist appropriately in the development of the infant or toddler" (sec. 635).

Under the law, goals are generated through a process of collaboration and mutual problem solving by a team that has the family as a central participant. Occupational therapists are called upon to think, work, and communicate in ways that support the reconfigured form and structure of the collaborative team. But how do therapists open their thinking to incorporate a family-centered approach to care? How do they ensure that they can positively affect a child's occupations as player? How do they move from the role of expert to one of collaborator? How do they embrace family members as equal partners? How do they design interventions that address the family as a unique social and cultural unit? To begin, therapists will need to broaden their thinking about families and expand their repertoire of communication skills. Play assessments and family narratives will allow therapists to develop new and innovative approaches to intervention.

PROBLEMS OF CURRENT-DAY PRACTICE

In pediatric practice today, therapists observing and assessing children use many formal and informal instruments to understand deficit states such as limited play interactions, sensory integration dysfunction, gross and fine motor delays, and difficulties in acquiring social, cognitive, and adaptive skills. After assessment, therapists are faced with the formidable challenge of transforming their findings into intervention plans. Not uncommonly, however, therapists find that their intervention plans are unsuccessful. Primary caregivers are often overwhelmed with their already full schedules, families are unable to work with their fussy and uncooperative child, or families try to implement plans but cannot seem to do it "the right way." In turn, therapists may become disheartened when parents do not follow their home programs and may label the parents as noncompliant, resistant, or lacking follow-through.

The therapist's failure to consider the child within the context of the family may be a reason for this lack of connection between the therapist's assessment of the child's problem and the parent's concerns. The therapist must recognize the family's values, goals, and aspirations for the child, his or her siblings, and the family as a whole, as well as the realities of the family's life. Without fully exploring these concerns, the therapist has created an intervention plan in a vacuum and has failed to address the problems that truly have meaning for this child and this family, given the context of their lives. According to Degrace (2003), practitioners need to learn how family members interact with each other and share time, space, and life experiences. Only then will the practitioner be able to "name the things to which [they] will attend" and "frame the context in which [they] will attend to" (Schon, 1983, p. 40). This is an important ingredient that is missing from the traditional occupational therapy assessment and intervention plan. First, it must be remembered that the primary membership for children is that of family and that each family has its own system of communicating, behaving, and setting priorities and goals. When therapists fail to interview parents and other key family members as part of their assessment, they have excluded critical information. Second, these authors believe that children must be considered within their occupational roles (player and family member). By viewing the child as a member of a family and as a player, the therapist is more likely to deliver a relevant and useful assessment. But how are these viewpoints transformed into a useful approach to assessment?

In this chapter storytelling is proposed as a strategy for therapists who wish to address physical, psychosocial, and cognitive needs of the child while placing these needs within the context of the realities of that child's family. Storytelling provides the platform for the therapist to ask: Who is this family? Who is this child? What is this family asking for? What can I do to help this family and child?

We believe that the most effective approach to assessment is for therapists to identify the key issues for any given child and family and design an effective plan to address those issues. This means providing the most relevant and meaningful therapy possible given the issues and intervention needs. We further propose that a focus on play is a particularly insightful mechanism for understanding and interacting with families and children while recognizing, respecting, and emphasizing the family's cultural, ethnic, and social values.

CENTERING THE FAMILY IN CARE

The family-centered legislation directs therapists to see the child as part of a family unit. Dunst, Trivette, and Deal (1994) identified the basic tenets of family-centered services, which include the following:

- Adopting a social systems perspective
- Placing the family as a unit of intervention
- Empowering families

- Promoting growth-producing behavior rather than treatment of problems
- Focusing on family-identified needs
- Building on family capabilities
- Strengthening the family's social network
- Expanding professional roles and the way the roles are performed

Congruent with a focus on the family, occupational therapists are finding great utility in the view of the child as an occupational being with definable roles and with skills that permit successful enactment of those roles. Thus, instead of being seen through her diagnosis, "a 3-year-old with Down syndrome and moderate retardation," the child is cast in her occupational roles as "Marie, the youngest child in a family of four, player, and preschooler in an early intervention center."

The broadened view of role behavior within a family unit is complemented by the use of narrative. The narrative approach calls for understanding a person within the context of his or her life story (Figure 6-1). It is a valuable strategy for developing a fuller picture of the kinds of behaviors and activities that are most important for children to learn given their particular life situations. Marie, for example, is now seen in the context of her family and the occupational roles she holds in it. She is the youngest member of a large extended family. The children in the family are valued for their playfulness and enthusiasm for fun. The family cherishes their time spent together and frequently uses weekends and holidays for such outings as trips to the zoo, picnics at the beach, and walks to the park.

USING NARRATIVE TO UNDERSTAND INDIVIDUAL EXPERIENCE
How Humans Make Meaning

Each person develops a set of meanings about people, places, and things based on his or her experiences, developmental background, and cultural and family circumstances. As life goes on, the individual gives more importance to some people, places, and things and far less significance to others. In this way the person constructs a perspective or a story that allows him or her to move about the world with certain expectations and orientations, responding to the people, places, and things he or she finds most important and paying less attention to or ignoring other situations, actions, or encounters that have less meaning and significance. This approach allows individuals to develop their own stories and "organize their views of themselves, of others, and of the world in which they live" (Bruner, 1990, p. 137).

When working with families and young children, occupational therapists have a significant role in assisting them to interpret their experiences and shape their stories. Holzmueller (2005), a parent of two children with special needs, believes that narrative and storytelling are important because they give the family an opportunity to identify their own view of strengths and weaknesses.

Therapists can draw out the meaning of significant events through the family's stories. Parents who are able to tell a therapist about their shock and disappointment on first learning that their newborn child was disabled, as

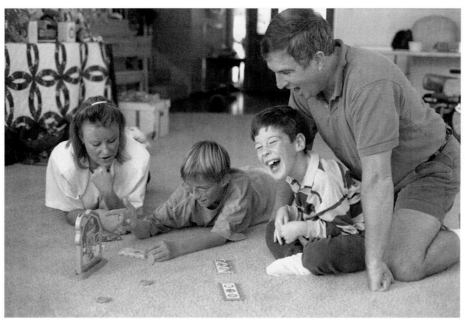

Figure 6-1

A family-centered, narrative approach entails seeing the child as a family member and player, rather than as a diagnosis. (Courtesy Shay McAtee.)

well as their surprise and hope when the child later learned to sit up, played peekaboo, or showed his or her awareness of music, are supplying the richly detailed information that allows the therapist to understand how families construct their lives, the kinds of behaviors that they hold in highest regard and are most meaningful, and what they look for and value in their children (Figure 6-2). This is important information for the therapist to use in selecting assessment strategies and developing interventions.

Stories provide ways to understand a person as an individual with a social and culturally constructed structure (Denzin, 1989). They offer opportunities to see the culturally specific actions, behaviors, and reciprocity of motives that drive individual meanings (Burke, 1993a). The next section examines the role of the therapist in understanding meaning.

Connected Knowing as a Way to Uncover Meaning

Within the feminist stream of literature, authors have looked at the types of knowledge that different groups of people value. One type has been termed "connected knowing." Connected knowing refers to a way of understanding a person as a person, "an attempt to achieve a kind of harmony with another person in spite of difference and distance, ...to enter the other person's frame to discover the premises for the other's point of view" (Belenky et al., 1986, p. 101). This way of knowing is differentiated from an impersonal, autonomous, or separate orientation, which is termed a "separate knowing."

It is the notion of connected knowing that stimulates scholars to become intrigued with alternative ways of understanding the world, relying on individual experience and thought rather than traditional "hard" or positivist logic. "Connected knowing builds on the subjectivists' conviction that the most trustworthy knowledge comes from personal experience rather than the pronouncements of authorities" (Belenky et al., 1986, p. 113).

Connected knowers seek to uncover methods for "gaining access to other people's knowledge" (Belenky et al., 1986, p. 113). The centerpiece for this process is the belief that "to understand another person's ideas is to try to share the experience that has led the person to form the idea" (Belenky et al., 1986, p. 113). In a connected knower dialogue, talk is "intimate rather than impersonal, relatively informal and unstructured rather than bound by more or less explicit rules" (Belenky et al., 1986, p. 114). Connected knowers spend more time listening to others and are nonjudgmental.

When occupational therapists incorporate such ideas as connected knowing into their practice, they move away from the professional authority role, in which they impose a quantitative view on the child and family, and move toward an orientation that asks: How is this family unit special? What matters most to this family? What occupational therapy information, skills, and techniques may be helpful to this family as they move toward their goals? One family may value mealtime because both parents have always considered this to be a nurturing and emotionally enriched interaction. In another family the

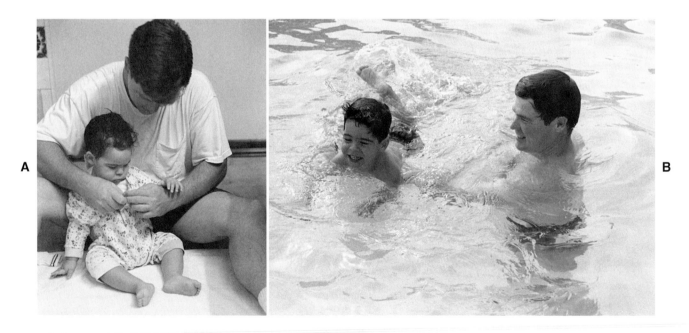

Figure 6-2
*Narratives capture the moments that leave marks on people's lives. These moments, **A,** may be part of the everyday routine or, **B,** may emerge in novel or unstructured situations, as when a child performs a new skill for the first time. (Courtesy Shay McAtee.)*

members may eat separately, little valuing the social and emotional quality of mealtime, but the family may instead appreciate the playful interactions that occur in the evening after bathtime and before bed. Yet another family may value weekly worship services, holidays, and similar special occasions as a time for the family to gather as a unit.

The use of narratives and life stories provides a way to understand children and families in the context of their physical, social, economic, political, and cultural world and allows therapists to move beyond their stereotypical views of how family life is constructed and enacted, leaving behind value judgments about who should be in a family and what a family should do with its time (Figure 6-3). For example, a common stereotype is that families have two parents, they spend time together in the evenings and weekends, they go on vacations to the mountains and to the grandparents for Thanksgiving, and they like to go camping in the summer and sledding in the winter. A family story perspective invites a positive, value-free inquiry that asks: Who is this family? What do they like to do? What kind of activity is the most meaningful? What activities are the most important? The most fun?

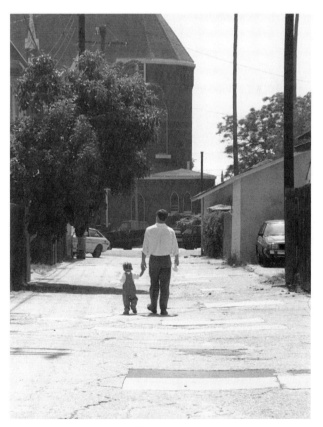

Figure 6-3
Use of narratives allows therapists to move beyond their stereotypical views of family life. One kind of nontraditional family, for example, consists of father and child. (Courtesy Shay McAtee.)

Play provides a unique window into the life of the child and family (D'Eugenio, 1986; Knox, 1996; Schaaf & Mulrooney, 1989). Given that people interact in patterns of behavior that are culturally meaningful, the ways a family engages in play can be expected to reflect their culturally driven values and purposes. Inquiries about play offer opportunities to understand the specific ways a family spends time; how it defines fun; the types of interactions, toys, and play materials that are most valued; and the availability and use of play environments (Figure 6-4). This culturally oriented glimpse into a family's life also provides a way to understand the environmental forces that shape play.

WITHIN OCCUPATIONAL THERAPY: A VIEW OF PLAY

In a modernized interpretation of occupational therapy, Mary Reilly (1971) urged her contemporaries to move beyond the medical orientation toward pathology so as to get at the real problems of their clients—the occupational dysfunction experienced when a person becomes disabled or chronically ill. For Reilly, such a proposal "would include not only the concerns for pathology correction but also for habit restructuring and for the environmental engineering of the opportunities and rewards associated with life adaptation" (p. 245).

Using the organizing principle of role behavior, Reilly conceptualized the unique and vital focus for the profession as the occupational behavior of persons with disability and disease. Early in the development of this concept Reilly (1962) suggested that humans have "a vital need for occupation and that [their] central nervous system demands the rich and varied stimuli that solving life problems provides…This is the basic need that occupational therapy ought to be serving" (p. 5) to facilitate the healing process in their clients.

Reilly envisaged occupational roles along a continuum associated with various stages in an individual's development, for example, the occupational roles of player, student, worker, and retiree. Each role provides opportunities for important learning and practice to ensure success in each of the subsequent roles to be acquired. Reilly wrote, "A child's ability to play, to explore his environment, to exercise his motor skills are the foundation for his later school experiences. The problem-solving processes and the creativity exercised in school work, craft and hobby experiences are the necessary preparations for the later demands of the work world" (p. 6). For Reilly and her associates (Bailey, 1971; Florey, 1971; Matsutsuyu, 1971; Shannon, 1972; Sundstrom, 1972; Takata, 1969), play is a primary occupation of childhood that not only ensures human adaptation but also provides the critical foundation for later childhood, adolescent, and adult successes.

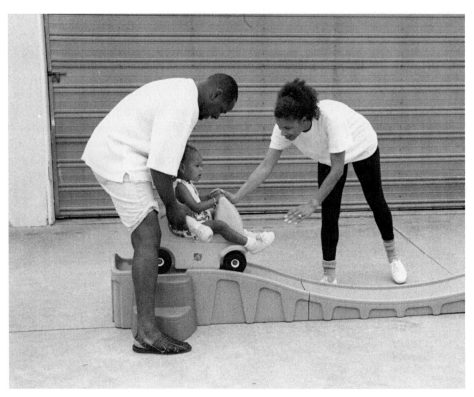

Figure 6-4
Inquiries about play lead to greater understanding of the family's values and goals by revealing how the family defines fun, how its members spend time together, and what play environments and materials they access. (Courtesy Shay McAtee.)

Play as a Marker in Childhood Role Behavior

In numerous exploratory studies and through assessments developed by occupational behaviorists, exemplars of successful player role enactment have been uncovered. These include the importance of human interactions, play with nonhumans, and the physical environment, as well as creativity and individual style as demonstrated in preferences and experiences (Bundy, 1997; Burke, 1993b; Florey, 1981; Hurff, 1974; Knox, 1974; Michelman, 1974; Takata, 1974).

Play is an avenue through which children learn social norms (Greene, 1997). Children achieve success in play when they are able to initiate contact and respond to the initiatives of others during the course of interaction (Figure 6-5). For a child with a disability, this important component to development may be difficult to achieve (Tanta, Dietz, White, & Billingsley, 2005).

DISABILITY AND FAMILY STORIES

People reflect their everyday experiences, their hopes for the future, and their memories of the past through stories. Storytelling is a basic human way of dealing with reality. All people form stories about their past, present, and future. Through stories, people chronicle their lives, remembering and reminiscing about the past, marking significant events

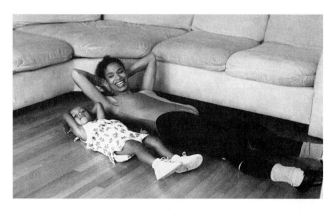

Figure 6-5
Stories concerning the child's role as player reflect the values, interests, and meanings of the family. A favorite story for the mother in this photograph is how one day her toddler spontaneously and enthusiastically joined in with her exercise routine. This is a particularly meaningful occupation for this mother, who is a performing dancer. (Courtesy Shay McAtee.)

as life unfolds, and spinning the dreams of their future (Burke, 1993a). Families are immersed in the storytelling process as they plan and ready themselves for a baby's birth. An expectant parent remembers the birth of sisters and brothers, cousins, and neighbors and begins to construct

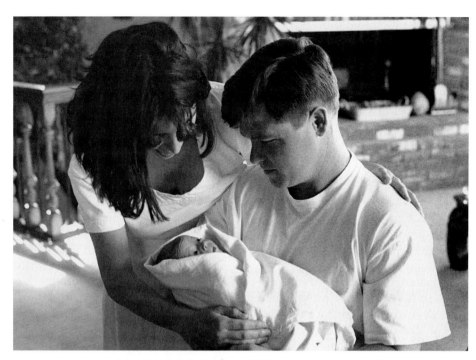

Figure 6-6
For many parents, a storyline about who their child will be is already established by the time the child is born. (Courtesy Shay McAtee.)

a tale about the soon-to-occur birth of his or her own child. Using culturally, ethnically, and socially constructed value systems, the parent tells himself or herself stories about who this child will be, what special qualities the child will have, and how the child's life will unfold (Burke, 1993a). Such stories as "My little girl will love her older sister; they will do everything together and be best friends" or "My son will love to play with cars and trucks, and when he is old enough, we'll make models together and race them" are typical of how parents begin to picture the future.

For some people the storyline may already be established when the child is born (Figure 6-6). Although minor modifications may be in order when the child is not the imagined sex, size, or temperament, these parents for the most part hold to the storyline they have created about their child and family life, and they work hard to see that the story unfolds as expected (Burke, 1993a). At the other end of the continuum, some expectant parents have only a vague notion about their child's story but find it is quickly filled in as the baby is born and moves into their lives.

The reality of the birth of a disabled, premature, high-risk, or otherwise ill baby wreaks havoc on both ends of the storyline continuum. Parents are typically unprepared for the dramatic changes in plot and storyline and have few experiences to draw on as they search for clues to how to think about and respond to the situation. In ways that are similar to the dilemmas of adults who recount their own struggles with illness and disability (Frank, 1991; Price, 1994), parents search for ways to understand what is happening to their family and how their experiences will

have an impact on their life story. Questions as basic as whether the child will live or die, be able to walk and talk, play with other children, dress herself or himself, and go to school dominate and threaten their life world. In such instances parents are faced with the task of constructing a new, tentative, or interim story about their child so as to begin to integrate the experience into their lives (Burke, 1993a).

The birth of a baby with health problems creates even greater complexity for parents who have little experience with the issues they are facing, have never known an infant with a similar diagnosis, and have had few interactions with people who are disabled or with health care professionals. Some parents expect that their child will be like another person they know to whom the term "disabled or special needs" also applies; they do not realize the great variation inherent in such a label. Parents may be at a loss when it comes to generating storylines and scenarios for family life with a child who has special needs. Parents and caregivers may ask, "Will I ever play with my child? Will he or she be able to climb on the jungle gym or ride on the carousel?"

STORYTELLING AS A STRATEGY FOR OCCUPATIONAL THERAPISTS

Storytelling gives therapists a strategy for entering into and assisting a family as it begins to construct a vision for the future. Stories have been documented as an effective clinical strategy for problem solving among therapists and between therapists and clients. "The narrative nature…manifests itself not only in the work therapists do to understand the effect of a disability in the life story of a particular patient, but also in the therapist's need to structure therapy in a narrative way, as an unfolding story" (Mattingly, 1991, p. 1000).

A narrative storytelling approach requires that therapists take the time to examine two points of view, one of the person receiving the care, and the other of the professional delivering it. From the client's point of view the therapist would ask, "What does this person want?" to gain a greater understanding of needs, motives, and individual meanings. Taking the practitioner's perspective the therapist would ask, "What can this person give?" This opening to the narrative process may provide the tools for examining and charting the boundaries that encircle treatment (Burke & Frank, 1994).

The use of settings, materials, or props may help to elicit the client's story. In her work with children and families Shirley Kramer devised an assessment tool called "A 'Snapshot' and 'The Developing Picture'" (Hanft et al., 1992). Using a piece of paper to represent a page from a scrapbook, the therapist asks parents "to close their eyes and capture the very first visualization which comes to them when they think about [their] child." In the second part of the assessment, the parent is asked to "think about the 'snapshot' you just took. How would you like to see [it] change or develop?" In both situations Kramer uses the scrapbook page as a physical prompt to evoke a story of family life, goals and dreams, and fears and problems as they are experienced now and as they look in the distant future. Through this family story therapists may find a prime entry point for assisting the family as it struggles with a particular dilemma the members wish to resolve in order to reach their future dream (e.g., my son is sitting in his high chair drinking from a cup; my daughter is riding a trike by herself; he's holding a pencil and writing his name). Because this assessment focuses on a picture that the family selects as meaningful, the therapist is more assured that they consider intervention, consultation, and collaboration to be valuable. In the instance of working with children and their families, two primary stories emerge: the story for the family and child, and the story for the therapist. The family and child story is considered the same unit, especially during the early years, since young children are thought to follow the story as it is constructed by the family.

Having gained an expanded view of the person's story, the therapist begins to infer, examine, and understand motives; works to understand how the person feels; and forms a realistic picture of the person's illness experience, as well as the therapist's own experience of treating the person. This ability to move closer to the intimacy of the illness experience and away from the sterility of the pathology focus so prevalent in medicine allows a "sympathetic accompaniment" (Frank, 1991) with the client that further legitimizes the illness experience (Kleinman, 1988).

Narrative and storytelling provide occupational therapists with an opportunity to develop a family-centered plan for intervention. Using such an approach, the therapist moves away from seeing each treatment interaction as an individual experience where skill acquisition is noted within the occupational therapy setting. In contrast, the use of narrative allows the therapist to focus on interactions and interventions as a series of events that tie together within the occupational therapy environment and beyond. The therapist in this instance moves away from seeing Joey as a participant in occupational therapy, showing gains in fine motor skills as evidenced by a more mature pincer grasp when using the therapy putty, or showing gains in attention as demonstrated by an increase in concentration to 5 or 6 minutes while balancing on the surfboard. Instead, the therapist sees this child as developing play skills to support age appropriate play behaviors and family roles that require fine motor and attention skills. Given this orientation, the therapist talks regularly with the family to gain its members' perceptions of whether the skills noted in the treatment are becoming generalized to valued family activities at home. This view provides an opportunity to see interactions with clients as unfolding (Joey is becoming more of a neighborhood player) rather than fixed and to some extent predictable (Joey holds objects using an unrefined three-finger grasp and will improve to a mature grasp within 6 weeks). In this way, storytelling allows health care providers to acknowledge how much they rely on stories to understand the children and families they treat, how profound the effect of illness and disability is on a family's life and on the way children play, and how illness affects the meaning and purpose of everyday lives.

Establishing Startpoints in Assessment

Occupational therapists traditionally have used both formalized and nonformalized methods of assessment. An important adjunct to traditional types of data gathering can be found in play observations and dialogues with the child and family in their natural environments. Through nonintrusive observation and documentation of play in a child's natural environment, valuable information regarding the child's ability to enact player and family roles is collected (Burke, 1993b). Information such as the use of play objects, play spaces, play interactions, and play opportunities is easily derived through such play observation and dialogues. By approaching the concept of play as a view to a child's competence, therapists are able to enter a child's world for the purpose of collecting important information that will contribute "to design[ing] and develop[ing]

Box 6-1 *Putting It All Together in Play*
Attention: Is the child able to attend to stimuli in the environment? Sustain attention? For what amount of time?
Exploration: Does the child explore objects and people in the environment?
Manipulation: How does the child manipulate objects?
Initiation: Does the child demonstrate intrinsic motivation to initiate play? In what type of situations? With whom?
Demonstrating variety: Does the child play with a variety of toys?
Diversity: Does the child demonstrate diversity in play? Does the child use toys and objects in different ways?
Interaction: Does the child include others in play? Who are the others? When does this occur?
Creativity: Does the child create play spaces and objects from the environment?

Box 6-2 *Skill Development and the Environment*
Skills
Does the child have the skills to support play?
• Gross motor skills?
• Fine motor skills?
• Visual skills?
• Language and cognitive skills?
Environment
What kinds of people are present and available for play?
What kinds of nonhuman factors are present or available for the child?
What is the relationship between the internal (motivation) and the external (environmental press)? How does this affect this child's play?
Do the child's play spaces facilitate or stifle play?
Do the available toys facilitate or stifle play?
Is the environment safe for play?
Is the environment organized for play?

activities that will be role-specific and address underlying areas of need" (Schaaf and Burke, 1992b, p. 1).

Play observation and history taking (dialogues) have proved to be valuable tools for occupational therapy. Takata (1969) recommended taking a play history to gain information regarding the materials, actions, people, and settings that are part of the child's play environment. Findings from the history can be analyzed by the use of a taxonomy that classifies play behaviors according to ages and stages of play (see Chapter 2). D'Eugenio (1986), Schaaf and Mulrooney (1989), and Schaaf and Burke (1992) have elaborated on the concept of play observation as a "window" that allows the therapist to collect information on both a child's competence in occupation and the underlying obstacles to successful occupational role enactment. Schaaf and Mulrooney (1989) developed a systematic framework for assessment of young children that used play observation as a way of gaining insight into the child's strengths and needs, as well as a means of assessing the environmental issues that affected the child's ability to play. They recommended incorporating play into both assessment and intervention to enhance overall development and skills. Such occupational therapy–based approaches to play provide a suitable foundation for incorporating family narratives into both assessment and treatment.

Observing play and hearing the family stories about play provide cues to the child's interests and ability to socialize, attend to others, use manipulative and large motor skills, and interact with objects and people in the environment. Information in these areas can be gained by considering the child's skills, habits, routines, and interests. Box 6-1 is a compilation of inquiries about these aspects of the child's play.

Additional areas to consider when collecting information about a child's play include issues related to skill development and the environment (Box 6-2). Further guidelines for appraising the impact of the human and nonhuman environments on a child's play are included in Box 6-3.

The child's story unfolds as the therapist becomes acquainted with the child and family and uses assessment instruments that collect and analyze traditional performance-based information (Figure 6-7). Similarly, a family story is formed as a result of interactions with the family. Key factors related to family stories are reviewed with the use of the schema in Figure 6-8. This type of framework provides a method for prioritizing observations made of the child with the concerns of the family. In this way, areas such as strengths and needs of the child as observed in human and nonhuman environments are combined with the priorities and values from the family story to identify plans for occupational therapy input.

Information about the child's story, as gained through play observation, is considered with the family story to create a plan for intervention. The goal is to provide a useful way for the therapist to address issues that have meaning to the family. Therapists consider this information but also look to the future (Mattingly, 1991), asking, "Who will this child and family be in 3 years? In 5 years?" The family, the child, play, and the environment are all considered in planning intervention. The information is initially organized by the therapist as illustrated in Figure 6-7. Figures 6-7 and 6-8 provide a framework for developing a synthesis of the family and child stories, which

Box 6-3 *Play Environment*

Nonhuman Factors

Are the basic needs of the family being met in terms of adequate food, clothing, housing, nurturing, and caring?

What are the child's main play environments, including the home, day-care, or school?

Is there adequate physical space for play?

Are there safety hazards in the play environment?

Is there any organization to the play environment in terms of toys or play spaces?

Are toys accessible to the child?

Are developmentally appropriate toys available to the child?

Is there freedom to explore the environment?

Is the level of stimulation in the environment conducive to play? Is there overstimulation? A lack of stimulation?

Are there established routines for sleeping and feeding?

Human Factors

Do the people in the child's environment (parents, teachers, caregivers) value play? What kind of play?

Are play interactions and synchrony (i.e., responsiveness to child's cues, availability to the child) evident?

Are there opportunities for the child to interact with or play with others?

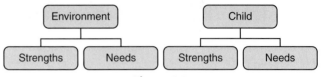

Figure 6-7
A schema of the child's story.

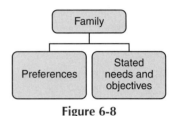

Figure 6-8
A schema of the family's story.

will be used, in turn, as a basis for a meaningful treatment plan focusing on play skills and interactions. In a sense, this framework is the beginning of a storyboard for the family, sketching out a picture of who this child and family are now and who they may become in the future, a story that the family may very well take up and continue to develop after therapy has ended.

Sample Clinical Storylines About Play

In developing storylines to serve families and children, therapists integrate clinical knowledge with family narratives to create their own storylines about children with whom they work. To illustrate this process, the following sections present types of clinical storylines. These storylines show how therapists might relate theory and research from occupational therapy and other fields to children's play behaviors and family narratives. Each demonstrates the profound effects of neurobehavioral functioning on the development and enactment of occupation and also illustrates how play may be used in evidence-based practice. These storylines are incorporated into two case examples later in the chapter.

Storyline 1: Play and Sensory Processing Issues

The viewpoint of play as a reflection of the child's ability to process and integrate sensory information for adaptive behavior was introduced by Ayres (1972) in her description of the sensory integrative process. She set forth the supposition that play is reflective of the child's sensorimotor systems and that difficulty in integrating and processing sensory information will result in difficulty interacting in the environment in such activities as play. A child with normal sensory integration, Ayres believed, would seek play experiences to further growth and development, whereas a child with dysfunction in sensory integration would often avoid or not know how to engage in normal growth-perpetuating play experiences. A child with a dysfunction may seek ways to fulfill the intrinsic need for environmental and sensory input, but these may be maladaptive in nature. These concepts were further explored by Schaaf and associates (1987) in two case studies that examined the relationship of play behavior to sensory integration. These studies found that when children whose disability included sensory integrative dysfunction were involved in a therapeutic program that addressed their underlying sensory integrative needs, they demonstrated positive changes in play behavior over the course of therapy.

A narrative approach can broaden the occupational therapist's application of sensory integrative theory. Specifically, it assists the therapist in formulating a story about a child that incorporates specific sensory processing information into a broader perspective of the child as a player and family member (Box 6-4).

Storyline 2: Play and Temperament Issues

Building on the notion that play reflects neurobehavioral substrates, the assessment of individual temperament as an important influence on play is a critical part of the examination of a child's story. Play observation can provide a valuable means for gaining information about factors related to temperament, such as the capacity for self-regulation,

Box 6-4 *Collecting Sensory Processing Information*

During daily family activities, does the child:
- Tolerate various types of sensory input?
- Crave certain types of stimulation?
- Avoid specific sensory inputs?
- Use self-stimulating behaviors?
- Seem fearful of movement?
- Avoid balance activities?
- Use hands for tactile exploration?
- Show variety in types of activities in terms of sensory input?

What is the family's definition of this child's problem?

What are the family's beliefs about the origins or reasons for the problem?

What are the typical interactions that occur within the everyday life of this family?

How does this child respond to these interactions?

How would the family like things to be different?

Which specific interactions are identified as suitable for change?

What are the times, preferences, and points in the day that the family finds appropriate to work on specific interactions they have identified?

Box 6-5 *Temperament, Play, and Behavior*

Is there an inherent rhythmicity in this child's play, or is the play scattered and disorganized?

Does this child appear comfortable and confident in play environments? How is this enacted?

How does this child make the transition from one activity to the next?

How does this child make the transition from quiet play to active play?

What level of arousal does this child demonstrate during play?

Does this child demonstrate strategies for self-calming or self-organization to regain composure after a period of disorganization?

Does the child stay organized during changes in the levels of environmental stimuli? During periods where multiple stimuli are present?

Does the environment support or inhibit playful interactions?

engagement, attention, and action (Anzalone, 1994). Authors such as Porges (1993), Brazelton and Lester (1983), Als (1986), Bates (1989), and Carey (1983) have directed attention to the relationship of temperament to later behavioral styles such as those observed in play. Using a model developed by Chess and Thomas (1989), these authors conceptualize temperament as an expression of an underlying reactive or self-regulatory process. The child demonstrates either maladaptive responses (avoidance) to environmental-sensory input or adaptive responses (approach) toward the people and objects in the environment.

The impact of sensory processing and temperament on play is implied in the term "goodness of fit," which refers to the match between the child and the environment. A goodness of fit occurs when "capacities, motivation, and temperament are adequate to master the demands, expectations, and opportunities to promote positive development," whereas a poorness of fit occurs when the "child's characteristics are inadequate to master environmental challenges and lead to maladaptive functioning and distorted development" (Chess & Thomas, 1989, p. 380). This concept of fit suggests a strong relationship between the child's temperament and his or her ability to interact with the environment in positive, growth-perpetuating ways, such as through play. Because play is related to temperament, observations of the child's capacity for self-regulation, engagement, attention, and action provide valuable cues about the child's areas of strength and need.

To understand the impact of temperament on the child's story, the therapist can use play observation and interviews to collect specific information (Box 6-5). This information is integrated with other assessment findings to provide a fuller understanding of the child as player and family member.

CASE EXAMPLES

The following case examples demonstrate the use of storytelling by two occupational therapists. These stories incorporate the collection of assessment information about a child's play, the family's story, and the therapist's synthesis of clinical assessment data with theory and research from the fields of occupational therapy and child development. The cases illustrate two different ways of constructing child and family narratives.

CASE EXAMPLE 1

Carmen: Finding My Place

Carmen lives with both parents in an urban setting. His mom, Wanda, works as an assistant in a city housing office. His father, Joe, is a carpenter. Both parents are friendly and talkative. Their original story of family life has been modified somewhat because of their son's complicated medical and developmental picture. For example, Wanda had planned to return to work full time with a babysitter at home for her child but changed that plan in response to her son's many needs. Both parents are actively involved in their family story, using their parenting roles to help them understand their son and make sense of their future.

Carmen is seen by an occupational therapist in his home as part of his early intervention program. He is considered to have significant sensory processing difficulties, as well as developmental disability. Three days a week he attends a program at an early intervention center. Two other days are filled with visits from his therapists.

During a typical home visit Natasha (the occupational therapist) and Wanda talk at length about why Carmen may be acting as he is, changes each has seen, and ways that interactions may be modified. Their conversation is filled with ideas about using playful situations, toy objects, songs, and jingles that would spark Carmen's attention and curiosity about his world. For example,

Wanda: I just bought several more of these squeaky toys, he seems to really recognize them.

Natasha: I know he really likes them. He plays with them a lot at school.

Wanda: Let's try the "Find It game" to see what he thinks.

Natasha: Good. Do you want to hold him or shall I?

In their interactions Wanda and Natasha engage in a constant give and take of ideas. Equally interesting is the way they share responsibility for initiating treatment sequences and playful interactions with Carmen. How did they get to this point? And how similar are their stories for Carmen?

The following stories have emerged over the course of informal conversation and direct inquiry between the parents and therapist. The stories are told by the therapist.

How Wanda Tells Her Story to Carmen's Therapist

Wanda views her 2½-year-old son as having the ability to engage at a much higher level than his present behavior demonstrates. She sees his difficulties as problems with hearing and seeing, understanding sensory information, and balancing when seated. Wanda and her husband are confident that given time and the right kind of intervention their son will have far more ability than it now appears. They expect that Carmen will talk, go to school, play, and have friends. Although they see Carmen as "always having some problems," their story for him is fairly close to a typical childhood with minor modifications (e.g., he will need a speech therapist, perhaps tutors; he may not be great in sports).

Both parents enjoy their interactions with Carmen, which includes feeding, bathing, dressing, and playing with him. Carmen has favorite toys, including rattles that make noise, soft rubbery toys that squeak, and toys with vibration such as the Bumble Ball. He enjoys being sung to and playing social games such as pat-a-cake and peekaboo. He likes being in water and is enrolled in a swimming program at the local community pool.

Thoroughly enjoying the mothering role, Wanda is very optimistic about Carmen. She feels she knows how to work hard for success and believes that if she is diligent in researching her son's problems, finding the best resources and therapists, and providing a stimulating home environment, she and her husband can help Carmen "overcome" his difficulties. Although Wanda expects this to take time (up to 3 more years), she is willing to work hard for the end result.

Wanda says that she never even considered the possibility of having a child with a problem. She had a typical pregnancy, labor, and delivery. There is no history of this type of problem in her family. Her only sister, Sue, is married with three healthy, active children.

Wanda considers herself to be the type of person who is used to struggle. She always had to work hard for what she earned. Although a good student in school, Wanda needed to study hard. She was social and active in high school and college but again needed to try hard and to look for second chances and special breaks to get what she really wanted. Her work career has unfolded in a similar pattern of hard work and payoff. She is pleased with her job, and although she puts in many long hours, she feels the fruits of her efforts are well worth it.

How Joe Tells His Story to Carmen's Therapist

Joe was and continues to be overwhelmed by the complexity of issues that surround his son's health. He is repeatedly surprised that in spite of their attention to prescriptive orders from doctors and specialists, Carmen's problems persist, and he is concerned at what he calls "a lack of progress." Joe views his wife as the emotionally stronger one and counts on her to deal with the medical care and therapy needs for their son. He is eager to support his wife as she increases her involvement in therapy with their son and decreases her work responsibilities. He feels his greatest contribution is in support, encouragement, and just plain manpower whenever possible.

Joe has had minimal exposure to people with disabilities. He grew up across the street from a boy who was mentally retarded. For the most part Joe remembers his neighbor as slow mentally but normal physically. Joe feels frightened for his wife and son and wishes there were something he could do to protect them both from the ongoing pressures of Carmen's problems. He is hoping that eventually all will work out and has his fingers crossed that the next several years will make a difference for his family.

The Therapist's Story

Natasha's story for Carmen contains some additional information compared with the family story. Natasha has been monitoring her evolving story in an effort to keep from moving too quickly to a view of Carmen's future needs and thus overshadowing the parents' concerns and focus on the present.

In Natasha's eyes, Carmen is a child who is "severely involved." She sees him as a boy who may have vision deficits, significant sensory integration dysfunction, and definite cognitive limitations. Natasha expects that Carmen will require specialized care and schooling as he gets older and that he probably will always depend on adults to initiate and follow through in all aspects of his behavior, including play, learning, and social interactions.

Natasha has worked with many children who have ability levels similar to Carmen's. She has also worked with other families who are deeply resolved to work hard and solve their child's problems; however, she respects the unique history and special concerns of each family. In this instance, Natasha sees the family as having some very definite overall characteristics, including a high level of expectation, a history of success and perseverance, little experience with physical or cognitive disability, and limited emotional support and resources from families and friends. Although Wanda and Joe have been very open and candid regarding some of their difficulties with the constant demand of Carmen's care, Natasha does not feel she knows whether or not these parents have deeper questions and concerns about his future and whether their sense of the future is realistic.

In considering Carmen's sensory processing characteristics, Natasha has considered the questions listed in Box 6-4. Natasha feels that Carmen has definite sensory processing deficits. He is hypersensitive to light touch and seeks proprioceptive and vestibular input. Natasha has noticed that Carmen enjoys rocking when left alone, and she has observed several other self-stimulatory behaviors, including head shaking and seeking visual input by pressing on closed eyes. Questions regarding visual and hearing abilities are still unanswered, although Natasha suspects that Carmen has serious limitations in these areas that, when combined with his cognitive and sensory deficits, will present challenges to the child and family throughout his life.

As Natasha asks herself questions regarding this family's story, she begins to formulate a picture of their beliefs, hopes, and dreams. To Natasha, it seems that Carmen's parents define his problem as a deficit state, something that with the right amount of treatment and care can be fixed or overcome. Carmen's parents enjoy many playful interactions with their son over the course of the day. This family values closeness—being able to talk with, be with, and play with one another. They are affectionate with one another and enjoy kissing and hugging. Carmen is very responsive to his parents; he smiles and laughs in response to their playful touch and voices. Both Joe and Wanda would like to be able to go on outings with their son. They have long dreamed of typical family trips to amusement parks, zoos, and similar attractions. Both are interested in Carmen's looking like other children and responding appropriately when faced with new yet safe and secure situations, such as petting a dog, holding a kitten, and being friendly when meeting new children and visiting friends and relatives.

Taking these priorities into account, Natasha collects information about Carmen's play behaviors and social interactions. When Natasha considers the questions listed in Box 6-5 (temperament, play, and behavior), she gains insight into how Carmen's play and social interactions are affected by his temperament. Natasha notes that Carmen's play is organized as long as an adult structures the interaction and provides the rhythmicity for it. In addition, Carmen has strong preferences for specific play spaces and play materials and exhibits disorganization in his behavior when new toys or different spaces are used. Teachers reported similar behaviors at school, characterizing Carmen as liking things his way. Similarly, his teachers noted that Carmen has difficulty changing from one activity to the next (playtime to snacktime, quiet play to noisy group play), even when those activities follow a prescribed order. Unscheduled and atypical situations present considerable difficulty for Carmen and can put him out of sorts for the rest of the day. These would be important details to share with Carmen's parents and to consider when moving toward play and social goals.

In making observations and inquiries into the specific qualities of Carmen's play, Natasha has found that Carmen has difficulty maintaining attention to his play because of environmental distractions, such as sounds from others; noises outside of the room, such as a car sound or children singing; and touch, including being touched by others who are playing nearby or who walk by, as well as touching the textures of play materials. Typically Carmen spends up to 10 minutes in play with repeated breaks in his attention over that period. Exploration, manipulation, and initiation are all limited by temperament and self-organization characteristics. Carmen's play is guided by his strong and narrow preferences for certain people, settings, and materials. He is most content when he is playing with a familiar adult.

Carmen's limitations in play are influenced by his deficits in gross motor, fine motor, and language and cognitive skills. Many of his skills are typical for a child who is between 15 and 18 months old. Although Carmen has the opportunity to function in several rich and varied environments (home, early intervention center), he maintains a distance from unfamiliar objects, situations, and people. To some extent his own limited preferences have kept him from experiencing variety in his play repertoire, including play companions, play spaces, and play materials.

Figures 6-9 and 6-10 summarize the therapist's view of Carmen and his family's story. They provide some footing for the therapist, who must now get down to the business of creating a viable plan for occupational therapy input to this child and family.

As Natasha considers her understanding of this child and his family, she acts on information that would facilitate the family story. Fortunately, she is able to provide intervention in the family home using the child's own toys and other familiar objects, as well as in the early intervention setting. Because of her experiences in both environments she is able to learn about and work toward goals and objectives that are valued by the family.

Based on her play assessments and interviews with both parents, Natasha has some particular issues to address in treatment: increasing play behaviors, including those that incorporate the parents' interest in having Carmen differentiate toys by touch (finding the ball when given a choice of a ball or a bottle) and increasing his responsiveness to simple commands ("Give me your hands," "Look over here"); developing strategies for family outings (ideas for places to go and ways to facilitate Carmen's participation); and increasing Carmen's spontaneous interactions with people and novel settings. Increasing social play, providing opportunities for modulated responses to new stimuli and situations, and problem solving with parents before outings and family events are all emphasized in the treatment plan. In addition, the therapist is interested in developing a long-term goal with the family in which their future picture of Carmen will take into account the nature of his cognitive, visual, and sensory deficits and the potential long-term impact of these deficits on their personal lives.

Natasha concludes her assessment with questions: Will Carmen be able to fulfill the occupational roles that his family anticipates for him? How will the family modify their occupations in response to Carmen's trajectory of development? How can the therapist best facilitate the family story and a goodness of fit in the evolving roles?

Summary

Priorities for Carmen's occupational therapy intervention were defined through several key avenues of input. The therapist developed an ongoing relationship with the family that allowed her to understand their family story as it related to their primary concerns for their child's needs. These needs were intimately tied to the family's social and cultural view of who they were themselves and what they would like their lives to be like. The therapist used those considerations to guide her assessment of Carmen in his primary occupational role of

player. She also used narrative strategies to create a picture of Carmen as a player and family member, which led her to ask how Carmen will fulfill his roles of player and of family member. Informed by the family story, the therapist designed treatment strategies that were based on the family's definition of their child, as well as on her professional knowledge of how play could be used as a focus for occupation-based intervention.

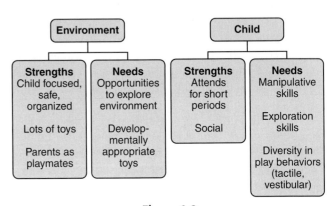

Figure 6-9
The therapist's view of Carmen.

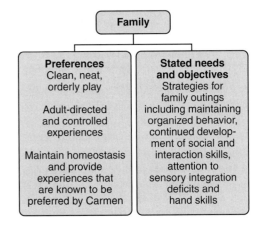

Figure 6-10
The family's story: Carmen, Wanda, and Joe.

CASE EXAMPLE 2

Monica: Rescue Me

The story of Monica demonstrates how the birth of a child with special needs reshapes the family storyline and its impacts on the family's routines and values. It also demonstrates how the telling of the story uncovers opportunities for further assessment and intervention and how play observation can provide a window into the child's and family's strengths and needs. Furthermore, this story demonstrates the effects of reshaping the play environment to enhance the competence of the child and the family as they perform their daily routines and create a long-term vision for their life.

Monica is a child with pervasive developmental disorder. She is bright, beautiful, and energetic. Although she has a strong drive to engage in play, her actions are dominated by a variety of self-stimulatory behaviors, such as hanging upside down on furniture, placing inappropriate objects in her mouth, and making gestures with and talking to her hands. She has an intense and insatiable need for sensory stimulation, while simultaneously seeming to beg for someone to rescue her from her driving urges so that she may play in the world of objects and people.

The Family Story

The story begins with Monica and her family. Monica is the second child of a middle-class, Caucasian family who live in a suburban neighborhood. Her medical and early developmental history were unremarkable with the exception of her sleep patterns, which were irregular at best. Mrs. C, Monica's mother, reports that as an infant, Monica would bang her feet into the wall forcefully in an attempt to get to sleep. This intense banging caused Monica actually to break through her crib one evening. Monica's irregular sleep patterns and frequent waking episodes during the night disrupted the family's sleep routines and placed them under enormous stress. The older child would awaken frequently because of the disruption that Monica caused during the night. Mrs. C felt increasingly tired and irritable because of lack of sleep, and Mr. C's work began to suffer.

The family was concerned about Monica's sleep behavior, but the family pediatrician assured them that there was no cause for worry and advised Mrs. C to calm down, saying that the baby and the rest of the family would in turn be able to calm down. This advice did not comfort the family. By the time Monica was 18 months old, the family had become overwhelmed by her increasingly difficult behaviors. They began to notice her delays in acquiring both language and social interaction skills.

By actively networking through the community, Mrs. C was able to access community support systems and to contact a citywide program that would provide a comprehensive evaluation for Monica. Based on this evaluation at 20 months of age, pervasive developmental disorder with borderline developmental delay and severe language delay was diagnosed. Although the diagnosis was troubling, it provided a degree of relief for Mrs. C because she no longer felt that Monica's behavior was a result of something she was doing wrong. She remembers feeling positive that now she had a

direction for addressing Monica's needs and enrolled her daughter in a local preschool program for children with special needs.

Monica's problem behaviors and intense sensory needs continued to dominate this family story. Although the preschool program offered some assistance with Monica's care, the family still felt stressed about her behavior at home. Left unsupervised, Monica was a danger to herself and her older brother. She quickly learned to unlatch the front door and run out to the street. She would scream, hit, pinch, or bite when her brother tried to prevent her from leaving the house or engaging in other dangerous play. Although the family fenced in the yard to provide a safe play area for Monica, she quickly mastered climbing the fence. Mrs. C was no longer able to work outside the home, which created considerable financial stress for the family.

Daily family routines were also significantly altered by Monica's behavior. Family mealtime was one of many battlegrounds for Monica. She refused all but a limited variety of foods and resisted remaining seated at the table. She disliked having clothing on her body, so dressing became a wrestling match that often ended in a tantrum. Brushing her teeth was impossible unless Mrs. C physically restrained her.

Despite the chaos created by Monica, the family remained committed to helping her in any way possible. Because of a close extended family, the grandparents offered considerable assistance with both children and provided periods of respite for the parents. Mrs. C continued to pursue any services that she felt would be helpful for Monica, including behavioral and speech therapy in the home and occupational therapy at a local clinic.

The family has always been able to look past Monica's disability and see her as a bright, beautiful, energetic youngster, with special needs. They continue to maintain a strong hope that once her behavior is under control and her language emerges, Monica will be able to function independently. Using the snapshot exercise described earlier in this chapter, Monica's parents talk about their future vision for her. They hope to see Monica grow up to be self-sufficient, use language with a true communicative intent, be able to socialize with others, and have a life that does not include special education.

Listening to the family story gives the therapist the opportunity to engage in connected knowing and to enter the family's frame to "discover the premises for the other's point of view" (Belenky et al., 1986, p. 101). The therapist is able to gain insight into how Monica's special needs shape the family storyline. It is obvious that the family values children and is willing to make the children the focus of their lives. The physical and emotional home environment echoes this value. Although the family is overwhelmed with the situation that Monica's needs have created, they continue to seek answers and solutions. Aware of the needs of their other child as well, the family seeks balance and stability in their lives, as well as ways to enhance Monica's behavior and functioning. As noted earlier in this chapter, families establish patterns of behavior that are culturally meaningful, and the ways a family engages in play reflect their culturally driven values and purposes. Although Monica has significantly disrupted this family's patterns, they continue to engage in an active process of redefining their patterns, seeking a fit between values and behaviors.

The following section describes how play observation is used to guide adaptations of the play environment in order to assist the family in meeting their valued goals for Monica and to reestablish a degree of stability and balance in the family.

The Therapist's Story

The therapist enters the story with a deep understanding and appreciation of the premises that Reilly (1962) set forth regarding human occupation. Monica is not able to realize the occupation of play. Her behavior is driven by her intense need for sensory input. Because the stimuli are not grounded in meaning, they simply perpetuate a vicious cycle of aggressive, sensory-seeking behavior. She is unable to use sensory input for adaptive, purposeful interactions with her environment. As a result, play, as we define it, does not exist for Monica.

Observation of Monica's unstructured time provides a valuable vehicle for interpreting her sensory processing play behaviors and other skills. In addressing the questions related to sensory processing as presented in Box 6-1, the therapist recognizes that Monica craves sensory input and uses self-stimulating behaviors to gain it. She uses her hands (and any other part of her body for that matter) not for exploration but merely for stimulation. She requires an extremely high and constant level of input. She is in perpetual motion. When deprived of this level of activity, Monica becomes aggressive and agitated and frequently throws tantrums and screams for long periods.

Examples of Monica's spontaneous behavior include running around the room and banging into a large upholstered chair, hanging upside down on the couch, walking across the top of the couch to the window ledge and jumping onto a large pillow on the floor, and finally running over to her mother and pulling up her shirt for a back rub. Monica also seeks oral stimulation using an object such as a plastic dinosaur or her fingers to provide the desired input. She enjoys playing outside on a swing set and running around the fenced yard using blades of grass to provide herself with visual self-stimulation as she runs in circles. Monica uses all types of sensory input for self-stimulation, including visual, tactile, vestibular, and proprioceptive. In contrast, Monica demonstrates a severe aversion to imposed stimulation such as her mother's combing her hair or the therapist's attempts to engage her in sand play.

A typical day for Monica begins after a night of interrupted sleep followed by difficulty waking in the morning. Breakfast is unpredictable, since Monica's tolerance for foods varies greatly on any given day. If presented with a food that is not tolerable, Monica has a tantrum and runs away. Dressing and grooming are also difficult because she dislikes putting clothes on and has severe aversive reactions to having her hair combed and her teeth brushed.

Monica rides the bus to school and returns each day at 3:15 PM. The afternoon and evening hours are characterized by the behaviors previously described. Monica enjoys watching videotaped movies. Bedtime often spans several hours. Monica is difficult to calm down at the end of the day, and once asleep she wakes at unpredictable times and remains awake and active for several hours. She often goes to her parents' bed and keeps them awake for several hours during the night.

Monica's behavior is characteristically driven by her sensory processing dysfunction and her temperament, which includes an extraordinarily high level of activity with little or no rhythmicity in her interactions. In reference to Box 6-5 and Box 6-1, which address issues of temperament and level of play, Monica's behavior is interpreted as in a constant state of overarousal. She is unable to maintain periods of focused attention for purposeful behavior, is guided by her own internal rhythms, and is driven by a need for a high level of stimulation. Monica is unable to engage in even the lowest level of play, since she cannot sustain her attention to materials or actions with the exception of self-stimulating objects and behaviors. Exploration, manipulation, variety, diversity, interaction, and creativity in play, as described in Box 6-1, are not possible at this point given Monica's preoccupation with sensory stimulation.

The next level of assessment gained through play observation is designed to clarify information regarding skill development (Box 6-2). Monica demonstrates highly developed motor skills, especially in the area of gross motor development. She is able to climb, balance, motor plan, and execute quite sophisticated motor activities such as pumping a swing, pedaling a bike, and climbing a metal fence. She demonstrates no fear of movement, and her coordination is excellent.

Fine motor and visual motor skills, although not formally assessed, appears age appropriate and certainly adequate for developmentally appropriate, functional behaviors such as feeding, dressing, and using crayons. Cognitively, Monica's abilities are more puzzling. Although she is limited by a severe language delay, she appears to be able to solve complex problems to have her needs met. Spontaneous language, although meaningless, demonstrates a wide range of skills. For example, Monica is able to verbalize intricate strings of words such as, "Stop it yellow, I'm coming over to get you." She can memorize long phrases and paragraphs from the videotaped movies she watches. Her potential for language seems excellent, but like her other behaviors, her language is inaccessible to the people around her.

An important area for assessment and intervention with Monica and her family is the environment. The environment is seen as providing the context within which behavior occurs, as well as supporting children's play (through exploration) and motor skill development (through movement and exercise). Consideration of the environment includes human and nonhuman characteristics that have an impact on the child's play. Use of the questions in Box 6-3 to structure the observation of Monica's environment reveals many positive characteristics of the play environment. There

is adequate space and time for play, and there are varied play objects and opportunities for different types of play (quiet play, active play, social play). Attention has been paid to safety and developmental appropriateness of play objects. In terms of the human environment, Monica has access to a variety of people (siblings, parents, grandparents, peers) to facilitate purposeful interactions. At this time Monica is unable to access these environmental supports. Her sensory processing dysfunction drives her intrinsic motivation toward activities that are self-stimulating rather than interaction oriented.

Summary

This unfolding of the story provides insight into Monica and her family that can be organized as shown in Figures 6-11 and 6-12. This organization provides direction for intervention, which addresses the sensory processing dysfunction that underlies Monica's extreme activity level, her inability to establish patterns of sleep, her self-stimulating behaviors, and her inability to sustain focused attention for purposeful behavior. Based on these findings, an approach combining traditional sensory integrative intervention with environmental adaptations in the home is initiated. Examples of intervention strategies are listed in Table 6-1.

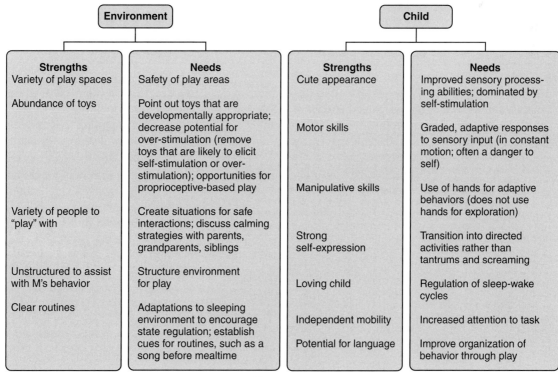

Figure 6-11
The therapist's view of Monica.

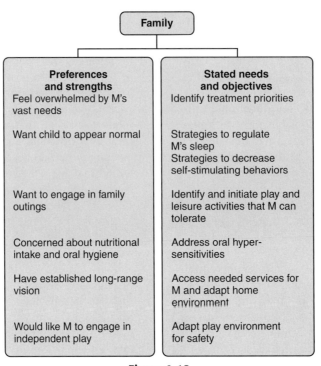

Figure 6-12
Monica's family's story.

Table 6-1
Intervention Strategies for Monica

Goals	Intervention Strategies	Play Activities
Short-Term Goals		
Decrease extreme activity level as a basis for improved ability to participate in play, learning, and social activities.	Use weighted vest in the home. Use weighted blankets at night combined with large pillows to create deep touch proprioceptive nest. Set up strategies for play with high levels of proprioceptive input.	Play cowgirl with child wearing weighted vest as she rides horsy and looks for stray cows. Play hide-and-seek under weighted blankets, or build a fort with large pillows and weighted blankets. Provide a secret hideaway for child to escape to when feeling overloaded; supply pillows, sleeping bags, comforters, towels, etc. for a hideout under a table or desk or behind a couch.
Establish regular sleep patterns as a basis for a regulated state needed for play, learning, self-care, and social participation.	Initiate predictable before-bed routines. Use comfort object (cuddly doll, blanket, pacifier, or chewy toy) to restore sleeping state when child awakens during the night. Use weighted blanket.	Establish quiet, calming playtime with parent before bed.

Continued

Table 6-1
Intervention Strategies for Monica—cont'd

Goals	Intervention Strategies	Play Activities
Decrease oral tactile hypersensitivity as a basis for improved ability to participate in play, learning, and social activities.	Use vibrating toothbrush to massage gums and cheeks. Provide crunchy foods, e.g., dry cereal, popcorn, chips, crackers, apples, celery, nuts, carrots, ice cubes. Offer chewing gum, gummy candy, or rubber tubing. Use Nuk Brush.	Introduce oral activities: blowing bubbles through a straw, blowing a whistle, licking stickers, drinking through "crazy" or regular straws. Allow child to safely explore mouth with Nuk Brush, and use a mirror to encourage playful interactions. Play peekaboo games with washcloths (wet, dry, cold, warm) with the goal of having her tolerate facial massage.
Decrease tactile sensitivity to improve manipulative exploration and play.	Participate in proprioceptive and pressure touch activities such as firmly toweling off after bath. Brush body.	Play hide-and-seek under a beanbag chair. Gradually increase tactile play as tolerated, e.g., play with water table, sandbox, play dough, clay, popcorn, rice, oatmeal, fingerpaint. Make a game of brushing with varied brushes. Play with textures (soaps, shaving cream, lotion). Draw with chalk on body and erase with varied textures (sponges, thick washcloths, plastic brushes).
Increase proprioceptive input and decrease excessive seeking of proprioceptive stimuli as a basis for improved self-regulation, attention, and play.	Provide opportunities for child to do "heavy work" in order to receive deep proprioceptive input at major joints in the body.	Practice crab walking or wheelbarrow walking in the yard. Bear walk under the table or through an obstacle course using couches and tables. Help child pull a wagon around neighborhood to deliver cookies to neighbors. Have her pull herself on scooter board to play human bowling.
Long-Term Goals		
Increase exploration of environment through play.	Encourage exploration, manipulation, initiation, diversification, and interaction.	Set up a fun, simple obstacle course with varied textures, motor challenges, and sensory rewards.
Develop play skills.	Introduce developmentally appropriate play objects.	Plant developmentally appropriate play objects around the house to entice child and encourage child-directed play.
Improve independence in self-care and routines of daily living.	Provide opportunities to develop dressing skills and grooming skills. Start a routine of always washing hands before snacktime.	Dress up a favorite doll. Play dress-up with mom's or dad's clothing.

SUMMARY

A great deal of information about a child can be gained as a therapist creates stories through assessment and observation of play, as well as informal dialogues and interviews with a family. Organization of this information into a usable format for analysis and synthesis provides the therapist with a structure for developing intervention priorities that flow from the integration of the therapist's view of the child with the interests and values of the family as expressed through the family's story. Assessment that is narrative in nature; focused on family-driven values, interests, and concerns; and oriented to the occupation of the child as a player yields useful and highly relevant data to guide successful occupational therapy interventions.

Review Questions

1. This chapter describes some of the current practice problems in pediatrics. Discuss these, considering implications for intervention and assessment.
2. Describe how therapists can use storytelling to assist families as they prepare to care for a disabled child.
3. Discuss the clinical storylines (1) play and sensory processing issues and (2) play and temperament issues. How can the therapist integrate these storylines into a broader perspective of the child?
4. What is a "family story"? What is a "therapist's story"? How does the therapist integrate these in an assessment to plan intervention?

REFERENCES

Als, H. (1986). *A synactive model of neonatal behavioral organization: Framework for the assessment of neurobehavioral development in the premature infant and for support of infants and parents in the neonatal intensive care environment.* New York: Haworth Press.

Anzalone, M. E. (1994, July). *Mother-infant play: Developmental level and exploratory style.* Paper presented at the Annual Conference of the American Occupational Therapy Association and the Canadian Association of Occupational Therapists, Boston.

Ayres, A. J. (1972). *Sensory integration and learning disorders.* Los Angeles: Western Psychological Services.

Bailey, D. (1971). Vocational theories and work habits related to childhood development. *American Journal of Occupational Therapy, 25,* 298-302.

Bates, J. E. (1989). Concepts and measures of temperament. In G. A. Kohnstamm, J. E. Bates, & M. K. Rothbart (Eds.), *Temperament in childhood* (pp. 3-26). Chichester, England: John Wiley & Sons.

Belenky, M. F., Clinchy, B., Goldberger, N., & Tarule J. (1986). *Women's ways of knowing: The development of self, voice, and mind.* New York: Basic Books.

Brazelton, T. B., & Lester, B. M. (1983). *New approaches to developmental screening of infants.* New York: Elsevier.

Bruner, E. (1984). The opening up of anthropology. In E. M. Bruner (Ed.), *Text, play, and story: The construction and reconstruction of self and society.* Washington, DC: American Ethnological Society.

Bruner, J. (1990). *Acts of meaning.* Cambridge, MA: Harvard University Press.

Bundy, A. C. (1997). Play and playfulness: What to look for. In L. D. Parham & L. S. Fazio (Eds.), *Play in occupational therapy for children.* St. Louis: Mosby.

Burke, J. P. (1993a). *Illness narratives* (Unpublished paper, University of Pennsylvania, Philadelphia).

Burke, J. P. (1993b). Play: The life role of the infant and young child. In J. Case-Smith (Ed.), *Pediatric occupational therapy and early intervention.* Andover, MA: Andover Publishers.

Burke, J. P., & Frank, A. (1994, July). *Narrative rehabilitation: The untaught half of occupational therapy.* Paper presented at the Annual Conference of the American Occupational Therapy Association and the Canadian Association of Occupational Therapists, Boston.

Carey, W. B. (1983). Intervention strategies using temperament data. In T. B. Brazelton & B. M. Lester (Eds.), *New approaches to developmental screening of infants* (pp. 245-257). New York: Elsevier.

Chess, S., & Thomas, A. (1989). Issues in the clinical application of temperament. In G. A. Kohnstamm, J. E. Bates, & M. K. Rothbart (Eds.), *Temperament in childhood* (pp. 377-386). Chichester, England: John Wiley & Sons.

DeGrace, B. W. (2003). Occupation-based and family-centered care: A challenge for current practice. *American Journal of Occupational Therapy, 57*(3), 347-350.

Denzin, N. (1989). *Interpretive biography.* Newbury Park, CA: Sage Publications.

D'Eugenio, D. (1986). Infant play: A reflection of cognitive and motor development. In C. Pehoski (Ed.), *Play, a skill for life.* Rockville, MD: American Occupational Therapy Association.

Dunst, C. J., Trivette, C. M., & Deal, A. G. (Eds.). (1994). *Supporting and strengthening families: Vol. 1: Methods, strategies and practices.* Cambridge, MA: Brookline Books.

Florey, L. L. (1971). An approach to play and play development. *American Journal of Occupational Therapy, 25,* 275-280.

Florey, L. L. (1981). Studies of play: Implications for growth, development, and for clinical practice. *American Journal of Occupational Therapy, 35,* 519-524.

Frank, A. (1991). *At the will of the body.* Boston: Houghton Mifflin.

Greene, S. (1997). Playmates: Social interaction in early and middle childhood. In B. E. Chandler (Ed.), *The essence of play: A child's occupation* (pp. 131-158). Bethesda, MD: American Occupational Therapy Association.

Hanft, B., Burke, J. P., Cahill, M., Swenson-Miller, K., & Humphry, R. (1992). *Working with families: A curriculum guide for pediatric occupational therapists.* Chapel Hill, NC: Frank Porter Graham Child Development Center.

Holzmueller, R. L. (2005). Therapists I have known and (mostly) loved. *American Journal of Occupational Therapy 59*(5), 580-587.

Hurff, J. (1974). A play skills inventory. In M. Reilly (Ed.), *Play as exploratory learning: Studies in curiosity behavior.* Beverly Hills, CA: Sage Publications.

Individuals with Disabilities Education Act Amendments of 1991 (IDEA). Oct. 7, 1991, PL 102-119, 105 Stat. 587.

Individuals with Disabilities Education Improvement Act of 2004 (IDEIA). Dec. 3, 2004, PL 108-446, Stat. 2647.

Kleinman, A. (1988). *The illness narratives.* New York: Basic Books.

Knox, S. (1974). A play scale. In M. Reilly (Ed.), *Play as exploratory learning: Studies in curiosity behavior.* Beverly Hills, CA: Sage Publications.

Knox, S. (1996). Play and playfulness in preschool children. In R. Zemke & F. Clark (Eds.), *Occupational science: The evolving discipline.* Philadelphia: F.A. Davis.

Matsutsuyu, J. (1971). Occupational behavior: A perspective on work and play. *American Journal of Occupational Therapy, 25,* 291-294.

Mattingly, C. (1991). The narrative nature of clinical reasoning. *American Journal of Occupational Therapy, 45,* 998-1006.

Michelman, S. (1974). Play and the deficit child. In M. Reilly (Ed.), *Play as exploratory learning: Studies in curiosity behavior.* Beverly Hills, CA: Sage Publications.

Porges, S. W. (1993). The infant's sixth sense: Awareness and regulation of bodily processes. *Zero to Three, 14,* 12-16.

Price, R. (1994). *A whole new life.* New York: Atheneum.

Reilly, M. (1962). Occupational therapy can be one of the great ideas of 20th century medicine. *American Journal of Occupational Therapy, 16,* 1-9.

Reilly, M. (1971). The modernization of occupational therapy. *American Journal of Occupational Therapy, 25,* 243-246.

Reilly, M. (1974). Defining a cobweb. In M. Reilly (Ed.), *Play as exploratory learning: Studies in curiosity behavior.* Beverly Hills, CA: Sage Publications.

Schaaf, R., & Burke, J. (Eds.)(1992a): *Sensory integration and play* (issues 1 & 2). American Occupational Therapy Association, Special Interest Section Newsletter, Rockville, MD: American Occupational Therapy Association.

Schaaf, R. C., & Burke, J. P. (1992b). Clinical reflections on play and sensory integration. *Sensory Integration Special Interest Section Newsletter, 15,* 1-2.

Schaaf, R. C., Merrill, S. C., & Kinsella, N. (1987). Sensory integration and play behavior: A case study of the effectiveness of occupational therapy using sensory integrative techniques. *Occupational Therapy in Health Care, 4,* 61-75.

Schaaf, R. C., & Mulrooney, L. (1989). Occupational therapy in early intervention: A family-centered approach. *American Journal of Occupational Therapy, 43,* 745-754.

Schon, D. (1983). *The reflective practitioner.* New York: Basic Books.

Shannon, P. (1972). Work-play theory and the occupational therapy process. *American Journal of Occupational Therapy, 26,* 169-172.

Sundstrom, C. (1972). The physiological aspects of work and play. *American Journal of Occupational Therapy, 26,* 173-175.

Takata, N. (1969). The play history. *American Journal of Occupational Therapy, 23,* 314-318.

Takata, N. (1974). Play as a prescription. In M. Reilly (Ed.), *Play as exploratory learning: Studies in curiosity behavior.* Beverly Hills, CA: Sage Publications.

Tanta, K. J., Deitz, J. C., White, O., & Billingsley, F. (2005). The effects of peer-play level on initiations and responses of preschool children with delayed play skills. *American Journal of Occupational Therapy, 59*(4), 437-445.

III

Play as a Means for Enhancing Development and Skill Acquisition

7

Power of Object Play for Infants and Toddlers

Veronique Munier, Christine Teeters Myers, and Doris Pierce

KEY TERMS

object play
occupational science
therapist design skill
occupational intactness
occupational appeal
occupational accuracy
spatial negotiation skills
temporal negotiation skills
social skills
motivational properties

TAPPING THE THERAPEUTIC POWER OF OBJECT PLAY

Object play is the predominant waking activity of the young child. Few are the pediatric occupational therapy sessions that do not rely on object play for their therapeutic outcomes. How, then, can object play be most effectively applied by occupational therapists to facilitate development in young children at risk for delays? This chapter offers a discussion of the sources of power in object play applications, the types of goals addressed in play-based interventions, and the use of object play in the treatment of young children.

An Occupational Science Approach to Object Play

The promise that occupational science has made to occupational therapy is that, through its contributions to the field's understanding of occupation, therapists will bring the applications of occupation to bear in increasingly potent ways (Clark et al., 1991). Recent research has called attention to some important aspects of childhood occupations: the relationship between memory and occupation (Lee, 2003), the role of culture in shaping occupational experience (Bazyk, 2003), and the realities of co-occupations (Pierce, 2000). This research highlights the relationship between the quality of occupational experience and important facets of human life. Focused study of the play of children with disabilities can yield further resources for application by teaching us how best to support occupation for these children (Baranek, 2005; Missiuna, 1991; Okimoto, Bundy, & Hanzlik, 2000).

A hallmark of human evolutionary adaptation is the reliance on alterations of the physical environment (Bechtel & Churchman, 2002; Chapple & Coon, 1942; Moore, 1992). Human occupations involve a striking variety of material culture: crops, shelters, domesticated animals, vehicles, tools and machinery, esthetic and ritual objects, clothing, information records, foods, medicines, and toys. Complex manipulations of physical objects in space and time are an essential aspect of the human occupational nature. Part of the scientist's fascination with children's object play stems from a desire to understand the interaction of humans with their physical environment. When therapists are supporting children's play with objects, they are encouraging the development of a profoundly human trait. It can be hypothesized that they also help establish the foundation for later mastery of objects.

Therapists are particularly familiar with stationary object play. Young children, however, also move with objects, incorporate objects into mobile play, and use objects to explore their environments. Children's interactions with their physical environment include the negotiation of space. Spatial skills are important in the consideration of object play. Henderson (1992) argued that occupational therapy has neglected examination of human spatial skills in near and far space. Her argument can be extended even further to propose that humans require spatial skills, not only for managing bodily movements in space, but also for managing complex relationships between themselves and a variety of physical objects. It is in object play that the early foundation is laid for constant adult interactions with the objects and spaces of the physical world.

Occupational Therapy for Infants and Toddlers at Risk for Developmental Delays

Pediatric occupational therapists often treat infants and toddlers at risk for developmental delays. These infants may have unclear diagnoses and a medical history that may or may not include prematurity, birth complications, irregularities of muscle tone, questions regarding hearing and vision, and respiratory and feeding problems. The play deficits of children with physical, developmental, intellectual, environmental, or psychological problems are also documented in the literature (Baranek, 2005; Dee, 1974; Gralewicz, 1973; Howard, 1986; Kalverboer, 1977; Mack, Lindquist, & Parham, 1982; Missiuna, 1991; Mogford, 1977; Okimoto et al., 2000; Vandenburg & Kielhofner, 1982; Wehman, 1977; Wehman & Abramson, 1976). In addition to the therapeutic needs of the child, the therapist is often dealing with a family in turmoil.

The unclear prognoses of these young children demand strong assessment, acute observation, and sensitivity to the many contexts of occupation to allow the establishment of treatment goals. The current expectation for early intervention services is the provision of occupational therapy within the natural environments of the child and family (Individuals with Disabilities Education Improvement Act of 2004). Natural environment settings are not just the home, but also any community or family settings where the child participates in activities, including the child care center, the library, the park, and relatives' homes. The environments incorporate a vast variety of contexts that support learning, such as engaging in water play at the child care center, choosing a book at the library, picking up rocks at the park, and helping a grandmother knead dough to bake bread (Dunst, Trivette, Humphries, Raab, & Roper, 2001; Hanft & Pilkington, 2000). Object play within this therapeutic approach creates unique opportunities for the occupational therapist to support and coach caregivers to assist in the child's learning of adaptive behaviors and developmental skills within naturally occurring occupations. To engage in truly family-centered therapy within the natural environment, however, therapists must shed their ties to the clinic and focus strictly on the affordances provided. In other words, the occupational therapist's bag of therapy toys must be abandoned for the objects already present in the natural setting (Hanft & Anzalone, 2001; Hanft & Pilkington, 2000). Creativity becomes even more important

as therapists concentrate on incorporating children's learning opportunities within the routines of the natural setting.

DESIGNING FOR POWER IN THERAPEUTIC OCCUPATIONS

How are the most effective object play interventions created? What are the sources of power in a successful therapeutic application of occupation? Occupational therapists are quite good at breaking down an activity into components or analyzing the weaknesses and strengths of a patient's performance. This facility is not surprising, considering its similarity to many forms of reductionist thinking in the medical milieu. Many therapists, however, do not understand how to creatively design occupations that will most effectively draw a patient toward goals. Often this critical ability is assumed to be acquired through practice or is dismissed as simple pragmatics or use of a "recipe book." Like very young children in object play, therapists are good at taking apart occupation but not yet so good at putting it together.

Occupational therapists currently create intervention activities by combining in-depth knowledge of a subskill area with a superficial grasp of the occupation to be used as an intervention. This is not the fault of the therapist but reflects the paucity of literature on the dynamics of everyday occupations. Generation of effective therapeutic occupations depends on the therapist's ability to consistently design activities that are intact, appealing, and custom fitted to the goals of the patient.

Therapist's Design Skill

The design skill of the therapist is essential to therapeutic outcomes (Pierce, 2001, 2003). Of course, the therapist also requires skills of empathy, assessment, goal setting, and management of the occurring treatment session. Recognizing naturally occurring activities that can be effective in reaching goals, however, is a demanding and poorly understood therapy skill. Occupational therapists working with children are required to do original problem solving for every treatment. The repeated effort to creatively adapt multiple activities the child may select throughout every treatment session can be extremely challenging, especially for a new therapist.

All treatment settings contain barriers to creative design. The effectiveness of play-based interventions can be limited by time pressures, a restricted choice of play objects, lack of understanding of normal play patterns, and a clinical culture that favors component level interventions over intact occupational applications. Some of these barriers are more easily overcome than others. The importance of identifying barriers to creative design is twofold. First, recognizing barriers to excellence in treatment design positions the therapist to change those barriers if the opportunity arises. Second, the therapist's realization that limited efficacy of treatment may not be entirely his or her fault reduces frustration and burnout.

Generating effective object play interventions is a design process (Pierce, 2001, 2003). The creative skills of occupational therapists require more nurturance and training than is often provided in our educational programs. The phases of the design process include self-motivation, analysis, problem definition, ideation, idea selection, implementation, and evaluation of the intervention's success. If therapists were to broaden their conceptualization of their own professional development to include these critical design skills, the skills could be easily developed to the professional levels required. The occupational design process offers many ways for therapists to enhance their creative design skills.

Sources of Power in Therapeutic Occupations

Occupational Appeal

The *appeal* of the therapeutic occupation is the attractiveness of the activity to the child. Appeal depends on the experience of a desirable blend of productivity, pleasure, and restoration during engagement. To create occupational applications with high appeal, the therapist depends on empathy for how the client sees the world. For children the interaction is usually the most valued aspect of the experience, emanating from sensations, fun, play, and novelty. Another factor in the appeal of an activity is its developmental fit to the child, or the degree to which the activity fits the child's current abilities and social identity. A strong understanding of normal object play is especially useful for creating play-based interventions that offer a good developmental fit to children at risk for delays. (See "Motivational Properties in Therapeutic Object Play" in this chapter.) Choosing play objects that are irresistible but not overwhelming requires both acute therapeutic judgment and a thorough assessment of the family's or community's resources. The therapist may collaborate with the family or other caregiver to choose among the objects available for therapy, but for a more authentic family-centered approach, the therapist should integrate therapy into activities and objects chosen by the child (Hanft & Pilkington, 2000).

Occupational Intactness

The *intactness* of an occupation is the degree to which the activity used as an intervention is whole. That is, it occurs in the natural condition in which it is to be found in daily life, rather than in some unnatural form created solely for use as an intervention. The natural conditions of an occupation include the patient's senses of usual choices, spaces, times, and social situations associated with that occupation. The importance of such self-direction to therapeutic gains is especially supported in pediatrics by the work of Ayres (1985). The usual spatial context of an occupation is rich with cues, opportunities, and affordances that can have positive effects on outcomes. The usual social context of an occupation similarly supports performance, as well as conferring a more positive identity than is conferred on a child by a medical setting. The wholeness of the temporal context of the occupation includes the tempo, length, sequence, time of day, and frequency of the activity. The intactness of an occupational application can be difficult to maintain in occupational therapy practice settings that are not the natural settings of the child and family to whom the therapist is providing services. Even in such unnatural settings the therapist can find ways to more closely approximate natural settings, such as the opportunity to offer the treatment in another place or time, to use usual play objects, or to normalize aspects of the clinical setting to which the therapist may be confined.

Having knowledge about occupations as they occur naturally will help therapists to design for intactness. Occupational science is producing increasing amounts of descriptive work on typical childhood play. As therapists learn more about children's play in the natural settings of the home, school, play yard, and day care, they will recognize ideas for interventions that are more complex, have a natural context, and appeal to the child and family. The complexity of natural occupations is a reflection of the many contexts involved and the subjectivity of occupational experience. Therapists must enlarge their understanding of occupation and of the dynamic relationship between occupational experience and context. Later in the chapter, resources are provided to help build this knowledge.

Occupational Accuracy

The accuracy of the therapeutic activity ensures that the application is clearly targeted on treatment goals. It is possible to design an intact and appealing occupation that does not result in any therapeutic gains. This can be a result of poor fit between identified goals and the selected intervention and reflects a failure in the therapist's design skills. The occupational therapist is required to perform a constant mental balancing act, blending occupations that will be engaging for the patient with those that will produce therapeutic gains. Therapists can feel, by their own satisfaction level at the end of the session, whether the correct balance has been struck. The accuracy of an occupational intervention also depends on the collaboration between the therapist and the family when identifying desirable goals. Therapists must combine their knowledge of typical infant occupations with excellent interview and observation skills to support the accuracy of family-centered interventions that make use of object play.

LITERATURE ON OBJECT PLAY

In the developmental interventions of pediatric occupational therapists, psychology and neurology form the extradisciplinary literature base, while play in the sessions is the active reality. Few descriptions of play development are available, leaving the more established theories of skill acquisition to predominate in the field. Thus, although pediatric therapists are convinced of the importance of play, they conceive of development mostly in terms of attaining motor and process skills (Couch, 1998). This fragmentary relationship between therapists' daily use of play and their training in development influences practice in two negative ways. Therapists are pushed toward reductionistic goal setting at the level of performance skills by the inadequacy of the play literature. They are also pushed away from interventions that use whole and developmentally typical play occupations as either the means or the ends of intervention (Gray, 1998).

The greatest challenge of using a play-based approach to occupational therapy for children at risk for delays is the creation of therapeutic applications primarily from a literature that does not describe children's play. In Western culture, play and development are related and intertwining concepts (Hutt & Hutt, 1970; Kalverboer, 1977; Kielhofner & Barris, 1984; Piaget, 1952, 1962, 1976; Rosenblatt, 1977). In classic texts "play" is a cultural and relatively amorphous term referring to the activities of children. It has been widely credited as a source of learning and a critical sphere for normal development (Florey, 1981; Piaget, 1962; Reilly, 1974; Robinson, 1977). On the other hand, "development" is a term that refers to the performance skills that support play actions (e.g., perception, movement, and cognition). Assessment tools currently used in the profession are congruent with this conception of development. To design interventions with therapeutic power requires the therapist to rethink development in terms of occupation: an intuitive leap from underlying performance skills to the creation of play applications. The growing literature on children's occupations can guide the therapist's thinking. When drawing from extradisciplinary knowledge, therapists must reformulate therapeutic goals to focus on occupations. Readers should keep this in mind as they become familiar with the basic theories on object play and spatial negotiation discussed in the following sections.

Theories on Object Play

Piaget's Play Theory
Piaget (1952, 1962) emphasized the development of cognition from play experience. According to Piaget (1962), practice games predominate before the age of 2 years. Within practice games, Piaget delineated three categories.

Mere practice games are reproductions of actions for the sake of exercising power over the environment. Later, they are replaced by fortuitous combinations, which are playful repetitions of discovered object combinations. Last in practice games are intentional combinations, in which the child deliberately designs action sequences that are repeated for the sake of play. The change from practice games to symbolic games at approximately 2 years of age is distinguished by the use of imaginary objects and settings (Piaget, 1962).

Occupational therapists working with very young children draw on Piagetian play theory primarily in their efforts to move the child from a passive lack of engagement with play objects to the simple production of effects on objects. Therapists with an interest in play theory may even attempt to facilitate advancement from one Piagetian play stage to the next. Piagetian theory, however, is used primarily to understand the cognitive skills supporting the childhood occupation of play. It is imprecise in describing the actual repertoire of play actions, the sequencing of those actions, or the influence of environmental characteristics on the child's play.

Pretend Play
Pretend activities begin to emerge during the second year, increase for 3 or 4 years, and then taper off (Fein, 1981). Although pretend increases over the early years, it is still a relatively infrequent play form, reaching a maximum of 37% of play acts in kindergarten children (Rubin, Maioni, & Hornung, 1976). At first, at around 12 months, pretend play is referenced only to the self (Piaget, 1962). Later pretend is directed toward another, such as a doll (Fein, 1981).

Pretend play is not a primary concern for occupational therapists working with infants and toddlers, since the youth and developmental delays of these children often place them at a less sophisticated play level than that of pretend. Therapists must recognize that children less than 2 years of age are generally playing in very concrete terms. Although pretend play acts, such as talking on a play phone, may hold the child's interest momentarily or stimulate some imitation, they are unlikely to produce the enthusiastic play engagement of a more developmentally appropriate activity. Recognition of the developmental complexity of pretend play will steer the therapist working with a very young child toward concrete object play strategies more likely to generate therapeutic gains.

Studies of Infant Play with Objects
As a group, the studies of infant object play confirm the existence of a variety of partial patterns in the development of infant-object interactions. Actions serving to explore the physical properties of objects (mouthing, handling, and others) increase in complexity, moving away from just mouthing and toward inclusion of vision, touch, and sound. Action fit becomes more specifically tailored to the

object (Palmer, 1989; Rochat, 1989; Ruff, 1984). Rochat (1989) studied the actions of 6- to 12-month-old infants who were offered hand-sized objects while being held in the mother's lap. The infants performed a broad range of actions: three types of fingering, mouthing, switching objects between hands, dropping, other releases, waving, banging on the table, banging between hands, slapping on table, dangling, pulling on a part of the object, scooting, pressing on the table, squeezing, and touching to face.

Developmental progression in object play can be seen in increasingly precise grasp, increasing appropriateness of object use, object separations and combinations, and the phases of pretense-symbolic object play. Fenson, Kagan, Kearsley, and Zelazo (1976) described changes in predominating play acts from close visual and tactual examination with mouthing at 7 months, to simple physical relating of objects at 9 months, to increasing diversity, symbolic activity, and sequential play by 20 months. Belsky and Most (1981), observing free play with standard objects in infants from 7 to 21 months old, found developmental progressions in the emergence of manipulation, use of objects in ways identified as their usual functions, object combinations, and increasingly complex pretend play.

Largo and Howard's (1979) laboratory study of children from 9 to 30 months old interacting with a standard set of toys demonstrated that exploration through mouthing, manipulation, and vision dominated at 1 year. Container play was most prevalent at 15 months. Functionally appropriate object play emerged at the beginning of the second year. Grouping behavior, the physical ordering of objects with like characteristics, began at 18 to 24 months of age. Representational doll play, such as pretend infant caregiving, predominated at 18 to 30 months.

Occupational therapists working with young children at risk for developmental delays must distill guidelines for treatment from this limited body of play research. Developmental trends in this group of studies can serve as ends, or goal targets, for play development, as well as means for designing developmentally appropriate therapeutic activities. This review clearly shows that changes gradually appear in the simple exploration of objects, from simple mouthing to very specific fit of action to object. Simple physical relating of objects begins at 9 months and then develops into the increasingly complex object relations of container play and other combinations. Use of objects in functional, or culturally expected, ways emerges at 12 months of age. The emergence of pretend and symbolic play is evident at approximately 18 months, at first directed toward the self and with real objects and then becoming directed toward others and completely imaginary objects. If the therapist can find the place on these play progressions that fits the at-risk child with whom he or she is working, the power of the treatment will be greatly enhanced.

Theories of the Development of Spatial Skills

The negotiation of space is a central skill in the development of the child. Most theories of infant perception and cognition attribute development to active engagement with the environment, yet research directly examining the development of infants' daily movements through and manipulations of their usual surroundings is rare (Haith, 1990). For infants the experience of object play is the training ground for understanding the relation of their bodies to their physical world, the arrangement of familiar terrains, and the potential combinations of objects in their world.

Specificity theory (Wachs & Gruen, 1982) describes the potential for the environment to offer particular types of objects at just the right place and time to have a positive impact on development. Providing the appropriate object experience, whether directly or indirectly, just as the child is ready to advance to more sophisticated levels is also the art of therapy. To use object play to address the skills of young children in negotiating the spatial environment, therapists require a basic understanding of the normal development of infant spatial abilities, as well as an understanding of how normal object play develops in spatial context.

Piaget: From Egocentric to Fully Coordinated Reference Systems

Piaget (1952, 1962) described developmental knowledge gained from the child's actions on the environment as moving from simple sensorimotor representations of action to more abstract complex representations. Piaget theorized that the child's spatial representations move from an egocentric reference system in the sensorimotor phase, relating object locations to his or her own body, to an allocentric system in the preoperational phase, representing space in terms of a layout of the environment that is abstracted from the location of the individual. Later, in the period of concrete operations, the child acquires representations of a few fixed regions of the environment. Adults hold a fully coordinated system of reference (Heft & Wohlwill, 1987).

More specifically, Piaget (1952, 1962) proposed that spatial understanding in infancy develops as follows. Up to 4 months of age, infants experience action in space as undifferentiated between themselves and the world around them (Acredolo, 1985). From 4 to 10 months, all observed changes in the surroundings of the infant are egocentrically attributed to the self as the causative agent. At this point, spatial understanding is concerned with how the object is related to the child, rather than how it may be related to other objects or persons. Piaget (1952) proposed that the infant begins physically relating objects to each other around the tenth month and proceeds from there to an increasingly internal representation of objects and their properties in relation to each other by 18 months of age. At 18 months of age the child is still performing most manipulations in the real world, rather than in the abstract (Piaget, 1952).

A part of the increasingly internal infant representation of the world is the acquisition of object permanence, the realization that an object continues to exist even though out of sight. Of all Piaget's theoretical contributions to an understanding of spatial cognition in infancy, object permanence has received the most research attention. Attempts to coordinate findings on this popular topic have been soundly criticized for the difficulty of drawing a meaningful synthesis from the wealth of object permanence studies, all using a variety of settings and test objects, different manipulations of the hidden object or the infant, and a great range of accompanying laboratory setting landmarks (Acredolo, 1985). In actuality, acquisition of object permanence is probably an isolated milestone along a developmental progression of spatial negotiation skills.

Gibson's Ecological Approach to Perception
James Gibson (1986), at the peak of a distinguished career in traditional visual perception research, proposed a revolutionary ecological approach to perception. His theory relies on the notion that it is not simply the passive acceptance of visual stimuli and its processing in the brain that results in our conceptions of the environment and its objects. Instead, Gibson proposed that people come to understand their surroundings through the active discovery of the objective properties of the physical environment. This claim has been supported by research (Acredolo, 1985; Benson & Uzgiris, 1985; Lockman, 1984; Sophian, 1986; Wellman, 1985).

Gibson's (1986) ecological psychology hypothesized that the meaningful environment is perceived in terms of medium, substance, surface, and affordance. *Medium* could be a liquid, solid, or gas. Each medium offers special characteristics in terms of breathing, locomotion, transmission of light and sound, chemical diffusion, and gravity. *Substances* are portions of the environment that are relatively solid and therefore do not easily transmit light, sound, or smell. The interface of one medium with another forms a *surface*, such as the ground surface at the meeting of solid earth and gaseous air. These surfaces are the areas of the environment at which most perception and action occur. *Affordances* are the opportunities the surfaces provide to the animal or human. For instance, a large and level piece of ground affords humans support. It can be stood upon upright, walked or run upon, danced upon. It cannot, however, be dipped into, poured, or swum through, as can an air-water surface. Objects are solid configurations that are detachable from the environment. These are the primary concepts of Gibson's (1986) theory of perception, in brief version.

In the field of ecological psychology, devotees of Gibson are pursuing research on various aspects of human interactions with the physical environment. For example, recent publications by E. J. Gibson (2003) and E. J. Gibson and Pick (2000) reflect on the infant's ability to differentiate between different features of the environment and its role in the perception of affordances.

Environmental and Ecological Psychology
Environmental psychology is "a multi-disciplinary approach to understanding person-environment interactions" (Cohen, 1987, p. 2). The discipline engages primarily in field research, studying the influence of the environment on individuals in context. One area of research in environmental psychology describes the internal representations, or cognitive maps, of the spatial dimensions of familiar large-scale settings (Bechtel & Churchman, 2002; Evans, 1980; Kaplan & Kaplan, 1981; Lynch, 1960; Neisser, 1976; Wellman, 1985). Most of these cognitive mapping studies have used methods inappropriate to infant research, such as analysis of adult directional narratives and sketch maps.

One exceptional environmental psychology study is Hart's (1979) examination of the way a group of elementary school–aged children in a small town negotiated their physical environment during their free time. Hart (1979) developmentally described the children's use of space throughout their neighborhoods, their knowledge of places, the values and feelings they associated with those places, and the activities they performed in different places.

The term "ecological psychology" most often refers to Barker and Wright's (1955) approach in their landmark study of the spatial and social aspects of childhood in a small midwestern town. They described the role of behavior setting in shaping the observed actions of the children. It is this somewhat greater emphasis on the dynamics of the environment in the person-environment interaction that distinguishes ecological psychology from environmental psychology (Wohlwill & Heft, 1987). Unfortunately, ecological psychologists usually limit their examination of the environment to social factors (Hart, 1979; Wachs, 1990).

Object Play Environments
Theorists and researchers have long touted the effects of the physical environment on development (Hebb, 1949). The consistent feedback available from the physical environment, in contrast to the more variable responses of the social environment, is important for the development of sensorimotor schemata (Piaget, 1952), for learning about the affordances of the environment (Gibson, 1986), and for development of a concept of the self (Neisser, 1991). In studies of the relationship between infant development and the home environment,

stronger predictive correlations were found between physical setting measures and developmental scores in later childhood than could be obtained between infant assessments and later developmental scores (Wohlwill & Heft, 1987). Several studies have shown that restrictions in floor freedom with playpens and other infant care equipment have negative effects on development (Ainsworth & Bell, 1974; Elardo, Bradley, & Caldwell, 1975; Tulkin & Covitz, 1975; Wachs, 1976, 1979).

Factors in the home and day-care environment that appear to have the greatest impact on development include both the characteristics of environmental objects and the ability to access the physical environment. Positive relationships have been found between infant development and object complexity, variety, and responsivity in the home (Bradley & Caldwell, 1984; Clarke-Stewart, 1973; Elardo et al., 1975; Jennings, Harmon, Morgan, Gaiter, & Yarrow, 1979; Wachs, 1976, 1978, 1979; Wachs, Uzgiris, & Hunt, 1971; Yarrow, McQuiston, MacTurk, McCarthy, Klein, & Vietze, 1982; Yarrow, Morgan, Jennings, Harmon, & Gaiter, 1983). These findings highlight the importance of the occupational therapist's object play interventions. She or he is altering the impact of the physical environment on the child's development, whether introducing the child directly to developmentally challenging objects, helping family members or day-care providers to understand how the home setting influences development, or initiating changes in the child's access to spatial experiences in the home and day care.

Theories of Play Motivation

The motivations proposed for play are as various as the theories of play. In psychoanalysis and gestalt psychology, play is seen as an attempt to reduce inner tension (Erikson, 1950; Slobin, 1964; Wehman & Abramson, 1976). Behavioral psychology views play as a response to environmental stimulation and reinforcement (Slobin, 1964). Piaget cites the equilibrium of ego assimilation and accommodation as a general motivator of behavior, functional pleasure as a motivation of play, and mastery as the desired result of learned schemata (Piaget, 1962).

Popular definitions of play usually associate play with fun and pleasure. Research shows, however, that interest is actually the predominant emotion in children's interactions with toys, with little variation. Joy is observed, but less often than would be expected from cultural representations of play (Phillips & Sellitto, 1990).

Optimal Arousal
Theories of optimal arousal view play as a strategy to maintain a pleasurable emotional state. Arousal is a measure of alertness (Berlyne, 1965). Novelty, complexity, and incongruity or surprisingness produce arousal (Berlyne, 1965, 1971; Fowler, 1965; Herron & Sutton-Smith, 1971;

Hutt, 1966; Look, 1977; Weisler & McCall, 1976). States of suboptimal and supraoptimal arousal are aversive. By engaging optimally arousing stimuli situations, the system is advanced upward along the scale of complexity as new concepts are explored and incorporated (Ellis, 1973). Resolution of these explorations is experienced as pleasurable. Hence the fun of play (Berlyne, 1971; Ellis, 1973).

Novelty-loving species learn to deal flexibly with a changing environment rather than use patterned behaviors. Ellis (1973) postulated that problem-solving skills are acquired through play, motivated by a drive to maintain an optimal arousal level. The potency of novelty in increasing attention span, activity level, exploration, and level of play in preschool children has been documented (Berlyne, 1971; Butler, 1977; Daehler & O'Connor, 1980; Eson, Cometa, Allen, & Hanel, 1977; Faulkender, 1980; Henderson, 1978, 1981; Henderson & Moore, 1980; Hutt, 1966; Lewis, 1978; Scholtz & Ellis, 1975; Sussman, 1979).

Flow Theory
Another useful perspective on the emotional qualities of the play experience is provided by Csikszentmihalyi's (1975, 1990) concept of "flow." The flow state is enjoyable and fully involving, a good match of perceived skills and action challenges. It is marked by five conditions: a merging of action and awareness, a centering of attention on a limited stimulus field, a loss of self-consciousness, control over actions and the environment, and unambiguous feedback from the environment (Csikszentmihalyi, 1975). This flow state is easily observed in normal infant object play.

Competence and Mastery
The urge for competency was proposed by Robert White in 1959 and adopted by occupational therapy as superior to then-current motivational theories of intra-ego tension reduction, instinct, and reinforcement (White, 1971). Leon Yarrow and colleagues have produced a body of research linking mastery motivation to cognitive development (Morgan & Harmon, 1984). Mastery motivation and the related concepts of intrinsic motivation and effectance motivation are rooted in the belief that humans naturally possess a motive to control the environment, master skills, and be effective. Standard sets of mastery motivation tasks follow a developmental hierarchy assessing object exploration, persistence tasks (effect production, combinatorial, means-ends, and multipart tasks), preference for challenging tasks (3 years and older), and self-initiated mastery (4 years and older). The strong relationships of infant mastery motivation to later cognitive skills support the importance of developmental progressions in infant play interactions with objects (Hrncir, Speller, & West, 1985; McQuiston & Yarrow, 1982; Morgan & Harmon, 1984; Yarrow et al., 1982, 1983).

INTEGRATING DEVELOPMENT, PLAY, AND OCCUPATION

Within the fields of occupational therapy and occupational science, there is shared knowledge about the occupation of play. As mentioned earlier in this chapter, several studies have already highlighted occupational characteristics of play (see "An Occupational Science Approach to Object Play"). Within this text are several contributions to the understanding of play. This should constitute a point of departure for therapists who wish to work beyond performance skills and use whole occupations.

Earlier scholars in occupational therapy had already stimulated thinking on this most important childhood occupation. Mary Reilly (1962, 1974) was one of the first occupational therapists to write about children's play. She hypothesized that children learn rules of people, objects, and movement during play. Reilly defined rules as symbols derived from and guiding interaction with the environment. Reilly's student, Robinson (1977), further elaborated on how rules are acquired in the arena of play.

Other scholars have sought to pursue the work of Reilly. Intrigued by Reilly's concepts and the central role that object play held in pediatric occupational therapy, Pierce (1991) completed a preliminary theoretical description of rules of objects. That study produced a descriptive taxonomy of three types of object rules learned in object play by children up to 2 years of age. Object property rules are the child's internal representation of the object's static and dynamic properties, such as shape or direct responses to action. Object action rules are the child's action repertoire, such as simple direct actions on objects and such strategies as repositioning an object to continue an interaction with it. Rules of object affect are the factors the child actively manages in selecting objects and keeping the emotional experience of play at an enjoyable level, such as novelty, sensory potency, and responsivity.

It is our responsibility, as therapists and scholars, to further the profession's knowledge about play so that Reilly's legacy can bear fruit. The following section presents original work designed to integrate knowledge of play and occupations. We hope that it can guide therapists toward integration of development, play, and occupation.

Infant Space Infant Time Study

Casual observation of children's play in a natural environment suggests that they interact with objects in a more complex and diversified manner than is supposed by laboratory studies. They play with toys, but also with household objects and with the space of the home itself. Any therapist working in pediatric practice is familiar with these examples, yet little description of this play has been provided so far in the literature. The Infant Space

Infant Time study constitutes the contribution of Pierce (1996) to the understanding of the way children play within the home environment and how they use space and objects. A study of 18 infants and toddlers at play in the home environment was performed to yield a description of interactions with objects and other aspects of the physical environment. The main findings of the study are outlined here. We hope that this description offers occupational therapists a clearer picture of normal, in-home patterns of infant-object play so they can generate strategies for intervention that are based in a developmental description of typical play. If therapists begin to base their play interventions on an understanding of the usual development of object play in a whole and natural context, those interventions may more effectively become generalized to changes in the everyday pattern of occupations.

Stationary Object Play

Infants develop an early interest in objects by exploring surfaces. Child development experts often neglect this aspect of object play, although it constitutes the foundation for further interaction with objects. Early on, infants sense surfaces with the mouth, hands, and feet. Infants quickly move to interactions between surfaces and free objects, such as pulling on a blanket to obtain an object. This type of blanket pull-in is the first instrumental use of one object to affect another and serves as a transition to more complex types of object play combinations. Over the following months, the infant progresses from sensing to grasping, batting, and shaking objects as his or her grasp becomes more proficient.

Between 5 and 7 months, infants are mouthing objects in succession. They are also interested in articulated toys such as busy boxes and articulating objects such as doors. The interest in parts of objects translates into a playful donning and doffing of clothes and accessories. Multiple object play progresses from bilateral hold of a single object to holding two objects in hand (not combining), to taking out or apart (including unloading cupboards), to putting in or together. The peak of this progression in using multiple objects is instrumentality, such as purposefully using a rolling pin on play dough.

Mobile Object Play (6 to 18 months)

Considering object play as an occupation implies a respect for the development of play within contexts. Within natural contexts, infants and toddlers engage in types of play that have rarely been described as play because they are often classified under the heading of mobility. However, mobile play patterns are frequent and important. Anyone who has spent time with children knows that they carry, push, and ferry objects all over their natural environments. Object play between 12 and 18 months is anything but static.

Surface play becomes more sophisticated once infants are mobile. At 11 months they love to dance to music and jump on beds, on trampolines, or into a pile of pillows. They also like getting under furniture, into other small spaces such as special corners, closets, or cupboards, or behind curtains and furniture. As infants begin to crawl, they quickly learn to climb over objects. They clamber over low surfaces such as couch pillows at 6 months. Later, they learn to climb stairs, couches, and other pieces of furniture. Children's parks offer great opportunities to climb up and slide down.

Infants' play patterns with free objects also evolve with age. By 6 months, infants are able to throw objects from bouncers, high chairs, and strollers. Often, this is part of an interaction with the caregiver, so long as he or she is willing to retrieve the object repeatedly! The sound of the object hitting the floor is frequently a compelling aspect of the game for the infant. As a toddler, he or she will seek out surfaces that offer more interesting sounds, such as moving from object play on a carpet to play on a tile floor. Toddlers will carry objects to their favorite place before throwing them with the full effect of hitting a louder surface.

Wheeled toys that can be pushed across the floor are a favorite of infants who are learning to pull to stand. This interest in driving toys across a surface is maintained even after the toddler has mastered walking. When the push toy can hold free objects, driving is sometimes combined with carrying and ferrying. Infants and toddlers will also carry objects in their hands or in containers while moving through space. The carrying becomes increasingly targeted, as toddlers transport objects from one place to another, distributing their toys across a wider space.

Movement Through Space

Between 1 and 18 months of age infants demonstrate several distinct patterns of space use. At the onset the nonmobile newborn, being dependent on others for movement through the home or day-care landscape, does not have an independent ranging pattern. By 18 months an infant's space use pattern appears relatively similar to an adult's.

Prone Fan
Between 2 and 4 months of age, infants begin to move slightly across a surface in prone position, trying to grab objects just out of reach. Because the infant frequently switches attention from one object to another, the pattern of movement is not a straight line. As the infant pivots back and forth on his or her stomach to reach for successive fresh objects, the overall pattern of movement resembles a fan shape.

Shifting Circles
Around 3 or 4 months, the infant becomes proficient at pivoting and the fan pattern evolves into full circles. As the infant gains mobility, slow travel forward moves the center of the circle through space. The result is a series of circles with shifting centers. This movement is often led by the infant's desire to maintain contact with an object that keeps falling out of reach.

Edge Crawling
Edge crawling is an early self-directed pattern. Infants engage in a series of brief pursuit lines along the edges of the room where they are playing. After making progress over a short distance by crawling on all fours or on their bellies, infants stop to engage an object or gaze around. The edges of a room offer the most interesting objects to explore: shelves, furniture, toy boxes, or even window drapes or blinds. Thus infants who have just begun crawling most often travel around the edges of rooms, rather than playing in the center of the room or on a blanket.

Roll Travel
A roll travel is repeated rolling to progress across a surface. It is common in typical infants between 4 and 8 months. After 6 months, it is most often used purposefully to attain an object, rather than just for the sake of movement.

Edge Cruising
Once infants begin to pull to stand, they spend time interacting with objects on low surfaces, such as coffee tables, couches, or toy bins. They work their way along the edges of a room, going from one surface to another.

Driving
Between the first supported stand and accomplished walking, infants become very interested in walking behind push toys. At first the toys support the child while walking, but the pattern remains frequent well after stable walking is acquired. Over time, the infant learns to negotiate the push toy around obstacles.

Roaming
When infants are able to walk without support, usually around 12 months, the space use pattern is no longer shaped by room edges. The space itself becomes the most compelling object for play, and infants will spend time going from room to room, or from one end of a room to another. At this point the pattern is not intended to reach a particular destination but is simply for the joy of traveling through the space.

Targeted Travel
As infants reach 18 months and roaming fades, the patterns of space use are less clearly associated with emerging motor skills and more targeted. Rather than exploiting objects that happen to be available to them as they enjoy moving through space, they select destinations for travel with the environment. Their choice is influenced by such things as the presence of the mother, siblings, or playmates in other rooms, the location of play objects, and

the possibility of accessing the outdoors. They are also using the space to transport, carry, and ferry objects to new locations.

Motor Lens: Integrating Play and Development

One of the characteristics of the development of space use patterns in infants is its close relationship with the emergence of motor skills. It is the coexistence of motor capacities and of the infant's desire for novel experiences, however, that guides development. This is the *motor lens* (Pierce, 1996). The infant's incremental changes in motor development provide him or her with constantly novel interactions with surrounding objects, which in turn activate curiosity. This concept is related to Ayres's description of *drive* and its importance for sensory development in the child.

Object Play Across Space: Integrating Play and Occupation

In the previous description of infant and toddler play, mobile play and stationary play are considered as complementary and co-occurring. The infant's intention, motor development, and environmental opportunities are an integral part of that description. Such a global approach distinguishes the description from what can be found in most motor development literature, which presents infant movement as an unfolding maturational process that is largely context free and uninvolved with objects.

This ongoing line of research can stimulate scientists' and therapists' thinking about the clinical use of object play as an occupation, as well as the promotion of occupational health. The following sections explore some possibilities for the application to therapy of such knowledge about object play.

Therapeutic Uses of Object Play

Occupational therapists have used object play in four ways. These are described only briefly here, from the simplest to the most wholistic level of play-based intervention, illustrating the uses of occupation as the means and end of therapy.

The simplest use of object play in treatment is as a therapy lure or reward for performance of the activity that generates the therapeutic change. For example, a therapist brings out a favorite ball at the end of each session to reward the child's participation. The play does not directly generate changes but serves only to keep the child engaged in the activities the therapist has prepared. The play is not an intact occupational application, since the object interactions occur separately from the therapeutic occupation. When using play to hold children's interest in therapy, therapists are drawing on the appeal of play and relying, explicitly or not, on the theories linking play and motivation.

In occupation-based practice, however, all aspects of effective therapeutic intervention (appeal, intactness, and accuracy) should be integrated. (See "Using Object Play's Motivational Properties" in this chapter.)

The most common use of object play is to facilitate acquisition of performance skills underlying play. For example, a small table might be used as a means for developing upright stability. In keeping with the fragmented developmental literature on which they depend, pediatric occupational therapists tend to focus on the isolated skills that underlie successful engagement in childhood occupations: primarily sensory, motor, and process goals. Knowledge of appropriate developmental milestones can strengthen an intervention's accuracy (the extent to which the intervention benefits a child). However, the achievement of performance skills is not an occupational goal. Similarly, focus on performance skills can undermine the potential of child-driven occupations for addressing developmental needs within natural environments.

Less often, therapists think in terms of facilitating the child's ability to negotiate the spatial, temporal, and social dimensions of the environment. Those who set goals that are addressed by object play in this sophisticated way are usually more experienced therapists who have immersed themselves in an understanding of play. They emphasize interaction between the children at play and the environment; the importance of context therefore represents a move toward intact occupations. (See "Using Object Play to Develop Environmental Negotiation Skills" in this chapter.)

Most creative of all is the pediatric occupational therapist who construes treatment goals in terms of desired patterns of occupational engagement. Occupational engagement patterns are the enactment of typical activity patterns (patterns that most typical infants exhibit) within a particular environment and by a particular child. For example, although most infants around 8 months carry objects while crawling, the type of object, the duration of the carry, and what the child does with the object after it is carried are part of the occupational experience. It all depends on the circumstances of the interaction. Therapists whose interventions draw on all three sources of therapeutic power will use their knowledge of typical play to create therapeutic occupations that are as close to the real thing as possible. They will also perform a thorough assessment of a child's abilities and environment, including the parents' values. Examination of an individual's occupational performance can reveal competence, developmental delay, strengths in some types of occupations and weaknesses in others, a poor fit between individual and contexts, or other insights. Furthermore, the motivational properties of play will be called upon throughout the session. Therapists who are setting goals and designing play-based interventions at the level of occupational pattern engagement are rare master therapists who are treating within the complexity of whole, naturally occurring occupations without completely reducing them to a performance skill perspective (Box 7-1). It is this approach that offers the greatest cohesiveness to providing family-centered services in natural environments. (See "Using Object Play to Alter Occupational Engagement Patterns" in this chapter.)

PUTTING INTO PRACTICE THE DIFFERENT USES OF OBJECT PLAY: USING OBJECT PLAY'S MOTIVATIONAL PROPERTIES

An understanding of the motivational properties of play objects can be used to increase the appeal of play-based activities. The competence of the therapist in fostering the child's motivation to play is critical to successful intervention for children with disabilities, who are often considered unmotivated. The most draining treatment sessions are those in which the child is lethargic and uninterested.

Selecting Objects to Enhance Motivation

The characteristics that endow an object with motivational power are subjectively perceived. That is, the past environmental experiences of the child determine the relative play value of any object. A toy or household object can motivate a child to engage it through its novelty, independent responses, responsivity, complexity, or sensory properties.

Novelty

Essentially, novelty is newness. Novelty is most powerfully compelling at the developmental age of about 5 to 9 months. At this peak phase for novelty almost any new object that can be picked up and explored provides a challenge. Following that period, novelty continues to hold some motivational power but the object must offer other characteristics that bring it up to the level of developmental challenge that best fits the child.

Box 7-1 *Introducing Roberto*

I met Roberto during his initial assessment at 5 months corrected age. He was a small male infant, born 6 weeks prematurely and displaying the features of Nager acrofacial dysostosis syndrome: deafness, micrognathia, preauricular tags, atresia of external ear canals, hand and arm malformations, and cleft palate. The thumb of his right hand showed no active movement. The musculoskeletal structures of his left shoulder, arm, and hand were irregularly formed: missing and incompletely developed portions of the rotator cuff, shortened humerus, synostosis and shortening of the radius and ulna, and a missing left thumb.

Beyond Roberto's upper extremity movement limitations, he also exhibited overall weakness, no functional grasp, and a strong tendency toward a right asymmetrical tonic neck reflex position. He was not holding up his head, reaching, or sitting without full support. He was considered to be at risk for cognitive delays (Figure 7-1). Because of his micrognathia, cleft palate, and tracheostomy, he was completely dependent on gastrostomy feedings. He was also chronically ill because of his bronchopulmonary dysplasia and required frequent suctioning.

In-home occupational therapy was initiated twice weekly shortly after Roberto's evaluation. Over the course of treatment, Roberto moved from very hesitant engagement to enthusiastic and creative play with objects. After a year of treatment he also underwent hand reconstructions. He was discharged when he moved away, at 2 years of age, with only minimal developmental delays.

In each of the remaining boxes in this chapter, examples are provided from Roberto's treatment sessions to illustrate how the concepts discussed in the chapter can be translated into practice.

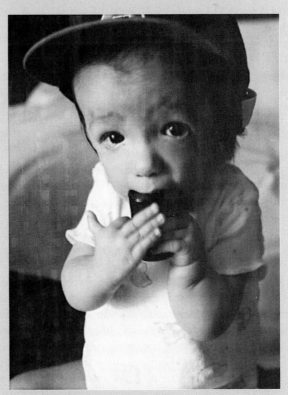

Figure 7-1
Introducing Roberto.

Independent Responses

Independent responses are qualities of action the object exhibits independent of any action on it by the child. For example, a wind-up toy can display independent responses. The object's movements or sounds call the child's attention. Therapists and parents often unconsciously use independent responses to attract children to activities, for instance, by rolling a ball or giving a swing a little push. Animals provide many independent responses.

Responsivity

Responsivity is the ease with which the child's action produces some reaction in the object. The response could be a sound, a light, a shape change, or a movement. The classic example of high responsivity is the rattle. The busy box, a multisite responsivity toy, is a modern technological expansion of the same concept. Again, a child of higher developmental level will not be motivated by rattles or busy boxes. The therapist must offer activities of the appropriate developmental challenge. However, any object that responds with a quick and easily observed reaction to the child's action is likely to be more motivating than an object that is unresponsive, is difficult to trigger, or offers a muted response.

Complexity

Complexity refers to the challenge to understanding that the object offers to the child. Even for a simple lure, the developmental fit of the play object to the child's current level of play development influences how motivating it is.

Sensory Properties

Sensory properties are the relatively constant and inactive aspects of objects, such as smell, taste, temperature, and texture. The sensory properties of an object can be highly motivating for children. However, the degree to which specific properties motivate specific children varies widely. For example, some children will climb barriers to play with sticky or messy substances, whereas others will climb barriers to avoid them. A wide variety of inexpensive objects of high sensory potency can be found in the kitchen or grocery store (Box 7-2).

Motor Lens

In addition to characteristics of play objects, the child's ability to play with a given object is an important aspect of motivation. In the first 18 months of life the combination of quickly developing motor skills and a strong attraction to novel experience creates for the infant a constantly opening realm of opportunities for play. Curiosity about the environment can press motor development, while the acquisition of new motor skills creates new ways of engaging the physical environment. The motor lens,

---

Box 7-2   *Maintaining Play Motivation with Roberto*

The effort to keep Roberto maximally engaged in goal-targeted play activities required constant attention. We selected activities carefully, and I remarked on their effectiveness in my notes. The family always had great ideas for intervention, which made the sessions very enjoyable, even though they could not afford a lot of toys. We used many household objects in treatment. Often, I would record recommendations for the next session while they were fresh in my mind and then review them when I planned my next visit to Roberto's home (Figure 7-2).

Novelty was maintained by choosing many activities to address the same goal areas and using them only briefly in treatment. This was especially important when Roberto was younger. Many similar toys would be interacted with for short periods. We would continue to use the same activity as long as it was compelling. Later, more challenging and complex offerings were required. I tried to keep all objects in the high-responsivity range throughout treatment. Sensory properties had to be used carefully because of Roberto's tactile defensiveness. The exploration of food tastes and textures was ongoing.

Although this sounds like a lot of design work, it was actually not. Once I had identified a large set of play objects along the normal developmental play progression, it was easy to select several for each session that addressed play development as well as other goals. In working with Roberto, I also began to notice the strong tie between how motivated he was during treatment and how satisfied I felt as I left. The effort to provide Roberto with intriguing activities not only enhanced the efficacy of his treatment but made treatment much more enjoyable for me.

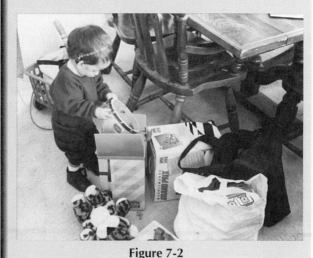

Figure 7-2
Motivational properties: keeping novelty high requires choices.

an ever-widening window on fresh interactions with the environment, can help therapists understand the preference for certain objects at certain stages of development. Unlike theories of motivation that focus uniquely on the object, the concept of the motor lens dynamically combines characteristics of infant play and objects.

Choosing objects that correspond to a particular stage in play development is crucial for engaging infants. For example, infants who are learning to crawl are often motivated to carry an object in one hand. Offering objects that can fit easily in the hand and be carried away can be enticing for such an infant. Therapists can ask parents about their infant's current use of objects and the types of objects they prefer. The therapist can also inquire about the child's previous and current use of objects and begin to write an object play history. Questions should refer specifically to the child's interaction with the physical environment and objects. This can help establish the developmental sequence and level for that particular child.

USING OBJECT PLAY TO ADDRESS COMMON PERFORMANCE SKILLS: SUPPORTING PLAY SKILLS THROUGH OBJECT PLAY

Pediatric occupational therapists most commonly use object play to address goals targeting development of sensory processing, movement, or cognition. Occupational therapists are comfortable at this level of intervention for several reasons. Their training emphasizes a breakdown analysis of performance skills, followed by setting goals in weak areas of performance. Most assessment tools perpetuate this fragmentation of occupational performance.

Many excellent resources exist within occupational therapy for using play as a means of skills acquisition. Occupational therapists must remember, however, that occupational engagement is the end goal of treatment. Trunk stability matters to occupational therapists because it creates unique possibilities for a child to interact with the environment. This reconstitution of occupations, from performance skills to participation, is an important tool of the therapist. It allows the integration of two different uses of occupation: occupation as means and occupation as end.

Object play is a wonderful medium for the practice and treatment of many performance skills. The skills involved in pushing a wheeled cart across the living room carpet include balance, motor planning and control, and stability, as well as the process skills involved in orienting the cart and distinguishing between different surfaces. But considered at the level of whole occupations, pushing a cart is also interesting. It is enjoyed by most children around the same age (about 10 months); allows a more complex, independent, and interesting exploration of the home space; can trigger new social interactions; and

constitutes a typical play milestone. In itself, pushing a cart (or other object) across the home space is a worthy occupational therapy goal for infants who are not displaying typical play patterns.

Sensation and Perception

Infant development of sensory and perceptual processes is often of concern to occupational therapists. The infant's processing of visual, tactile, auditory, vestibular, kinesthetic, proprioceptive, and gustatory information is essential to interactions with the physical environment (Ayres, 1985; Neisser, 1976). For example, children whose sensory processing skills are impaired may not benefit from typical childhood activities such as swinging and may suffer at many levels, including social interactions and acceptance. In general, therapists writing goals in the area of sensation and perception try to make changes in sensation tolerance, perceptual accuracy, and interpretation of perception in the production of an active response.

Thanks to the work of A. Jean Ayres (1972, 1985) and others, occupational therapists are the premier professionals for remediation of perceptual problems in childhood. Amelioration of problems of processing tactile and movement information through interactions with the physical environment is especially strong in the field. Some therapy supply companies are focused almost entirely on offering therapists objects for remediation of sensory processing problems. Some clinical settings are completely designed around offering these challenges. Amelioration of sensory processing difficulties should not be the only therapeutic approach. Given the importance of addressing family needs and priorities in early intervention, therapists must also be ready to adapt various properties of the child's usual environments to support the child in occupational engagement. Since therapists are already so resourceful in the area of sensory processing, several types of sensory processing are only briefly mentioned here as a spur to thinking about the range of play objects to which therapists have access in their practice.

Tactile Perception
Object play challenges tactile processing skills by providing a wide variety of textures. Therapists should survey the child's environment for objects that easily offer complexes of these textures: dry, wet, smooth, rough, moldable, solid, stretchy, particulate, and variations of density and softness of pile fibers. Types of object play used to interact with these textures include simple texture exploration, seeking and matching by touch games, art production, food preparation, and pretend. Textures can also be added to objects used frequently to address other goals, such as balls, swings, and large containers. Infants begin to test textures very early with many body parts, such as sensing a surface with the foot or the mouth. In some

homes the "messiness" of some of these potential activities prevents them from being frequently used. This is an unfortunate triumph of housekeeping concerns, or parent sensitivities, over the needs of the child. Therapists may also find that some households are more reluctant to let children engage in messy activities. In such households therapists can suggest engaging in clean-up activities before the end of the session, such as assisting the child with the broom or vacuum cleaner. Adaptation of objects may also be necessary for a child to participate in an activity. For instance, a group activity in a child care center may involve finger painting. For the child with tactile defensiveness, participation in the activity may be more important than addressing desensitization to paint textures. The therapist can creatively adapt the activity through the use of paint brushes, sponges with handles, or other tools. Play clean-up is a wonderful way to integrate heavy work. In addition, therapists must never forget that providing a tool with which to manipulate a material can present a graded approach to full contact with an intimidating texture. Rotating different objects for combining with a frequently used textured material also increases the novelty and potential repertoire of actions with which it can be used.

Vestibular Processing and Balance

Processing of movement sensation has been addressed in the past primarily through object play involving suspended equipment, such as the variety of swings and platforms typically used in a clinic specializing in the sensory integration approach. Simply staying positioned on these during movement could have been the primary activity, or they could be used as the surface on which another type of object play occurs. The challenge for a therapist working in the natural environments of the child is to find vestibular challenges for the child who may benefit from this type of occupation. Swings and hammocks are not uncommon in home settings, although less so at schools. Object play demanding vestibular processing can also use nonsuspended unstable surfaces, such as a ball, a snow disk, a scooter board, an incline, skates, riding toys, or surfaces that have give (trampoline, waterbed, piles of cushions). The therapist must control the level of demand the activity places on vestibular input to the child. Safety is always a concern with the use of unstable surfaces. Object play facilitating vestibular processing without using unstable surfaces includes games in which the young child must use extremities to reach, catch, hit, or kick objects without losing balance.

Proprioceptive and Kinesthetic Perception

Processing information about limb position is most often challenged in object play incorporating movement. Infants naturally enjoy dancing, jumping, and climbing. Many opportunities can be created around these occupations. Object play involving heavy work, such as lifting, carrying, pulling, or pushing, also provides input to the proprioceptive system. As described in the preceding section on the development of natural infant play, infants will be interested in a variety of movement activities depending on their developmental stage. They will carry objects, at first light and easy to fit in the hand, and gradually heavier and bulkier. They love to ferry objects or push them around in carts. Therapeutic interventions can easily reflect these natural occupations. Play in darkness or in which vision is occluded is especially useful for work on proprioception: walking under a blanket, for example. Very fine kinesthetic demand can be provided in games or art projects requiring carefully graded control, such as drawing within a limited area or placing a small object through an aperture.

Visual Perception and Coordination

Effective gaze is the base for visual perception. Infants must master gaze localization, fixation, pursuits, and shifts (Erhardt, 1986). Use of object play to work on goals of visual perception with very young children usually involves visual seeking of some type of target, whether that be the therapist's face, a place to throw or place another object in a simple game, or an attempt to locate a desired object. The child must have achieved object permanence to play any seeking games in which the target is largely obscured. Visual perception can also be challenged in combinational play, in which the accurate placement of an object is required. Visual perception of objects in motion is often used when gaze coordination is an issue. Finer visual perception in older children is tapped in many tabletop paper-and-pencil activities, such as mazes, hidden pictures, writing, and drawing.

Auditory Perception

Object play challenging auditory processing includes games of seeking by sound, simple direction following, sing-alongs, playing simple instruments, childhood chants that cue action (such as ring-around-the-rosy), and objects that give pleasurable auditory responses. For many infants the problem of auditory defensiveness requires the therapist to monitor closely, and possibly limit, the degree of auditory input in the infant's environment.

Arousal

Therapists addressing goals of sensory processing often also set goals addressing arousal levels in children who appear chronically underaroused or overaroused. Object play to address goals of arousal draw on the same activities just described within the areas of sensory processing. In working on arousal, however, the therapist is more interested in the effects on alertness and its stability than in the accuracy of perception.

Using Object Play to Address Development of Motor Skill

Families highly value movement goals. Occupational therapists often struggle with the need to address motor performance while their professional identity stresses whole occupations. The concept of motor lens presented in a preceding section can help therapists reconcile these two imperatives. The drive to play is supported both by the discovery of new objects and by the experience of new skills. They occur together, fueling the desire to play. In this perspective the development of new motor skills is not only a preliminary to play. It is part of the play experience itself and part of a child's motivation to engage in play.

For the purpose of discussing how object play can be used to facilitate movement goals, we have used the traditional categories used to create goals: stability and locomotion, and object contact and manipulation. These skills, however, are often integrated in natural play. In addition, some areas of the following discussion can be used to adapt the child's environments or occupations to better accommodate the child's and family's capacities, sensitivities, and goals.

Stability and Locomotion

With very young children, movement goals focusing on stability and locomotion can be framed in two ways. One approach is to target qualities of performance, such as strength, endurance, or coordination. The other way is to move the child along a familiar developmental progression: head control, turning over, prone propping, sitting, supported standing, pulling up, combat crawl, crawling, cruising, standing, clambering, walking, climbing, and running. Therapists can use the description given in the preceding section on play development to understand how each stage is tied to a particular use of objects. For example, propping the head is encouraged by the desire to see and reach for a new object. Linking object use, spatial exploration, and motor milestones can help support occupation-based practice.

Goals of stability, in which the therapeutic interaction requires the child to remain relatively stationary, require sufficiently engaging object play to incite the child's endurance. Therapists need to be aware of a variety of naturally occurring play activities at the child's developmental level that challenge the targeted stability skill. For instance, playing within an area that has boundaries and is surrounded by interesting media, such as a sandbox or small pool, can provide many interesting options for object play while addressing proximal stability in sitting. Motivation to stand supported is enhanced by the possibility of unloading a cupboard, basket, or other container. Unloading is more motivating and occurs earlier in the developmental sequence than loading. In addition, infants and toddlers sometimes prefer to play at the edge of a room, rather than in the center, where most therapy tends to occur.

Goals of locomotion use surfaces or media, special spaces, or transportable objects. "Surfaces" or "media" appeal to infants because they can move over (surface) or through them (media). Examples are crawling in very shallow water or walking on a trampoline. Special spaces are large stationary objects that offer the child opportunities to go in and out, go under, or go on top of the object. Examples are pools, sandboxes, blanket forts, appliance boxes, and corners behind furniture.

Transportable objects are those that the child can enjoy pushing, pulling, riding, or carrying across a surface. Pushing and riding toys are found in most households with young children. The therapist, however, needs to have a developmental progression, both in the motor complexity and in the size of the toy. This is problematic for children who are working on locomotion goals at a chronological age when they are significantly larger than the children for whom the toy industry has designed these toys. The therapist must be sensitive to these issues, using object adaptations and shopping savvy when recommending to families the appropriately challenging pushing and riding toys. Many objects can also be pulled, such as a light wagon, a blanket with a stuffed animal rider, or a long tail of light fabric. Push or pull toys that are also containers offer additional play possibilities.

Carry objects can be anything the child is interested in transporting in his or her arms. Sometimes, this can be made into a game of carrying a series of objects to a container or can be incorporated into the getting out or picking up phases of the treatment session. Containers with handles, such as purses or buckets with bails, are especially useful for encouraging object transport.

When viewing movement development goals from the perspective of sensory integrative theory, the therapist must consider the degree to which offered object play challenges self-directed praxis (Ayres, 1985). The therapist needs to work from the child's current level of ability, offering actions of high appeal to draw out just slightly more sophisticated performances each time. Ayres (1985) emphasized the importance of action sequencing and timing in her work on praxis. Often, a spontaneous game of sequence repetition and sequence expansion can be generated from the child's initially simpler actions. Therapists must always remember that working on praxis requires object play that is novel, not routine, and that children should be allowed to select activities.

When working with families in the home and other natural environments, therapists can teach caregivers how to adapt the physical environment to promote novelty and encourage environmental exploration that supports motor planning. For example, a toddler playing with a doll can be encouraged to have the doll "sleep" in a bed to support the learning of a new skill, climbing.

Object Contact and Manipulation

Like locomotor goals, goals for hand skills can specify attainment of qualities of performance, such as strength or degree of dexterity, or can follow a developmental sequence. The development of object contact and manipulation skills is familiar for most pediatric therapists. Furthermore, many assessment tools support the evaluation and treatment of manipulation and eye-hand coordination.

Infant development of reach and grasp passes through these phases: early reflexive grasp that is extinguished by 24 weeks (Gesell, 1940), reaching beginning as early as 8 weeks, object contact at 20 weeks, and successful gross grasp of a cube at 24 weeks (Gesell, 1940; White, Castle, & Held, 1964). As infants gradually gain control over the many degrees of freedom in upper extremity movement, reaching becomes more continuous and precise (Elliot & Connolly, 1973; Gesell, 1940). By 18 months of age, reaching is highly automatic.

Development of eye-hand coordination has been widely described (Bushnell, 1985; Erhardt, 1982; McDonnell, 1979; White et al., 1964; Williams, 1973). Along with the earlier acquisition of visual fixation and tracking skills, prehension is initially accomplished with gaze at the hand, later with gaze primarily for grasp adjustments, and finally with vision fixed only on the object of interest. Increasing differentiation in bimanual coordination is often attributed to the normal development of brain lateralization (Bresson, Maury, Pieraut-Le Bonniec, & De Schonen, 1977; Fagard & Jacquet, 1989). Exner (2005) has described the wide variety of in-hand object manipulations used by children, although how these emerge in infancy is not yet known. There is also evidence of the infant's adjustment of hand orientation to object characteristics as early as 18 weeks of age and becoming increasingly sophisticated over time (Lockman, Ashmead, & Bushnell, 1984; Newell, Scully, McDonald, & Baillargeon, 1989).

Many play activities of infants and toddlers necessitate reaching and grasping ability for optimal participation. The same activities typically support the development of eye-hand coordination. For an occupational therapist working in the home environment, the focus should be on coaching caregivers to incorporate opportunities for practicing these skills within daily routines, such as playfully encouraging an infant to reach for and grasp a small washcloth during a bath or encouraging blanket pull-ins while lying on the floor. Rattles, teething rings, and linked shapes support reaching and grasping for hand-to-mouth exploration during stationary play, and for more mobile children, object contact and manipulation are facilitated when the child grasps small knobs on cabinets, doors, and drawers or moves obstacles that have been placed in the child's path as he or she navigates around the home.

Connolly and Dalgleish (1989), in an innovative videotape study of the acquisition of spoon feeding, found the following pattern across development: increasing consistency in type of grasp and in use of the preferred hand, increasing involvement of the contralateral hand in the eating task, changes in patterns of movement, action smoothing, increased visual monitoring of the spoon, and decreased time required to bring the spoon to the mouth.

The specificity and multiplicity of goals for hand skills preclude a more detailed discussion here of the possible object play interventions to reach those goals. The interface of the human hand and the physical environment is such a crux of human occupation that object play addressing goals of object contact and manipulation can be generated from nearly any activity that is of interest to the child. The key is to follow the child's lead, making small adaptations as the child is engaging in play that will both facilitate the development of skills and support participation in the chosen occupation.

Using Object Play to Address Process Skills

Because Piagetian theory is the premier window on both infant cognitive development and play development, the relationship of play and cognition is deeply woven for therapists. The following discussion of using object play to facilitate cognition is based on the Piagetian stages found in the sensorimotor period (birth to 2 years). Although it is not possible to discuss Piagetian theory fully within this chapter, Piaget's work is recommended to all pediatric therapists who find themselves frequently addressing cognitive development.

The first stage (birth to 1 month) of the sensorimotor period is elementary sensorimotor adaptations. This stage is characterized by simple reflexes, uncoordinated movements, and the first discrimination and recognition of human and nonhuman objects. Selection of play objects for goals at this level of cognition strives simply to focus attention on an interesting object, produce reactions that demonstrate recognition, and provide experiences of reflexive grasp. Objects to attract visual gaze should offer visual contrast or high responsivity. For grasp, the objects must be of hand size.

The second stage (1 to 4 months) involves acquired adaptations. The first primary circular reactions, the child's retention of chance results in play, are seen in this stage. Object play facilitating cognition in the second stage uses visual observation of stationary and moving objects, early sound play turn taking, reflexive holding of an object and moving it within the visual field, and mouthing of objects in hand or not in hand. This is a stage at which a large variety of rattles, balls, and other small graspable objects are most useful.

Stage three (4 to 8 months) of the sensorimotor period, intentional sensorimotor adaptations, is dominated by the repetition of discovered patterns. The child begins distinguishing means and ends. Parts of an action are linked in time, but a series of actions is not. At this stage, objects that produce a clear direct response to the child's actions are useful, such as busy boxes, infant keyboards, and percussion toys. The child spends a long time simply grasping, handing from one hand to the other, and releasing objects, often until all objects within reach are beyond reach. If the infant is crawling, he or she pursues objects within close visual range. Discovering objects that are partially obscured leads to establishment of object permanence.

The fourth stage (8 to 12 months) involves further formation of concepts regarding the properties of objects. Time, causality, and space relationships begin to form as the child travels through the setting. The child begins to circumvent barriers to reach a desired object, further demonstrating emerging object permanence. Intermediary objects are used to reach goals, as in climbing on something else to get up on the couch, or pulling on a blanket to get a toy that is on it. The child more clearly anticipates outcomes from indicators in the environment. Play strategies from one toy are tried out on another toy. At this age objects begin to be used in simple combinations, such as banging a spoon on a tray and dumping things out of containers.

The fifth stage (12 to 18 months) is the stage of experimentation. Much time may be spent in what appears to be repetition but is actually subtly varied action. Large numbers of objects are typically engaged over time, yielding what can seem to the parent to be an explosion of toys, pots and pans, clothing, and other objects scattered through the house. Putting in, taking out, transporting, and early matching of parts (pans and lids often) are constant. Children's understanding of how objects can be combined becomes so much more sophisticated that by the end of this stage they begin simple tool use, such as drawing with chalk, stirring with a spoon, or other functional uses of one object on another.

The sixth stage (18 to 24 months) of the sensorimotor period is characterized by the use of mental combinations to invent new means of acting on objects. The child now encounters many of the "problems" of reaching an end and accommodates to them internally through mental combinations. This results primarily in a difference in speed of invention in comparison to the previous stage, as well as an abbreviation of object manipulations leading to invention. Object combinations become even more complex as the child begins simple constructions, continues to develop tool use, and enters fully into imitation of others as a mode of exploring objects.

The sensorimotor period is followed by the preoperational period, which lasts from 2 to 7 years of age. The preoperational period is characterized by the egocentrism of the child, demonstrated in attitudes of animism, realism, and magical thinking. Games of make-believe predominate from 2 to 4 years, giving way to interactive games with increasingly complex shared rules (Box 7-3).

USING OBJECT PLAY TO DEVELOP ENVIRONMENTAL NEGOTIATION SKILLS

Occupational therapists working with children are most accustomed to thinking of goal setting in terms of a series of intraindividual skills, such as movement, perception, and cognition. Since occupations are interactions between child and environment, however, both internal developmental skills and skills for negotiating the environment are required of children. Object play is a natural medium for the acquisition of skills for negotiating the spatial, temporal, and social dimensions of the environment.

Negotiating Infant Space

Henderson (1992) argued that visual-spatial ability in children is poorly understood in occupational therapy. Furthermore, she stated that most evaluations of spatial abilities in children are confined to examination of figural spatial tasks in cognitive space, neglecting evaluation of the role of spatial abilities in the negotiation of the real spaces of daily environments. Henderson (1992) offered a useful typology of spatial abilities and disabilities: real space includes peripersonal space (within the range of grasp), near space (space through which a person moves), and far space (seen in the distance). Cognitive space includes "mental images of places and things in places" (Henderson, 1992, p. 4). Grasping this differentiation of types of spatial abilities offers therapists an excellent beginning for understanding infant skills for negotiating space.

As occupational therapists working with infants and toddlers are now expected to provide services within the natural environments of the home, child care center, playground, and other locations, the argument for increased focus on spatial negotiation is even more salient. Rather than simply working within the confines of the clinic, therapists have an opportunity to address the spatial negotiation aspects of occupations within their natural contexts, while simultaneously training caregivers to take advantage of relevant infant and toddler learning experiences within daily routines.

Using Object Play To Enhance Spatial Negotiation
It is time for occupational therapy, in working with young children at risk for developmental delays, to go beyond helping them master the simple challenges of moving their own bodies smoothly through space. The spatial skills required for living in today's technological culture far exceed balance and coordination. Performance of everyday actions requires spatial skills for precise manipulations of object combinations, for understanding of large and detailed spatial layouts, and for movement of objects through environmental space. Therapists should now extend their grasp of

Box 7-3   *Facilitating Performance Skills Goals with Roberto*

In the area of sensation and perception, Roberto's goals were primarily focused on reducing his tactile defensiveness. For this, play objects of a variety of textures were used, beginning with less potent textures and working toward more challenging textures over the treatment period (Figure 7-3). Food textures were explored in play and in brief feeding sessions just before gastrostomy feedings. In addition, treatment activities initially supported visual development. Auditory experience was also included in many activities, since the degree of Roberto's deafness was not clear. The sensory goals were addressed through simple variety in play objects that offered a good developmental fit for Roberto.

Roberto's needs in the area of movement primarily involved upper extremity skills because of the malformations of his hands and left arm and shoulder. Both before and after his hand reconstructions, we selected activities that would challenge the emergence of his ability to grasp and manipulate objects. For this reason, we often spent much of the session seated on the floor playing with small manipulable objects. Treatment also supported the emergence of movement and locomotion skills (Figure 7-4). Although consistently delayed, they were acquired in a relatively normal sequence. The exception to this was crawling, which was difficult because of Roberto's

left shoulder malformation. He resisted all but the most interesting activities if they required efforts to crawl. We continued to work with activities that yielded shoulder strengthening, even after he was walking well. Roberto did eventually learn to crawl.

Roberto's cognitive development was at risk because of his deafness, chronic illness, physical limitations, and restrictions to environmental exploration. Cognition was easily supported in this case, simply by assisting Roberto to progress through the developmental sequences of normal object play (Figure 7-5). The object interactions used were too numerous to describe here. However, they roughly included the early use of multiple hand-sized objects for

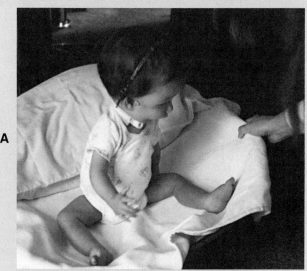

A

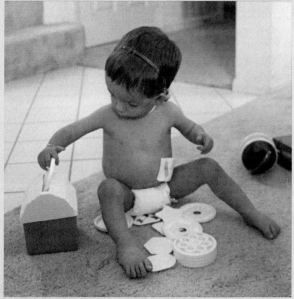

B

Figure 7-4

A, *Early work on motor goals: postural stability on a snow disk.*
B, *Later work on motor goals: grasp and dexterity.*

Figure 7-3
Early work on tactile defensiveness.

exploration, then objects that provided strong direct or challenged object permanence, later the simplest object combinations, and then container and construction play and more complex tool use.

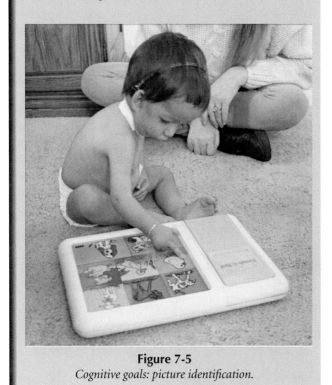

Figure 7-5
Cognitive goals: picture identification.

infant spatial skills beyond the blend of visual processing and sensory integration concepts on which they have previously depended for these interventions. The ways in which infants acquire these skills within object play suggest a wealth of therapeutic interventions facilitating spatial negotiation skills. The following indications of the development of spatial skills are derived from the Infant Space Infant Time study (Pierce, 1996).

Simple Movement Through Object Space
In conquering surrounding space, the infant's earliest explorations are visual. Active negotiation of space during play begins with the child's simple movements across level surfaces, perhaps in an attempt to move toward a toy or move off a blanket spread on the floor. The developmental progression of this travel is described in a previous section that outlines the work done through the Infant Space Infant Time study. These simple negotiations across surfaces bring lessons about traction, differences between level and inclined surfaces, and ways of circumventing or clambering over low obstacles. For this phase, sofa cushions, small hills, ramps, recumbent individuals, single steps, and other low objects are useful. In the home environment, it

might be helpful to explain this progression to caregivers, encouraging them to support their child's motivation for moving toward objects of interest, particularly those that are not "toys."

A more three-dimensional sense of how the infant's body is spatially related to the environment emerges as the child begins to pull up, clamber, and climb up on objects. The child then starts going around, behind, and under furniture, doors, walls, and anything else of interest. An appliance box with holes cut out can be highly motivating in this phase of spatial development. Infants may discover favorite child-sized spaces in the home, such as behind a couch or in a blanket fort built by an older sibling. At some point most children become intrigued with trying to move through space with vision obscured by a blanket or a bucket over the head. In the second year infants usually become interested in removing, and later donning, their own and others' clothing. As infants gain more of an interest in others, the therapist working in natural environment settings can engage other children, especially siblings, in occupations that promote spatial awareness.

As the child becomes more adept at locomotion, the distance traveled independently around the home increases. At first, all play is within arm's reach, then mostly within a single room, usually close to a family member. By 9 months of age, a child ranges easily over the whole house if allowed, usually following or leading a companion. By 18 months, the child quite comfortably goes to other rooms of the house without being accompanied. The sum of all of this simple movement experience is spatial skill, as well as the development of cognitive maps of the home landscape.

Object Transport
Once the child becomes mobile, he or she transports objects about the environment. Mothers will testify that this seems like a centrifugal process, as objects spread inevitably outward from their starting point but only rarely back. With development, the child's object transports become increasingly intentional and aimed to a specific destination.

The earliest object transport is crawling with an interesting small toy in hand. At times, objects are carried in the mouth. Later, the infant more intentionally carries, pushes, pulls, and rides objects through space. Seeking objects out of sight and occasional placing of objects in a space associated with them emerges around the end of the first year. Propelling objects begins with dropping, then unloading objects off of surfaces and out of cupboards. Later, infants throw, and then kick, objects. Last, the infant player uses one object on another to propel it through space, such as hitting a ball with a bat, and uses containers (purse, wagon, bucket with handle) to transport groups of objects.

Box 7-4   *Working on Spatial Development with Roberto*

Roberto's weakness and need for frequent suctioning limited the development of his spatial skills. The family kept him close to the suction machine instead of allowing his exploration of home spaces. However, with my encouragement and attractive play objects, Roberto began to venture out and explore, although his skills were delayed. His resistance to crawling, because of his shoulder weakness, also impeded his early experiences of space use. We incorporated a lot of upright spatial exploration, supporting the creation of play activity sites in some of the rooms. Roberto was encouraged to spend time in cruising and supported standing play and in unloading a small kitchen cupboard full of hand-sized toys and plastic ware. This exploration allowed Roberto to acquire knowledge about features of the home space and opportunities for play.

Roberto spent time unloading small toys out of bags, boxes, and crates, and later placing pegs and stickers and other objects on, in, and through other objects. To foster increased awareness of the home space, we played in transition spaces such as stairways and encouraged visual and physical pursuit of objects throughout the house. We pushed balls around the house, climbed up and down the stairs, and clambered over disassembled couches. We also spent time outside when the weather permitted, despite Roberto's fears of the texture of the grass, thus expanding Roberto's mapping of the home environment to include paths within the home and to and from outside. The family became receptive to the therapist's encouragement. This supported the creation of a wider and more mature neighborhood map, as well as increasing the variety of Roberto's occupational experiences.

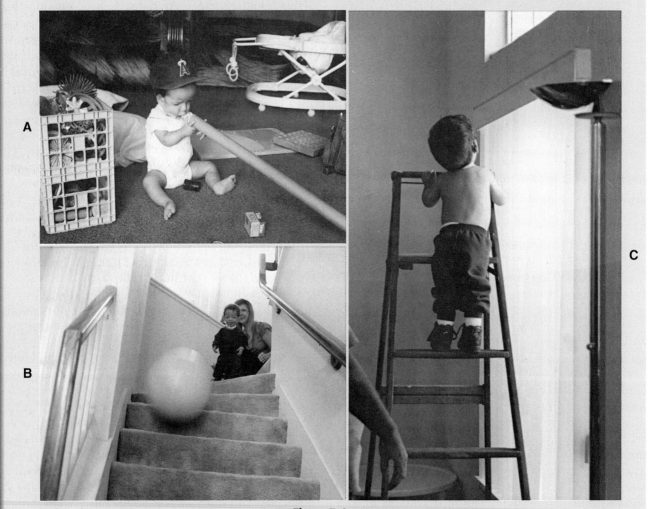

Figure 7-6
*Exploring home space. **A,** Roberto watching a bearing roll down a tube. **B,** Roberto rolling a ball down the stairs. **C,** Roberto up a ladder.*

In Roberto's case, the goals that primarily addressed spatial negotiation skills included everyday spatial object play with an increased variety and number of objects and activities, broader and more frequent independent ranging in home space, initiation of horizontal and then three-dimensional movements in space, and a development progression through object combinations and tool use (Figure 7-6).

Object Manipulations in Peripersonal Space

Some objects afford fine manipulation within the immediate reach of the child. Earliest are exploratory interactions, which often include mouthing and handling of surfaces at hand, small hand toys, foods, drinks, and straps and strings. Many of these simple toys are interesting in their high responsivity, producing sounds or movements in reaction to the child's actions. Pounding small objects on available surfaces is probably the earliest object combination. Later, approximating two objects in hand, the classic pounding together of blocks is seen. Also in this period, infants may spend time interacting with busy boxes, multisite toys that offer simple responses to simple actions.

Developmental progressions in object combinations emerge following simple pounding and object release. Occupational therapists would do well to note that, in combinational play, the developmental phase of learning to put together is always preceded by and depends on the taking apart phase. Thus there will be unnesting and then nesting, disassembling puzzles long before assembling, and knocking down or struggling to take apart block structures before interest in construction. Most complex is tool use, or using one object to affect another: using drawing and eating utensils, for example (Box 7-4). In the home the most common play space for a wide variety of object combinations is a kitchen cupboard full of light pans and lids or plastic ware.

Negotiating Infant Time

In occupational therapy the most poorly understood skills for successfully negotiating the environment are those used to organize actions within time. Time is the invisible, and often forgotten, dimension of the context of our actions. Temporal negotiation skills in infancy include the establishment of a biotemporal base rhythm, differentiation between simultaneity and succession, recognition of the temporal sequences in environmental events, and action timing and sequencing. Occupational therapists often intuitively challenge these skills in treatment through the use of object play. Temporal negotiation skills, however, are rarely acknowledged as goals. Infants' and toddlers' acquisition of skills for sequencing interactions with the physical environment is foundational to almost all childhood and adult occupations.

Infant Biotemporal Rhythms

Most research on infants' experience of time is concerned with physiological processes, or biotemporality. The oscillation durations of biological rhythms include short (heartbeat, respiration), circadian (day length), monthly, circannual, and lifespan.

Little is known regarding differences between adult and childhood biotemporal rhythms or their entrainment to environmental zeitgebers, or time givers. In the human infant, circadian regularity is thought to precede the capability of entraining to environmental cues. In utero, the infant is subject to the circadian rhythms of the mother. The sleep-wake pattern is rhythmic and repetitive at birth. However, the child does not immediately entrain to environmental zeitgebers. Infants alternate between periods of wakefulness and napping around the clock. The periods of sleeping and waking lengthen over the first few months. This free-running rhythm may appear in the early months to reach synchrony with the rest of the family, with the baby sleeping at night. In actuality, it is often merely a congruent free-running oscillation that matches for a few nights to the entrained family's sleep-wake cycle. Then the oscillations continue into completely incongruent patterns, to the despair of the baby's parents. By about the twentieth week of life, the infant begins to achieve true synchrony through entrainment to light and social cues (Moore-Ede, Sulzman, & Fuller, 1982).

Later in infancy and toddlerhood, a rhythm of daytime sleep and activity is established within the activity patterns of the family. By 9 months of age, this pattern is clearly settled into between one and three predictable nap periods each day. As the child matures, the awake periods lengthen and the nap periods decrease in number. Typically, the midday nap is retained until about 4 years of age. This midday slump in energy level is also typical of adults and is retained in many cultures as a usual rest time for all ages (Moore-Ede et al., 1982).

Temporal Cognition in Childhood

Research on temporal cognition in childhood has focused on children old enough to articulate their perceptions of the world around them. The perception of time in the most immediate sense includes differentiation between simultaneity and succession, perception of order and interval, and estimation of duration. Memory processes are inseparably tied to these perceptual abilities (Fraisse, 1963). Piaget (1971) envisioned children's growing capacities as internal representations emerging from their actions on the world, changing from simple reflexive action to anticipation of future events and a practical series of actions to reach an envisioned end. Piaget (1971) and Fraisse (1963) detailed the older child's abilities to manage abstract estimations of time, recalling the order of events, estimating duration, and understanding order and duration separately. Once the child is able to reverse constructions, a more complex set of logical operations can be used to access time. All of these abilities contribute to a developmental expansion of temporal horizons, that is, the lengths of time to which the child can project events into the past or into the future from the present.

Research on temporal skills of older children provides a framework for describing the antecedent understandings of time that may be held by infants and toddlers. A newborn seems to live in the moment, with little awareness of the sequences in which his or her experience is embedded. In the early months, infants begin to differentiate between simultaneous and successive events. They demonstrate recognition of the sequences observed around them by their responses, such as turning to see an approaching person appear around a corner, or attempting to escape the approach of a washcloth. At 6 months of age, the infant clearly demonstrates intentional action sequences, such as wriggling toward a desired object or pounding an object repeatedly on a surface. The infant holds in mind a desired object for a short period after it disappears but then can be distracted by another interesting object. Later, the infant shows frustration when anticipated outcomes fail to materialize and persists in searching for desired objects out of sight.

At later ages, infants progress to increasingly complex sequences of action. By 1 year of age, the infant is using fairly sophisticated sequences of instrumental planning, such as transporting an object to use as a step to reach a counter, or handing pieces of laundry out of the dryer for mother to fold. Ayres (1985) discussed some aspects of action sequencing and timing in her work on praxis, primarily in relation to movement skills. Piaget (1952) also discussed the infant's evolving complexity of action in the progression in the first 2 years from primary to tertiary circular reactions. This literature, however, does not begin to describe the sophistication of the 2-year-old's understanding of household routines and the potential series of object combinations available in play.

Research on infant understandings of temporality is limited at this time. Infants do demonstrate a maturing understanding of the temporal context of their own actions and the actions of those around them. Occupational therapists working with children at risk for developmental delays need to consider a child's skills for negotiation of time when setting goals for facilitating development through object play.

Object Play in Enhancing Temporal Negotiation Skills

Although occupational therapists are not accustomed to thinking in this way, object play is easily used to improve temporal skills in young children. The place to start is at the base of temporal skill development: biotemporal rhythms.

Establishing Regular Biotemporal Rhythms

The therapist should begin by checking with the family about their interest in establishing improved sleep-wake routines. Having an infant who sleeps and wakes in a predictable and healthy way can be critically important to parents who are suffering from a lack of sleep. This is especially important for children recently discharged from the hospital, where they may not have been exposed to the normal light and activity cues that usually entrain the infant biological clock.

The first step is for the family to record a log of a minimum of 1 week of the child's sleep-wake rhythm. This will sensitize the parents to the biotemporal rhythm and provide the therapist with information. If no pattern is recognizable, the immediate goal becomes to facilitate the solidifying of a pattern. If there is a pattern in need of change, the therapist should select with the infant's caregivers the pattern toward which they wish to aim.

Changes must be made in very small increments and in the direction of lengthening awake periods and moving them later rather than shortening them or moving them earlier. The primary tools that can be used to influence the sleep-wake pattern are exposure to light, hunger-satiation, activity context, and object play. Exposure to light at the beginning of the child's day and during active play times and limitation of light exposure at sleep times assists entrainment of temporal patterns. A predictable schedule of feedings also helps, especially the avoidance of hunger during desired sleep periods. The family can create a sleep routine, including favorite toys or blankets, feedings, music, rocking, or sequencing ties to other activities, such as bathing or dinner. The activity context of the family's actions surrounding the child also influences the child's sleep-wake pattern. For example, if the family is busily engaged in energetic actions around the child, he or she is more likely to remain awake. Keeping motivating play objects until the end of the desired awake period can be used to extend the length for the awake period toward the goal pattern.

Facilitating Temporal Awareness

Infants first acquire awareness of temporal sequences by recognizing temporal patterns in the activities surrounding them. For this reason, it is important that infants at risk for delays be included as much as possible in these patterns. During everyday household activities the family can include the infant by placing him or her at a good vantage point for observation, allowing the infant to handle and play with the objects involved, and encouraging participation in other simple ways. Family members can accentuate the temporal pattern of the activity by making eye contact or doing a simple repetitive play action with the child at repeating points in the activity. For instance, every time that the mother reaches for another T-shirt to fold, she may momentarily drape it over the baby's face and then pull it away, creating a repeating game of peekaboo.

Box 7-5 *Facilitating Temporal Negotiation with Roberto*

Roberto's early months of life in a neonatal intensive care unit and his chronic respiratory problems resulted in a completely unpredictable sleep-wake schedule. The establishment of a regular biotemporal rhythm was an immediate goal when therapy began. This process included keeping periodic logs, discussing with the family desired temporal patterns and strategies to reach them, gradually building up a sleep routine, and introducing changes in Roberto's sleep space. Transition from a completely unpredictable to a settled sleep-wake pattern took approximately 6 months. After that, there were gradual maturational changes in his sleep-wake pattern.

Temporal cognition goals for Roberto included extending his temporal horizons in the anticipation of environmental sequences, learning turn taking, and independently sequencing play actions of increasing lengths (Figure 7-7). For this, a wide variety of play activities was used, especially games that had strong ending points, such as the collapse of a block structure or production of music. When working with object play of sequences longer than Roberto could maintain on his own, I used chaining, encouraging Roberto to assume a larger and larger portion of the sequence until he performed it all on his own. We often used these sequence-chaining play objects several times during a treatment session before Roberto conquered them. At times, we would try favorite objects from earlier months to check on how he was remembering the previously learned uses of those objects. I deliberately gave many cues about upcoming portions of the session by picking together a series of activities and laying them out within view, saying that I was leaving after a certain play object, and using a shared arrival and leave-taking ritual that we developed together (Figure 7-7, *B*).

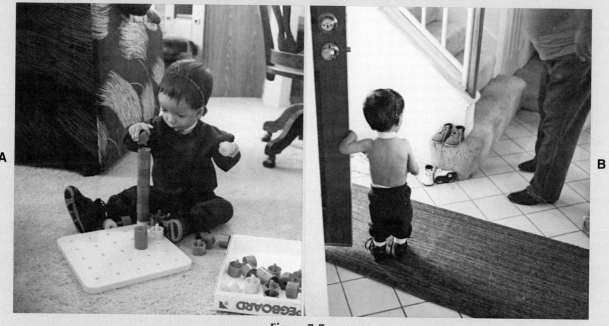

Figure 7-7
A, Roberto in sequencing play. B, Roberto participating in a leave-taking.

The infant's anticipation of events can be facilitated through cuing. The therapist or the caregiver can call the infant's attention to impending events, such as a toy that is about to produce a sound or a bottle that is going into the microwave. Selection of toys that lend themselves to demonstrating strong repeating patterns also assists in acquisition of temporal awareness. An example of a strong repeater is an old-fashioned toy called a jack-in-the-box. Involving the infant in a pattern of turn taking also facilitates this skill.

Facilitation of normal patterns of play sequences in therapy is difficult because of the lack of literature describing these developmental patterns. It is not difficult to create activities for the simple pattern of a single action and response, but the patterns beyond that are not well understood. At 6 to 9 months old, the infant plays with a series of small hand-held toys, grasping, mouthing, banging, passing them from one hand to the other, and dropping them. Often the infant returns to the same objects over and over, as long as they remain within reach. For this phase the sequence requires a large number of small objects with which to repeat similar actions. As infants mature, they appear to play longer with an object, performing a related series of actions on it. By 18 months, they are performing longer instrumental combinations of objects. Research describing these lengths and sequences in play is needed to support therapeutic facilitation of temporal skills in infants and toddlers (Box 7-5).

Negotiating the Infant Social Environment

The third dimension of the environment that the young child must learn to negotiate is the social dimension. Object play can be used to facilitate the child's social skills, to draw the family into involvement in treatment, and to establish interactive play in the home.

Sociocultural Impacts on Development

The social dimension of the child's play environment has a strong impact on the infant's development. Research indicates that cultural and socioeconomic status differences shape the daily experience of infants, especially through the pattern of the mother-infant relationship (Bornstein, Azuma, Tamis-LeMonda, & Ogino, 1990; Bornstein, Toda, Azuma, Tamis-LeMonda, & Ogino, 1990; Bornstein, Tamis-LeMonda, Pecheux, & Rahn, 1991; Rubin et al., 1976). Infants of specific groups of mothers, such as teenagers or depressed women, are at high risk for compromised development (Coll, Vohr, Hoffman, & Oh, 1986; Lyons-Ruth, Zoll, Connell, & Grunebaum, 1986). Infants' referencing to maternal facial expressions has been shown to influence their actions with toys (Cohn & Elmore, 1988; Gunnar & Stone, 1984; Hornik, Risenhoover, & Gunnar, 1987; Klinnert, 1984; Walden & Ogan, 1988). In a factor analytical study of the predictive validity for intelligence of a home physical environment inventory, the highest dependence was on measures of the learning materials provided and the mother's facilitation of her child's development (Stevens & Bakeman, 1985). This research on the impact of the social dimension on infant development supports the importance of the therapist's attention to the infant's social environment and social skills.

Facilitating Infant Social Skills Through Object Play

The social skills of infants and young children generally include the ability to establish bonds with family members, to communicate with others, and to enjoy developmentally appropriate shared activities. All of these are learned through interactions with family members during play or caregiving activities. The most valuable action the therapist can take in facilitating the infant's social skills is to impress on the family the importance of interactive play to the child's development. Families of children at risk for developmental delays are often dealing with critical health issues, in which concerns for the child's health may override the desire to interact in usual, playful ways with the child. Loss of opportunities for play because of a demanding care schedule can also have a negative impact on the child's social and play skills, the family members' enjoyment of the child, and the strength of the emotional bonds between the child and family members. Beyond reiterating to caregivers the importance of social play in the home, the therapist can facilitate social skills in the following ways.

In direct treatment the therapist can use object play as the basis for his or her interactions with the child or for interactions between the child and any willing family member or day-care staff. The therapist should always include any interested others in interventions. Some explanation of the specific gains that can be expected from play activities may encourage them to join in, regardless of how nonserious the activity may seem. Interactions require the child to communicate with, alternate action with, and anticipate the actions of others. The therapist must focus on understanding and responding to the child's smallest attempts at communication. She or he must also have great patience, repeatedly awaiting the child's action in the shared play sequences. By 15 months, a typically developing child is able to request objects, bring adults to desired objects out of reach, ferry objects to an adult, and bring objects to an adult for play.

Social object play is easily facilitated in the home. For interventions in the absence of the therapist, every effort should be made to frame all aspects of family or caregiver participation in terms of play. Optional ideas for play interactions should be provided frequently and updated regularly. The therapist should always inquire about play between treatment sessions by asking such open-ended questions as "What has been the favorite play object or action this week?" and should find positive things to say about the value of that play. If the family requests holiday or birthday gift ideas for the child, the therapist can suggest challenging play objects. If the caregivers and therapist are fortunate enough to share the aims of treatment clearly among them, the family may begin to discover and invent play objects that meet the needs of the child, proudly showing their creations to the therapist (Box 7-6).

USING OBJECT PLAY TO SUPPORT ENGAGEMENT IN OCCUPATION

The most sophisticated level at which occupational therapists set collaborative goals and attempt intervention is in the promotion of developmentally appropriate occupational engagement. This section offers

---

Box 7-6 *Using Object Play to Facilitate Roberto's Social Negotiation*

In Roberto's case, the family was very much involved in his treatment. His mother was young, his father was out of the country, and there were concerns that his mother would not be able to provide his care while continuing as the sole support of herself and her parents. Institutionalization was a possibility. Roberto was the only young child in the home. He was cared for during the day by his grandparents, both active despite some disabilities.

I was hoping that, during intervention, I could also make the mother more comfortable with her child. She seemed afraid to play with Roberto because of his fragility. At first, we focused on small, quiet, playful interactions that she could share with Roberto. Some of these included holding his gaze on her face or on slowly moving objects that interested him, gentle touching games, and gentle movements to music.

At times, the family was so intent on observing Roberto's interactions with me that it felt like a performance. I was able to draw the family into play at some times and not at others, depending on other household activities. I also found that, when Roberto was feeling uninterested in treatment activities, especially when he was ill, pulling a family member into play would support his motivation nicely. I was pleased that the family was always trying to understand how Roberto could improve his skills. I often suggested objects for play, and the family would proudly report his exploits with them upon my return.

In home programs and in discussions with the family, I tried to provide as many different play ideas as possible. I jotted them down on notes that I stuck on the refrigerator at regular intervals. I encouraged the family to problem solve with me over times when Roberto was not progressing in some area. Roberto's grandfather was especially creative in finding and inventing objects to encourage Roberto's progress (Figure 7-8).

As is not unusual with children at risk, there was a point at which questions of discipline and limit setting were confronted. After several brief discussions prompted by eruptions of problematic behavior, Roberto's mother established a successful approach to discipline. Roberto's social skills were excellent by his second birthday, despite his limited language.

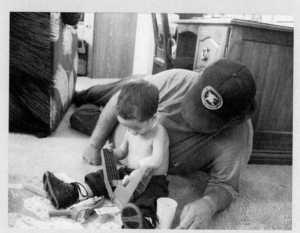

Figure 7-8
Roberto and his grandfather playing with play dough.

---

theoretical and empirical perspectives on normal play development to support therapists' interventions at this master level of practice within the daily activities of their young patients. Developmentally appropriate self-care and play are the occupational pattern areas most often addressed in occupational therapy with very young children.

Occupational Pattern Goals for Young Children at Risk for Delays

Setting goals to change occupational engagement first requires an examination of current performance. The therapist can use family interview, observations, or more formal play assessments. From this initial picture and discussions with the family, the therapist can then begin to discuss a plan for treatment with the family.

For a young child at risk for delays, the acquisition of normal patterns of play is both an important goal and a powerful means through which to reach other goals.

The foregoing review of primary areas of research on object play offers both new and experienced therapists perspectives from which to draw in generating goals and interventions.

Goals for Establishing Developmentally Appropriate Play Patterns

Goals that are intended to facilitate developmentally appropriate play in the child's daily life can range from the broad to the specific. Of course, what a desirable goal is depends on the judgment of the family. It may be helpful to describe to family members the usual patterns of play at the age of their child and to inquire as to the importance of these patterns to them. Usually this is a goal area that is valued by both family and therapist. Goals for establishing developmentally appropriate play can address the frequency or amount of the child's play time, the types or developmental complexity of the child's play content, and the availability of play objects that facilitate the type of play toward which the family wishes the child to move.

Developmentally appropriate play is established through facilitated play progressions. The child's play competencies must be accepted as they are initially found. If the child is not playing, the goal will be for the child to engage briefly by showing interest in objects and interactions. The therapist, with help from the family or day-care staff, facilitates the child's gradual progress along aspects of developmental play complexity. These aspects are described in the foregoing review of primary theoretical and empirical perspectives on play. The object play research suggests several continua along which to advance: increasing specificity of exploration of a single object, learning object functions, changing ways of physically relating objects, and, at later ages, developing different types of pretense. The occupational therapy research line started by Mary Reilly suggests other areas to consider: building a broad repertoire of object uses, moving through a variety of increasingly complex object combinations, using strategies to maintain play with an object, and increasing independence in play initiation and discontinuation (Box 7-7).

Box 7-7   *Establishing Play Patterns for Roberto*

At the time of initial evaluation, Roberto was not playing. The first step was to coax him into simple, brief exploration of objects. Early exploration of textures and shapes in the infant leads to free object play such as grasping and batting. Encouraging this exploration of objects and surfaces can facilitate progression along the typical developmental sequence. This required a volume of novel, responsive, and mostly hand-sized objects. These were not all toys. We also used some household objects, which were equally interesting to Roberto. Later, use of large objects in simple motor play was incorporated, such as pulling up, supported standing play (Figure 7-9), reaching for and pursuing objects short distances, and, last, climbing. Taking advantage of the widening motor lens, or the increased opportunities for object play that accompany motor skill development, is crucial to stimulate motivation to play. With Roberto, play activities were introduced to meet and challenge emergent skills and to fill the new horizon with interesting objects to explore. Mobile play and surface play, such as climbing, are important experiences in infant object play and were encouraged with Roberto. Developmental changes in stationary object play were facilitated: from simple single-object exploration and object pounding to interactions with articulating toys such as busy boxes, to object pounding and other single-object movements within reach, to multiple-object play including disassociating objects in provided combinations (taking out or apart), intentional combinations of objects (putting in or together), and, lastly, appropriate use of one object on another in a simple tool pattern (instrumentality).

The objects used in Roberto's play progression are too numerous to describe. A thorough knowledge of the typical development of play and of play patterns is useful in incorporating objects and features from the home environment in therapy. For example, the importance of activity sites for typical infants (a cupboard, a shelf) and the almost universal fascination for certain shapes, such as strings, can guide the therapist's choice. Roberto's family was very creative in identifying and inventing challenging play objects for Roberto, and I always talked with to them about why I was encouraging Roberto to engage in particular types of play.

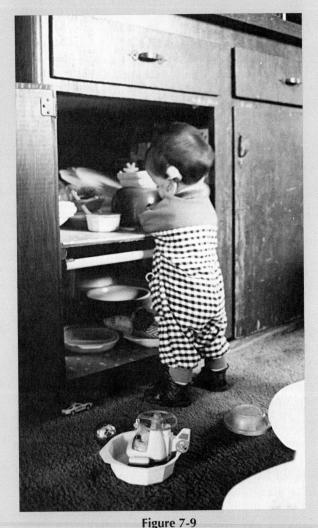

Figure 7-9

A normal play pattern: unloading a cupboard in a supported stand.

Box 7-8 *Establishing Self-Care Patterns for Roberto*

Because of Roberto's age and fragility, toileting and dressing were not a focus of treatment in his case. Feeding was a primary concern. Roberto's micrognathia, cleft palate, tracheostomy, and severe bronchopulmonary dysplasia prevented him from having normal feeding experiences. He was fed by gastrostomy. During the course of treatment, the approach to feeding went through several phases: chewing on safe food and nonfood objects, taking small bites of puree with his gastrostomy feedings, sipping liquids, and eating some small bites of soft solids. Roberto was very interested in experimenting with spoon use, helping with the gastrostomy feedings (Figure 7-10), and tasting a variety of flavors. Play was used by including feeding objects in treatment sessions, playing with food, encouraging play at home with feeding tools and foods, and working with a variety of toys to desensitize Roberto to textures. This treatment approach was not aggressive in establishing independent self-feeding because of concerns regarding the impact of feeding on Roberto's respiratory status. However, it was aggressive in including Roberto as fully as possible in the occupation of feeding.

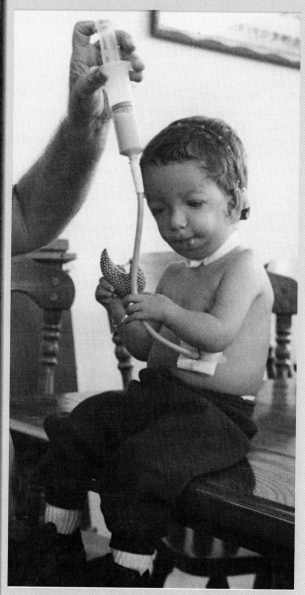

Figure 7-10
Roberto assisting with his gastrostomy feeding.

The Infant Space Infant Time study suggests that infants and toddlers are negotiating space as they play and that object play development is inseparable from environmental exploration. The different varieties of mobile object play showcase the relationship between mobility and object manipulation: carrying, ferrying, and playing with riding and push toys, among others. Furthermore, the study highlights how the motivation to play is fueled both by the emergence of greater mobility and by the discovery of new objects with which to engage.

Object Play and Establishing Patterns of Self-Care
Object play can be used to establish more normal occupational patterns in self-care for children at risk for developmental delays. Generally, object play is used to facilitate childhood self-care by blurring the markers that identify an activity as either play or self-care. Objects associated with the desired self-care arena can be included in playtimes. This familiarizes the child with them and provides a gradual approach to what may be an anxiety-provoking experience. An example of this is food play, in which the child is encouraged, but not required, to taste a food as it is manipulated for the sake of play alone. If the child is willing to engage in the self-care activity only briefly, it may be tried in alternation with a play activity. If the child is an unenthusiastic participant in the self-care activity, infusing the activity with a playful spirit can make it more enjoyable. This can be done by including play objects in the activity (e.g., tub toys or a musical potty chair) and placing an emphasis on just having fun with the activity (Box 7-8).

Review Questions

1. Consider what the chapter means by "sources of power in therapeutic occupations." What elements of intervention may or may not contribute to this power?
2. Generating effective object play interventions is described as a "design process." Consider ways the therapist can develop her or his design skills.

3. Describe ways the therapist can enhance the occupational appeal of a treatment activity.
4. Describe ways in which occupational therapists currently use object play. Consider the strengths and limitations of these modes of use.
5. Identify ways occupational therapists can use object play to alter occupational engagement. Consider perspectives on normal play development as you formulate your response.
6. Discuss environmental negotiation skills. Consider spatial, temporal, and social negotiation skills in your answer. Suggest specific therapeutic strategies that can be used to address each of these areas.
7. How do occupational therapists use object play to address sensory, perceptual, motor, and process goals? Describe specific therapeutic strategies in your answer.
8. Consider play motivation. How can occupational therapists design effective play experiences with high appeal by better understanding play motivation?

REFERENCES

Acredolo, L. P. (1985). Coordinating perspectives on infant spatial orientation. In R. Cohen (Ed.), *The development of spatial cognition* (pp. 115-140). Hillsdale, NJ: Lawrence Erlbaum.

Ainsworth, M. D. S., & Bell, S. M. (1974). Mother-infant interaction and the development of competence. In K. J. Connolly & J. S. Bruner (Eds.), *The growth of competence* (pp. 97-118). New York: Academic Press.

Ayres, A. J. (1972). *Sensory integration and learning disorders.* Los Angeles: Western Psychological Services.

Ayres, A. J. (1985). *Developmental dyspraxia and adult onset apraxia.* Torrance, CA: Sensory Integration International.

Baranek, G. T. (2005). Object play in infants with autism: Methodological issues in retrospective video analysis. *American Journal of Occupational Therapy, 59,* 20-30.

Barker, R. G., & Wright, H. F. (1955). *Midwest and its children: The psychological ecology of an American town.* New York: Harper & Row.

Bazyk, S. (2003). Play in Mayan children. *American Journal of Occupational Therapy, 57,* 273-283.

Bechtel, R., & Churchman, A. (2002). *Handbook of environmental psychology.* New York: John Wiley & Sons.

Belsky, J., & Most, R. (1981). From exploration to play: A cross-sectional study of infant free-play behavior. *Developmental Psychology, 17,* 630-639.

Benson, J. B., & Uzgiris, I. C. (1985). Effect of self-initiated locomotion on infant search activity. *Developmental Psychology, 21,* 923-931.

Berlyne, D. E. (1965). *Structure and direction in thinking.* New York: John Wiley & Sons.

Berlyne, E. E. (1971). *Aesthetics and psychobiology.* New York: Meredith.

Bornstein, M. H., Azuma, H., Tamis-LeMonda, C., & Ogino, M. (1990). Mother and infant activity and interaction in Japan and in the United States: I. A comparative macroanalysis of naturalistic exchanges focused on the organization of infant attention. *International Journal of Behavioral Development, 13,* 267-287.

Bornstein, M. H., Toda, S., Azuma, H., Tamis-LeMonda, C., & Ogino, M. (1990). Mother and infant activity and interaction in Japan and in the United States: II. A comparative macroanalysis of naturalistic exchanges. *International Journal of Behavioral Development, 13,* 289-308.

Bornstein, M. H., Tamis-LeMonda, C., Pecheux, M., & Rahn, C. W. (1991). Mother and infant activity and interaction in France and in the United States: II. A comparative study. *International Journal of Behavioral Development, 14,* 21-43.

Bradley, R. H., & Caldwell, B. M. (1984). The relation of infants' home environments to achieve test performance in first grade: A follow-up study. *Child Development, 55,* 803-809.

Bresson, F., Maury, L., Pieraut-Le Bonniec, G., & De Schonen, S. (1977). Organization and lateralization of reaching in infants: An instance of asymmetric functions in hand collaboration. *Neuropsychologia, 15,* 311-320.

Bushnell, E. W. (1985). The decline of visually-guided reaching during infancy. *Infant Behavior and Development, 11,* 419-430.

Butler, K. B. (1977). *The effects of novelty on the young child's exploration of objects* (PhD thesis, University of Houston, Houston, TX).

Chapple, E. D., & Coon, C. S. (1942). *Principles of anthropology.* New York: Henry Holt.

Clark, F. A., Parham, D., Carlson, M., Frank, G., Jackson, J., Pierce, D., et al. (1991). Occupational science: Academic innovation in the service of occupational therapy's future. *American Journal of Occupational Therapy, 45,* 300-310.

Clarke-Stewart, K. A. (1973). Interactions between mothers and their young children: Characteristics and consequences. *Monographs of the Society for Research in Child Development, 38* (6-7, Serial No. 153).

Cohen, D. (1987). *The development of play.* New York: New York University Press.

Cohn, J. F., & Elmore, M. (1988). Effect of contingent changes in mothers' affective expression on the organization of behavior in 3-month-old infants. *Infant Behavior and Development, 11,* 493-505.

Coll, C. G., Vohr, B. R., Hoffman, J., & Oh, W. (1986). Maternal and environmental factors affecting developmental outcome of infants of adolescent mothers. *Developmental and Behavioral Pediatrics, 7,* 230-236.

Connolly, K., & Dalgleish, M. (1989). The emergence of a tool-using skill in infancy. *Developmental Psychology, 25,* 894-912.

Couch, K. J. (1998). The role of play in pediatric occupational therapy. *American Journal of Occupational Therapy, 52,* 111-117.

Csikszentmihalyi, M. (1975). *Beyond boredom and anxiety.* San Francisco: Jossey-Bass.

Csikszentmihalyi, M. (1990). *Flow: The psychology of optimal experience.* New York: Harper & Row.

Daehler, M. W., & O'Connor, M. P. (1980). Recognition memory for objects in very young children: The effect of shape and label similarity on preference for novel stimuli. *Journal of Experimental Psychology, 29,* 306-321.

Dee, V. (1974). *An investigation into the play behaviors of mentally retarded and normal children* (Unpublished master's thesis, University of Southern California, Los Angeles).

Dunst, C. J.,Trivette, C. M., Humphries, T., Raab, M., & Roper, N. (2001). Contrasting approaches to natural learning environment interventions. *Infants and Young Children, 14,* 48-63.

Elardo, R., Bradley, R. H., & Caldwell, B. M. (1975). A longitudinal study of relation of infants' home environment to language development at age three. *Child Development, 46,* 71-76.

Elliot, J., & Connolly, K. (1973). Hierarchical structure in skill development. In K. Connolly & J. Bruner (Eds.), *The growth of competence* (pp. 11-48). New York: Academic Press.

Ellis, M. J. (1973). *Why people play.* Englewood Cliffs, NJ: Prentice Hall.

Erhardt, R. P. (1982). *Developmental hand dysfunction: Theory, assessment, treatment.* Tucson, AZ: Therapy Skill Builders.

Erhardt, R.P. (Producer and Director). (1986). *Normal visual development: Birth to 6 months* [videotape]. (Available from Erhardt Developmental Products, 2109 Third Street North, Fargo, ND 58102).

Erikson, E. H. (1950). *Childhood and society.* New York: W.W. Norton.

Eson, M. E., Cometa, M. S., Allen, D. A., & Hanel, P. A. (1977). Preference for novelty-familiarity and activity-passivity in a free choice situation. *Journal of Genetic Psychology, 131,* 3-11.

Evans, G. (1980). Environmental cognition. *Psychological Bulletin, 88,* 259-287.

Exner, C. (2005). Development of hand skills. In J. Case-Smith (Ed.), *Occupational therapy for children* (5th ed.). St. Louis: Mosby.

Fagard, J., & Jacquet, A. (1989). Onset of bimanual coordination and symmetry versus asymmetry of movement. *Infant Behavior and Development, 12,* 229-235.

Faulkender, P. J. (1980). Categorical habituation with sex-typed toy stimuli in older and younger preschoolers. *Child Development, 51,* 515-519.

Fein, G. (1981). Pretend play in childhood: An integrative review. *Child Development, 52,* 1045-1118.

Fenson, L., Kagan, J., Kearsley, R. B., & Zelazo, P. (1976). The developmental progression of manipulative play in the first two years. *Child Development, 47,* 232-236.

Florey, L. (1981). Studies of play: Implications for growth, development, and for clinical practice. *American Journal of Occupational Therapy, 35,* 519-524.

Fowler, H. (1965). *Curiosity and exploratory behavior.* New York: Macmillan.

Fraisse, P. (1963). *The psychology of time.* Translated by Jennifer Leith from French, 1976. New York: Harper & Row.

Gesell, A. (1940). *The first five years of life: A guide to the study of the preschool child.* New York: Harper & Brothers.

Gibson, E. J. (2003). The world is so full of a number of things: On specification and perceptual learning. *Ecological Psychology, 15,* 283-287.

Gibson, E. J., & Pick, A. D. (2000). *An ecological approach to perceptual learning and development.* New York: Oxford University Press.

Gibson, J. J. (1986). *The ecological approach to visual perception.* Hillsdale, NJ: Lawrence Erlbaum.

Gralewicz, A. (1973). Play deprivation in multihandicapped children. *American Journal of Occupational Therapy, 27,* 70-72.

Gray, J. M. (1998). Putting occupation into practice: occupation as ends, occupation as means. *American Journal of Occupational Therapy, 52,* 354-364.

Gunnar, M. R., & Stone, C. (1984). The effects of positive maternal affect on infant responses to pleasant, ambiguous, and fear-provoking toys. *Child Development, 55,* 1231-1236.

Haith, M. M. (1990). Progress in the understanding of sensory and perceptual processes in early infancy. *Merrill-Palmer Quarterly, 36,* 11-27.

Hanft, B. E., & Anzalone, M. (2001). Issues in professional development: Preparing and supporting occupational therapists in early childhood. *Infants and Young Children, 13,* 67-79.

Hanft, B. E., & Pilkington, K. O. (2000). Therapy in natural environments: the means or end goal for early intervention? *Infants and Young Children, 12,* 1-13.

Hart, R. A. (1979). *Children's experience of place.* New York: Irvington.

Hebb, D. O. (1949). *The organization of behavior.* New York: John Wiley & Sons.

Heft, H., & Wohlwill, J. F. (1987). Environmental cognition in children. In D. Stokols & I. Altman (Eds.), *Handbook of environmental psychology* (pp. 175-203). New York: John Wiley & Sons.

Henderson, A. (1992). A functional typology of spatial abilities and disabilities. In S. McAtee (Ed.), *Symposium '92 Proceedings: Current topics in sensory integration* (pp. 1-19). Torrance, CA: Sensory Integration International.

Henderson, B. B. (1978). *Exploratory behavior of preschool children in relation to individual differences in curiosity, maternal behavior and novelty of object* (Thesis, University of Minnesota, Minneapolis).

Henderson, B. B. (1981). Exploration by preschool children: Peer interaction and individual differences. *Merrill-Palmer Quarterly, 27,* 241-255.

Henderson, B. B., & Moore, S. G. (1980). Children's responses to objects differing in novelty in relation to level of curiosity and adult behavior. *Child Development, 51,* 457-465.

Herron, R. E., & Sutton-Smith, B. (1971). *Child's play.* New York: John Wiley & Sons.

Hornik, R., Risenhoover, N., & Gunnar, M. (1987). The effects of maternal positive, neutral, and negative affective communications on infant responses to new toys. *Child Development, 58,* 937-944.

Howard, A. C. (1986). Developmental play ages of physically abused and non-abused children. *American Journal of Occupational Therapy, 40,* 691-695.

Hrncir, E. J., Speller, G. M., & West, M. (1985). What are we testing? *Developmental Psychology, 21,* 226-232.

Hutt, C. (1966). Exploration and play in children. *Symposium of the Zoological Society of London, 18,* 61-81.

Hutt, S. J., & Hutt, C. (1970). Direct observation and measurement of behavior. Springfield, IL: Charles C Thomas.

Individuals with Disabilities Education Improvement Act of 2004. DOCID: f:publ446.108, 20 USC 1400. Public Law 108-446.

Jennings, K. D., Harmon, R. J., Morgan, G. A., Gaiter, J. L., & Yarrow, L. J. (1979). Exploratory play as an index of mastery motivation: Relationships to persistence, cognitive functioning, and environmental measures. *Developmental Psychology, 15,* 386-394.

Kalverboer, A. F. (1977). Measurement of play: Clinical applications. In B. Tizard & D. Harvey (Eds.), *Biology of play. Clinics in Developmental Medicine,* No. 62. Philadelphia: J.B. Lippincott.

Kaplan, S., & Kaplan, R. (1981). *Cognition and environment: Functioning in an uncertain world.* New York: Praeger.

Kielhofner, G., & Barris, R. (1984). Collecting data on play: A critique of available methods. *Occupational Therapy Journal of Research, 4,* 150-180.

Klinnert, M. D. (1984). The regulation of infant behavior by maternal facial expression. *Infant Behavior and Development, 7,* 447-465.

Largo, R. H., & Howard, J. A. (1979). Developmental progression of play behavior of children between nine and thirty months. I. Spontaneous play and imitation. *Developmental Medicine and Child Neurology, 21,* 299-310.

Lee, C. J. (2003). The contributions of activity and occupation to young children's comprehension of picture books. *Journal of Occupational Science, 10,* 146-149.

Lewis, M. (1978). Attention and verbal labeling behavior in preschool children: A study in the measurement of internal representations. *Journal of Genetic Psychology, 133,* 191-202.

Lockman, J. J. (1984). The development of detour ability during infancy. *Child Development, 55,* 482-491.

Lockman, J. J., Ashmead, D. H., & Bushnell, E. W. (1984). The development of anticipatory hand orientation during infancy. *Journal of Experimental Child Psychology, 37,* 176-186.

Look, K. S. (1977). *An occupational therapy view of play and skill in primates and humans* (Unpublished master's thesis, University of Southern California, Los Angeles).

Lynch, K. (1960). *The image of the city.* Cambridge, MA: M. I. T. Press.

Lyons-Ruth, K., Zoll, D., Connell, D., & Grunebaum, H. U. (1986). The depressed mother and her one-year-old infant: Environment, interaction, attachment, and infant development. *New Directions for Child Development, 34,* 61-82.

Mack, W., Lindquist, J. E., & Parham, L. D. (1982). A synthesis of occupational behavior and sensory integration concepts in theory and practice, part 1. Theoretical foundations. *American Journal of Occupational Therapy, 36,* 365-374.

McDonnell, P. M. (1979). Patterns of eye-hand coordination in the first year of life. *Canadian Journal of Psychology, 33,* 253-270.

McQuiston, S., & Yarrow, L. J. (1982, August). Assessment of mastery motivation in the first year of life. Presented at the annual meeting of the American Psychological Association, Washington, DC.

Missiuna, C. (1991). Play deprivation in children with physical disabilities: The role of the occupational therapist in preventing secondary disability. *American Journal of Occupational Therapy, 45,* 882-888.

Mogford, K. (1977). The play of handicapped children. In B. Tizard & D. Harvey (Eds.), *Biology of play. Clinics in Developmental Medicine,* No. 62. Philadelphia: J.B. Lippincott.

Moore, A. (1992). *Cultural anthropology: The field study of human beings.* San Diego, CA: Collegiate Press.

Moore-Ede, M. C., Sulzman, F. M., & Fuller, C. A. (1982). *The clocks that time us.* Cambridge, MA: Harvard University Press.

Morgan, G. A., & Harmon, R. J. (1984). Developmental transformations in mastery motivation: Measurement and validation. In R. N. Emde & R. J. Harmon (Eds.), *Continuities and discontinuities in development* (pp. 263-292). New York: Plenum Press.

Neisser, U. (1976). *Cognition and reality.* New York: W.H. Freeman.

Neisser, U. (1991). Two perceptually given aspects of the self and their development. *Developmental Review, 11,* 197-209.

Newell, K. M., Scully, D. M., McDonald, P. V., & Baillargeon, R. (1989). Task constraints and infant grip configurations. *Developmental Psychobiology, 22,* 817-831.

Okimoto, A. M., Bundy, A., & Hanzlik, J. (2000). Playfulness in children with and without disability: measurement and intervention. *American Journal of Occupational Therapy, 54*(1), 73-82.

Palmer, C. F. (1989). The discriminating nature of infants' exploratory actions. *Developmental Psychology, 25,* 885-893.

Phillips, R. D., & Sellitto, V. A. (1990). Preliminary evidence on emotions expressed by children during solitary play. *Play and Culture, 3,* 79-90.

Piaget, J. (1952). *The origins of intelligence in children.* New York: International Universities Press.

Piaget, J. (1962). *Play, dreams, and imitation in childhood.* New York: W.W. Norton.

Piaget, J. (1971). *The child's conception of time.* New York: Ballantine.

Piaget, J. (1976). Symbolic play. In J. S. Bruner, A. Jolly, & K. Sylva (Eds.), *Play—Its role in development and evolution.* New York: Basic Books.

Pierce, D. (2000). Maternal management of the home as a developmental play space for infants and toddlers. *American Journal of Occupational Therapy, 54,* 290-299.

Pierce, D. (2001). Occupation by design: dimensions, therapeutic power, and creative process. *American Journal of Occupational Therapy, 55,* 249-259.

Pierce, D. (2003). *Occupation by design: Building therapeutic power.* Philadelphia: F.A. Davis.

Pierce, D. E. (1991). Early object rule acquisition. *American Journal of Occupational Therapy, 45,* 438-449.

Pierce, D. E. (1996). Infant space, infant time: Development of infant interactions with the physical environment, from 1 to 18 months. *Dissertation Abstracts International, 57.* A AG 9705160.

Reilly, M. (1962). Occupational therapy can be one of the great ideas of twentieth century medicine. *American Journal of Occupational Therapy, 16,* 1-9.

Reilly, M. (1974). *Play as exploratory learning.* Beverly Hills, CA: Sage Publications.

Robinson, A. (1977). Play, the arena for acquisition of rules of competent behavior. *American Journal of Occupational Therapy, 31,* 248-253.

Rochat, P. (1989). Object manipulation and exploration in 2- to 5-month old infants. *Developmental Psychology, 25,* 871-884.

Rosenblatt, D. (1977). Developmental trends in infant play. In B. Tizard & B. Harvey (Eds.), *Biology of play. Clinics in Developmental Medicine,* No. 62. Philadelphia: J.B. Lippincott.

Rubin, K. H., Maioni, T. L., & Hornung, M. (1976). Free play behaviors in middle- and lower-class preschoolers: Parten and Piaget revisited. *Child Development, 47,* 414-419.

Ruff, H. (1984). Infants' manipulative exploration of objects: Effects of age and object characteristics. *Developmental Psychology, 20,* 9-20.

Scholtz, G. J., & Ellis, M. J. (1975). Repeated exposures to objects and peers in a play setting. *Journal of Experimental Child Psychology, 4,* 59-79.

Slobin, D. I. (1964). The fruits of the first season: A discussion of the role of play in childhood. *Journal of Humanistic Psychology, 4,* 59-79.

Sophian, C. (1986). Developments in infants' search for invisibly displaced objects. *Infant Behavior and Development, 9,* 15-25.

Stevens, J. H., & Bakeman, R. (1985). A factor analytic study of the HOME Scale for infants. *Developmental Psychology, 21,* 1196-1203.

Sussman, R.P. (1979). *Effects of novelty and training on the curiosity and exploration of young children in day care centers.* Unpublished thesis, University of Chicago.

Tulkin, S., & Covitz, F. (1975, April). *Mother-infant interaction and intellectual functioning at age 6.* Paper presented at the meeting of the Society for Research in Child Development, Denver, CO.

Vandenburg, B., & Kielhofner, G. (1982). Play in evolution, culture, and adaptation: Implications for therapy. *American Journal of Occupational Therapy, 36,* 20-28.

Wachs, T. D. (1976). Utilization of a Piagetian approach in the investigation of early experience effects: A research strategy and some illustrative data. *Merrill-Palmer Quarterly, 22,* 11-30.

Wachs, T. D. (1978). The relationship of infants' physical environment to their Binet performance at 2½ years. *International Journal of Behavioral Development, 1,* 51-65.

Wachs, T. D. (1979). Proximal experience and early cognitive-intellectual development: The physical environment. *Merrill-Palmer Quarterly, 25,* 3-41.

Wachs, T. D. (1990). Must the physical environment be mediated by the social environment in order to influence development? A further test. *Journal of Applied Developmental Psychology, 11,* 163-178.

Wachs, T. D., & Gruen, G. E. (1982). *Early experience and human development.* New York: Plenum.

Wachs, T. D., Uzgiris, I. C., & Hunt, J. McV. (1971). Cognitive development in infants of different age levels and from different environmental backgrounds: An exploratory investigation. *Merrill-Palmer Quarterly, 17,* 283-317.

Walden, T. A., & Ogan, T. A. (1988). The development of social referencing. *Child Development, 59,* 1230-1240.

Wehman, P. (1977). *Helping the mentally retarded acquire play skills.* Springfield, IL: Charles C Thomas.

Wehman, P., & Abramson, M. (1976). Three theoretical approaches to play. *American Journal of Occupational Therapy, 30,* 551-559.

Weisler, A., & McCall, R. B. (1976). Exploration and play: Resume and redirection. *American Psychologist, 31,* 492-508.

Wellman, H. M. (1985). *Children's searching: The development of search skill and spatial representation.* Hillsdale, NJ: Lawrence Erlbaum.

White, B. L., Castle, P., & Held, R. (1964). Observations on the development of visually-directed reaching. *Child Development, 35,* 349-364.

White, R. W. (1971). The urge toward competence. *American Journal of Occupational Therapy, 25,* 271-274.

Williams, H. G. (1973). *Perceptual and motor development.* Englewood Cliffs, NJ: Prentice Hall.

Wohlwill, J. F., & Heft, H. (1987). The physical environment and the development of the child. In D. Stokols & I. Altman (Eds.), *Handbook of environmental psychology* (pp. 281-328), New York: John Wiley & Sons.

Yarrow, L. J., Morgan, G. A., Jennings, K. D., Harmon, R. J., & Gaiter, J. L. (1982). Infants' persistence at tasks: Relationships to cognitive functioning and early experience. *Annual Progress in Child Psychiatry and Development 1,* 217-229.

Yarrow, L. J., McQuiston, S., MacTurk, R. H., McCarthy, M. E., Klein, R. P., & Vietze, P. M. (1983). Assessment of mastery motivation during the first year of life: Contemporaneous and cross-age relationships. *Developmental Psychology, 19,* 159-171.

8

Play Occupations and the Experience of Deprivation

LISA A. DAUNHAUER AND SHARON CERMAK

In play a child is always above his average age, above his daily behavior; in play it is as though he were a head taller than himself.
L. S. VYGOTSKY, MIND IN SOCIETY, 1978

Developmentalists have proposed that a child's environment nurtures or restricts a cycle of learning and development (Ainsworth, 1965; Bandura, 1978; Rogoff, 1990). Rogoff specifically theorized that children learn and develop through participation in routine daily activities with the guidance of a skilled partner, even if those activities are not explicitly instructional. Therefore time spent in such activities as playful interaction with a responsive caregiver may be a developmental asset, whereas time missed in these experiences may be a detriment. When children experience adverse caregiving environments such as institutionalization in an orphanage, they are typically deprived of both maternal interaction and developmental stimulation. Play, often dubbed the job of childhood, provides a unique window for understanding and assessing the effects of deprivation and for providing intervention to children who have experienced such conditions.

This chapter has the following objectives:

- To describe typical orphanage life and the time-use patterns and developmental outcomes of children living in institutions as a basis for understanding how occupations, particularly play, may be affected in these environments
- To review the state of inquiry on play behaviors of children experiencing deprivation

- To describe a humanitarian partnership with a Romanian orphanage using a play-based developmental stimulation program
- To provide a case study of a child targeted in this humanitarian effort
- To give readers an example of a study to assess play behaviors in an institutional environment
- To make suggestions for practice with this population

ENVIRONMENTS OF DEPRIVATION

After the fall of Romanian dictator Nicolae Ceaucescu in 1989, the media inundated the Western world with footage of undernourished and poorly developing orphans rocking in cribs or banging their heads on walls for stimulation. Humanitarian relief quickly flooded the country. Although many of the initial charitable efforts from the 1990s have subsided, Romania continues to actively improve conditions for children in the state's care through foster care, group homes, and in-country adoptions. The number of children living in public and residential care in Romania has grown, however. The percentage of children in the state's care from newborn to age 3 has increased 35% to 45% since 1989 (Dunn, Jareg, & Webb, 2003). Furthermore, more than 2% of the country's total child population from birth through 18 years of age resides either in institutions or in foster care (National Authority for Child Protection and Adoption, 2004).

Romania placed a moratorium on international adoptions in December 2000 and banned them in 2004 (McGeown, 2005). The number of adoptions from other countries by Americans, however, has continued to increase since the early 1990s (U.S. State Department, 2005). American parents adopt large numbers of children from other Eastern European countries, the former Soviet Union, China, and to a lesser extent India and some South

American countries. The majority of these children have spent at least some time in an orphanage (Gunnar, Bruce, & Grotevant, 2000). Unfortunately, children in many countries around the world live in environments of deprivation, including children in group care in institutions such as orphanages. These institutions often struggle to meet children's physical, emotional, and developmental stimulation needs. Although institutions across the world are diverse, common problems include understaffing, insufficient developmental stimulation, abuse, neglect, malnutrition, and inadequate medical care. Not surprisingly, institutionalization has been associated with delays in all areas of development—growth, language, intellect, motor skills, and behavior—as well as with abnormal stress reactions and increased risk of infectious disease (Ames et al., 1997; Gunnar et al., 2000; Miller, 2005; O'Connor, Rutter, Beckett, Keaveney, Kreppner, & the English-Romanian Adoptees [ERA] Study Team, 2000; Rutter & the ERA Study Team, 1998).

EXPERIENCE OF DEPRIVATION

It seems logical that minimal interactions with an attuned caregiver and low amounts of stimulation would affect a child's ability to engage with people and objects. A description of an ordinary day of a child's life in this setting can provide further insight.

Typical Orphanage Day

It's around 7:00 in the morning and the air is heavy with humidity, ripe diapers, and industrial-strength cleaning solution. The orphanage is located in a concrete, block-shaped building hours outside of Romania's capital of Bucharest. Nicolae, a 15-month-old toddler with a face framed in dishwater blond curls, is lying on his back, rocking to and fro. Like him, many of the children have been awake for some time. His clothing and sheets are damp with urine because expenses limit disposable diapers to special occasions such as christenings. In the past, the children woke to bare walls and cribs devoid of the accoutrements typical of Western baby life: stuffed animals, busy boxes, and mobiles. Some orphanages are now making the living areas more homelike with wall paintings, pictures, toys, and colorful children's furniture.

Valerica, one of the caregivers, picks up a baby to start the changing routine. The babies are changed in an assembly-line fashion that allows little give and take between Nicolae and his caregiver. Valerica, like many of the caregivers, has one or two favorites. Even though she tries to give Nicolae attention, she rarely has the time to coo to him, play peekaboo, or distract him with a favorite toy while she changes and dresses him. The infants and younger toddlers are often fed in their cribs while lying on their backs with a bottled propped in their hands. The older children like Nicolae are usually fed hot cereal in mugs reminiscent of Dickens's *Oliver Twist* while sitting in ill-fitting patio-style furniture. After breakfast, children who can walk toddle out of the living area to spend 30 to 45 minutes sitting on toilet training bowls in the bathroom.

After toileting, the children vie to play with the scant toys and miscellaneous objects such as discarded snack wrappers from a caregiver or a common article such as a comb. Nicolae attempts to reach for a bright red porcupine squeaky toy, only to draw his hand away before he makes contact. This approach and withdrawal action is often referred to as the "orphan salute." Nicolae seems overwhelmed by the sights and sounds created by the 15 or so other toddlers with whom he shares a living area. Instead of continuing to compete for the high-demand toys or Valerica's attention, he manages to scoot under a crib where he rocks his head back and forth. Competition for toys is so high that a child lucky enough to get an object usually holds it close to the body or inspects it while keeping a strong grasp on it. If the child puts it down to manipulate or explore, another youngster is likely to swipe it.

When the caregivers are done cleaning up, the children participate in circle time, led by one or two of the caregivers. The women sing songs and direct the children in a game of kicking over large cardboard blocks. Valerica and the other caregivers appear more directive with the children than caregivers in child care centers in the United States. For example, Valerica moves Nicolae through the activity even though he is unable to stand alone, much less kick. Nicolae, predictably, cries through this session, smearing his face with tears and mucus. In an environment where it really helps to be cute and endearing to get coveted affection and attention, Nicolae is a hard sell. In fact, when the caregivers are asked, they say, *"Nimeni iubeste Nicolae"* ("Nobody loves Nicolae"). From about 10:30 until lunchtime the children have "free play." In the summer this means that Nicolae and the others sit outside on a blanket, explore the littered orphanage lawn, or sometimes play with a small number of battered toys, most of which no longer work. The caregivers supervise at a distance. During cooler or rainy weather this time is spent in a large room with few toys.

Lunch, the largest meal of the day, is a hurried process. Nicolae can sit but cannot feed himself. He is fed from a spoon held high above his head so that he has to open his mouth while tilting his head back like a baby bird. The meal is followed by another toileting or changing session. The babies and children are then put down for an approximately 3-hour nap regardless of whether they sleep or not. After naptime the children have a snack and more free play. Then they eat a simple dinner and it is lights out until morning. Nicolae is left rocking in his crib once more.

Clinical Vignette

The case of Nicolae, the toddler described above, demonstrates how play can be used both in assessment and in intervention in an institutionalized setting. Nicolae could visually track an object and reach for it, but he rarely voluntarily picked up an object or toy. He could pick up only large items such as a pliable tennis ball–sized object. Picking up or releasing a small building block was too challenging for him. He could crawl and would view toys and people from a quadruped position. As described above, Nicolae was overresponsive to touch, light, and sounds. The "orphan salute," a withdrawal of the hand when offered toys, was a frequently observed behavior of his. This occurred even when he initiated an exploration for toys on his own, not just when he was offered a toy. Sometimes a cruel loop of behavior would result in which he reached and withdrew and reached and withdrew his hand repetitively for the same toy, making little or no contact. During free play, which was sometimes noisy with a radio blaring while caregivers talked and did chores, he could be observed responding to sensory input on the extreme ends of the gamut. He tended to cry egregiously or to withdraw and shut down. Frequently he could be seen crawling under the cribs to sit in the shadows and rock. He cried and withdrew in response to light touch, and when he did make contact with toys, he would often lie on top of them or press himself against them, suggesting that he was seeking them out for pressure rather than play.

One intervention goal for Nicolae was to decrease his sensory overresponsiveness so that he could more effectively interact with the caregivers, peers, and play opportunities in his environment. The intervention plan included facilitating the caregivers' interactions and rapport with him. Although the caregivers were dedicated and hardworking, the ratio of adults to children was low. Other than a child's smile or giggles in response to the caregivers' efforts, they had little incentive to work harder. It is easy to see how a fussy child like Nicolae, who almost never smiled, could become just a face in the melee. Cultural issues were also at the forefront of this intervention. A child-led approach was novel to the caregivers, whose primary reward would be personal satisfaction in helping this particular child.

The first step was to get the caregivers invested in Nicolae and his progress so they would be more likely to give him the extra attention and interaction he required. In addition, the caregivers needed the skills to provide calming sensory input and opportunities for play. The therapist introduced a program of playful touch pressure with brushing, gentle bouncing, linear rocking, swaddling, and soft singing. The caregivers started seeing that Nicolae was capable of responding with smiles and coos. They learned the techniques quickly, but needed a great deal of help in recognizing that they had to monitor Nicolae's response instead of administering the program in a cookbook fashion. For example, the caregivers were encouraged to stop brushing and try more calming activities such as joint compression if he began crying. After approximately 2 weeks of the use of therapeutic activities and education of the caregivers, Nicolae was able to seek and maintain more eye contact and actively look for a person to hold him. During free play he was now crawling after a toy instead of hiding under a crib. The ability to seek out a caregiver and chase a toy is important for a child growing up in an environment with limited resources. Although Nicolae's play skills were still below age expectations, he was beginning to imitate play actions and explore small objects such as building blocks.

Time-Use Patterns of Children Residing in Institutions

Classic field studies have described orphanages as offering less stimulation and interaction than other child care environments (Bowlby, 1953; Provence & Lipton, 1962). Researchers empirically investigating the time-use patterns of children residing in an orphanage in Romania compared with children attending child care in the United States found results congruent with these classic descriptions (Daunhauer, Bolton, & Cermak, 2005). In this study, Romanian institutionalized children spent significantly less time with caregivers and participated in a smaller variety of daily activities than children in a U.S. child care group. The Romanian children spent almost twice as much time alone (70% of waking hours) as the U.S. child care group (37%). In addition, the caregivers in the orphanage structured only 24% of the Romanian institutionalized children's activities, compared with over half (53%) of the U.S. child care group's activities. The study documented that both daily activities and caregiver-child interactions may be affected when a child lives in an orphanage, possibly contributing to the developmental delays observed in this population. Interestingly and unexpectedly, the amount of time engaged in play was similar for the Romanian institutionalized children and the U.S. child care group. It should be noted that for the purpose of this time-use study, play was operationalized to be any playful or exploratory activity in which a child engaged (Daunhauer et al., 2005). Consequently, play was not limited to scheduled "playtime" or just play with toys. If a child was patting and crinkling a plastic wrapper while her peers slept, she was coded as "playing." Bruer (1999) proposed that young children need only an approximation of the normal environment for brain development; the process by which the brain is shaped by experiences in early life is called "experience-expectant plasticity." Therefore the similar amounts of play recorded between these two groups may reflect a biological drive for stimuli that facilitates development.

Informal observations of play behavior (e.g., exploratory or symbolic play) indicated that the U.S. child care group may have employed more developmentally competent levels of play. Numerous investigators (Gunnar, 1998; Gunnar et al., 2000) have suggested that the quality of the environmental stimulation is critical for development. Therefore the small amount of time that institutionalized children spent playing while engaged with a caregiver may be associated with the developmental delays often described in this population.

STUDIES OF DEVELOPMENT AND PLAY IN INSTITUTIONALLY REARED CHILDREN
Early Studies

Institutionalization and the Wide-Ranging Effects of Deprivation

Research on children institutionalized in orphanages from the 1940s through the 1960s described how institutions were associated with children's delayed growth and development in general, and delayed play behaviors in specific. Converging lines of research from primate studies (Harlow, 1958; Harlow & Harlow, 1966; Harlow & Suomi, 1970) and studies with children in institutions (Bowlby, 1951, 1953) supported the concept that a mother (or a maternal figure) is critical for typical infant development. Much of the early research on the effects of institutionalization emphasized maternal deprivation. Casler (1961) proposed that institutionalization was characterized not only by maternal deprivation but also by reduced handling, reduced opportunities for interaction, and decreased stimulation. Casler (1961, 1968) stated that insufficient stimulation in these institutions contributed to the developmental delays previously reported to be associated with maternal deprivation. Infants residing in institutions did not have a consistent mother to provide the touch and movement experiences essential for emotional and physical growth and development.

Institutional environments were typically described as sensory deprived, providing infants with limited sensory experiences (Provence & Lipton, 1962). In studying children in an orphanage over a period of time, Provence and Lipton stated, "As one walked along the halls to reach the rooms where the infants and children lived…an unusual degree of quietness was an outstanding feature" (p. 25). Infants were fed in their cribs with a propped bottle, thus missing the opportunity for the touch, smell, position sense, and sight provided by a primary caregiver (Provence & Lipton, 1962). These authors, like Casler (1961), underscored the concept that maternal care includes sensory stimulation, particularly tactile and kinesthetic stimulation. Describing infants' experiences in the orphanage, Provence and Lipton (1962) observed the challenges of routinized care, describing how infrequently infants' needs were met by a caregiver at the actual time the infants expressed a need (e.g., by crying). As a result, infants had fewer opportunities to learn about what and who

brings comfort or pleasure. The authors noted that infants appeared passive in feeding, play, and other contexts.

Bowlby (1953) stated that infants less than 6 months of age who have been institutionalized for some time present a well-defined picture characterized by listlessness, quietness, relative immobility, and unresponsiveness to stimuli such as a smile or coo. He reported that an institutional environment may contribute to sleep disturbances, delayed language development, and poor concentration. Institutionalized infants also demonstrated lack of appetite, absence of good sucking habits, frequent stools, and failure to gain weight properly despite the ingestion of adequate diets. According to his observations, infants had an appearance of unhappiness, emaciation, and pallor and were prone to febrile episodes.

Institutionalization and Developmental Foundations

Extensive research on the relationship of institutionalization to developmental outcomes took place from the 1900s through the 1960s. These studies, conducted in England, the United States., and other countries, have provided evidence that maternal and environmental deprivation in orphanages is associated with delays in children's language, intellectual, physical, emotional, and social development. Findings from these early studies are highlighted below.

Spitz (1945, 1946) studied the effects of social class and experience on the developmental quotients of infants at the beginning and end of their first year. A group of urban children whose mothers were absent was compared with three other groups whose mothers were present: children of professionals, peasant children, and children of unmarried delinquents. Children in the mother-absent group showed the greatest decline in developmental quotient ($M = 100$, $SD = + 15$), dropping from 124 in their first through fourth months to 72 in the ninth to twelfth months.

Goldfarb (1945) reported converging evidence for the link between institutionalization and developmental status. The mean IQ score of a group of 15 children who had spent their first 3 years in an institution was 72 compared with 95 for the noninstitutionalized control group. Social maturity, as measured on the Vineland Scale, was 79 for the institution group compared with 98 for the control group. Only 2 to 3 of the 15 children in the institution group were rated positively on such factors as ability to keep rules, guilt in breaking rules, and capacity for relationships. This investigation highlighted the relationship between institutional care and outcomes in cognition, social skills, and adaptive behavior.

In comparing the development of 75 institutionalized infants with 75 infants raised in families, Provence and Lipton (1962), like their colleagues, found that institutionalized children exhibited delays in motor development, social skills, language development, and discovery of the body. Like Goldfarb (1945), they found that the longer lengths of institutionalization were associated with lower developmental quotients. In addition, Provence and Lipton proposed that sensory stimulation is important in building a repertoire of experiences from which an individual can organize and interpret external stimulation to produce voluntary motor actions—called *action units*. The institutionalized infants they observed demonstrated poor modulation of movement in comparison with their home-reared peers.

Institutionalization and Play Behaviors

In their longitudinal study of institutionalized children, Provence and Lipton (1962) described the evolution of play behavior, highlighting the relationship between stimulation and social interaction. The researchers noted that although young infants in institutions appeared to be able to interact with toys initially, this behavior dissipated as they grew older. Provence and Lipton described the reaching behavior of infants 5 to 6 months of age as appearing normal when they reached and grasped for toys. From 8 to 9 months of age onward, however, infants became increasingly less attracted to and less likely to work for toys, and their movements became less coordinated when reaching for a toy. As a result, they had little playful interaction with toys. Provence and Lipton (1962) stated, "The baby who is not playful should arouse concern. An infant who has not had enough nurturing is often apathetic; he does not enter vigorously into or initiate playful interchanges with others" (p. 10).

Provence and Lipton (1962) noted that institutionalized infants were less likely than their home-reared peers to use exploratory actions such as looking, banging, mouthing, shaking, poking, and dropping toys. Also notable was the observation that the institutionalized children in their first year of age did not appear upset when a toy was taken away, typically did not try to recover a lost toy, and usually did not show preference for one toy over others. Most important, Provence and Lipton (1962) observed that, "What the babies missed was not the presence of the toy itself, but something that makes a toy interesting and worth while" (p. 49). In reviewing the research, Ainsworth (1965) suggested that the most detrimental aspect of institutionalization is the lack of handling and interaction with a maternal figure. "As a result a child grows unresponsive to the toys provided for him to play with and to the opportunities for activity that even the restricted life-space of an institution offers" (p. 231).

Provence and Lipton (1962) pointed out that the infant needs to perceive, organize, and integrate stimuli with other experiences and that a maternal figure contributes to this organization. They noted that a caregiver's joy and pleasure in a child's action with a toy encourage the child to explore and act on his or her environment. They stated that children need balance between attachment to a caregiver and time to explore and use toys on their own. Provence and Lipton (1962) also observed that the infants who were labeled as caregiver "favorites" typically seemed more interested in toys. Furthermore, they suggested that the typically large number of caregivers who are responsible for various duties in institutions may contribute to the infants' difficulty in developing a sense of self and the environment.

Summary of Early Studies of Deprivation

As highlighted by the early studies of deprivation, two factors play a role in the developmental delays and problems in play observed in this population: an environment deprived of adequate stimulation and a lack of a primary caregiver. Research and early descriptions of children in institutions indicate that opportunities for interaction with the physical, sensory, and social environment coupled with the presence of a responsive, consistent, caregiving figure are essential components of child development. These findings are supported by animal research indicating that interaction with both the human and the nonhuman environment results in structural and functional changes in the brain, which allow animals to experience and interpret information from the environment more effectively (e.g., Diamond, 1967; Diamond, Ingham, Johnson, Bennett, & Rosenszweig, 1976; Liu et al., 1997; Sapolsky, 1997; Schanberg, Kuhn, Field, & Bartolome, 1990). Thus the way the brain in humans organizes or reorganizes information reflects the developmental experiences of animals.

Recent Studies

Research conducted on participants who have experienced an event that would be unethical to deliberately create for investigation, such as deprivation, are referred to as experiments of human nature. The fall of communism in Eastern Bloc countries and the subsequent adoption of many institutionalized children into Western families has permitted the use of newer, empirical methodologies to study the effects of deprivation on human development.

As in the classic field studies, delays have been observed in all areas of development for children recently adopted from institutions around the world. For example, Albers and colleagues (1997) found that 82% of previously institutionalized children studied exhibited delays in fine motor skills, 70% in gross motor skills, 59% in language, and 53% in social-emotional skills. Although children exhibited delays while institutionalized or on arriving in their newly adopted family, many of these previously institutionalized children continued to catch up developmentally for years following their adoption (Ames et al., 1997; Miller, 2005; O'Connor et al., 2000; Rutter & the ERA Study Team, 1998). Using sophisticated sampling and a longitudinal model, a group of researchers in England was able to demonstrate the effects of length of time institutionalized and progress over time once adopted. Upon adoption to English families, previously institutionalized Romanian children under 2 years of age demonstrated significant delays in both physical growth and cognitive skills when compared with

British-adopted children (Rutter & the ERA Study Team, 1998). At 4 years of age, however, the Romanian adoptees who were adopted before 6 months of age (spending less time in institutions) were performing similarly to the British adoptees, whereas Romanian adoptees who were adopted *after* 6 months of age made less progress. Another follow-up of this study when the children were 6 years of age demonstrated that the Romanian children adopted *after* 6 months of age continued to exhibit catch-up but still demonstrated smaller cognitive and physical gains than children adopted from Romania before 6 months of age (O'Connor et al., 2000).

There is little recent information regarding daily occupations such as play among institutionalized and previously institutionalized children. When studying a small group of children institutionalized in a Romanian orphanage, Kaler and Freeman (1994) found that the children's play skills appeared low for their chronological age, yet seemed appropriate considering their mental age. In fact, they found that the children's level of play behaviors was positively correlated with performance on the mental domain of the Bayley Scales of Infant Development ($r = .64$) (Kaler & Freeman, 1994).

Another investigation found evidence that the effects of institutionalization on play behaviors are far reaching. In this study 4-year-olds who had been adopted from Romanian orphanages by families in the United Kingdom at least 2 years previously were compared with British adoptees who had never been institutionalized (Kreppner, O'Connor, Dunn, Andersen-Wood, & the ERA Study Team, 1999). The British adoptees demonstrated significantly more developmentally competent levels of pretend play, role play, and referencing of others' mental states than the Romanian adoptees. Again, this occurred at least 2 years *following* adoption. Unlike Kaler and Freeman's (1994) orphanage study, however, this study found little relationship between general cognitive status and play behaviors for the sample ($r = .19$).

Lyons (2003) found that an institutionalized group demonstrated different play actions (often related to ideational praxis) than their home-reared peers. The institutionalized group in this study played with significantly fewer toys, used a smaller variety of actions, and employed significantly fewer actions during play sessions than did age-matched, home-reared children. These play skills, however, were not examined in relationship to other developmental measures such as general cognitive status and the children were not matched for developmental age.

Project Loving Arms: Promoting Play and Caregiver-Child Interaction

In 1995, as part of a humanitarian relief effort in conjunction with an organization of parents who had adopted children from Romania, the second author Dr. Cermak, with colleagues and graduate students from Boston University, began work in Center #1 in Buzau, Romania. This group equipped the orphanage with playrooms and provided caregiver training to enhance the development of children birth through age 3 residing in the orphanage. After the team's 1995 visit to Buzau, two members stayed on to continue work in the orphanage. After the main team departed, the new play areas set up for the children initially went unused. While both the children and the caregivers appeared to enjoy and benefit from the developmental stimulation and stress relief afforded by playful interaction in the new play areas, the caregivers appeared to lack the confidence and know-how to help the children engage on their own with the variety of play opportunities and objects in the space. Furthermore, playtime in these areas had not yet become part of their daily schedule. With these observations and further input from the orphanage staff, subsequent team efforts focused on specific instruction for the caregivers in understanding child development, facilitating development through grading activities, and providing social-emotional and task support. Hands-on activities similar to aspects of fieldwork activities completed in many therapeutic professions were included throughout this training. Later teams made up of professors and students provided ongoing caregiver training, toys, and other supplies annually.

In 1998, the team built an outdoor playground for the children. With an appropriate outdoor play space, caregivers began to take the children outside, resulting in a decreased incidence of rickets. In 1999, with funding assistance from Orphan Reach, a nonprofit foundation, the team hired and trained five additional Romanian educators to provide the children with added caregiver attention. The following year, a Romanian psychologist was hired with funding from the Pediatric Therapy Network. There are several ongoing projects. The first is the Elise Gilbert Family Connection, named in memory of a graduate student who served on Dr. Cermak's 1995 team. In this project, women from the community spend two afternoons a week with two children. This allows the children to experience family-like interactions. In the past several years the Romanian government has emphasized placing more children in foster care instead of orphanages. Consequently the team started a program to support this effort, the Cranaleith Child Development Center. The project, funded in part by the Cranaleith Foundation, provides support to children in foster care, many of whom had at one time been institutionalized. Other current programs include a preschool language program, a school-readiness program, and a toy lending library. Across all of its efforts, the mission of Project Loving Arms continues to be enhancement of children's development through meaningful caregiver-child interactions and playful activities.

DESIGNING A STUDY TO OBSERVE PLAY AND CAREGIVER-CHILD INTERACTIONS

Through the initial efforts of Project Loving Arms, this chapter's first author designed a study to examine play behaviors in a naturalistic context for the children residing in orphanages. Play behaviors have been related to both cognitive and social development (Fisher, 1992; Piaget, 1951; Vygotsky, 1978). The occupation of play was chosen for two reasons. First, it provided a supplemental picture of the children's development in addition to the Bayley Scales of Infant Development, 2nd edition (BSID-2, Bayley, 1993), an assessment that, while having evidence of cross-cultural validity, was standardized on home-reared children. Through participating in the play sessions, the children would have the opportunity to explore objects without having to follow the standardized directions or work within time constraints typical of developmental assessments. It was thought that play might elicit higher levels of motivation and perhaps skill than would be evident on standardized assessments of general cognitive status. Second, the play sessions provided an occupation-based observation of the children's performance. This was viewed as important, given the previously mentioned time-use study findings indicating that when the institutionalized children were engaged in an activity, it was most frequently play (Daunhauer et al., 2005). Informal observations made during data collection for the time-use study indicated that in the Romanian institutionalized group, the range of play appeared less developmentally competent than was observed in the U.S. child care group.

The goal was to study the children's play behaviors both in independent play and in collaborative play with a known caregiver. The collaborative play condition was selected based on Rogoff's (1990) theory that interactions between more and less skilled members of a culture (guided participation), particularly in routine daily activities, facilitate children's development. Supporting this theory, researchers (e.g., Doctoroff, 1996) have found that both typical children and children with developmental delays exhibit more developmentally competent play when interacting with a caregiver. Further support for examining the children and caregivers in collaborative play comes from child care research indicating that low child-to-adult ratios in child care, which presumably fosters more frequent caregiver-child interactions, are associated with better cognitive and language outcomes (Burchinal, Roberts, Nabors, & Bryant, 1996; Burchinal, Roberts, Riggin, Zeisel, Neebe, & Bryant, 2000; National Institute of Child Health and Human Development Early Childcare Research Network, 1999). Two of the primary study questions were: (1) did a relationship exist between the children's play behaviors and their general cognitive status? and (2) would the children exhibit more developmentally competent play behaviors when interacting with a known caregiver than when playing alone?

Pilot Testing to Determine Challenges and Solutions: Lessons Learned

Rather than placing a child in a high chair or in a chair at a table and recording the child's exploration with a toy handed to him or her for a specific time as done in some studies (Hatwell, 2003; Ruff & Lawson, 1990; Streri, 2003), this study was pilot tested to ensure that the children were observed in the most naturalistic way possible. The orphanage had four living areas, typically organized by the child's age and mobility. Change appears to be far more upsetting to institutionalized children than to home-reared children. Quite often, for a child living in an orphanage, leaving his or her room may mean getting an injection or having an abrupt change of living circumstances. Not surprisingly, pilot testing of both the BSID-2 and the play observations indicated that children were better able to engage in the activities if they remained in the living areas known to them.

When study space is set up in an environment of deprivation, it is useful to remember that a child living in these conditions rarely has an uncontested opportunity to explore and play with novel objects. Children compete for both limited caregiver attention and play objects. To limit interruptions from other children in the living area who were attracted to the testing activities, one of the research team members was assigned the job of helping to entertain the other children and keeping them from interfering in the testing area, which was partially blocked off with chairs or benches from that room. This provided the additional benefit of ensuring that no extra workload was imposed on the caregivers.

A study of typical children found that just the supportive presence of a child's mother, without any interaction, could increase the child's time spent in exploration (Sorce & Emde, 1981). Other researchers (e.g., Belsky, Goode, & Most, 1980; Fiese, 1990; Lawson, Parrinello, & Ruff, 1992; Slade, 1987) have demonstrated that, more important, it is the mothers' interactions that lead to higher levels of play than the child could produce independently. Not surprisingly, during pilot testing the children were better able to remain in independent play if either the examiner or a caregiver sat near them. Although the children were able to remain in independent play with a known caregiver, the caregivers were unable to reliably follow the independent play protocol and refrain from actively engaging the children in play or scaffolding play for them. Ultimately, since the examiner had developed a rapport with the children while assessing them with the BSID-2, it was decided to use her as a warm presence during the independent play condition and then incorporate the known caregiver into the collaborative play condition. The examiner did not initiate interactions during the independent play condition and simply responded to a child's bids for interaction by saying warmly, "Yes," "That's nice," or "I have work, you play here."

How Play Was Observed

To participate, the children, 10 to 38 months of age, had to pass the BSID-2 motor item requiring them to sit alone while playing with a toy. Two sets of toys were used for the play sessions. The first set consisted of sensorimotor and cause and effect toys similar to those that had been donated to the institution over the years. These included a toy key ring, bumpy squeak toy, tambourine, stacking busy tower, ball drop, multisensory toy, toy hammer, and spoon from the children's everyday utensils. Since the children seemed eager to explore any object, the second set of toys was weighted with symbolic toys to provide ample opportunity for eliciting the children's optimal pretend play. This procedure has been used by other researchers as well (Hill & McCune-Nicolich, 1981; McCune, 1995). The symbolic toys represented aspects of daily life typical of the children's experience. These included a baby doll with a cap, play crib, crib blanket, towel, brush, comb, magic bottle, two stackable toy mugs, bowls and spoons similar in shape to the children's everyday utensils, and three magnetic train cars, one with small blocks. Both toy sets could be used for a variety of play.

The play sessions followed the developmental testing using the BSID-2. The child participated in the independent play condition first. This consisted of 6 minutes of free play with the sensorimotor toys and 6 minutes of play with the symbolic toys. Then the child participated in the collaborative play condition with a known caregiver. The primary investigator instructed the caregivers to play with the child as they normally would. She also asked them to set up the toys from the sensorimotor and symbolic toy sets in a way that would work best for that child. The caregivers could select one or all of the toys. They could elect to store some of the toys within reach to be offered as the session progressed. The caregivers' decisions about how they set up the collaborative play session reflected an aspect of scaffolding or guided participation skills described by Vygotsky (1978) and Rogoff (1990), respectively.

In a synthesis of the literature, Varga (1991) proposed that childhood researchers in the 1920s and 1930s influenced the use of play as a tool to manage, supervise, and facilitate development. Gesell and other childhood authorities converted play observations of typical children into scales of normal play. According to Varga, this idea of using play to manage a child's progression in successful developmental tasks led to an idealization of the concept of play and consequently a creation of new criteria for early childhood teaching, the environmental setup of preschools, and the materials they use. Based on the literature

(e.g., Belsky & Most, 1981), a play scale was constructed for this study to score the gamut of play behaviors from the most basic exploratory behaviors, such as mouthing, to symbolic or pretend play with a doll. The children's highest level of play demonstrated in 10-second intervals was recorded for both the independent and the collaborative play sessions (Daunhauer, Coster, Tickle-Degnen, & Cermak, 2007).

Play Behaviors Observed

Typically the children in the upper half of the age range (20+ months) would explore two to three objects in both the exploratory and symbolic sessions. Many of the younger children, however, would often focus on just one object, particularly the balls, during the exploratory session. Many appeared to find pleasure in just picking one ball up and setting it or dropping it on a metal tray, which made an audible bang. They also banged the balls together or on other objects over and over. Some of the younger children would bang or mouth the balls for the entire session. Sometimes it was difficult to tell whether this was exploratory behavior or self-stimulatory behavior. Many of the older children were drawn to the ball drop or stacking tower, dropping the balls or replacing the stacks repeatedly during the session. This drive to do a play action repeatedly was noted with use of the test items during the Bayley testing as well. On one end of the gamut of responses was a young girl who barely touched a ball two or three times, preferring to gaze alternately at the examiner and the toys. On the other end was an older boy who frenetically explored all of the toys.

Notable in the play sessions was how the children's strength and motor skills affected their exploration, particularly for the children under age 2. While all of the children could sit and play with a toy, many did not have the postural stability needed to shift and reach comfortably. Many younger children would move into a modified quadruped position to explore the toys farther away from them. Others would make several attempts to pick up or swipe an object for exploration.

Social bids from the children were an almost ubiquitous behavior in the play sessions. They frequently made eye contact with the examiner, who provided a warm, supportive presence during the independent sessions, and they socially referenced her many times during these sessions. Many children also attempted to engage the investigator in play by handing her a toy—some quite persistently. While they generally appeared interested in the toys, the children's affect was typically neutral. They rarely smiled or looked surprised. When they did smile, it was usually in an attempt to engage the investigator or occasionally in a response to mastering an aspect of one of the toys such as putting a ball in the ball drop. Children often grew wide eyed or looked behind them in response to sounds such as crying or toys thrown by their peers who were blocked from the play session.

Outcomes

In the independent play sessions the children demonstrated play skills below expectations for their actual (chronological) age, but on par with their developmental age as measured by the BSID-2 (Daunhauer, 2004). In general, the higher a child's general cognitive abilities as measured by the BSID-2, the more developmentally competent the play skills he or she demonstrated. These findings suggest that standardized developmental assessments, even though normed on home-reared children, may accurately reflect the children's cognitive performance, although not necessarily their potential. Conversely, if an institutionalized or previously institutionalized child is unable to participate in standardized testing, play observations might provide helpful insights into the child's development.

In the collaborative play condition the children as a group demonstrated more developmentally competent play behaviors when interacting with a caregiver than when playing in the independent condition. This finding was notable given that these caregivers are responsible for large groups of children and may not get to know what motivates a child in the same way that a parent with daily interaction does. The collaborative play condition supported Rogoff's (1990) theory that more skilled members of a culture can guide the participation of children, which enhances their participation in daily life. Vygtosky (1978) proposed a concept called the zone of proximal development. This zone describes the difference between what children can actually do on their own and what they can do with scaffolding (social-emotional and task support) from an adult. Thus the difference between the children's play capacities in the independent session and their play competence in the interaction session would be their zone of proximal development in this study. Vygotsky proposed that the zone of proximal development may provide a way to predict how children will progress in a developmental area. Further investigation is needed to understand whether the zone of proximal development may be useful in determining how a child will progress or how the increased skills elicited through a caregiver-child interaction may be incorporated in subsequent independent play.

SUMMARY: PLAY AS MEANS AND ENDS

Unfortunately, children around the globe continue to experience degrees of both maternal (caregiver) and environmental deprivation. Play and playful interaction in environments of deprivation can facilitate development, can serve as a supplementary observation of developmental status, and certainly can provide relief from boredom and stress. There is growing evidence that improving caregiver-child interactions and providing regular engagement in occupations such as play will lead to more optimal developmental outcomes for institutionalized children (Groark, Muhamedrahimov, Palmov, Nikiforova, & McCall, 2004; Sparling, Dragomir, Ramey, & Florescu, 2005). Two occupational therapy approaches that are relevant in this environment are the education process and the therapeutic use of activities and occupations (Barnekow & Kraemer, 2005). Through the education process, occupational therapy practitioners can promote caregiver-child interactions and knowledge about the developmental processes. Through the use of therapeutic activities and occupations, regularly scheduled amounts of time with age-appropriate objects and responsive caregivers can begin to assist children's development and well-being.

Review Questions

1. Define the following key words and concepts:
   Deprivation
   Guided participation
   Zone of proximal development

2. In the time-use study cited in the chapter, how did the institutional group and the U.S. child care group compare in (a) the amount of time spent in play and (b) the amount of time spent alone? Are these findings congruent with early field studies describing life in an orphanage?

3. If a therapist is unable to engage a recently adopted child in a standardized developmental assessment, is there evidence to suggest that play observations can be used as a supplemental tool?

REFERENCES

Ainsworth, M. D. (1965). Further research into the adverse effects of maternal deprivation. In J. Bowlby, *Child care and the growth of love* (2nd ed., pp. 191-251). London: Penguin Books.

Albers, L. H., Johnson, D. E., Hostetter, M., Iverson, S., & Miller, L. (1997). Health of children adopted from the former Soviet Union and Eastern Europe. *Journal of the American Medical Association, 278,* 922-924.

Ames, E. W. (1997). *The development of Romanian orphanage children adopted to Canada.* Burnaby, BC, Canada: Simon Fraser University.

Bandura, A. (1978). The self system in reciprocal determinism. *American Psychologist, 33,* 344-358.

Barnekow, K. A., & Kraemer, G. W. (2005). The psychobiological theory of attachment: A viable frame of reference for early intervention providers. *Physical and Occupational Therapy in Pediatrics, 25,* 3-15.

Bayley, N. (1993). *Bayley Scales of Infant Development second edition: Manual.* San Antonio, TX: The Psychological Corporation.

Belsky, J., Goode, M. K., & Most, R. K. (1980). Maternal stimulation and infant exploratory competence: Cross-sectional, correlational, and experimental analyses. *Child Development, 51,* 1163-1178.

Belsky, J., & Most, R. K. (1981). From exploration to play: A cross-sectional study of infant free play behavior. *Developmental Psychology, 17,* 630-639.

Bowlby, J. (1951). *Maternal care and mental health.* Geneva, Switzerland: World Health Organization.

Bowlby, J. (1953). *Child care and the growth of love.* Baltimore: Penguin Books.

Bruer, J. (1999). The myth of the first three years: A new understanding of early brain development and lifelong learning. New York: The Free Press.

Burchinal, M. R., Roberts, J. E., Nabors, L. A., & Bryant, D. M. (1996). Quality of center childcare and infant cognitive and language development. *Child Development, 67,* 606-620.

Burchinal, M. R., Roberts, J. E., Riggin, R., Jr., Zeisel, S. A., Neebe, E., & Bryant, D. (2000). Relating quality of center-based childcare to early cognitive and language development longitudinally. *Child Development, 71,* 339-357.

Casler, L. (1961). Maternal deprivation: A critical review of the literature. *Monographs of the Society for Research in Child Development, 26*(2), 1-64.

Casler, L. (1968). Perceptual deprivation in institutional settings. In G. Newton & S. Levine (Eds.), *Early experience and behavior* (pp. 573-626). Springfield, IL: Charles C Thomas.

Daunhauer, L., Bolton, A., & Cermak, S. (2005). Time-use patterns of young children institutionalized in Eastern Europe. *OTJR: Occupation, Participation & Health, 25,* 1-8.

Daunhauer, L. A. (2004). The developmental status and play occupations of young children institutionalized in Eastern Europe (Doctoral dissertation, Boston University, 2004). *Dissertation Abstracts International, 65,* 6274.

Daunhauer, L. A., Coster, W. J., Tickle-Degnen, L., & Cermak, S. A. (2007). The effects of caregiver-child interactions on play occupations among young children institutionalized in Eastern Europe. *American Journal of Occupational Therapy, 61,* 429-440.

Diamond, M. C. (1967). Extensive cortical depth measurements and neuron size increases in the cortex of environmentally enriched rats. *Journal of Comparative Neurology, 131,* 357-364.

Diamond, M. C., Ingham, C. A., Johnson, R. E., Bennett, E. L., & Rosenszweig, M. R. (1976). Effects of environment on morphology of rat cerebral cortex and hippocampus. *Journal of Neurobiology, 7,* 75-86.

Doctoroff, S. (1996). Parents' support of infants' object play: A review of the literature. *Infant-Toddler Intervention, 6*(2), 153-166.

Dunn, A., Jareg, E., & Webb, D. (2003). *A last resort: The growing concern about children in residential care.* International Save the Children Alliance. London, UK. Retrieved August 24, 2007 from http://www.scslat.org/search/publieng. php?_cod_19_lang_e.

Fiese, B. H. (1990). Playful relationships: A contextual analysis of mother-toddler interactions and symbolic play. *Child Development, 61,* 1648-1656.

Fisher, E. P. (1992). The impact of play on development: A meta-analysis. *Play and Culture, 5,* 159-181.

Goldfarb, W. (1945). Psychological privation in infancy and subsequent adjustment. *American Journal of Orthopsychiatry, 15,* 247-255.

Groark, C. J., Muhamedrahimov, R. J., Palmov, O., Nikiforova, N., & McCall, R. B. (2004). Improvements in early care in Russian orphanages and their relationship to observed behaviors. *Infant Mental Health Journal, 26,* 96-109.

Gunnar, M. R. (1998). Quality of early care and buffering of neuroendocrine stress reactions: Potential effects on the developing brain. *Preventive Medicine, 27,* 208-211.

Gunnar, M. R., Bruce, M., & Grotevant, H. D. (2000). International adoption of institutionally reared children: Research and policy. *Development and Psychopathology, 12,* 677-693.

Harlow, H. F. (1958). The nature of love. *The American Psychologist, 13,* 673-685.

Harlow, H. F., & Harlow, M. K. (1966). Learning to love. *American Scientist, 54,* 244-272.

Harlow, H. F., & Suomi, S. J. (1970). The nature of love— Simplified. *American Psychologist, 25,* 162-168.

Hatwell, Y. (2003). Manual exploratory procedures in children and adults. In Y. Hatwell, A. Streri, & E. Gentaz (Eds.), *Touching for knowing* (pp. 67-02). Philadelphia: John Benjamins Publishing.

Hill, P. M., & McCune-Nicolich, L. (1981). Pretend play and patterns of cognition in Down syndrome children. *Child Development, 52,* 611-617.

Kaler, S. R., & Freeman, B. J. (1994). An analysis of environmental deprivation: Cognitive and social development in Romanian orphans. *Journal of Child Psychiatry, 35,* 769-781.

Kreppner, J. M., O'Connor, T. G., Dunn, J., Andersen-Wood, L., & the ERA Study Team. (1999). The pretend and social role play of children exposed to early severe deprivation. *British Journal of Developmental Psychology, 17,* 319-332.

Lawson, K. R., Parrinello, R., & Ruff, H. A. (1992). Maternal behavior and infant attention. *Infant Behavior and Development, 15,* 209-229.

Liu, D., Diorio, J., Tannenbaum, B., Caldji, C., Francis, D., Freedman, A., et al. (1997). Maternal care, hippocampal glucocorticoid receptors, and hypothalamic-pituitary-adrenal responses to stress. *Science, 277,* 1659-1662.

Lyons, J. (2003). *Play behaviors of typically developing and institutionalized children* (Unpublished master's thesis. Boston University, Boston).

McCune, L. (1995). A normative study of representational play at the transition to language. *Developmental Psychology, 31,* 198-206.

McGeown, K. (2005). *Romanian adoptees struggle to adapt July 13, 2005.* Retrieved February 17, 2006 from http://www.news.bbc.co.uk/1/hi/world/europe/4649383.stm.

Miller, L. C. (2005). *The handbook of international adoption medicine: A guide for physicians, parents and providers.* New York: Oxford University Press.

National Authority for Child Protection and Adoption (Romanian) (2004). *Specialised [sic] public services for child protection August 21, 2004.* Retrieved February 17, 2006 from http://www.copii.ro/1e.htm.

National Institute of Child Health and Human Development Early Childcare Research Network. (1999). Child outcomes when child care center classes meet recommended standards for quality. *American Journal of Public Health, 89,* 1072-1077.

O'Connor, T. G., Rutter, M., Beckett, C., Keaveney, L., Kreppner, J. M., & English-Romanian Adoptees (ERA) Study Team (2000). The effects of global severe privation on cognitive competence: Extension and longitudinal follow-up. *Child Development, 71*, 376-390.

Piaget, J. (1951). *Play, dreams and imitation in childhood.* London: Routledge & Kegan Paul.

Provence, S., & Lipton, R. C. (1962). *Infants in institutions.* New York: International Universities Press.

Rogoff, B. (1990). *Apprenticeship in thinking.* New York: Oxford University Press.

Ruff, H. A., & Lawson, K. R. (1990). Development of sustained, focused attention in young children during free play. *Developmental Psychology, 26*, 85-93.

Rutter, M., & English-Romanian Adoptees (ERA) Study Team (1998). Developmental catch-up and deficit following adoption after severe global early privation. *Journal of Child Psychology and Psychiatry, 39*, 465-476.

Sapolsky, R. M. (1997). The importance of a well-groomed child. *Science, 277*, 1620-1621.

Schanberg, S., Kuhn, C., Field, T., & Bartolome, J. (1990). Maternal deprivation and growth suppression. In N. Gunzenhauser (Ed.), *Advances in touch: New implications in human development. Pediatric Roundtable 14* (pp. 3-10). Skillman, NJ: Johnson & Johnson.

Slade, A. (1987). A longitudinal study of maternal involvement and symbolic play during the toddler period. *Child Development, 58*, 367-375.

Sorce, J. F., & Emde, R. N. (1981). Mother's presence is not enough: Effect of emotional availability on infant exploration. *Developmental Psychology, 17*, 737-745.

Sparling, J., Dragomir, C., Ramey, S. L., & Florescu, L. (2005). An educational intervention improves developmental progress of young children in a Romanian orphanage. *Infant Mental Health Journal, 26*, 127-142.

Spitz, R. (1945). Hospitalism: An inquiry into the genesis of psychiatric conditions in early childhood. In O. Fenichel, P. Greenacre, H. Hartman, E. B. Jackson, E. Kris, L. S. Kubie, et al. (Eds.), *The psychoanalytic study of the child* (Vol. 1, pp. 53-74). New York: International Universities Press.

Spitz, R. (1946). Hospitalism: A follow-up report. In P. Greenacre, H. Hartmann, E. B. Jackson, E. Kris, L. S. Kubie, B. D. Lewin, et al. (Eds.), *The psychoanalytic study of the child* (Vol. 2, pp. 113-117). New York: International Universities Press.

Streri, A. (2003). Manual exploration and haptic perception in infants. In Y. Hatwell, A. Streri, & E. Gentaz (Eds.), *Touching for knowing* (pp. 51-66). Philadelphia: John Benjamins Publishing.

U.S. State Department. (2005). *Immigrant visas issued to orphans coming to the U.S.* Retrieved February 19, 2006, from: http://travel.state.gov/family/adoption/stats/stats_451.html.

Varga, D. (1991). The historical ordering of children's play as a developmental task. *Play and Culture, 4*, 322-333.

Vygotsky, L. S. (1978). *Mind in society.* Cambridge, MA: Harvard University Press.

9

Play and the Sensory Integrative Approach

ZOE MAILLOUX AND JANICE POSATERY BURKE

Sensory integration unfolds in a predictable pattern as part of central nervous system development in infancy and childhood, as well as throughout the lifespan. The development of sensory integrative skills and behaviors is observed in all aspects of children's lives, including their abilities to maintain a calm and alert state; to develop new skills such as picking up, holding onto, and examining a fuzzy stuffed animal (Figure 9-1); and to learn about interacting and relating to others. Similarly, play skills develop in concert with a child's physical, cognitive, and motor abilities that support their emergence. For occupational therapists, interest in and attention to both sensory integration and play provides a complex and intriguing framework for structuring intervention for children who exhibit deficits and related problems in these domains.

The sophisticated relationship of sensory integration to play is dependent on the development of a number of neurobehavioral capacities, including the drive for receiving, perceiving, and integrating sensory information with motor responses (Miller & Miller-Kuhaneck, 2006a, 2006b). The opportunity to practice and refine sensory integrative behaviors provides the scaffolding for the more complex thinking and doing that emerge in the everyday play of a child. In turn, these play behaviors fuel further sensory integrative development. The interrelatedness

of these systems is discussed in this chapter, which is designed to illustrate the role of sensory integrative behaviors in normal play development, to discuss how sensory integrative deficits affect play, and to describe how play provides a useful construct for addressing sensory integrative deficits.

SENSORY INTEGRATIVE CONTRIBUTIONS TO PLAY DEVELOPMENT
Infancy: The Sensory Beginnings of Play

In typical development, early sensorimotor play is strongly influenced by the drive for sensory and motor experiences. During this stage of play development, basic sensory functions dominate behavior, with infants spending a great deal of time in exploratory play, seeking and experiencing tactile, vestibular, proprioceptive, olfactory, gustatory, visual, and auditory input. Infants are captivated by these sensations, and they spend their time searching for new and interesting, as well as known and comforting, sensory experiences. Self-regulation, which involves varied physiological and culturally influenced patterns of sleep-wake cycles, feeding, emotions, and behavior, also emerges as an important aspect of development that overlaps with sensory processing during infancy (National Research Council and Institute of Medicine, 2000).

Along with a natural drive for a variety of sensory experiences, infants begin to experiment with moving their bodies in novel ways (Figure 9-2). As infants develop voluntary, controlled movement, they begin to form ideas about what to do and ways to plan that action. This drive is evident in every purposeful action that is initiated by the young child. Ben, a 9-month-old infant, illustrates how the drive for sensation blends with the ability to plan new motor actions. This little boy generally spends his mornings at home with his mother, engaging in play embedded within their regular

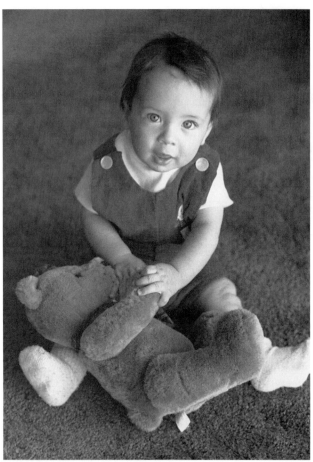

Figure 9-1
Simple acts such as picking up and holding a fuzzy stuffed animal depend on the integrity of sensory integrative functions. (Courtesy Shay McAtee.)

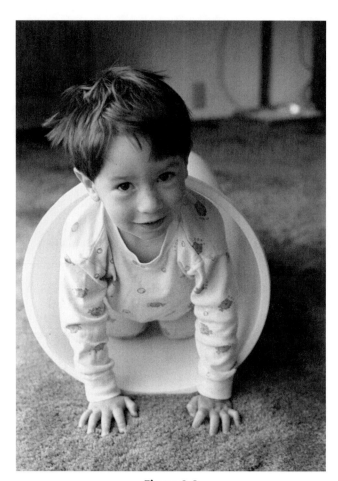

Figure 9-2
With increasing mobility, infants begin to experiment with moving their bodies in novel ways and in novel places. (Courtesy Shay McAtee.)

daily routines. Using his newly developed mobility, Ben spends most of his waking hours moving in search of sensory experiences. On this day, he climbs the couch to reach the shutters, which provide a visual bonanza of light and shadow (Figure 9-3). As he approaches them, he becomes intrigued by the smooth texture of the wood and the rounded edges of each slat and the vertical bar that holds them together. He discovers the clicking sounds that occur as he opens and closes the slats and is intrigued with his homemade sight and sound machine, which also has an appealing feel to it. While standing on the couch to enjoy his new toy, Ben begins to bounce and sway on the cushions. A rhythm emerges blending motion with sights, sounds, and touch. Every aspect of this experience feeds his sensory drives to engage, experiment, and explore.

While Ben is motivated to receive, perceive, and integrate the sensory experiences inherent in this type of activity, his basic sensory systems are also using the experience to lay the groundwork for more complex tasks of the future. The movement and kinesthetic

experiences Ben receives through bouncing and swaying on the cushions are contributing to a fundamental sense of knowing where his body is in space. This affects his balance, his muscle tone, and the coordination of his head and eye movements and contributes to his ability to use his hands together in a coordinated manner. His motivation to run his fingers along the wooden slats provides an opportunity to manipulate a foreign object and gain sensory information. As this occurs, he begins to integrate what he sees with what he feels, thus laying a foundation for mastering and understanding the properties of objects, how they work, and how his body can use them to experience and effectively interact with them.

Preschool Years: A Focus on Directing Play Toward Interaction

During the preschool years, constructive play predominates, with imaginary and social play skills emerging (Caplan & Caplan, 1974; Knox, 2005). The drive for

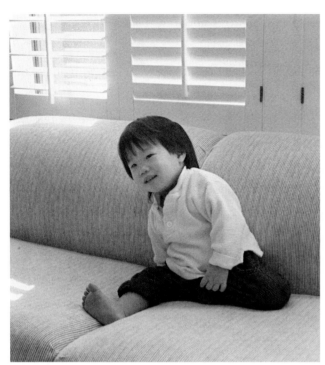

Figure 9-3
The shutters above the couch provide a visual bonanza of light and shadow that can be manipulated by the exploring infant. (Courtesy Shay McAtee.)

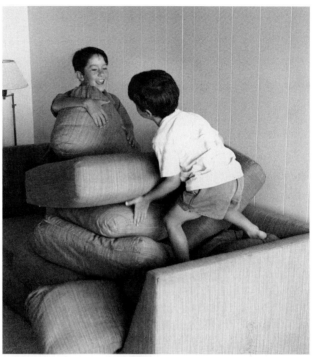

Figure 9-4
For older children, play with objects such as pillows, cushions, and blankets continues to provide sensory experiences, but it also carries symbolic and social meanings. Well-developed, automatic sensorimotor abilities free the child to transform the materials imaginatively into a den, a cave, a wall, or a castle without having to attend to more primitive functions such as maintaining standing balance. (Courtesy Shay McAtee.)

sensory experiences continues but no longer directs virtually every action the child makes in play. In this stage of development the child continues to seek and enjoy basic sensory experiences, but now the child incorporates more complex interactions into play, with language and symbolic thought making increasingly significant contributions to the intricacies of play. The sensory integration experiences that occur within this more complex stage of play continue to provide a base for skills that will be needed later in life. For example, Mark, age 4, and Tricia, age 3, are next-door neighbors who participate in play interactions that fluctuate between parallel play and an early form of cooperative play. One afternoon, their individual play with a bevy of stuffed animals flows into a cooperative experience in which they construct a deep, dark den for the animals using blankets, cushions, and pillows. The sensory aspects of the scene are found in the number of tactile and proprioceptive sensations that are inherent in the cozy den and in the children's being surrounded by the stuffed animals that inhabit it. But this is no longer primarily a sensory activity, as it might have been for Mark and Tricia as infants. The construction of the den becomes very important as the children concern themselves with how the cushions should be arranged. How much light should be allowed inside? How will they get to the den from across the room? Which animals belong to each child, and who is in charge? As the cushions are

placed, pathways are built, and negotiations take place, the sensory and motor aspects of this play experience are making a significant foundational contribution to the children's ability to make things happen. They also set in motion new neuronal models for how things work. However and perhaps most important, because the sensory and motor functions occur automatically, they allow more complex conceptual and social functions to emerge (Figure 9-4).

School Years: More Sophisticated Play with Rules and Skills

During the school years, play in which rules and skills are important becomes more predominant (Caplan & Caplan, 1974; Knox, 2005). Motor skills that depend on efficient sensory integration and praxis become important and can influence a child's social status, motivation, and self-esteem. Although games and activities involving conceptual thought, language, and problem solving make up a great deal of play for some children, the emphasis in this age group is clearly on sports and skill-based play activities.

Some play activities common in the school-age group, such as roller-skating, roller-blading, jumping rope,

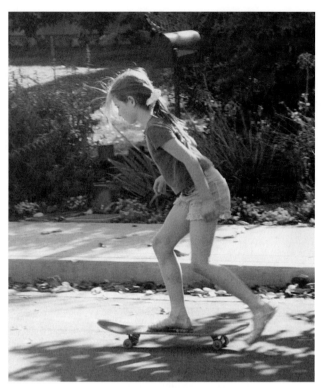

Figure 9-5

School-age children typically spend some portion of their play in sensorimotor activities that challenge the vestibular and proprioceptive systems.(Courtesy Shay McAtee.)

playing ball sports, and constructing models with detailed patterns, require a high level of praxis, which entails timing, sequencing, and anticipatory motor skills. The very nature of many rule-generated games and sports reveals a continued emphasis on sensory and movement experiences. Most children at this age continue to enjoy spending at least some portion of their play in sensorimotor activities. The basic functions of the nervous system that ensure optimal sensory integration must be intact and efficient for a child to continue to enjoy activities that depend highly on these functions, especially given that self-consciousness and peer evaluation of performance become increasingly important during this stage (Figure 9-5). The contribution of sensory integrative functions to other developing abilities continues, but by school age, children are able to rely on alternative approaches to accomplishing a task, such as using a strategy to make an activity easier, compensating with other skills, avoiding difficult activities, and practicing components of skills. For example, Patrick is an 8-year-old who finds balance-related activities such as bicycle riding, roller-skating, roller-blading, ice-skating, and surfboarding easy to master. He enjoys the sensory experiences they provide, as evidenced by his motivation to ride or skate fast, to turn circles, and to go up and down hills. The efficient vestibular and proprioceptive functions that these play activities

require may also be supporting his above-average skills in academic tasks such as writing, reading, and organizing his work. His participation in these activities provides an arena for engaging in social interactions with other children. In contrast to these areas of prowess, Patrick finds ball skills and organized sports more challenging and less interesting. It is difficult for him to maintain the eye-hand or eye-foot coordination needed for many of the ball skills required in these sports, and when he attempts them, he feels self-conscious about his performance. For Patrick these skill areas are perceived as weaknesses that are uninteresting compared with his areas of strength and enjoyment. For the most part he is able to compensate for his limitations by practicing and developing strategies to improve his performance, but he prefers to select play activities at which he excels. These provide an adequate outlet for receiving continued sensorimotor experiences appropriate to his age level.

Beyond Childhood: Play to Recreation

In older childhood, adolescence, and adulthood, sensory integrative aspects of play behavior are bound by factors such as individual skills and interests, environmental constraints, the necessity of incorporating play into more complex schedules, and associated role requirements and responsibilities (Caplan & Caplan, 1974; Knox, 2005). Although the drive for some types of movement probably decreases (Ayres, 2005), other forms of sensory experience continue to be essential. Even at older ages, play is a vehicle for experiencing sensations that are necessary for the nervous system to function well. Blanche (2001) studied play and leisure preferences in adults and found that sensory qualities of activities were salient aspects of choices.

HOW SENSORY INTEGRATIVE DEFICITS AFFECT PLAY

An understanding of the central role that sensory integrative functions have in the development of normal play illustrates how important it is that these functions operate in an efficient manner. When this does not occur, one of the most devastating results is a disruption in play. Parents of children who demonstrate sensory integrative disorders often bring these problems to a therapist, expressing such concerns as, "He doesn't know how to play with toys," "She won't play by the rules," "He breaks his toys and destroys others' games," and "No one wants to play with him."

Decades of research incorporating various measures of sensory integration functions (Ayres, 1989; Mulligan, 1998; Parham & Mailloux, 2005) have revealed several patterns of sensory integration disorders that appear in study after study. These dysfunctional sensory integrative patterns may occur as discrete issues or in conjunction with other sensory integration patterns. Moreover, sensory integration deficits are often identified in children who already have other educational or medical diagnoses, as well as in children who do not have other recognized disorders. Within the range of the ways in which sensory integration problems occur, there is a great deal of overlap in how various subsets of problems can affect play. For illustrative purposes some of the most common sensory integrative disorders are discussed individually here in relation to ways that they may affect play behavior.

Problems in Sensory Modulation

In early factor analyses (1964, 1965, 1966a, 1966b, 1969, 1971) and in early writing on sensory integration theory (1972), Ayres described unusual responses to sensory experiences under specific sensory system headings such as "tactile defensiveness" and "gravitational insecurity." The terms "sensory defensiveness" and "sensory modulation disorders" describe unusually heightened, diminished, or fluctuating responses to sensation (Lane, 2002; Parham & Mailloux, 2005).

Sensory modulation disorders can occur in relation to one type of sensory experience or to multiple sensations. Parham and associates found factors based on sensory systems when evaluating 5- to 8-year-old children on a sensory modulation measure in which parents and teachers rated the children's responses to various sensory experiences (Parham, Ecker, Miller-Kuhaneck, Henry, & Glennon, 2007). Dunn and Brown (1997) have reported cross-modal patterns such as sensory seeking. An individual's response to the sensation(s) may vary depending on the time of day, time of year, type of specific sensation, and individual state (e.g., illness, fatigue, hunger). Such common sensory modulation problems as tactile defensiveness, auditory sensitivities, and gravitational insecurity may limit play behavior in children by restricting ease of participation and creating a tendency toward social withdrawal and isolation (Ayres, 2005; Bundy, 2002; Bundy, Shia, Qi, & Miller, 2007; May-Benson & Koomar, 2007).

Tactile Defensiveness
"Tactile defensiveness" is the term Ayres (2005) used to refer to an unusual sensitivity to touch. Tactile defensiveness is commonly characterized by hypersensitivity in areas of the body with a high concentration of tactile receptor sites, especially the hands, feet, and face.

Tactile defensiveness is a sensory integrative disorder that affects children's play behavior at a very early age and in a pervasive manner. Because early stages of play are characterized by tactile exploration, particularly through hand and mouth manipulation of objects, a tendency to avoid certain textures limits the scope of experiences the child has and the range of skills the child develops. Children with tactile defensiveness may not put objects into their mouths in typical ways during

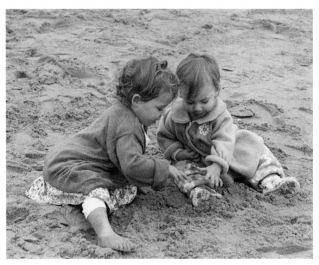

Figure 9-6
Playing in sand at the playground or beach depends on a well-modulated tactile system. This type of play activity is usually disturbing for a child with tactile defensiveness, who will tend to avoid it. (Courtesy Shay McAtee.)

infancy, so parents of these babies usually do not have to deal with this common source of worry. However, these children are likely to resist and withdraw from many forms of play if tactile input is involved. They may lack prerequisite skills for eating solid foods, forming words, and handling and manipulating toys and play materials (Parham & Mailloux, 2005). Limitation of tactile experiences in infancy can contribute to deficiencies in visual and manipulative skills.

As children grow, there is a continuum of play experiences that are based on tactile play (Figure 9-6). Such common activities as playing with sand, grass, mud, water, finger paints, and play dough are likely to be considered aversive by children with tactile defensiveness. As social play emerges, these children may react negatively if other children brush lightly against their skin when sharing materials, touch them when moving about, or bump into them unexpectedly. Engaging in imaginary play activities such as dress-up can be disconcerting, as can participating in special events such as donning a Halloween costume for a school party, having the face painted at a carnival, or visiting a petting zoo. In older grades, contact sports such as soccer, football, or baseball may create discomfort and hinder participation in these play activities, as does the need to wear a uniform and helmet.

CASE EXAMPLE 1

Jillian: Tactile Defensiveness

Jillian's problems with tactile defensiveness illustrate the interruptions in normal play that often occur for children who experience a tactile disorder. As an outgoing, talkative 4-year-old, Jillian has a lot of friends and generally enjoys spending time with them. Jillian experiences periods of extreme tactile defensiveness, often associated with changes in the weather or alterations of her daily sleeping patterns. When this occurs, Jillian starts off the day in an unstable or vulnerable state, which becomes exacerbated by the many tactile-based behaviors that she needs to enact, including finding clothes and shoes that feel comfortable, getting through the morning routines of having her hair combed and her teeth brushed, and deciding on a breakfast that includes textures she finds tolerable. By the time she arrives at preschool, she is irritable and uncomfortable. The challenge of sitting next to other children at play who brush lightly against her skin as they exchange toys proves unnerving, and she responds by taking her toys to her own space. Doing this makes her feel sad and confused. She would like to be playing with the other children, but simultaneously she feels the need to retreat.

Over time, tactile defensive behavior sets Jillian apart and limits the kinds of play experiences in which she is able to participate. The impact of her tactile limitations on her ability to participate in social play is an example of how a sensory processing problem hampers further skill acquisition and satisfaction in a young life.

Auditory Sensitivities

Some children are overly sensitive to sounds that are not normally disturbing or uncomfortable. The implications for difficulties in play are clearly significant, since many toys, play activities, and play interactions involve some type of predictable or spontaneous noise.

Many toys have inherent sound capabilities (horns, bells, and other musical instruments), are designed to use sound as an incentive for play (cause and effect toys), or use sound to teach skills (electronic games). When sound that is meant to comfort, encourage, or reward is perceived as irritating, disturbing, or frightening, a child may withdraw and refuse to participate. Equally significant is the incidental noise that arises from play interactions; children who are having a good time are typically noisy and generate sudden bursts of intense sound that match the action of the play. Children with auditory defensiveness often withdraw from informal activities such as play in groups and from more formal social events such as birthday parties.

Auditory sensitivity is a processing problem that limits the child's play experiences in the here and now. The concern is that such curtailment of activity may have long-term sequelae in more complex social, physical, and cognitive skills.

CASE EXAMPLE 2

Derrick: Auditory Defensiveness

Derrick is a 3-year-old boy with a diagnosis of autism. He is hypersensitive to many types of sensory input but especially to sounds. Noises that are barely detectable to most people (e.g., an air conditioner shutting off or a horn blowing in the distance) send Derrick into a state of panic; he withdraws from the task at hand, places his hands over his ears, and rocks back and forth. In Derrick's case, sensory issues characterized by extreme auditory hypersensitivity override his ability to tolerate even the most basic types of play experiences. Reactions to sounds constantly interrupt his attention to toys and drive him away from the kinds of environments where play occurs. Derrick's oversensitivity to sound severely hinders his acquisition of skills and concepts that are part of the early play experiences from which children his age learn and gain pleasure.

Gravitational Insecurity

Gravitational insecurity is a condition in which an individual feels irrational fear, anxiety, or distress in relation to movement or a change of position (Ayres, 2005; May-Benson & Koomar, 2007; Parham & Mailloux, 2005). Young children typically derive pleasure from their experiences with movement. Because moving and using the body to explore are such important parts of play in the early years, it is easy to imagine how a disorder such as gravitational insecurity can disrupt many kinds of play experiences.

Parents of children who demonstrate signs of gravitational insecurity frequently remember the early signs of distress in relation to movement when their children were small infants. Because of their reactions, these children are less likely to be swung, rocked, or otherwise moved through space, which in turn reduces the amount of vestibular sensation they receive. Since stimulation of the vestibular system normally contributes to neurologically based functions such as development of muscle tone (especially of the extensor muscles), coordination of head and eye movements, balance and equilibrium reactions, and bilateral coordination (Lane, 2002; Parham & Mailloux, 2005), children who do not engage in movement activities are at risk for suboptimal development of these functions. This is another example of the recursive cycle that occurs when a sensory processing problem interferes with play behavior, which in turn affects sensory processing. Finding movement unpleasant, a child engages infrequently in the kind of play that generates a great deal of movement sensation. Without this sensation the child's nervous system does not receive the stimulation needed to develop more complex movement skills used in play and other aspects of the child's life.

On a more generalized level, being in a frequent state of fear or anxiety limits the desire to participate in social

Maggie: Gravitational Insecurity

Maggie is an 8-year-old girl with a learning disability. Maggie demonstrates significant signs of gravitational insecurity. As a young child, she cried if she was lifted high into the air, and she has resisted climbing and swinging activities from an early age. She has always appeared distrustful and has tended to withdraw from people other than her parents. Her mother painfully recounts early play group experiences when Maggie clung to her while the other toddlers in the group scampered through the park. Now, at age 8, Maggie has significant difficulties maneuvering through the world. She feels uncomfortable in open spaces where she has less feedback about the location of her body in relation to the rest of the world. She avoids the playground and prefers to sit on a bench close to the classroom buildings during recess. Many of the activities the other girls in her class enjoy, such as bicycle riding, jumping rope, roller-blading, and roller-skating, are frightening or simply unappealing to Maggie. Her playtime is limited by the sedentary nature of the activities she chooses, further compounding her already compromised base of skill. Her parents are worried about her self-consciousness and what they perceive as possible signs of depression. Maggie has the drive to engage in the play activities that would attract any girl her age, but reactions within her nervous system do not allow her to pursue them.

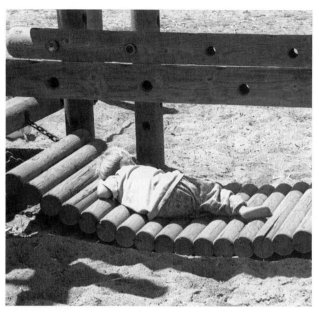

Figure 9-7

Children with gravitational insecurity typically have limited play experiences because of anxiety regarding movement through space. This will have a negative effect on social relationships, as well as motor skills. (Courtesy Shay McAtee.)

interactions and explore new situations (Figure 9-7). According to Ayres (2005), "If the child-earth relationship is not secure, then all other relationships are apt to be less than optimal" (p. 81).

Vestibular-Bilateral and Sequencing Disorders

Ayres (1979, 1989, 2005) described vestibular-bilateral and sequencing disorders as characterized by poor postural mechanisms, inadequate bilateral integration, underresponsive vestibular systems, and difficulties with sequencing. Although these types of problems can severely hinder a child's ability to perform academic tasks and certain physical skills, they are relatively more subtle than other sensory integration disorders. Similarly, the relationship between vestibular-bilateral and sequencing disorders and play can be subtle and difficult to identify.

Because children with underresponsive vestibular systems probably do not perceive the same type or intensity of sensation as other children unless they receive more intense motion, they have a tendency to seek activities that involve a great deal of movement (Ayres, 2005; Parham & Mailloux, 2005). Parents sometimes describe children

with this disorder as always being in motion and not showing the usual signs of dizziness or other reactions to spinning, swinging, and turning.

Vestibular deficits may be less obvious in the play of young children, since refined skills are not usually required for success and a great deal of movement during play is still considered normal. In the school-age years, however, difficulties in mastering bicycle riding, roller-skating or roller-blading, and throwing and catching a ball are more likely to emerge (Figure 9-8). Confusion about directionality (right versus left) often accompanies bilateral integration problems (Ayres, 2005); therefore situations where players must know which way to run (e.g., on the soccer field or basketball court) may result in feelings of embarrassment and failure. Difficulties with bilateral integration and sequencing are also likely to interfere with construction-oriented play activities that involve cutting, pasting, folding, and building. Low muscle tone and poor extensor tone associated with this disorder may make a child lethargic and sluggish in many physical activities because of difficulty maintaining a readiness to act.

Jason: Vestibular-Bilateral Integration and Sequencing Disorder

Jason is a 9-year-old boy who is representative of many children with vestibular-based bilateral and sequencing problems. From the time he was a young child, he has loved merry-go-rounds, roller coasters, and other fast-moving playground and carnival rides. For a 9-year-old these types of activities are still acceptable, but he is beginning to be aware that he craves more of this type of movement than others do. He sometimes covers up his drive to engage in moving activities by forming themes around action play that involves motion. With limited skill for ball sports, Jason is attracted to such sports as karate and gymnastics that provide a great deal of proprioceptive feedback for his sensory needs. Jason is talented in drawing and often incorporates action figures into his artwork. However, he has trouble coordinating his hands together when building with interlocking blocks and other construction and manipulative playthings. Although his friends spend time together playing with these types of toys, Jason does not. Overall, Jason's sensory integrative disorder interferes with some aspects of his play, but he does have other skills and opportunities that contribute to his feeling good about himself as he engages in age-appropriate play experiences.

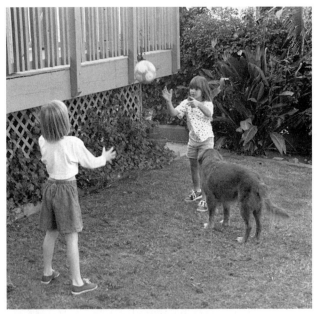

Figure 9-8

Skill in throwing and catching a ball depends on vestibular-proprioceptive functions and bilateral integration. Difficulty with this kind of activity is common among children with vestibular-based bilateral integration and sequencing deficits. (Courtesy Shay McAtee.)

Dyspraxia

Ayres (1985) described developmental dyspraxia as a disorder characterized by difficulty in ideation, planning, and execution of unfamiliar actions. Praxis is involved in enacting new and unfamiliar tasks, and children must call upon this process as they confront the many activities that are part of their day. For adults the subroutines of daily tasks are familiar and with repetition have become automatic; therefore they do not require as much praxis. Perhaps nowhere in the spectrum of human activity is praxis more critical than in the play of children, which involves constantly changing themes, actions, sequences, and possibilities of outcome.

Dyspraxia often occurs in conjunction with sensory processing disorders, probably because the nervous system depends on appropriate, efficient, and predictable sensory information to form action plans (Reeves & Cermak, 2002). If the incoming information is not perceived or processed accurately, efficiently, and effectively, acting on it is difficult.

Praxis begins with ideation, which is an especially important aspect in enacting play behavior. Forming a notion about what to do, based on the possibilities for action that exist, is fundamental to the creative aspects of play behavior. Ideation is closely linked to the planning component of praxis, in that forming the idea of what to do leads directly to the process of knowing how to do it (Ayres, 2005; May-Benson, 2001). Consequently, when a child has problems coming up with an idea for a plan or forming a plan of action, the actual performance of the action is likely to be difficult as well, and many aspects of meaningful occupation, including play, can be affected (May-Benson & Cermak, 2007) (Figure 9-9).

CASE EXAMPLE 5

Jeremy: Autism with Praxis Problems

Jeremy is a 5-year-old boy who has a diagnosis of autism and has significant sensory processing problems. He is often overwhelmed by his environment and tends to engage in ritualistic behaviors and routines. When he is presented with a piece of play equipment such as an inner tube swing, it appears to have no meaning to him. Whereas most 5-year-olds readily imagine sitting, lying, standing, or kneeling on the swing and may compose elaborate play themes in which they star as the hero or villain sweeping through the town in flight, Jeremy merely pushes the tire away as it is swung in his direction. When he shows little interest in imitating a child who is lying prone in a tire nearby, he is placed in this position by his therapist. Because this is something new, his first response appears to be dislike. As the tire is gently swung and bounced, however, he seems to enjoy the sensation. For now, this is the most complex practic interaction Jeremy can have with this piece of play equipment; he demonstrates very little ideation or planning ability in using it.

CASE EXAMPLE 6

Rita: Dyspraxia

Rita is an 8-year-old girl with a speech and language disorder. She has low scores on tests of praxis and presents many signs of dyspraxia when she is observed trying to do something new or novel. Rita's problems with ideation are different from Jeremy's in that she often appears to be forming an idea of what she wants to do but struggles with putting a plan together. She was observed to place her rag doll on one side of a seesaw and then attempt to mount the other side. As she tried to push off from her side, her doll fell off and she tilted backward, appearing unaware of and unable to control the reduced force she needed to use to compensate for the light weight of the doll. In a subsequent attempt she appeared frustrated when she attempted to tie the doll's legs around the seat. She was unable to master securing the doll in this way. When another child approached and asked to join Rita on the seesaw, Rita replied, "No thanks, my doll not like it." Although Rita had some concept of what she wanted to do, she could not fully put the plan together. Her poor sensory integration contributed to poor planning and execution of the intended action, and at her age, her self-consciousness about her difficulties kept her from engaging in a social play experience. Unfortunately, each day Rita has many similar experiences that make play an often frustrating and embarrassing experience.

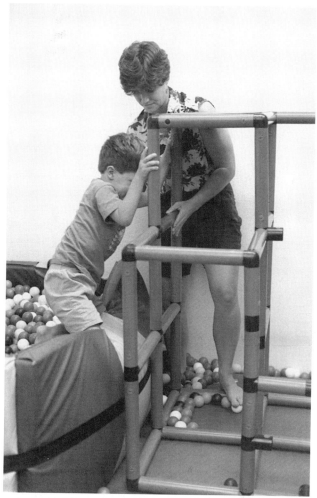

Figure 9-9
Children with dyspraxia have difficulty enacting simple plans for action and consequently may need assistance to experience success in negotiating the physical environment. (Courtesy Shay McAtee.)

HOW DEFICITS IN PLAY AFFECT SENSORY INTEGRATIVE FUNCTIONS

Although occupational therapists more commonly encounter problems in play that can be explained by underlying inefficiencies or difficulties in sensory integrative functions, disruption of typical play can also affect the development of sensory integration. The large and varied literature on the effects of experience and early environments on brain development (Black, Jones, Nelson, & Greenough, 1998; Greenough & Black, 1992; Guralnick, 1997) provides a platform for understanding how limited play opportunities could lead to disrupted development of sensory integrative functions. A developing child within a family represents a multidimensional dynamic in which playfulness, play resources, attitudes about play, and routines and customs affect how time is spent and what activities are valued and made priorities (Knox, 2005; National Research Council and Institute of Medicine, 2000). Variations in play experiences and opportunities resulting from cultural, socioeconomic, and individual differences can influence how the sensory integrative functions develop as much as sensory integrative abilities and dysfunction can affect play.

PLAY IN THE CONTEXT OF OCCUPATIONAL THERAPY USING A SENSORY INTEGRATIVE APPROACH

The difficulties and disruptions that sensory integrative dysfunction imposes on play experience and that play experience can impose on sensory integrative development are of concern to occupational therapists as they consider childhood occupations. The domains addressed by occupational therapists include engagement in occupation in areas such as play, leisure, and social participation, as well as a concern for underlying client factors that include the body structures and functions involving sensory and motor functions (American Occupational Therapy Association, 2002). Therapists using a sensory integrative approach in treatment have access to a special environment and set of tools that enable them to address the play experiences of the children with whom they work.

Many of the fundamental principles guiding the sensory integrative approach in treatment converge with occupational therapists' understanding of play activity and behavior. Parham, Cohn, et al. (2007) identified 10 core principles of occupational therapy intervention with a sensory integration approach: provision of sensory opportunities, provision of "just right" challenges, collaboration in activity choice, guidance toward self-organization, support for optimal arousal, creation of a context of play, maximization of the child's success, assurance of physical safety, room arrangement that engages the child, and fostering of a therapeutic alliance. These principles reflect the importance of play in the sensory integration framework and furthermore suggest that intervention that does not emphasize play would not be considered a true application of a sensory integration approach.

The relationship between sensory integration and play in treatment is not a simple, linear one. Knox & Mailloux (1997) described play as a means, as well as an end product, within the sensory integration approach. Bundy (2002) also highlighted the dynamic aspect of play in relation to sensory integration as she discussed the potential for both an improved ability to play through enhanced sensory integration and improved sensory integration through the incorporation of play in treatment. Coster, Tickle-Degnen, and Armenta (1995) suggested that play may give both meaning and structure to treatment using a sensory integration approach. In a related study, Tickle-Degnen and Coster (1995) noted the association between playfulness on the part of the therapist and a tendency for the child to use playful language and show signs of enjoyment and success. Bundy et al. (2007) found that relationships between playfulness and sensory integration disorders differed between children who had sensory modulation issues and those who had dyspraxia, although all of the children in this study had relatively high levels of playfulness. These findings might reinforce the idea that even children with identified sensory integration problems can bring a playful style into the therapeutic relationship. All of these explanations and findings on the relationship between play and sensory integration in treatment suggest a dynamic interplay that occurs between therapist and child within a therapy session.

The next section discusses ideas about play in relation to the components of the treatment process, namely the preparation period, therapy session, and follow-up phase.

Getting Set for Treatment

Preparing for a treatment session is important in all types of occupational therapy. To make the most of the time spent with a child, the therapist must have (1) a clear understanding of the child based on assessment; (2) a plan for what areas need to be addressed, articulated through treatment goals; (3) an idea of appropriate activities to achieve these goals; and (4) the equipment and materials required during the treatment session. When the therapist is working with a child, the preparation phase is particularly critical, since the child cannot be relied on to wait while activities are set up and arranged. Preparation is especially important to allow a natural flow that encourages the possibility of play during the treatment session.

Occupational therapists evaluate sensory integration functions, as well as play skills and play style, through a wide variety of assessments and observations (Knox, 2005; Smith Roley, 2006a). The process of establishing meaningful goals can be especially challenging for the occupational therapist working with children who have sensory integrative disorders because the relationship between the problem presented and the underlying issue is often not obvious (Mailloux, 2006). This dilemma is often seen in the relationship between sensory integration and play. The goals of a parent or teacher for a child often relate to social participation and play skills, which actually can often be best understood and addressed in relation to the underlying sensory integrative issues that are interfering with the child's success in making and keeping friends.

Preparation for intervention using a sensory integrative approach incorporates the role of the environment as providing an enticement to the child, allowing imaginary themes to prosper, and encouraging social interaction and challenges similar to those that may be part of games or sports. Because novelty enhances exploration and play (Bundy, 2002; Smith Roley, 2006b), selecting new or different toys and pieces of equipment and devising unexpected combinations and arrangements are part of preparing for a treatment session (Figure 9-10).

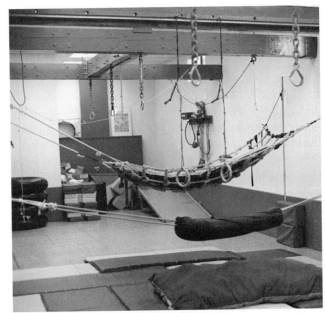

Figure 9-10

The classic sensory integrative treatment setting is rich in objects and materials that can be set up and combined in an infinite number of novel arrangements. (Courtesy Shay McAtee.)

In addition to readying the environment and objects within it, the pediatric occupational therapist must prepare for the treatment session. Occupational therapists who wish to instill play in a therapy session need to be ready to play as well. To "communicate playfulness," as suggested by Parham (1992), the therapist must check her or his own mood and state of playfulness to set the tone for the emergence of a playful situation.

Like therapists, some children require a form of preparation themselves to be ready to play. Children who have high or low responsivity to stimuli in the environment may first need to engage in specific inhibitory or facilitatory types of activities before they are ready to enter into a play experience. Lethargy, fear, anxiety, irritation, and agitation are among the feelings that are not conducive to play and therefore must be addressed before play can occur in any setting.

CASE EXAMPLE 7

Emily: Preparation of the Environment and the Therapist

Emily is a 5-year-old girl who has autism. Although she scores above the average range on IQ tests, she is socially withdrawn and does not have any friends. When she plays with toys, she tends to use them in a ritualistic manner, such as placing her dolls in specific positions and locations within a dollhouse. Emily has sensory defensiveness that is characterized by hypersensitivity to touch, sounds, and movement. Her occupational therapist, Mary, is hoping to encourage Emily to engage in imaginary play as a step toward her being able to interact socially with other girls her age.

While observing Emily in her first few visits to the occupational therapy room at school, her therapist saw that she tended to pace around the room and avoided playing with any of the toys or equipment while delivering rambling monologues about her plans for the day. She appeared anxious, uncomfortable, and unable to settle into play interactions.

To provide an appropriate play experience for Emily, Mary prearranged the environment, setting up an area where the child could start with activities that provided calm and organizing sensory experiences. Using large pillows, dim light, and a rocking chair, Mary found she could help Emily to become relaxed and organized before other, more challenging activities were introduced. In separate areas, Mary arranged toys and equipment that encouraged imaginary play and challenged Emily to experience a greater variety of sensory experiences. For example, since Emily was extremely interested in unicorns, Mary found a stuffed unicorn and placed it atop a piece of moving equipment to serve as an enticement during vestibular challenges.

Mary found that Emily first was relaxed by the initial calming stage of the therapy session and then was enticed by an object of interest to her, thus becoming more open to challenging movement and touch experiences. Because Mary had prepared the therapy environment and helped Emily to become ready to accept challenging experiences in therapy, the therapist found that she could begin to introduce dramatic and imaginary play themes into the sessions. As Emily began to gain meaning from these experiences, she was also able to engage in more challenging activities for longer periods of time. Mary also found that the better she prepared herself emotionally and mentally for the sessions with Emily, the more successful they were. In this case, Mary had to take time to remind herself not to become sidetracked by Emily's verbal maneuvering to avoid activity and, instead, to remember to read it as a sign that Emily needed help to become organized. By planning to avoid power struggles and by preparing for a playful experience, Mary was able to be more successful at helping Emily reach her therapy goals

---

The Session

The therapy session offers a broad range of opportunities for merging play with sensory integrative goals of treatment. As Bundy and Koomar (2002) described it, during an effective therapy session an interactional effect takes place in which the incorporation of play can enhance sensory integrative processes and, in turn, improved sensory integration allows more elaborate play abilities to emerge (Bundy & Koomar, 2002; Smith Roley, 2006b).

At a basic level, incorporation of play themes can make many challenging activities more enticing and can encourage longer duration of involvement in activities for children with sensory integrative dysfunction. For example, the child who is fearful of movement may better tolerate a swinging platform if it is presented with a favorite theme of interest such as a space ship on its way to the moon. The child may be able to stay on the swing longer if motivated by involvement in the play theme, for instance, to reach for a planet or catch a falling star (Figure 9-11). At a more complex level the dynamic relationship between sensory integrative function and play can serve the development of skills in ideation, imagination, and socialization within the context of the therapy session. Ayres (1985) described ideation as a cognitive process that involves understanding the possibilities for actions of the self in relation to objects or other people. She stated that ideation is "basic to most child's play

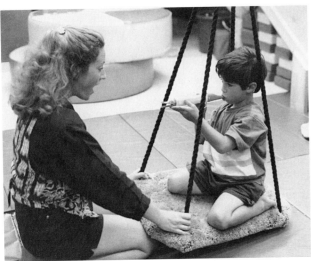

Figure 9-11

An imaginative theme will often lead to more complex interactions and longer durations of involvement with a challenging activity. (Courtesy Shay McAtee.)

and to many adult occupations" (Ayres, 1985, p. 20). As the key that can unlock the door of possibilities, ideation allows the child to begin to plan what to do. Ideation is almost palpable when a normal 5-year-old is observed in a typical therapy room in which a sensory integrative approach is practiced. A novel piece of suspended equipment brought into the room can easily elicit a series of experiments that test the possibilities of interaction between the child and the toy. A child who has a sensory integrative disorder, however, may lack the basic body percept and awareness of the properties of objects that are vital to initiating the ideation process.

The therapy experience is designed to help a child be able to initiate ideas and plans. Although a principle of sensory integrative theory is that activity is more meaningful if it is "child directed" (Parham & Mailloux, 2005; Smith Roley, 2006b), a child who has poor ideation may not be able to self-direct his or her actions. Ayres stated, "If ideation is limited, the therapist must help the child select a simple task and help the planning and execution of it" (1985, p. 67). In most instances, choosing activities that are simple enough for a child to be successful requires more skill and attention on the part of the therapist than thinking of complex activities.

The therapist's initial work in helping a child get started in a "just right" activity is likely to be organizing the activity for the child to ensure that a playful experience occurs. For play to continue to develop, the child needs to build on these experiences, recognizing new possibilities and generating new ideas; otherwise, actions remain limited and are likely to become rote and routinized.

William: Stimulation of Ideation

William is a 4-year-old who tends to move aimlessly from one piece of equipment to another. Although he occasionally stops to push a swing or knock over a bolster, he does not appear to know "what to do." At preschool, he often pushes other children and is beginning to be seen as a behavior problem.

Julie, William's occupational therapist, has found that she needs to help him engage in very simple interactions with equipment. As William approaches a large inner tube and appears to get ready to kick it, Julie gently places one of his feet on the inner tube and presses it up and down, saying, "Jump, jump, jump." She then holds onto his hands while he stands on the mat, and she steps up into the inner tube and begins jumping herself. When William begins to move his torso up and down in a jumping motion, Julie helps him to step up onto the inner tube and they jump together.

Over the next several weeks, William always goes to the inner tube first when he comes to therapy. After a few sessions he seems to have mastered the concept of one of the things he can do on this piece of equipment. Seeing that this has occurred, Julie tries to incorporate play into the activity by saying "I'm a frog. Ribbit! Ribbit!" while jumping from a squatting position from the inner tube onto the mats. William initially needs help getting his body into a squatting position, but the idea of being a frog seems to entice him. Once he has mastered this action, he continues to be interested in playing "frog" and says, "I'm a frog, I catch flies." Julie then introduces beanbag "flies" for William to catch as he jumps through the air. For William, emerging ideation allows him to come up with new ideas of how to play. Playful interactions with the therapist, in turn, motivate him to keep trying actions that are challenging yet organizing to him.

Although imagination is a basic element of typical childhood play, it develops only after a child masters a primary understanding of the properties of his or her own body, of objects, and of people. Probably much of imagination is related to ideation, or the conceptualization of possibilities for action. Some children who have poor sensory integrative functions feel threatened by imaginary themes. This often occurs in children with autism, who appear, for example, unable to cope with consideration of a slide as anything other than a slide and certainly not as a drawbridge in a castle. This tendency is also seen in some children with severe dyspraxia, who seem to have the need to deal with objects in concrete terms, with little room for experimentation or ambiguity. The therapist may need to begin treatment for these children by helping them feel secure enough with their own bodies to experiment with pretending that they or some object is something that it is not. For other children, use of imaginary play in therapy can be an important motivator to try difficult or unusual movements to enact a story. Parham (1992) noted that superhuman figures are often appealing to young children and stated, "The superhuman theme may be especially salient to the child with sensory integrative problems who experiences feelings of power-lessness daily" (p. 3).

As discussed earlier in this chapter, imaginary play often helps a child to stick with a difficult activity and to attempt more and more challenging actions. A young girl with extreme gravitational insecurity was once observed to use a fantasy scenario of hanging Christmas lights for an entire treatment session. So motivated was she by the idea of decorating her imaginary house that she hardly noticed the heights to which she was climbing or the precarious surface on which she stood while securing her decorations. Thus, helping a child feel comfortable in using imagination and knowing how to use imaginary play in treatment are essential parts of the sensory integrative approach.

Even the most elementary aspects of social play can be difficult for a child with a sensory integrative disorder. Tolerating another child nearby is hard for a child with sensory defensiveness, just as maneuvering through an area without knocking down another child's building may be difficult for a dyspraxic child. The therapy environment offers a safe haven for trying out social skills under the guidance of a therapist who can help the child enter into, negotiate, and retreat from interactions with peers. This support for social interaction is often facilitated during treatment when a therapist works in a one-to-one situation with a child while other therapist-child pairs work nearby (Figure 9-12). This model creates a fairly unique opportunity for social interaction in which relationships can be introduced gradually, monitored closely by the therapists, and repaired or redesigned as needed. Therapist-child teams may begin by playing near each other, with one or the other therapist commenting about the other child's play or use of a piece of equipment. A natural progression includes the use of turn taking, with two or more children engaging in the same activity. Often another child can motivate a child to try something that he or she might not otherwise have been willing to attempt. Children can gradually be encouraged to engage in cooperative, interactive play with common goals and purposes. Since each child usually has her or his own therapist, it is possible to retreat from the interaction should one of the children become disorganized, maladaptive, or nonpurposeful.

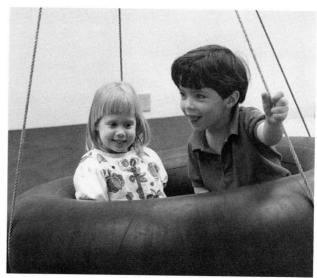

Figure 9-12
Tandem therapy allows close individual monitoring by a therapist; at the same time it provides opportunities for the child to develop tolerance for close proximity to other children and to build more sophisticated social skills. (Courtesy Shay McAtee.)

CASE EXAMPLE 9

Sean and Andy: Working on Social Play

Sean and Andy provide an example of emerging social play in therapy. Sean is 6 years old and has speech and language delays, as well as dyspraxia. He attends a special education class, where he works well in small groups in class but tends to play alone on the playground. Andy is an 8-year-old who has some mild learning problems but attends a regular second grade. He has tactile defensiveness and signs of an under-responsive vestibular system. At school he is considered to have a behavior problem, and most of the children avoid him because he tends to be a bully. Neither Sean nor Andy has experienced any true cooperative play experiences with peers.

In a carefully designed effort to increase play skills in these two children, their therapy appointments were scheduled at the same time because their therapists saw the boys as having the potential for being able to play together. As the older child, Andy was at first encouraged to show Sean how to climb through an obstacle course he had constructed. Maneuvering through various textures of the pieces of equipment and keeping his balance on the unstable sections of the course were challenging for Andy, but he seemed motivated to show Sean how to do it. Sean, on the other hand, was challenged by the motor planning demands of the task, but he was enthusiastic about being like "the big kid."

Sean and Andy played together in this way for several sessions, with Andy usually showing Sean how to do an activity. Sean had actually had generally more positive interactions with other children than Andy had and was the first to suggest that they build something together. Although he had become used to having Sean follow him through activities, Andy still seemed somewhat surprised that Sean did not appear afraid to work with him on a project, since this was the typical response he had from children at school.

The therapists planned this therapy session carefully to make sure the cooperative task was successful. Andy's therapist helped him prepare by using some calming activities that decreased his tactile defensiveness. Both therapists arranged the therapy room before the boys arrived to ensure that the materials they would need were accessible. At one point when Sean began to look frustrated because he could not express what he wanted to add to the fort structure they had decided to build, Andy's therapist asked if he had any idea about what Sean wanted, since he and Sean had all the master plans locked away in their secret hiding place. Although there were no real secret plans, Sean appeared to like this idea and readily accepted Andy's suggestion. This was one way that the therapists attempted to give the boys the message that they were capable of being successful and that it was natural for them to be able to work as a team. Experiences such as this one helped both boys begin to have positive, cooperative play experiences, first in the therapy setting and later at home and school.

Therapeutic Importance of Follow-Up

In addition to promoting play through preparation for and enactment of therapy sessions, an occupational therapist can facilitate play in the follow-up component of treatment. Including the family in the therapy process is one important way this can occur. The more family members understand the difficulties a child is having and the types of activities that are helpful to the child, the better equipped they become to help the child in other settings (Figure 9-13). Schaaf and Burke (1992) noted several ways the therapist can involve the family in the therapy process to facilitate play, including planning activities that help the family to feel competent as caregivers, helping the family members know how to be role models for play behavior, and assisting in making environmental adaptations and suggestions for toys that can enhance sensory integration and play at home.

Including siblings is often a productive way to ensure carryover of therapy activities at home and to make the siblings feel a part of the process. Home programs that are not overwhelming to a family but involve activities that

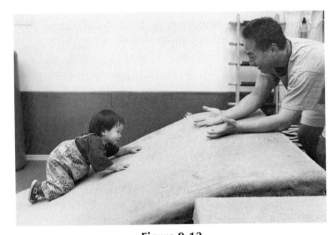

Figure 9-13
Inclusion of family members in the therapy process helps them gain insight into their child's sensory processing characteristics, which in turn better prepares them to find ways to help the child in other settings. (Courtesy Shay McAtee.)

can be incorporated into everyday family experiences are more likely to be followed than those requiring additional effort in an already busy family routine. The therapist can play an important role in helping to ensure carryover at school and in other community settings by assisting those who work with the child in arranging environments and experiences likely to facilitate sensory integration and play.

CASE EXAMPLE 10
Deborah: Follow-Up at Home

Deborah is a 3-year-old who has a diagnosis of autism. She does not seem to know how to play with toys and tends to spend her time twirling strings. Her parents have tried to provide a variety of toys, but because she seems to like puzzles, this is the type of toy they most commonly buy for her. Sara, Deborah's therapist, suggests that the family consider a piece of suspended equipment for Deborah to use at home. Sara begins to feel frustrated when the family continues to report that they are buying their daughter puzzles and they do not seem to be making progress on installing any suspended toy.

When Sara offers to make a home visit, her expectations for home intervention change dramatically. Witnessing the hectic picture she finds at Deborah's home, she begins to understand why the family may not have followed up on her suggestion. With a 6-month infant, a 6-year-old, and a 12-year-old, Deborah's mother has her hands full at home. There does not appear to be any obvious place that a swing can be hung, and although Deborah's behavior is fairly rote and nonpurposeful, she does remain quietly entertained by her strings and puzzles. Sara needs to rethink the home plan in a way that is feasible for the family.

Following several sessions at Deborah's home, Sara creates a sensory enriched environment in the child's room with beanbag pillows, a quiet corner, and lots of blankets and pillows. She covers an old mattress that was in the garage and places it in the backyard for Deborah to use for jumping. Sara also develops a plan for using a neighborhood park that is within walking distance. She works out an arrangement with the family whereby the 12-year-old sister can take Deborah to the park every day after school. Here they are able to use the swings and several other pieces of moving equipment. This gives the 12-year-old a break before beginning her homework and allows Deborah's mother to get dinner started. This plan provides the possibility of capitalizing on the gains Deborah is making in therapy in a way that is manageable and satisfying for her family.

SUMMARY

Sensory integration as a normal process occurring within the nervous system is woven throughout development into a foundation from which play skills emerge. Occupational therapists can benefit from understanding how sensory integrative processes contribute to play, as well as how sensory integrative disorders hinder play. Fostering sensory integration naturally leads to enhanced play skills, just as encouraging play inherently promotes sensory integration. Application of both play and sensory integration concepts is therefore a natural and perhaps essential component in occupational therapy programs for children.

Review Questions

1. Describe the development of sensory aspects of the play experience from infancy to adulthood.
2. During the preschool years, play becomes increasingly influenced by language, symbolism, and social relationships. How do these affect the ways that preschoolers play? In what ways do sensorimotor aspects continue to play a role?
3. During the school years, play begins to be dominated by rules and skills. How do sensory integrative components contribute to a child's success in play during these years?
4. Describe how sensory defensiveness may have an impact on the child's play development. Include issues related to tactile defensiveness, auditory defensiveness, and gravitational insecurity in your answer.
5. How do vestibular-bilateral integration difficulties typically interfere with play development?
6. How do problems with praxis typically interfere with play development?
7. In the sensory integrative approach to individual treatment, how may the therapist prepare for a treatment session in a way that encourages productive play?
8. How can play be incorporated directly into individual occupational therapy using a sensory integrative approach? Describe specific intervention strategies in your answer.

REFERENCES

American Occupational Therapy Association (2002). Occupational therapy practice framework: Domain and process. *American Journal of Occupational Therapy, 56,* 609-639.

Ayres, A. J. (1964). Tactile functions: Their relation to hyperactive and perceptual motor behavior. *American Journal of Occupational Therapy, 18*(1), 6-11.

Ayres, A. J. (1965). Patterns of perceptual-motor dysfunction in children: A factor analytic study. *Perceptual and Motor Skills, 20,* 335-368.

Ayres, A. J. (1966a). Interrelations among perceptual-motor abilities in a group of normal children. *American Journal of Occupational Therapy, 20*(6), 288-292.

Ayres, A. J. (1966b). Interrelationships among perceptual-motor functions in children. *American Journal of Occupational Therapy, 20*(2), 68-71.

Ayres, A. J. (1969). Deficits in sensory integration in educationally handicapped children. *Journal of Learning Disabilities, 2*(3), 44-52.

Ayres, A. J. (1971). Characteristics of types of sensory integrative dysfunction. *American Journal of Occupational Therapy, 25*(7), 329-334.

Ayres, A. J. (1972). *Sensory integration and learning disorders.* Los Angeles: Western Psychological Services.

Ayres, A. J. (1979). *Sensory integration and the child.* Los Angeles: Western Psychological Services.

Ayres, A. J. (1985). *Developmental dyspraxia and adult onset apraxia.* Los Angeles: Sensory Integration International.

Ayres, A. J. (1989). *Sensory integration and praxis tests.* Los Angeles: Western Psychological Services.

Ayres, A. J. (2005). *Sensory integration and the child, 25th Anniversary Edition.* Los Angeles: Western Psychological Services.

Black, J. E., Jones, T. A., Nelson, C. A., & Greenough, W. T. (1998). Neuronal plasticity and the developing brain. In N. E. Alessi, J. T. Coyle, S. I. Harrison, & S. Eth (Eds.), *Handbook of child and adolescent psychiatry. Vol. 6. Basic psychiatric science and treatment* (pp. 31-53). New York: John Wiley & Sons.

Blanche, E. (2001). Transformative occupations and long-range adaptive responses. In S. Smith Roley, E. I. Blanche, & R. C. Schaaf (Eds.), *Understanding the nature of sensory integration with diverse populations* (pp. 421-432). San Antonio, TX: Therapy Skill Builders.

Bundy, A. (2002). Play theory and sensory integration. In A. Bundy, S. Lane, & E. Murray (Eds.), *Sensory integration—Theory and practice* (pp. 228-240). Philadelphia: F.A. Davis.

Bundy, A., & Koomar, J. (2002). The art of therapy. In A.Bundy, S. Lane, & E. Murray (Eds.), *Sensory integration—Theory and practice* (pp. 252-262). Philadelphia: F.A. Davis.

Bundy, A. C., Shia, S., Qi, L. & Miller, L. J. (2007) How does sensory processing dysfunction affect play? *American Journal of Occupational Therapy, 61*, 201-208.

Caplan, F., & Caplan, T. (1974). *The power of play*. Garden City, NY: Anchor Books.

Coster, W., Tickle-Degnen, L., & Armenta, L. (1995). Therapist-child interaction during sensory integration treatment: Development and testing of a research tool. *Occupational Therapy Journal of Research, 15*, 17-35.

Dunn, W., & Brown, C. (1997). Factor analysis on the Sensory Profile from a national sample of children without disabilities, *American Journal of Occupational Therapy, 51*(7), 490-499.

Greenough, W. T., & Black, J. T. (1992). Induction of brain structure by experience: Substrates for cognitive development. In M. R. Gunner & C. A. Nelson (Eds.), *Developmental behavior neuroscience, Vol. 24* (pp. 155-200). Hillsdale, NJ: Lawrence Erlbaum.

Guralnick, M. J. (1997). *The effectiveness of early intervention*. Baltimore: Paul H. Brookes.

Knox, S. (2005). Play. In J. Case-Smith (Ed.), *Occupational therapy for children* (5th ed., pp. 571-586). St. Louis: Mosby.

Knox, S., & Mailloux, Z. (1997). Play as treatment and treatment as play. In B. Chandler (Ed.), *Play in occupational therapy* (pp. 175-204). Rockville, MD: American Occupational Therapy Association.

Lane, S. J. (2002). Sensory modulation. In A. Bundy, S. Lane, & E. Murray (Eds.), *Sensory integration—Theory and practice* (pp. 101-122). Philadelphia: F.A. Davis.

Mailloux, Z. (2006). Setting goals and objectives around sensory integration concerns. In S. Smith Roley & R. C. Schaaf (Eds.), *Sensory integration: Applying clinical reasoning to practice* (pp. 63-70). San Antonio, TX: Psychcorp.

May-Benson, T. (2001). A theoretical model of ideation. In S. Smith-Roley, E. I. Blanche, & R. C. Schaaf (Eds.), *Understanding the nature of sensory integration with diverse populations* (pp. 163-182). San Antonio, TX: Therapy Skill Builders.

May-Benson, T., & Cermak, S. A. (2007). Development of an assessment tool for children with gravitational insecurity (GI) along with preliminary reliability and validity studies differentiating children with GI from typical peers and examining developmental trends in preschoolers. *American Journal of Occupational Therapy, 61*, 148-153.

May-Benson, T., & Koomar, J. A. (2007). Identifying gravitational insecurity in children: A pilot study. *American Journal of Occupational Therapy, 61*, 142-147.

Miller, E., & Miller-Kuhaneck, H. (2006a). The relationship among sensory preferences, play preferences, motivation, and mastery in guiding children's play: A review of the literature, Part 1. *Sensory Integration Special Interest Section Quarterly 29*(2), 1-3.

Miller, E., & Miller-Kuhaneck, H. (2006b). The relationship among sensory preferences, play preferences, motivation, and mastery in guiding children's play: A review of the literature, Part 2. *Sensory Integration Special Interest Section Quarterly 29*(3), 1-4.

Mulligan, S. (1998). Patterns of sensory integration dysfunction: A confirmatory factor analysis. *American Journal of Occupational Therapy, 52*(3), 819-828.

National Research Council and Institute of Medicine (2000). *From neurons to neighborhoods*: The science of early childhood development. Committee on Integrating the Science of Early Childhood Development. J.P. Shonkoff & D.A. Phillips (Eds.). Board on Children, Youth and Families, Commission on Behavioral and Social Sciences and Education. Washington, DC: National Academy Press.

Parham, L. D. (1992). Strategies for maintaining a playful atmosphere during therapy. *Sensory Integration Special Interest Section Newsletter, 15*, 2-3.

Parham, L. D., Cohn, E. S., Spitzer, S., Koomar, J. A., Miller, L. J., Burke, J. P., et al. (2007). Fidelity in sensory integration intervention research. *American Journal of Occupational Therapy, 61*(2), 216-227.

Parham, L. D., Ecker, C., Miller-Kuhaneck, H., Henry, D. A., & Glennon, T. J. (2007). *The sensory processing measure*. Los Angeles: Western Psychological Services.

Parham, L. D., & Mailloux, Z. (2005). Sensory integration. In J. Case-Smith (Ed.), *Occupational therapy for children* (5th ed., pp. 356-411). St. Louis: Mosby.

Reeves, G. D., & Cermak, S. A. (2002). Disorders of praxis. In A. Bundy, S. Lane, & E. Murray (Eds.), *Sensory integration—theory and practice* (pp. 71-100). Philadelphia: F.A. Davis.

Schaaf, R., & Burke, J. P. (1992). Clinical reflections on play and sensory integration. *Sensory Integration Special Interest Section Newsletter, 15*, 1-2.

Smith Roley, S. (2006a). Evaluating sensory integration function and dysfunction. In S. Smith Roley & R. C. Schaaf (Eds.), *Sensory integration: Applying clinical reasoning to practice* (pp. 15-36). San Antonio, TX: Psychcorp.

Smith Roley, S. (2006b). Implementing intervention. In S. Smith Roley & R. C. Schaaf (Eds.), *Sensory integration: Applying clinical reasoning to practice* (pp. 71-90). San Antonio, TX: Psychcorp.

Tickle-Degnen, L., & Coster, W. (1995). Therapeutic interaction and the management of challenge during the beginning minutes of sensory integrative treatment. *Occupational Therapy Journal of Research 15*, 122-141.

10

Play in Middle Childhood

LINDA L. FLOREY AND SANDRA GREENE

Clinical Vignette

An occupational therapy student with 6 weeks' experience is in charge of a group of three 6-year-old boys who are impulsive and have difficulty paying attention. She has decided to have the group make animal masks in preparation for a play they are going to perform later in the week. The masks involve typical cutting, pasting, drawing, and painting activities. The goals for the group are to work together to share materials and space, to attend to the task, to persist with the activity to see it through to completion, and to encourage imaginative play. The children have been working productively for about 20 minutes. During the group session, the kids begin talking about characteristics of the different animals they are making and start to get "silly." The occupational therapy student, encouraging play and creative behavior, joins in the fun, asking, "Does anyone know what sound a pig makes?" One child jumps from his seat and begins snorting and acting like a pig, much to the delight of the other children. One by one they leave the table and begin to imitate animals. The student supports this because she believes that she is encouraging creative and imaginative play behavior based on the theme of making the masks. The children begin to escalate. The occupational therapy student attempts to calm the children down and get them back to task, but the children ignore her and get more and more out of control.

In the preceding clinical vignette, the goals set by the occupational therapy student for the group were reasonable, as was the task selected and the manner in which it was introduced. The student had carefully planned the group, pacing the activity according to developmental level, providing supplies, and making the activity meaningful, relevant, and fun for the children. She thought that by allowing the children to engage in imitating animals, she was encouraging creativity and imagination and she herself was becoming more flexible in working with the group. What she did not anticipate or recognize was that this group of children did not have the skills to engage in unstructured creative play in this situation. She was unable to view and read the situation as escalating and out-of-control behavior. Children with problems in controlling impulses and focusing attention tend to be highly reactive to their settings. They have few internal controls to monitor their behavior. When they begin to act "silly," the experienced therapist begins to set limits and watches the reactions of the group. When one child leaves his or her seat and the activity, the therapist definitely intervenes to prevent the rest of the group from following. The ability to read, interpret, and adjust therapeutic strategies in the ever-changing clinical situation is the hallmark of a seasoned therapist. In this situation the student was demonstrating the behavior of a therapist inexperienced in working with children who have problems in focus and attention. Situations such as this are typical in clinical settings with students and new clinicians, as well as with experienced clinicians who change practice areas and begin working with children exhibiting behavior problems.

The impetus for this chapter comes from our interest in the play and social interactions of children with behavior and emotional problems during the period of middle childhood. Its intent is to provide clinical information to assist in working with these children, and it is written with a model of clinical reasoning in mind. As such it acknowledges and is drawn from both the explicit theoretical conceptions of play and the everyday information gained from clinical practice. The information gleaned from clinical practice reflects the profession's ongoing interest in clinical reasoning, guided by the pioneering work of Schön (1983), Mattingly (1991, 1998), and Fleming (1991) and continued in the work of Schell (2003) and Schell, Crepeau, and Cohn (2003). Their writings detail the process of identifying and analyzing the tacit or embodied knowledge that becomes part of the therapist's habitual way of doing things. This is everyday knowledge that practitioners acquire, as well as the language they use to impart information to professional peers in the course of clinical experience. The importance and scope of such knowledge may not be readily apparent to them. Practitioners tend to discount informally acquired clinical knowledge as less significant than knowledge acquired in a more formal manner, yet it is the practical reasoning based largely on clinical knowledge that guides therapists' practice. Mattingly (1991) stated, "Whereas theory directs us to what is generally true, action always occurs in a unique context given…the complexities and idiosyncrasies of the concrete case, any theoretical knowledge is bound to be crude and approximate, giving a starting place but not a rule book for action" (p. 982). Practitioners go through several stages in the process of gaining experience and reflecting on that experience: novice, advanced beginner, competent, proficient, and expert (Schell, Crepeau, & Cohn, 2003). The occupational therapy practice framework (American Occupational Therapy Association [AOTA], 2002) supports this approach to embedded clinical reasoning, with emphasis on how clients engage in occupation in the context of their everyday lives.

Clinical practice mediates conceptual and theoretical knowledge. A categorization process helps explain how this occurs; incoming information is sorted and categorized based on similarity to memories of the present situation or strict rules for interpretation of information. The process of clinical reasoning—selecting what to think about in the course of identifying and addressing clinical problems—becomes more complex as the clinician becomes more experienced (Burke & DePoy, 1991). To find out how clinicians actually employ clinical knowledge, we asked questions of experienced occupational therapy practitioners working with children. The therapists were asked about their experiences in clinical situations in which students and new practitioners experienced the most difficulty and were asked to speculate what piece of the puzzle the new practitioners were missing. Two major themes emerged. One is that novice practitioners have difficulty when they are dealing with children who manifest "scattered" performance because the inexperienced clinician does not yet firmly understand models of hierarchical development, particularly with respect to observing and analyzing play activities as they are occurring. A child with the

cognitive and physical skills of a 7-year-old but the social skills of a 4-year-old is difficult for them to conceptualize. Consequently, new practitioners often select and pace activities according to one set level and have problems downgrading or upgrading expectations based on individual variation. Novice therapists may not know where they have been (past developmental markers) or where they are going (future markers) and often become mired in having children engage in making or doing a product rather than engaging in a process. The other common difficulty for inexperienced therapists lies in determining how psychiatric symptoms are manifest in functional performance. Therefore they miss the initial signs of behavior problems and fail to identify the problems. Throughout the chapter we emphasize both developmental markers in play and examples of how psychopathology is manifest in functional performance.

This chapter is derived from knowledge acquired through theoretical constructs as mediated by clinical experience and is divided into three main sections. The first section, characteristics of play in middle childhood, addresses the developmental markers in play observed when the therapist is working with children in this age period. The second section, children with behavioral and emotional problems, focuses on typical symptoms of these problems and how symptoms are manifest in daily play performance. The term "behavioral and emotional problems" refers to the gamut of problems reflected in the behavioral manifestations children exhibit in expressing affect and in their relations with others. The third section, clinical guides to assessment and treatment, details assessment and treatment of play in middle childhood with children exhibiting behavior and emotional problems.

PLAY IN MIDDLE CHILDHOOD

Clinical Vignette

"GaGa" is a group elimination game resembling kickball. It is played with a large rubber ball in a space about 20 × 25 feet, surrounded on four sides by a 3-foot wall. Children are eliminated by being hit with the ball, by picking up a "hot" ball before it has bounced three times, or by hitting someone with the ball above the knee. A 6-year-old girl explains the rules. "There are millions of people and someone starts out and they toss up the ball. They say 'Ga, Ga, Ga' three times and you start pushing. When you get hit, you tell the counselor and you have to leave." She then goes on to explain that there are different kinds of GaGa. There are "silly face GaGa," "freeze GaGa," and "honest GaGa." Two 9-year-old girls say, "It's like this—no hits above the knee; you can block the ball with your hands but you can't touch it twice in a row; if the ball goes out, it is thrown in and it has to bounce three

times before someone touches it and you say 'Ga' for each bounce. When you get down to two people, you start countdown and the last person to touch the ball loses. You can only join at the beginning and then as many as want to play join in. That's about it." A 10-year-old boy who has just been eliminated during countdown loudly says, "If I've ever seen cheating at its highest rate, I've seen it here. The countdown is too fast, way too fast."

The above rules of GaGa were learned during naturalistic observation of children at a summer day camp. These rule explanations according to age level illustrate some of the changes in children's abilities to understand and process rules, which are characteristic of changes that occur during middle childhood. To the 6-year-old girl, playing GaGa puts you in the center of a group. She describes most of the rules in general action terms—"throwing" the ball "up," saying "Ga, Ga" when others say it, and "pushing." The counselor is the mediator of rules. GaGa is going with the group, yelling, and pushing until you get hit and then telling the counselor that you have been hit. You have to tell because this is the whole point of "honest GaGa." The 9-year-olds can detail the main points of the game, and the 10-year-old not only knows the rules but is into a defense strategy. He does not refuse to obey the rule as if countdown did not apply to him, as might a child of 6 or 7, nor does he argue that he was not the last one hit. He has an understanding of rules and suggests that they may be manipulated by "cheaters," implying that the countdown cadence is what really has beaten him. The understanding of rules, the planning of strategy in games, the increasing complexity of the social network, and the number and complexity of physical and social environments in which play occurs are all characteristic of changes in play that occur during middle childhood. This section reviews major changes that take place during middle childhood and characteristics of play behavior of children during this period. Suggestions for constructing a play environment are provided.

DEVELOPMENT DURING MIDDLE CHILDHOOD

Middle childhood is generally regarded as encompassing the ages of 6 to 12 years (Collins, 1984). Classic theorists contributing to an understanding of development during this period include Piaget, Erikson, and Havighurst. Jean Piaget (1962) outlined the importance of middle childhood as the period in which a new form of thought is crystallized. This is the period of concrete operations, in which logic begins to structure the way children perceive relationships around them. Erik Erikson (1963) proposed eight stages in personality development, which included concern for the demands that society makes on

an individual at different times in the life cycle. At each stage he identified a crisis that has to be resolved, the resolution of which will add either a positive or a negative dimension to the ego. The crisis that must be resolved during middle childhood he termed industry versus inferiority. Industry involves making and doing things beside and with others and doing things well. Erikson believed that socially middle childhood is a most decisive stage because a first sense of division of labor occurs. Robert J. Havighurst (1973) identified developmental tasks that must be mastered. He characterized middle childhood as representing three major thrusts: a thrust out of the home and into the peer group, a physical thrust into games and work requiring neuromuscular skills, and a mental thrust into adult concepts, logic, symbols, and communication.

In 1981, the Committee on Child Development Research and Public Policy selected a panel of experts to identify significant aspects of social, emotional, cognitive, and physical development that occur during middle childhood (Collins, 1984). They identified three major themes: greater complexity in intellectual problem solving and the capacity to maintain intimate friendships, marked changes in overall capacity and behavior, and a continuity suggesting that development during this period has great significance for behavioral orientations, success, and adjustment in adolescence and adulthood (Collins, 1984).

A variety of theorists and researchers have continued to show interest in middle childhood, which is also called the school-age period (Combrinck-Graham & Fox, 2002; Davies, 2004). This is the time when children learn to adapt to elementary school routines and new people in authority and learn to function more autonomously (Davies, 2004). Independent learning is facilitated by increasing capacities to pay attention, understand and respond to rules, and maintain self-control (Cincotta, 2002).

MAJOR HALLMARKS OF MIDDLE CHILDHOOD

1. Skills and modes of thought and behavior are characterized by *greater complexity in intellectual problem solving and the capacity to develop and maintain friendships.* Changes in cognition influence changes in social behavior. Children show growth in reality testing and cognitive development, with a clear understanding of the difference between fantasy and reality. At the beginning of this period children are able to see and acknowledge another person's viewpoint, and at the end of the period they are able to hold different viewpoints in their head at the same time. They can keep different perspectives in mind, which in turn permits better abilities to communicate and to consider the views of others. Children move from a view that rules are externally imposed and governed to a view that rules are negotiated among individuals (Collins, 1984; Davies, 2004; Piaget, 1962).

2. *Capacities and behavior change markedly.* Major transformations in skills and abilities take place during middle childhood such that this period cannot be viewed as a time of homogeneous functioning (Collins, 1984). Children experience growth in the physical and neuromuscular realms and are able to use more tools and to refine their skills in hobbies, sports, and games. They generally show an increased ability to restrain impulsive behavior. They become more able to monitor their own activities. Children develop increasing skill in organizing tasks and organizing time (Collins, 1984; Davies, 2004).

3. The *physical environment becomes more complex* temporally and spatially (Havighurst, 1973). During this period children spend the majority of the day engaged in activities that are conducted away from home—in school and in organized and spontaneous after-school activities. The biggest transition is in leaving home for a substantial period of the day and going to school. Children spend most of their waking hours in school. A major achievement of children during this period is viewing themselves as members of society (Combrinck-Graham & Fox, 2002). In addition to the classroom, there are other environments to master—the lunchroom, the playground, clubs, parks, and baseball and soccer fields.

4. The *social environment becomes more complex* with respect to adults and, more important, with respect to peers. Children are involved with teachers, coaches, and other adults with authority who are judging and grading them with regard to standards or outcomes such as grades or not making the team. School is the central arena for both success and failure. Academic skills and diverse social skills must be mastered (Epps & Smith, 1984). The emotional pitfalls of middle childhood are inferiority and defeat because of the difficulty and importance of mastering complex skills in multiple environments (Combrinck-Graham & Fox, 2002).

The biggest change occurs in children's allegiance to the peer group. It is estimated that children spend over 40% of their waking time with peers (Cincotta, 2002; Cole & Cole, 1989). In the peer group, children learn to interact with age mates, deal with hostility and dominance, relate to a leader, and be a leader. They learn to work with a group and to form close friendships. They learn to cooperate and to compete (Figure 10-1). In the beginning of middle childhood, friendships are characterized by sharing of interests. Toward the end of this period, children tend to organize around common values, commitment, loyalty, and mutual support (Davies, 2004). During this period, children develop a peer culture (Corsaro & Schwarz, 1991; King, 1987). As more and more of their allegiance is transferred to the peer group, they derive from this group their sense of self-worth and sense of being respected and valued. This is the age in which children

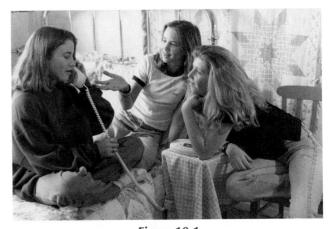

Figure 10-1
The peer culture emerges as a prominent aspect in the lives of children during middle childhood. (Courtesy Shay McAtee.)

compare themselves with others and develop images of themselves based on how they "measure up" to others. For children who struggle with social interactions, there is little place to hide (Cassidy & Asher, 1992; Mussen, Conger, & Kagan, 1963). Among themselves, children decide who can play in a game, codes for inclusion and exclusion, how to deal with cheaters and troublemakers, and how to manipulate the situation to their own and their friends' advantage (Knapp & Knapp, 1976; Slukin, 1981).

Social skills development is an area that is often taken for granted until the child begins to have difficulty. Hartrup (1992) proposed that children's interactive skills are the best predictor of adult success, more important even than educational achievement and intelligence, and that the ability to get along with other children is the single best indicator of future success as an adult, more than educational ability, intelligence, or classroom behavior.

Socially able, positive children are more accepted and sought out both by other children and by teachers. Social acceptance is an indicator of current and future academic success. The ability to interact effectively and to adapt and cope with challenges results in a reserve of positive feelings from the approval of others, while children who do not have these abilities tend to amass a reserve of negative feelings and expectations from others (Ladd, Birch, & Buhs, 1999). A positive outlook, independence, empathy, humor, the ability to solve problems and handle negative emotions, and fairness are traits that tend to be looked on positively by others (Cassidy & Asher, 1992). Middle childhood is a distinct period of development and one that reflects a range of increasing skills and abilities in the physical, social, and cognitive spheres of children. It does not represent a homogeneous period and therefore is not a homogeneous population.

PLAY BEHAVIOR IN MIDDLE CHILDHOOD

Play assumes major importance in middle childhood as a processor of social relatedness and relationships. Peers and peer interactions are prominent during this time, and children become proficient in influencing one another through their cognitive, physical, and verbal skills. Changes in play development during this period are related to growth in the areas of cognition, language, moral reasoning, social understanding, and social-emotional mastery (Fromberg & Bergen, 1998). Play is more group focused and involves team sports, clubs, and other organized gatherings (Cincotta, 2002). Socialization among peers occurs largely in the context of play and games that are outside the direct supervision of an adult (Maccoby, 1984).

Play can be conceived of as an interactive process in which socialization is learned, practiced, and mastered. Play and socialization are inseparable concepts. In middle childhood the quality of the social interactions changes, as do the play activities themselves. There is increasing emphasis on games and on negotiating the rules of games. Play can be conceived of as an interaction process in which socialization is learned, practiced, and mastered and social interactions are embedded in play activities. For purposes of highlighting differences in play behavior during this period, characteristics of play have been selected and separated and are organized according to changes in peer relationships, rules and games, and play interests. The changes in play are drawn from classic descriptions of children's play by Hartley and Goldenson (1963) and Gesell, Ilg, and Ames (1977) and from recent descriptions by Manning (1998), Davies (2004), and Cincotta (2002), as well as from clinical practice. The changes, listed in Table 10-1, are presented in terms of differences between "younger" and "older" children. "Younger children" represent the beginning of middle childhood, from 6 through 8 years. "Older children" represent the end of the age period, from 9 through 12 years. These changes represent not normative changes but a progression from simple to more complex levels of behavior. The table does not provide a comprehensive list of play activities or materials during this period but simply a sampling.

In *peer relations*, the group is very important to younger children in middle childhood. They like to talk and look like one another. They are not necessarily interested in one another but just enjoy being together. Being accepted as part of a group is easier with the younger children, and popularity and leadership change rapidly. With older children of this period the group is still important, but they are becoming more selective as to who gets in (Figure 10-2). There are often secret clubs with secret codes and rules, and cliques start to form. Adherence to group standards—in dress or behavior—is important. Organized groups are popular. Children are beginning to socialize in smaller groups based on shared likes, dislikes, temperament, and skills and are establishing best friends. There are sustained cooperative and competitive social interactions.

Rule or *game* behavior in younger children is characterized by a view that rules are externally imposed, usually by an adult. They typically conceive of games such as baseball as actions, such as hitting the ball and running around the bases. The number of players on the field and the number of outs in an inning are "rules" imposed by adults, and children at this age have only a vague idea of how rules operate. They do not understand that rules apply equally to everyone and are often unable to put the rules of the game above the need to win. When children begin to understand that rules are agreements among the players as to how a game is to be played, they love to make up their own rules but change them rapidly to suit their own needs. Older children during this period are more conscious of rules and of obeying them. They can decide on rules and change them to suit different occasions and different players (Figure 10-3). For example, children observed in a neighborhood playing a game would alter the rules depending on the age of the children playing. One of the younger children was named Rosy, and the children in play would yell out "Rosy rules" to signal one another that they would be playing a different and less complex version of the game. Older children spend time arguing over what is fair and allowed according to agreed upon rules (Figure 10-4). At this age they are also able to accept majority decisions.

Play interests change during middle childhood. An intense interest in sports can begin to build. There is a great deal of physical play during this entire period—running, tumbling, climbing, roller-blading, skipping rope, and skateboarding, in addition to team sports and activities. Computer and video games are popular with younger and older children. Dramatic play is still popular with younger children; details in costume and realistic emblems of roles are important. Collecting is popular, but quantity is the key. In crafts, assistance is needed in figuring out the steps in an activity; the presence of an older child or an adult nearby is helpful. Without such guidance or instruction, younger children become frustrated and may abandon the effort. Older children engage in play that is more cognition based, such as word games and riddles. The dramatic play of older children often reflects events outside of home or school and involves more organization. It is symbolic of significant aspects of the child's life experiences. Older children may still need help with crafts materials or procedures, particularly if the activity is unfamiliar or difficult. This is a "sampling age" in which children try many different crafts and begin to narrow interests to form hobbies (Manning, 1998).

CONSTRUCTING A PLAY ENVIRONMENT

One of the reasons for reviewing the characteristics of children and of play during middle childhood is to help the occupational therapist construct a treatment environment

Table 10-1
Characteristics of Play During Middle Childhood

Characteristics of Younger Children	Characteristics of Older Children
Peer Relationships	
Group very important—adjusting to group controls	Groups very important—join many and establish cliques
Learning to work with others although little cooperation	Clubs with passwords, secret codes, and group-sanctioned rules of behavior—clubs may be formed by mutual interests or to exclude other children
Rapidly changing leadership of group	Conformance to peer codes and competition with others
Helping age mates, and fighting with them	Organized activities such as sports, Scouts, classes in specific areas of interest
Separation of sexes	Development of best friends
Rules and Games	
Unable to put rules of game above need to win	Desire to make and break rules
Lacking understanding that rules apply equally to everyone; desire to make and break rules	Deciding how rules and turns will be determined
Vague about how rules operate	Arguing over what's fair and opposed to cheating
Desire to make up own rules and go on until they win	More conscious of rules and of obeying them
Cheating, tattling common	Acceptance of majority decisions
	Rules becoming relative, not absolute; more flexibility with how rules are implemented
Play Interests	
Dramatic play—details in costume and realistic emblems of roles important	Dramatic play—done in groups and reflects events outside of home and school
Collecting—quantity important, nature items popular	Collecting and trading—big collections, although collecting declining; may collect based on current fads
Crafts—bogged down in the middle and need a clear notion of sequence of steps and reassurance to finish	Crafts—need for help with materials or procedures; exploring many crafts and hobbies; may take classes specific to a craft interest
Critical of own work and work of others	Beginning to achieve satisfaction in making things
	Desire to participate in activities popular with other children
	Separation into gender groups and interests
	Current trends toward more solitary game activities with advent of computer and video games

or approach based on key features of this developmental period. The goal is to capture the "kidlike" qualities of middle childhood and to incorporate these in treatment programs targeted to help children with identified deficits. For example, in our clinical practice children are taught social skills within the context of a club. Children make club T-shirts, wear them to the club meetings, and help establish club rules. Social skills curricula or content is used within the context of the club meeting. This format provides a normalizing context for the learning of social skills, and the children are usually eager to attend and participate. Just as the provision of dolls, dollhouses, and play furniture complete with toy dishes and housekeeping equipment encourages symbolic, imaginative play with younger children, certain "props" and elements

are necessary to evoke a play ambience characteristic of middle childhood. In working with children exhibiting problems in behavioral and emotional areas, therapists need to consider additional factors in developing an environment and a therapeutic approach. The following are suggestions for constructing a play environment for children exhibiting behavior and emotional problems in middle childhood.

1. *Populate the play environment with peers.* For children with significant behavioral issues, the therapist may choose to begin therapy in a one-to-one situation, but as soon as is feasible a peer should be included. Peers and peer groups are dominant during middle childhood, and it is in this arena that children who are immature or have emotional problems often have the most difficulty. In

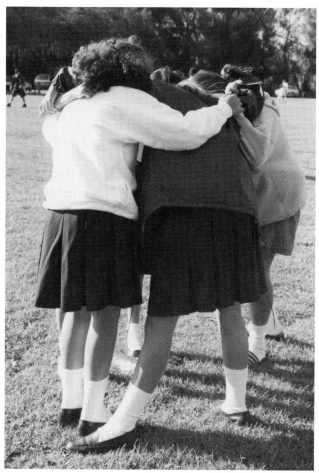

Figure 10-2
Belonging to a group is a hallmark of middle childhood.

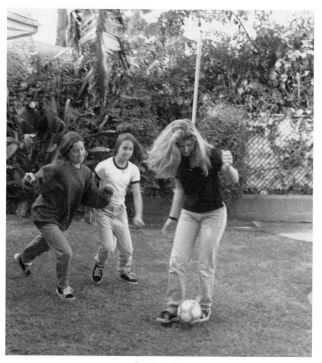

Figure 10-3
Through the middle childhood years, children develop a growing understanding of game rules as well as a willingness to abide by them. This is reflected in the ways they engage in sports and games. (Courtesy Shay McAtee.)

addition to sharing materials and equipment, children must share space and the attention of others. It is within a small group of peers that this can be learned and practiced.

2. *Use every opportunity in the occupational therapy intervention to model and teach social skills.* Numerous social skill checklists and training guides are available. Although the best interventions occur in daily interactions with others in a variety of settings, many children need to be explicitly taught and given the opportunity to practice social interactions in a therapeutic environment. The occupational therapist helps to model and frame interactions by giving feedback for both positive and negative interactions (e.g., "I like the way everyone is working together" or" How else could you have done that?"). The therapist may frame different groups around key peer issues, such as expressing anger appropriately, handling bullies, and entering and participating in groups. Developmental level must be considered in teaching social skills because children's capacities to communicate, solve problems, and take the perspective of others change. Younger or less mature children might have goals involving tolerating others in

their play environment, making eye contact, smiling, taking turns, sharing, and compromising. Goals for older or more mature children might include giving compliments, being tactful, and understanding and appropriately reacting to more nuanced social interactions (Cartledge & Milburn, 1995).

3. *Conduct programs within natural childhood activity models in which crafts and games are emphasized.* The occupational therapist essentially needs to examine the *process* of the activity and not get stuck on the *product* of the game or craft. Crafts and games should be viewed with respect to three major dimensions so that they can be rapidly upgraded and downgraded according to the level of the children within the group. The dimensions of cognitive, motor, and social complexity of an activity should be viewed separately with this population. *Cognitive complexity* refers to a mix of problem-solving processes that involve mastering steps and mastering the controls necessary to complete the steps. Activities should be examined for the number of steps they require, the sequence and complexity of the steps, and the amount of patience and persistence required in problem solving. Patience and persistence are control skills children are learning to develop. They are often critical of their own work and become frustrated when it does not look like the model. Children during this period are beginning to construct projects and need to be encouraged and cajoled

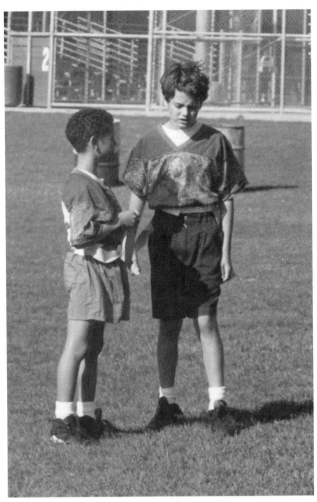

Figure 10-4

Skills in negotiating with peers are critical in middle childhood activities, such as sports.

into following the steps to completion. In terms of *motor complexity,* an activity should be examined with regard to how much motor or visual-motor control is required and whether the children have sufficient skills in this area. In addition to having problems in the social and emotional realm, the children we have seen over the years often manifested deficits in motor and visual-motor integration that were identified in assessment. Learning disabilities are a concurrent diagnosis with some psychiatric disorders of childhood (Gibbs & Priest, 1999; Lewis, 1991; Lewis & Yeager, 2002; Weiss & Weiss, 2002). *Social complexity* means the opportunities the situation affords for sharing and cooperating in the use of materials, space, and peer and adult attention and interaction. Children exhibiting emotional problems have the most difficulty with the social complexity of a situation. For that reason, therapists may downgrade or simplify the cognitive and motor components so that the social features of the situation can be learned and emphasized. For example, children often share and talk with one another more frequently when

engaged in simple repetitive activities such as stringing medium-sized beads because they easily master the physical requirements of the task. We do not mean to suggest that there be no activity complexity with this population. Rather, therapists must have knowledge of the different processes an activity requires so they can target particular social goals in the intervention.

4. *Vary activities to support the child's developmental skills.* Many children with psychiatric disorders engage in solitary activities such as playing computer and video games and watching television. They have a restricted repertoire of activities because of lack of interest, poor skill development, or repeated failure in attempts to participate in more socially based activities. Providing a variety of activities offers children a chance to learn skills in a safe situation under the guidance of a therapist. A safe starting point for most activities is to limit the steps and use easily controlled materials. For example, markers used for an art project are easier to control than paint. Simple, successful projects give children the opportunity to engage in a possibly unfamiliar activity, gain skills, and acquire a sense of competence. A sample of a completed project helps children anticipate steps and visualize the finished product. Activities can be made more complex and challenging, but it is difficult to simplify a task once a child is engaged in it. If a more complex activity is unsuccessful for the child, he or she may hesitate or refuse to participate in similar activities in the future and the therapeutic opportunity to help the child gain skills and competence is lost.

In middle childhood, activities should include an emphasis on group activities that have a distinctive identity to the children. Children of this age seek to "belong," to be a part of something, and organized groups serve that need. As an historical example, the University of California Neuropsychiatric Hospital had a Cub Scout den chartered under the Boy Scouts of America beginning in 1971. The boys wore scout uniforms to the meetings, which the hospital supplied; they began the meetings with the scout oath and worked on badges and activities typical of other scout troops. Social skills were emphasized in this den and were embedded within this naturally occurring childhood model. The children were registered in the scout den and could be referred to the scout program in their area after discharge. Not all occupational therapy programs at the Neuropsychiatric Hospital are conducted within a club format, but such "special" groups provide a bit of novelty in the treatment situation, as well as normalizing ties to neighborhood and community activities.

A club or group format can be used in almost any setting, including a school system, hospital practice, community practice, and private practice. It can be used with children who are seen on a limited or ongoing basis. No matter what the setting for treatment is, it is important that the child have an opportunity to experience being a group member, including working together with the other group members to make group decisions. Many children with emotional and behavioral difficulties have little experience with functioning within the context of a group. This description includes many children who have physical disabilities and concurrently experience emotional or behavioral problems.

5. *Establish rules for each treatment session or group.* The learning and processing of rules are a major focus in middle childhood. Expectations for how the children follow rules should be appropriate to their developmental level. For example, a child might have the cognitive ability to play a complex board game but not have the functional ability to follow the given game rules with a group of peers. The occupational therapist would adapt the game rules so that the child could successfully participate in the game activity while concurrently expanding the child's game and rule-following skills. Rules for safety and for general ways of proceeding should be established by the therapist, and the consequences of rule following and rule violation should be known to the children. Again, this must be done with the level of ability of the group members in mind. These rules have to do with the therapist's behavioral expectations for the way in which the group or session is to proceed. They may include such things as sitting at the table after entering the room, not touching materials until told to do so, or taking turns. The children should also have an opportunity to construct rules, and the therapist may suggest such areas as fairness, listening, and saying things nicely to others. "No touching others with your hands," "No horsing around," and "Feet have to stay on the floor" are examples of rules children have constructed to deal with respect for one another's personal space. Adherence to rules may be promoted by verbal praise or concrete symbols for good effort such as earning stickers. Children with behavioral or emotional problems often have trouble identifying when they have done something "right," and the reward of a sticker or other small prize often serves this purpose. We ask the children to identify their positive behaviors and those they need to work on so that they can begin to put their behaviors in perspective. This method also gives equal weight to positive behavior. The positive efforts of children with behavioral problems often go unacknowledged. It is imperative that the occupational therapist have a behavior management system in place for the group. This should include behaviors that constitute rule violation and subsequent consequences.

6. *Set up materials and space in advance of the treatment session.* This is particularly critical in working with a group of children who have difficulty focusing and attending to activities. Although straightforward and simple, this suggestion is one that students and novice practitioners often do not consider. If the therapist is unprepared and begins gathering the necessary supplies for the activity after the children have arrived, individual children or the whole group can become unfocused and more time is spent on regaining the attention of the members than on the planned activity.

The preceding suggestions form some parameters for establishing "structure" in therapy for children exhibiting problems in behavioral control. "Structure" is a term used in milieu therapy to describe social processes that affect patients therapeutically. It refers to the organization of time, space, and activity (Gibson & Richert, 1993). It is not a specifically defined process. Occupational therapists and other disciplines working in psychiatry credit structure in the environment when all goes well and refer to lack of structure or no structure in the environment when patients are unfocused or out of control. With children, structure has to do with capturing their attention and interest and targeting the activity to the skill level of the members of the group. This is accomplished within an environment that has established temporal and spatial boundaries, in which codes of behavioral conduct are explicit. Although structure is a term used in mental health settings, it is a useful concept in any context where the therapist is working with people with emotional or behavioral difficulties.

CHILDREN WITH BEHAVIORAL AND EMOTIONAL PROBLEMS

Clinical Vignette

Danielle is an 8-year-old girl attending sleep-away camp for the second year in a row. She is verbal and engaging and initiates games and conversation with her companions. She likes to be at the center of things and volunteers to be the walker in the dining room, the helper in the cabin, and the star of the evening skit. When she does not get her way, she does not want to do anything—she says she will not eat, she will not clean her bunk in the cabin, and she will not be in the skit at all. She has a hard time obeying rules. When everyone is asked to sit, she sits and then stands up. When asked to stand up, she stands and then sits. She accuses her peers of hitting her, messing with her food, and taking her things. She complains of stomach aches as well. The rest of the children deny her accusations, then they pretty much ignore her. She is not well liked.

Danielle displays problems in relationships with others and in her adjustment to the rules of camp life. She may be displaying immature behavior to mask an immediate crisis, such as homesickness or insecurity in a new situation, or her behavior may signify a psychopathological condition. Whatever the underlying cause, her behavior indicates an immediate problem in the social realm. The purpose of this section is to briefly review the different settings in which occupational therapists may encounter a population of children exhibiting behavior disorders and to describe typical manifestations in the play of children with psychiatric disorders.

Service Settings

Children with psychopathological problems are identified in five distinct types of public service systems: schools, the juvenile justice system, and child welfare, general health, and mental health agencies. Primary care and the schools are the major systems for the recognition of youth with psychosocial disorders (U.S. Department of Health and Human Services [DHHS], 1999). Occupational therapists working within the school system are most likely to encounter this population of children. Within the lexicon of special education, this group of children is referred to as emotionally disturbed (ED) and makes up the fourth largest group of children with disabilities under the Individuals with Disabilities Education Act (IDEA). In 2003, 5% of children ages 4 to 17 were reported by a parent to have definite or severe difficulties with emotions, concentration, behavior, or ability to get along with other people (DHHS, 2005). In addition to schools and mental health settings, the pediatric wards of hospitals and private practice are locations where occupational therapists encounter these children. In settings for treatment of physical disability the children may have suffered bruises, fractures, or head trauma as a result of their impulsive or aggressive behavior or as a result If abuse. Children with chronic medical conditions and brain damage are at high risk for psychiatric disorders (Offord & Fleming, 1991).

Psychiatric Disorders and Their Manifestation in Play

It is conservatively estimated that at least 9% to 13% of children and adolescents have diagnosable mental disorders (DHHS, 1999; Zigler, Finn-Stevenson, & Tanner, 2002). Incidence with respect to age and sex tends to vary with specific disorders. In general, disorders are less prevalent in preadolescence, more prevalent among boys than girls from ages 4 to 11 years, and more prevalent among girls than boys in the 12- to 16-year age range (Offord & Fleming, 1991). The causes of mental disorders are varied and include biological, psychosocial, and environmental factors. Risk factors that make children vulnerable

to psychiatric disorders include chronic medical conditions that limit participation in activities, brain damage, intrauterine exposure to toxins (e.g., lead and alcohol), severe parental discord, exposure to acts of violence, familial psychiatric illness, poor parenting, and family dysfunction (DHHS, 1999; Offord & Bennett, 2002).

Novice occupational therapists often fail to recognize psychiatric disorders. In other childhood disability areas, such as those involving neurological or orthopedic conditions, the types of functional problems that children usually manifest are relatively easy to identify or forecast. Behavioral problems are often less obvious at first, and the occurrence is less predictable. New practitioners frequently have difficulty distinguishing behavioral difficulties from the vast repertoire of children's actions and reactions typical of play at this age and may not identify the first stages of defiant or escalating behavior. For example, when children are experiencing difficulty in taking turns or agreeing on game rules, therapists may set limits too soon or too firmly and inadvertently turn the session into one in which the children perceive that no disagreement at all is tolerated. Conversely, if the therapist does not set any limits or boundaries, the children may manifest out-of-control behaviors as a result of poor impulse control and lack of ability to manage their own behaviors. Recognizing problems and intervening effectively are generally difficult areas for novice practitioners.

The fourth edition of the *Diagnostic and Statistical Manual of Mental Disorders* (*DSM IV*) is one of the current systems by which psychiatric disorders are assessed. It employs a descriptive approach for mental disorders in which identification is based on recognizable behavioral signs or symptoms. The prominent disorders in middle childhood, those with high incidence despite variations in epidemiological studies, are attention deficit hyperactivity disorder, conduct disorder, mood disorders, and anxiety disorders. Specific features of these disorders are available elsewhere (American Psychiatric Association [*DSM IV*], 1994; Florey, 1993).

CASE EXAMPLES

The following case examples are provided in an effort to describe the effect of psychopathological disorders on social, play, and task behaviors. They have been developed from composites of patients we have seen, and they are generalized for the purpose of illustration. The case situations portray a child with a particular psychiatric disorder playing a game with a peer and making a simple craft project in the presence of a peer. They are presented here to assist the practitioner in recognizing problems as they are manifest in play.

CASE EXAMPLE 1
Stevie: Attention Deficit Hyperactivity Disorder

Stevie tends to be loud and intrusive with peers but does not seem to be aware of this. He often expresses surprise and sadness at how other children treat him. He talks a lot and quickly, he tends to interrupt, and his body movements are rapid. He has difficulty waiting his turn during a board game and frequently grabs pieces of the game from other children. He often does not appear to be paying attention and is in an almost constant state of fidgeting—moving around in his seat, playing with objects, and getting in and out of his chair. He tends to complain that the game rules are not fair.

While doing a craft project, Stevie has difficulty listening to the sequential directions, has a lot of trouble completing the steps in the correct order, and often becomes frustrated. When an adult offers to assist him, the adult has to help him focus on each step of the project, including finishing each step before he goes on to the next one. He often grabs at tools and materials and tries to take his choice of items before anyone else has a chance to choose. He frequently interferes with the work of his neighbor. Peers often complain that Stevie does not listen to them and that he is "annoying" to be around.

CASE EXAMPLE 2
Tom: Oppositional Defiant Disorder

In peer situations, Tom takes over and gets his own way. He is directive and controlling with peers and is not well liked by them. Because he often makes veiled threats to other children when adults are not around, some of them say that they are afraid of him and just do what he says to avoid conflict and retribution. Tom does not give his peers a chance to choose a game and makes the choice for all of them. He tells them which color marker he is going to use and then tells them that they can take "the leftovers." If Tom is losing at a game, he often cheats and attempts to cover his cheating by accusing a peer. Although Tom understands the directions of a simple craft project, he is easily frustrated and quickly stops working, labeling the project "for babies" and "stupid." He needs coaxing to complete his project but does not show pleasure or pride in his work. On the way out of the door, he throws his project in the trash and makes a comment to the therapist that all she does is provide "baby" activities for children and that she does not know what she is doing. Although momentarily he appears quite upset, within a minute he is laughing and attempting to engage everyone in conversation.

CASE EXAMPLE 3
Annie: Mood Disorder, Manic Episode

Annie decides on a game and quickly begins to open the box, but another game catches her eye and she quickly takes that game out. After a brief look at that game, she enthusiastically grabs yet another game and begins to look at it. The three games and game pieces are now mingled together on the table. When the therapist attempts to help her focus her choices, she objects to this process and says that narrowing choices interferes with her "independence."

Once a single game is chosen, Annie is able to play the game with frequent reminders about the rules and taking her turn. She appears to be thinking of several things at once and often asks her peers or the therapist if they don't think it would be fun to try something new—many of these ideas seem quite grand and difficult to achieve. Annie rushes through projects and works impulsively. She easily tires of projects and asks for her tasks to be changed frequently, and she seems to take more pleasure from thinking about the next thing she is going to do than what she is doing at the moment. She does best with step-by-step instructions and reminders to take her time, focus, and slow down.

Annie has poor personal space boundaries and often invades the space of others. She asks for hugs from adults and is overly friendly to strangers. She sometimes has sexualized themes in her play and jokes, and at times she acts out sexually.

CASE EXAMPLE 4
Mary: Mood Disorder, Depressive Episode

Mary is generally very quiet and moves slowly and deliberately. She often complains that she has difficulty sleeping and that her body hurts. At times she is irritable. She does not seem to experience pleasure in activities, and when she does, it is short lived—only for the period of time that she is involved in the activity. In game play, she leaves the choice of game to her peers and does not seem to care what game they choose. She plays the game lethargically and is not invested in winning. She does not initiate many conversations with others but will usually respond when asked direct questions, although she does not readily participate in ongoing conversations. She is able to follow most directions on craft projects but usually will not ask for help if she does not understand something—she seems preoccupied and stares into space until someone comes along to help her. She appears to be "going through the motions" instead of fully participating.

CASE EXAMPLE 5
Paul: Anxiety Disorder

Paul is very concerned about doing the right thing and asks for further clarification in choosing a game, for example, "Is one better than another?" He frequently asks the therapist whether he is playing the game correctly and is concerned that he is moving game markers and pieces correctly. He is quick to point out any mistakes or instances of suspected cheating on the part of his peers. His concern with correctness carries over to craft projects. He asks a lot of questions, although he has a good grasp of the process. He needs reassurance and becomes visibly anxious when participating in the activity. He often states that he knows he is going to do something wrong, even before he attempts anything.

Paul does not appear to enjoy the process of engaging in activities or seem pleased with or proud of his craft projects. He is not well liked by peers and is often the target of name calling because of his anxious and somewhat rigid mannerisms.

CASE EXAMPLE 6
Pamela: Thought Disorder

Pamela does not respond to the opportunity to select a game but does not object when one is offered to her. Her interests are limited, and she is a physically inactive child. During the game she often seems distracted and sometimes leaves the table to go to the corner of the room. She is frequently heard softly speaking out loud when in the corner, but when asked what she is talking about, she quickly answers, "Nothing." She often stares into space and can seem to stare right through a person with whom she is playing a game, smiling or looking fearful of what she is perceiving. She sometimes responds to questions asked of her, but her answers have an odd, tangential quality to them. Her statements have this quality as well, making it difficult for others to respond to her.

Pamela can become enthusiastic about a certain interest that is not generally shared by the others in the group. She will participate in craft activities, but she rarely initiates this, although there are periods of time when she wants to make the same craft over and over again. She seems to lose focus as the steps of the activity go on and is not concerned about the end product.

CASE EXAMPLE 7
Nick: Asperger Syndrome

Nick has difficulty making eye contact, but this improves as he becomes more comfortable with the other children in his group. He has restricted interests, and at first when it is suggested that he play a board game, he says that the only games he likes to play are computer and video games. He suggests that the children use the therapist's computer to go on line and find a game. When he is directed back to helping choose a board game, he has difficulty negotiating with the other children in the group and becomes angry at them when they do not choose what he wants to play. When he speaks to the group, he talks about one of his interests and gives a great deal of technical detail. He does not notice when the other children start to give him signals that they are no longer interested. At times during the game he becomes caught up in his own game play and seems to forget that the other children are waiting to play. During the craft activity, Nick begins to cry because what he drew was not perfect and the lines were not at the correct angle. He has difficulty recovering from this and has a hard time with the therapist's attempts to help him with his drawing, insisting that he has to start over to make it "perfect." He has difficulty making "small talk" during both the game and the craft activities and often will not answer questions or participate in group conversations.

CLINICAL GUIDES TO ASSESSMENT AND TREATMENT

Clinical Vignette

An occupational therapist greets Nathan, a 9-year-old boy who has been referred to her because he is having trouble keeping up on the playground with other children, often gets into fights with other boys, and is slow to complete his work at school, even though his intellectual abilities have been measured at an above-average level. The physician who referred the child wonders whether he has some "motor impairments." Nathan's parents report that he often goes to his room and cries when he thinks no one is watching him and that ever since he started a new grade in school 3 months ago, he seems to be less interested in things than he used to be.

When Nathan enters the therapy room, he barely makes eye contact with the therapist. He compliantly sits in the chair the therapist offers him but mumbles answers to questions and does not brighten up even when asked about favorite toys, activities, or his pet. The therapist gives him a quick, untimed screening for eye-hand skills.

He completes this in a slow, deliberate manner, doing well on each item but making a negative comment about his abilities after each attempt. He asks the therapist repeatedly, "Did I do that right?" The therapist scores his test and finds that his score is above average. At a later time she assesses his visual-perceptual and motor skills because this has been the primary reason for referral, although she has not observed any signs of difficulty in this area. Again, she finds that Nathan is scoring at age level or a little above on everything.

The therapist continues the evaluation by interviewing Nathan, targeting areas of information about his family and where he lives, a self-report on activities of daily living skills, chores, school, friends, and play. As the session goes on, Nathan begins to make better eye contact and mumbles less, but the therapist notices that he often falls into a babyish way of talking and that he keeps asking her for approval. Nathan answers all of the questions in the interview, with a few responses that pique the therapist's interest. When asked whether he likes school, Nathan yells, "NO! I HATE IT! SCHOOL IS BORING AND THE WORK IS TOO HARD." When asked whether he has a best friend, he replies, "Yeah, I have hundreds of friends but just can't remember their names right now." In response to a question about who he likes to play with and what he likes to do when he plays, he responds, "I like to play with my dog—we go on walks." When pressed on this answer, he is unable to name any child with whom he regularly spends time after school. He also says that he comes home every day after school and does not do any after-school activities. Nathan is asked whether he ever gets into fights at school. He says that he does "sometimes" but that other kids pick fights with him and that it is not his fault.

The therapist asks Nathan to choose between two craft activities so that she can assess the process of completing the craft: the child's ability to make a choice, follow and sequence directions, solve problems, use materials, and pay attention. She is also interested in what Nathan's reaction will be to the finished product. Instead of showing interest in the two craft projects shown to him, he goes over and picks up a much simpler stencil project completed by a 4-year-old earlier in the day. "Can I do this one instead?" he asks and says that he likes the "easier" one better. The therapist reassures him and tells him that she will help him with his choice of the other two projects. He finally settles on a copper tooling project and has to choose his design from eight different tooling molds. He takes about 5 minutes to choose, finally settling on a lion mold. Although he is able to remember the multistep directions and does not need them to be repeated, he continues to ask the therapist whether he is doing the right thing, whether he should change the way he is doing the tooling, and whether she likes what he is doing. When the

project is completed and framed, Nathan refuses to take the project, stating, "I just want to keep it here so I can see it when I come back to this room."

During the next session, Nathan is paired with Robert, age 8 years, to assess their peer interactions. Because part of this evaluation involves observing the process the children go through in choosing and playing a game together, the occupational therapist steps back and does not intervene, only giving the boys directions to "choose a game that you like and then we'll all play it." The boys enter the room and immediately begin grabbing randomly at the many games stored on a bookshelf. They almost get into a fight over pulling on the same game box. After about 5 minutes of this kind of behavior, Robert finally chooses Candyland. Nathan retreats to the table and almost begins to cry, saying, "Why did he get to choose—it isn't fair. He always gets to choose," even though this is the first time the boys have met each other. When they sit down to play the game, they cannot organize the cards, fight over which marker they want, and do not wait their turns. Both of them are, in turn, angry when they get a "bad move" and repeatedly take themselves out of the game and then put themselves back in. When Nathan wins the game, he pumps his fists in the air and says "I won" over and over again, ignoring Robert, who is visibly angry and is on the verge of crying over losing the game.

What is happening here? Why is Nathan having such difficulty at school? Why does he keep making negative comments about himself when his physical and cognitive skills have been assessed as adequate? Why are an 8-year-old and a 9-year-old having such difficulty cooperating? Why did they choose Candyland, which is a game typically introduced to preschoolers as one of their first experiences with board games? Why are they having such difficulty getting organized?

The assessment and treatment of children with behavioral problems constitute a complex process. When working with children who have difficulty functioning with other people and doing what they should be doing at home, at school, at camp, and at soccer practice, therapists do not have the behavioral equivalent of a precise goniometer reading to measure these problems with function. What therapists do have are keen observational skills that improve and broaden over time and the acquired experience to recognize certain behaviors as red flags, indicating obstacles to success. These children have experienced many challenges. What is right cognitively for them is sometimes not right socially and emotionally. Some children with behavioral problems have learning disabilities, and some do not. Some have motor and perceptual problems, and some do not. Many children with average or above-average IQs who are doing well or who have the potential to do well in school have severe performance deficits when it comes to other life demands. The common denominator for these children is devastating experiences in social interactions that most children would not think twice about or would look forward to. This disability is often not visible, but it severely impairs their ability to function.

When a child who is having behavioral problems is referred to occupational therapy, where does the therapist start? What are relevant areas to assess? What does the therapist do, once he or she has obtained test results? What should the therapist do if the picture is complicated by other skill deficits, such as motor or perceptual difficulties?

Clinical Guide to Assessment

The areas chosen to assess must be directly tied to the identification of a child's functional abilities, to include both areas of strengths and problems. This is old news to occupational therapists. What is proposed here is that therapists take a more comprehensive look at the ways children are functioning. Currently many therapists feel tied to assessing and treating only how the child's motor, sensory, and perceptual skills influence his or her ability to function. Certainly these abilities critically affect the ways in which children are able to play, learn, and take part in everything in which children should take part. Yet if these are the therapist's only areas of concern, he or she has taken these skills completely out of the context of the child's life. From the perspective of a child who is experiencing problems in many areas of functioning, an improvement in social abilities and experiences may be as or more important than improving gross motor skills. The normal development of skills does not take place out of context—a child develops gross motor skills by playing, often in the company of other children. The motor skills are an avenue by which play with other children can develop into a budding friendship. Therapists cannot continue to work on basic skills in isolation from their social context, hoping that the skills will transfer to real-life situations and neglecting the child's social arena in which the skills will be put to use.

Task, play, and social and perceptual-motor skills are the target areas of assessment. Equal importance should be placed on standardized assessments, such as adaptive behavior scales, visual-perceptual tests, and motor tests; on information gathered from an interview with the child; and on structured observations of play, task performance, and social abilities. Children are seen individually and with a peer. They are seen individually for an interview in which they are asked to describe a "typical weekday" and "typical weekend day," for observation of task performance in a craft, and for specific testing of motor skills or adaptive behavior. Children

are seen with a peer for the assessment of social behavior in a game or a task. Ideally a child is evaluated within the context of his or her community, whether at school, at home, or on the playground. If this is not practical, the therapist can try to recreate these normal settings as nearly as possible and include other children currently being evaluated. Although this is an artificially constructed peer group, children with social skills deficits continue to evidence common problems with peers even when the other children are new to them. Often the problems are stable across any group in which the child participates.

Two guides for assessing play and tasks in a social context provide ways of structuring observations of the task, play, and social behaviors of children. The Activity Observation Guide in Box 10-1 was developed at the University of California Neuropsychiatric Hospital to provide an indication of the way children approach and carry through with activities in the context of a social setting. This guide has been extremely useful to everyone from new occupational therapy students, who need help in defining what they should look for, to experienced clinicians, who use it to add more experienced clinical knowledge to the emerging picture of the child being evaluated. Although the guide can be used with a wide age range, expectations for each item should be viewed developmentally. The Social Behavior Observation Guide in Box 10-2 was also developed at the University of California Neuropsychiatric Hospital and is adapted from Cartledge and Milburn (1995). This guide is used in conjunction with the Activity Observation Guide.

Several assessments measure the crucial area of adaptive behavior, including the social-emotional portion of the Miller First Step (First Step scale) and the Vineland Adaptive Behavior Scales (Vineland scales). These assessments are usually part of a more comprehensive evaluation and are useful if the therapist wants to establish an age level of adaptive functioning for the child. The adaptive behavior checklist on the First Step scale includes daily living skills, self-management, social interactions, and functioning within the community. A social-emotional scale is also part of this screening test and includes items on task confidence, cooperative mood, temperament and emotionality, uncooperative or antisocial behavior, and attention-communication difficulties. The First Step scale can be used for children from 2 years, 9 months of age to 6 years, 2 months. The First Step scale also includes screening items for cognitive, language, and motor abilities (Miller, 1993).

The Vineland scales assess adaptive functioning in the areas of daily living skills, communication, socialization, and motor skills. They can be used from birth through 18 years, 11 months and yield an adaptive level and an age-equivalent score. The evaluation is completed by an interview

Box 10-1 *Activity Observation Guide*

A. TIME
   1. How long does it take for the child to settle on an activity?
   2. How long does the child stay engaged in the activity?
   3. How does the child use structured versus unstructured (free-time) play?

B. TASKS
   1. Is the child able to make decisions when given choices?
   2. Is the child able to follow directions?
   3. Does the child use materials and tools correctly?
   4. Is the child able to tolerate frustration?
   5. Does the child attempt to solve problems independently before asking for help?
   6. Is the child able to ask for help when needed? Does the child ask for too much assistance?
   7. Does the child participate in cleanup?
   8. Is the child proud of his or her efforts?

C. STRUCTURED GAMES
   1. Does the child decide which game to play?
   2. Does the child know the rules?
   3. Does the child know the object of the game?
   4. Does the child take his or her turn in the correct sequence?
   5. Does the child follow rules?
   6. Is the child able to accept winning or losing?

D. PEOPLE
   1. Is the child able to play alone?
   2. Interaction with adults
      a. Does the child interact with adults?
      b. Is the child dependent on adult interaction?
      c. Is the child able to follow directions and rules?
      d. Is the child able to become involved in an activity through imitation and visual imitation?
      e. Is the child able to become involved in activities through verbal instructions?
      f. Is the child able to get attention from adults in an appropriate way?
      g. Does the child respond appropriately to praise?
      h. Is the child able to accept help from an adult?
   3. Interaction with peers
      a. Does the child interact with other children?
      b. What type of social play does the child engage in? Onlooker play, parallel play, associate play, cooperative play? Is this developmentally what you would expect?
      c. What kinds of play themes does the child propose to other children?
      d. Does the child imitate peers? Is this appropriate or inappropriate?
      e. Is the child possessive with toys or materials?
      f. Is the child aggressive to others?
      g. Is the child able to share?
      h. If the child is old enough, does he or she compete appropriately and accept winning or losing?
   4. Does the child express emotion and have fun in play?
   5. Does the child pick up social cues, use feedback from others, and learn from prior interactions?

with parents or caregivers. The Vineland scales are useful to occupational therapists because the questions asked all examine the child's ability to function in the real world. For example, such questions as "Does the child follow community rules?" "Does the child have a preferred friend of either sex?" and "Does the child play more than one board or card game requiring skill and decision making?" are asked. Scoring criteria are provided for each question on the Vineland scales (Sparrow, Bolla, & Circhetti, 1984).

Although perceptual and motor skills are not the focus of this chapter, they should be thoroughly assessed as a part of any full evaluation of children who are experiencing behavioral problems, not only to rule out deficits but also to explore whether concurrent deficits in these areas are contributing to difficulties with coping. It is documented in the literature that children with learning disabilities or emotional-social problems have concurrent physical problems (Kramer, Deitz, & Crowe, 1988). Therapists at the Neuropsychiatric

Hospital have found that at least 50% of the children admitted to the inpatient unit have deficits in visual-perceptual, visual-motor, or motor skills severe enough to limit their ability to participate in common play and work activities. In some cases the identification of problems in these areas, subsequent intervention, and structuring of activities so that the child consistently experiences success have helped children bring their behavior under control. For all children, it is important to establish whether they are having skill problems in these areas so that meaningful recommendations can be made for further occupational therapy intervention and for adaptations needed in community settings, including home and school. Some of the typical assessments used for this purpose include the Beery-Buktenica Developmental Test of Visual-Motor Integration (Beery, 1989), the Motor-Free Visual Perception Test (Gardner, 1982), and the Bruininks-Oseretsky Test of Motor Proficiency (Bruininks, 1978).

Box 10-2 *Social Behavior Observation Guide*

1. Eye contact
   Does the child establish eye contact when spoken to or when speaking to others?
2. Listening
   Does the child pay attention to the person who is talking and make an effort to understand what is being said?
3. Conversation
   Does the child initiate conversation? Does he or she talk to others?
4. Asking a question
   Does the child decide what information is needed and ask the right person for information?
5. Asking for help
   Does the child request assistance when he or she is having difficulty?
6. Joining and staying in
   Does the child have strategies for entering an ongoing group or activity?
7. Cooperation
   Does the child follow group rules? Does he or she comply to reasonable requests made by others? Does he or she take turns and share?
8. Apologizing
   Does the child tell others he or she is sorry after doing something wrong? Does the child overapologize or take responsibility for something he or she has not done?
9. Convincing others
   Does the child attempt to persuade others that his or her ideas are better and will be more useful than those of the other person?
10. Expressing feelings
    Does the child let others know how he or she is feeling?
11. Understanding feelings
    Does the child try to figure out what others are feeling? Does the child let others know that he or she appreciates favors?
12. Asking permission
    Does the child figure out when permission is needed to do something and then ask the right person?
13. Helping others
    Does the child give help to others who may need or want it? Does the child ask before giving help to another child?
14. Using self-control
    Does the child control his or her temper? Does the child respect the property of others?
15. Responding to teasing
    Does the child deal appropriately with being teased by others in ways that allow him or her to be in control? Is the child routinely teased by other children?
16. Avoiding trouble
    Does the child stay out of situations that may get him or her into trouble?
17. Likability
    Is the child sought out by other children to be played with?

Modified from Cartledge, G., & Milburn, J. (Eds.). (1985). *Teaching social skills to children.* New York: Pergamon Press.

Case Study Evaluation

To illustrate how an evaluation of a child actually takes place, the clinical vignette presented at the beginning of this section is used here as a model to describe how the evaluation progresses and what underlying problems an occupational therapist may pick up from the child's behavior. Each evaluation area is followed by a "reasoning" section that targets some of the conclusions and further questions the therapist poses in the evaluation process. Therapists must assess and target areas for intervention quickly, and this requires prioritization of assessment strategies and interpretation and synthesis of evaluation data. The following is an attempt to tease out a portion of the clinical reasoning process that therapists use in daily practice.

Motor and Perceptual Motor Skills

Although Nathan was referred by his physician because of a possible "motor impairment," in formal testing the occupational therapist could not find any sign of this. Visual-perceptual, fine motor, and gross motor evaluations are all at or above age level. In clinical observation, Nathan shows good skills, although he is a little slow at times. His perception of his skills, however, is not consistent with his performance. He constantly makes negative comments about himself and asks for reassurance.

Reasoning. Nathan may have anxiety about performing activities and tasks, or his self-confidence may be poor. What is the link among his skills, his perception of his skills, and his decreased ability to engage in play activities on the playground with other children? The therapist needs more observation of this behavior in a peer group to better assess what is going on.

Task Skills

Nathan initially chose a project immature for his age and one that did not match his cognitive, motor, or perceptual skills. He has some difficulty making a choice but shows good abilities in following directions and using the craft tools correctly. Again, he constantly asks for reassurance. He does not make any comments about the successful completion of his project, instead asking whether he can leave it with the therapist. He says that school is boring and too hard.

Reasoning. Nathan is showing some slowed decision making and motor skills but not enough to keep him from successfully completing his project in the allotted time. He spends much of his time simultaneously working and asking for reassurance—similar to the situation with his motor skills. He is very dependent on the therapist to structure his emotional environment for him and tries to ensure structure by asking over and over for reassurance and by using a babyish voice in an effort to get and keep the therapist's attention. The therapist wonders whether this kind of behavior is also present at school, thinking that he most likely does not get constant reassurance in a classroom situation and may have to be "quietly" anxious about himself in that situation. He does not outwardly show any pride in his completed project. He leaves the project with the therapist, saying, "I just want to keep it here so I can see it when I come back to this room." Sometimes children are relieved, even in evaluation settings, that the therapist is structuring the situation and presenting challenges at their level, and they will leave a project, toy, or an item of clothing as a kind of insurance that they will come back to the room for occupational therapy.

Play and Social Skills

Nathan's parents are concerned because he is looking sad, cries a lot, and shows less interest in things than he did previously. They wonder if this is tied to something that has happened or is happening at school. Nathan interacts socially in an odd way with the therapist. His eye contact is initially poor, he mumbles his words, and he shows no enjoyment when discussing activities that children usually enjoy. When he warms up in the session, he is anxious about how he is doing and speaks to the therapist in a regressed manner.

Nathan gives the therapist cues about his social life. He cannot remember his friend's name, says he has "hundreds" of unnamed friends, likes to play with his dog more than with other children, does not spend any time with children after school, and perceives that other children

often pick on him. When he is paired with Robert, the 8-year-old boy, the social situation is disastrous. He has difficulty handling the unstructured situation presented to him, resorting to random grabbing of different games on the shelf. He is unable even to attempt to negotiate with Robert about what game they are going to play, instead giving up and going back to the table, almost crying. He objects to Robert's choosing the game but readily accepts the choice, even though it is a very immature game for him. He has difficulty waiting his turn, cannot organize the game cards, and gets upset because he wanted the red marker, which Robert has taken. He cannot play cooperatively with Robert, shows poor frustration tolerance when he gets a "bad move," and takes himself out of the game. The concept that fortunes change in board games is not very apparent to him. He loses hope quickly and does not persist in trying to continue with the game. When Nathan finally does win the game, he gloats over his victory and fails to read Robert's cues of being angry and upset.

Reasoning. With the presence of a peer, Nathan's social problems that the therapist could only imagine suddenly become reality. Nathan's social and play skills are not only immature, they are maladaptive. He is choosing easier activities in a quest for success. Unfortunately, his play and social skills are so poor that choosing a simpler activity probably makes Nathan look even worse to other children, who by this time are playing fairly complex, competitive games with rules and teams. He does not have fun in the process of playing the game but somehow takes pleasure in winning it, apparently oblivious to the process. He does not show any skills in cooperating, compromising, or convincing Robert of his position. Instead, he copes by giving up or by becoming irritable and angry. Nathan is immature in his relations with others, in his ability to make decisions independently, and in his selection of tasks matching his motor and cognitive skills. When the therapist administers the Vineland scales to obtain age-equivalent scores, Nathan scores at the 5 year, 6 month level.

Summary of the Evaluation

What is right for Nathan cognitively is not right for him socially or emotionally. His cognitive, motor, and visual-perceptual skills are average or above average. His social skills are maladaptive. At 9 years of age, Nathan should be able to play a fairly complex board game in a cooperative way with a group of children. He should also be showing enjoyment over exploring new, multistep craft activities and striving to make his skills better and better. By this age, children no longer rely on adults to help them negotiate familiar social territory but have generally become quite independent. Nathan is an example of the child whose many good abilities are overshadowed by a lack of social competence. He attempts to cope with this by relying on adults, asking for reassurance, showing regressed behaviors, and withdrawing from situations in which he has to compromise or cooperate with peers. As a result of this, his self-esteem has suffered and he is experiencing performance anxiety. This may have started in social situations but is now also intruding on his other skills, such as academics, in which he has previously been successful. Nathan is often tearful and irritable, is motorically slowed, and does not enjoy activities as he once did. He could be suffering from dysthymia or depression.

Clinical Guide to Treatment

What does a therapist do with boys like Nathan and Robert? Children with behavior and emotional problems generally have poor self-esteem, reinforced daily when their lack of coping skills and abilities makes them unable to participate in normal peer, school, and community activities with any success. In addition, many of them have poor ability to read social cues, so feedback from the environment is impaired. Because of their behavior, their environment is often restricted and they miss out on normal daily activities that are the arena in which children learn how to interact in groups. This is the dilemma—most behaviorally disturbed children have an extremely hard time working in groups, but they have little opportunity to participate in group activities because of their behavior.

The purpose of the assessment is to identify areas of strength and weakness from which goals and treatment interventions may be developed. In targeting goals and interventions for children exhibiting behavior and emotional disorders, priority is given to the behaviors and situations that are causing the children the greatest difficulties in their social relations. Goals should be measurable, and they should address the who, what, when, and how of behavior expected in the occupational therapy practice framework (AOTA, 2002). The "who" and "what" identify the person and the behavior in which the person is expected to engage. The "when" and "how" identify how frequently the behavior is expected to occur and under what circumstances, such as how much assistance or prompting the therapist must give. The components of the treatment goals—the behavior, the frequency and duration, and the circumstances—may all be varied to reflect changes in the child's skills and abilities.

Agrin (1987) and Schultz (1992) both wrote of models of practice for children with behavioral problems. Small group activities, with a strong emphasis on cooperation, sharing, respect for one another and for materials, and participation as a group member, are recommended. In practice, this model is extremely effective. Children with social skills deficits require highly structured programs that emphasize the learning and practice of life skills in

context. As the child gains more appropriate skills, he or she can be integrated into less structured activities and spend more of the day in normal play and social experiences with other children. The word "structure" is often used without explanation of what it means or why it is important. As in the case study evaluation section, a "reasoning" section is included here to uncover some of the considerations a therapist makes in constructing an approach and environment for treatment. Elements of structure are discussed in this section.

Case Study Treatment
For Nathan, the quality of his interactional skills with peers and adults was a problem, as was his dependence on adults to select activities for him. These became the target areas for setting treatment goals and selecting interventions. Initial goals for Nathan were as follows:
1. Nathan will initiate and carry through a social interaction (e.g., asking a peer to play with him, sharing materials) four times a session.
2. Nathan will interact with others using his "regular voice" instead of his "baby voice."
3. Nathan will demonstrate more independence in school, play, and home activities by persisting and sticking with an activity to completion.

Initially all of these goals require reminders or prompts from the therapist. These form the "startpoints" for intervention. Nathan is involved in the process of goal agreement and monitoring. The therapist suggests to Nathan that he needs to learn to ask his companions to share materials or to play, using his regular voice, and that he needs to finish an activity. The therapist asks, "Do you think this is something we might work on?" and in treatment sessions says, "Remember what we're working on." To implement the goals, Nathan is involved in an ongoing social skills club and is the therapist's helper in occupational therapy sessions with younger children. The rationale and format of these groups are stressed to provide a snapshot of "how" and "why."

Social Skills Club and Therapist Helper
The Dinosaur Club is the name given to an occupational therapy social skills group by the children. The purpose of the group is to listen to others, to include others, to express positive and negative feelings, to identify feelings in others, and to think of consequences before acting. There are currently three children other than Nathan in the club, between the ages of 8 and 9 years. All members have club T-shirts that they made with their name and a Dinosaur footprint on the front. Because Nathan does not have a shirt, he is seen individually in an occupational therapy session to make his shirt and to learn from the occupational therapist about the purpose and general format of the club meetings. Each meeting has a routine format or sequence that is dependable for the children.

The club meeting begins with greetings to one another, followed by all members' putting on their club shirts, which are worn over their regular clothing. Following this the club rules are reviewed. Because Nathan is new, at his first meeting he is asked to contribute a rule to the club that can be followed by all but that will help him in working with other club members. His rule is "Talk right to others." The remainder of the club rules are read and include such things as taking turns and listening to others. The group then talks about what has happened since the last club meeting. The members are asked, "Anything going on?" and are also specifically asked about good or bad things that have happened. The club meeting then focuses on an activity—a game or craft that requires sharing materials with others, sequencing steps, and talking with one another. The games or crafts used are simple and initially stressed successful completion so that the social behavior could be targeted. As the group works together, the cognitive complexity—the number of steps and independence in steps—is increased.

Nathan is also involved as a helper to the therapist in a group with four younger children, ages 4 to 5 years. Nathan is responsible for providing initial verbal instruction in an activity, such as paper bag puppets, and for helping children share materials. In this way he can practice some of the skills he himself needs and gain more confidence in his ability to influence others in a nurturing way.

Reasoning

Nathan is placed in a group because it is with peers that he demonstrates the most difficulty. The goals for each child must be considered, as are the goals for the group as a whole. For example, one child may be timid, one aggressive, and one impulsive. Each child has individual goals in social interactions and for participating in the activity. The goal for the timid child may be to initiate interactions with one other peer, the goal for the impulsive child may be to listen and to respond to conversations initiated by a peer, and the goal for the aggressive child may be to use words and not actions to make feelings and needs known. Although these three goals are different and are implemented differently for each child, the common goal for everyone is better social interactions. An example of a group goal is "The children will be able to play together cooperatively for 20 minutes," with each individual goal being implemented and encouraged to further the group goal.

In all groups the therapist has a game plan. This involves not only selecting a particular activity, but also planning how to present and pace the activity and having a contingency plan in case the activity is not successful. Activities should be targeted to the social abilities of the group, with the cognitive and motor abilities downgraded initially. The game plan also includes the anticipation of problems that may occur and a plan for intervention before things get out of hand. If a child is having chronic behavioral problems, a consistent plan of action should be developed among all of those who come in regular contact with the child, including the parents, teachers, and therapists.

The process of providing structure to children encompasses consideration of the physical, social, and activity environments within the treatment session:

1. The therapist structures the physical environment to provide a challenging, interesting variety of toys and materials for the children. Too many items may cause the children to become disorganized, and for some children even tools such as hammers may become objects with which to test the safety rules.

2. The therapist structures the social environment as well. Rules are made and followed in the occupational therapy session. Older children can help make up their own rules, whereas younger children may need to have rules given to them. Rules help children "feel out" the boundaries of a situation and help them begin to gain independence by thinking in more positive ways of interacting and getting along with each other. Rules and consequences for transgressing rules should be consistent. Each child should have a good understanding of the rules of the setting.

3. The therapist structures the activity environment by carefully analyzing the level of skill needed to participate. Choices of activities can be provided that are slightly below the child's intellectual abilities to give the therapist and the child more freedom to work on the social aspects of the activity. As a result, children do not become anxious about not knowing how to perform a certain task or game. As children begin to gain skills in social play, they are provided with less structure and more options to choose and carry through activities with their peers.

Children benefit from participating in the structured activity as contextually as possible. This could take the form of occupational therapy sessions during free-play time in a classroom, on classroom outings, or in after-school activities such as sports, the YMCA, or scouts.

SUMMARY

This chapter illustrates clinical interventions in play with children exhibiting behavior and emotional disorders. The chapter is informed both by theoretical perspectives and by "hands-on" experiences we have had. The leading construct in designing clinical interventions is play.

Interventions may target a vast number of skills and behaviors in which the children are deficit, but the context is play. To embed the learning, unlearning, and relearning of skills in play is to construct a world that has meaning for the child and one in which he or she must function. Occupational therapists are interested in improving a child's ability to function in tasks and with others in school, in the family, and in community settings. We, however, take the view that the ability to function independently in tasks and with others is immeasurably fostered, nurtured, hampered, or squelched in the peer culture during times of free play. To help children with behavior and emotional disorders understand this culture and to assist them in achieving the necessary skills to fit in is a major goal of occupational therapy practice in this area.

Review Questions

1. In the first clinical vignette of this chapter, how might the occupational therapy student have tailored the group intervention to be more effective?
2. What is middle childhood? What are the major hallmarks of development in middle childhood?
3. Describe the nature of peer relations, rules, and play interests in middle childhood. Differentiate between younger and older children within middle childhood in your answer.
4. How may the occupational therapist construct play environments to enhance social skill development of children in middle childhood?
5. Discuss the impact of childhood psychiatric disorders on the development of play.
6. Describe the process of play assessment for a child in middle childhood who has a psychiatric diagnosis. What does the assessment entail, and how are data interpreted? How are assessment results then used to guide treatment?
7. The chapter suggests four broad domains for guiding activity observation of children in middle childhood. What are these domains? Provide examples of questions you might ask in an assessment within each domain.
8. Discuss the variety of ways in which a therapist may provide structure to children within a treatment session.

REFERENCES

Agrin, A. (1987). Occupational therapy with emotionally disturbed children in a public elementary school. *Occupational Therapy in Mental Health, 7,* 105-113.

American Occupational Therapy Association. (2002). Occupational therapy practice framework: Domain and process. *American Journal of Occupational Therapy, 56,* 609-639.

American Psychiatric Association. (1994). *Diagnostic and statistical manual of mental disorders* (4th ed.). Washington, DC: Author.

Beery, E. (1989). *The Developmental Test of Visual-Motor Integration* (3rd ed.). Cleveland: Modern Curriculum.

Bruininks, R. H. (1978). *Bruininks-Oseretsky Test of Motor Proficiency examiner's manual.* Circle Pines, MN: American Guidance Service.

Burke, J. P., & DePoy, E. (1991). An emerging view of mastery, excellence, and leadership in occupational therapy practice. *American Journal of Occupational Therapy, 45,* 1027-1032.

Cartledge, G., & Milburn, J. (Eds.). (1995). *Teaching social skills to children* (3rd ed.). Boston: Allyn & Bacon.

Cassidy, J., & Asher, S. R. (1992). Loneliness and peer relations in young children. *Child Development, 63,* 350-365.

Cincotta, N. (2002). The journey of middle childhood: Who are latency-age children? In S. Austrian (Ed.), *Developmental theories through the life cycle* (pp. 68-122). New York: Columbia University Press.

Cole, M., & Cole, S. (1989). *The development of children.* New York: Scientific American Books.

Collins, W. (1984). Conclusion: The status of basic research on middle childhood. In W. Collins (Ed.), *Development during middle childhood: The years from six to twelve* (pp. 398-421). Washington, DC: National Academy Press.

Combrinck-Graham, L., & Fox, G. (2002). Development of school-age children. In M. Lewis (Ed.), *Child and adolescent psychiatry: A comprehensive textbook* (3rd ed., pp. 324-332). Philadelphia: Lippincott, Williams & Wilkins.

Corsaro, W., & Schwartz, K. (1991). Peer play and socialization in two cultures. In B. Scales, M. Alm, A. Nicolopoulou, & S. Ervin-Tripp (Eds.), *Play and the social context of development in early care and education* (pp. 243-354). New York: Teachers College.

Davies, D. (2004). *Child development: A practitioner's guide.* New York: Guilford Press.

Epps, E., & Smith, S. (1984). School and children: The middle childhood years. In W. Collins (Ed.), *Development during middle childhood: The years from six to twelve* (pp. 283-334). Washington, DC: National Academy Press.

Erikson, E. (1963). *Childhood and society.* New York: W.W. Norton.

Fleming, M. (1991). The therapist with the three-track mind. *American Journal of Occupational Therapy, 45,* 1007-1014.

Florey, L. (1993). Psychiatric disorders in childhood and adolescence. In H. Hopkins & H. Smith (Eds.), *Willard and Spackman's occupational therapy* (8th ed., pp. 503-519). Philadelphia: J.B. Lippincott.

Fromberg, D., & Bergen, D. (1998). Perspectives on play development. In D. Fromberg & D. Bergen (Eds.), *Play from birth to twelve and beyond* (pp. 133-134). New York: Garland Publishing.

Gardner, M. F. (1982). *Test of Visual-Perceptual Skills (Non-Motor).* San Francisco: Children's Hospital of San Francisco.

Gesell, A., Ilg, F., & Ames, L. (1977). *The child from five to ten.* New York: Harper & Row.

Gibbs, M., & Priest, H. M. (1999). Designing and implementing a dual diagnosis module: A review of the literature and some preliminary findings. *Nurse Education Today, 19,* 357-363.

Gibson, D., & Richert, G. (1993). Section 1F, The therapeutic process. In H. Hopkins & H. Smith (Eds.), *Willard and Spackman's occupational therapy* (8th ed., pp. 557-566). Philadelphia: J.B. Lippincott.

Hartley, R., & Goldenson, R. (1963). *The complete book of children's play*. New York: Thomas Crowell.

Hartrup, W. W. (1992). *Having friends, making friends, and keeping friends: Relationships as educational contexts*. Urbana, IL: ERIC Clearinghouse on Elementary and Early Childhood Education.

Havighurst, R. (1973). *Developmental tasks and education*. New York: David McKay.

King, N. (1987). Elementary school play: Theory and research. In J. Block & N. King (Eds.), *School play* (pp. 143-165). New York: Garland Publishing.

Knapp, M., & Knapp, H. (1976). *One potato, two potato: The secret education of American children*. New York: W.W. Norton.

Kramer, L., Deitz, J., & Crowe, T. (1988). A comparison of motor performance of preschoolers enrolled in mental health programs and non-mental health programs. *American Journal of Occupational Therapy, 42*, 520-525.

Ladd, G. W., Birch, S. H., & Buhs, E. S. (1999). Children's social and scholastic lives in kindergarten: Related spheres of influence? *Child Development, 70*, 1373-1400.

Lewis, D. (1991). Conduct disorder. In M. Lewis (Ed.), *Child and adolescent psychiatry: A comprehensive textbook* (pp. 561-573). Baltimore: Williams & Wilkins.

Lewis, D., & Yeager, C. (2002). Conduct disorder. In M. Lewis (Ed.), *Child and adolescent psychiatry: A comprehensive textbook* (3rd ed., pp. 670-681). Philadelphia: Lippincott, Williams & Wilkins.

Maccoby, E. (1984). Middle childhood in the context of the family. In W. Collins (Ed.), *Development during middle childhood: The years from six to twelve* (pp. 184-239). Washington, DC: National Academy Press.

Manning, M. (1998). Play development from ages eight to twelve. In D. Fromberg & D. Bergen (Eds.), *Play from birth to twelve and beyond* (pp. 154-161). New York: Garland Publishing.

Mattingly, C. (1991). What is clinical reasoning? *American Journal of Occupational Therapy, 45*, 979-986.

Mattingly, C. (1998). In search of the good: Narrative reasoning in clinical practice. *Medical Anthropology Quarterly, 12*, 273-297.

Miller, L. J. (1993). *First Step Screening Test for Evaluating Preschoolers manual*. New York: Harcourt, Brace, Jovanovich.

Mussen, P., Conger, J., & Kagan, J. (1963). *Child development and personality*. New York: Harper & Row.

Offord, D., & Bennett, K. (2002). Epidemiology and prevention. In M. Lewis (Ed.), *Child and adolescent psychiatry: A comprehensive textbook* (3rd ed., pp. 1320-1335). Philadelphia: Lippincott, Williams & Wilkins.

Offord, D., & Fleming, J. (1991). Epidemiology. In M. Lewis (Ed.), *Child and adolescent psychiatry: A comprehensive textbook* (pp. 1156-1168). Baltimore: Williams & Wilkins.

Piaget, J. (1962). *Play, dreams and imitation in childhood*. New York: W.W. Norton.

Schell, B. (2003). Clinical reasoning: The basis of practice. In E. Crepeau, E. Cohn, & B. Schell (Eds.), *Willard and Spackman's occupational therapy* (10th ed., pp. 141-146). Philadelphia: Lippincott, Williams & Wilkins.

Schell, B., Crepeau, E., & Cohn, E. (2003). Professional development. In E. Crepeau, E. Cohn, & B. Schell (Eds.), *Willard and Spackman's occupational therapy* (10th ed., pp. 141-146). Philadelphia: Lippincott, Williams & Wilkins.

Schön, D. (1983). *The reflective practitioner: How professionals think in action*. New York: Basic Books.

Schultz, S. (1992). School based occupational therapy for students with behavior disorders. *Occupational Therapy in Health Care, 8*, 173-196.

Slukin, A. (1981). *Growing up in the playground*. London: Routledge & Kegan Paul.

Sparrow, S., Bolla, D., & Circhetti, D. (1984). *Vineland Adaptive Behavior Scales manual*. Circle Pines, MN: American Guidance Service.

U.S. Department of Health and Human Services. (1999). *Mental health: A report of the surgeon general*. Rockville, MD: Author.

U.S. Department of Health and Human Services. (2005). *Summary health statistics for U.S. adults: National health interview survey, 2003*. Centers for Disease Control and Prevention, National Center for Health Statistics. Hyattsville, MD: Author.

Weiss, M., & Weiss, G. (2002). Attention deficit hyperactivity disorder. In M. Lewis (Ed.), *Child and adolescent psychiatry: A comprehensive textbook* (3rd ed., pp. 670-681). Philadelphia: Lippincott, Williams & Wilkins.

Zigler, E., Finn-Stevenson, M., & Tanner, E. M. (2002). National policies for children, adolescents and families. In M. Lewis (Ed.), *Child and adolescent psychiatry: A comprehensive textbook* (3rd ed., pp. 1340-1352). Philadelphia: Lippincott Williams & Wilkins.

11

Play, Leisure, and Social Participation in Educational Settings

YVONNE SWINTH AND KARI J. TANTA

All I really need to know about how to live and what to do and how to be I learned in Kindergarten. Wisdom was not at the top of the graduate-school mountain, but there in the sandpile at Sunday School. These are the things I learned...Live a balanced life—learn some and think some and draw and paint and sing and dance and play and work every day some...
ROBERT FULGHUM in *All I Really Need to Know I Learned in Kindergarten*

━━ *Clinical Vignettes* ━━

Tyler, a 3-year-old in a developmental program, sits by himself during free choice. He engages in activities only when directed by an adult. He never initiates interactions with peers or models what his peers are doing.

Rebekah, a first grader, enjoys climbing and swinging during recess. When she can participate in such activities, she is able to go back to class and attend to classroom tasks until lunchtime. Her school, however, recently removed all swinging and climbing equipment from the playground because of liability issues.

Reagan, a fourth grader, stands by herself during recess. When asked why she does not go and play with her peers, she shrugs her shoulders and walks away.

Henry, a junior high student, is getting into trouble during "free time" at school and at home. His latest activity of choice is to wander into empty classrooms at school or the rooms of other family members at home and "borrow" small objects. He states he does not know what else to do.

Greg, a 20-year-old in high school, will be graduating in 6 months and plans to live in a group home. His parents and teacher are worried about his lack of leisure skills: "All he does is sit in front of a TV, whether it is on or off. He will wait until someone else turns it on for him."

All of these students lack the ability to participate in activities that are part of the occupational performance areas of play, leisure, and social participation. In turn, this inability is affecting their participation in meaningful school, home, and community routines. Occupational therapists who work in educational settings typically feel that they are limited to addressing academic needs, such as literacy and functional academics, or skills that directly influence academic achievement, such as visual-perceptual, visual-motor, or fine motor skills. Contrary to this more traditional approach to occupational therapy in educational settings, however, occupational therapists should be considering all areas of a student's occupational performance, including participation in play, leisure, and social participation. Play is powerful and deserves a place within each child's educational program.

Robert Fulghum's simple, yet profound poem "All I Really Need to Know I Learned in Kindergarten" strikes a chord for the power of play, which is in harmony with the belief that not only do children learn through play, but play, leisure, and social participation are important areas of occupation throughout a person's life. The skills that are gained and mastered through play are essential for the roles, habits, and routines individuals perform throughout life as members of society.

Other chapters in this book have defined play and leisure and have discussed the role of the occupational therapist in such areas as assessment, intervention, and the use of assistive technology to address play and leisure. In this chapter we do not repeat these definitions or strategies. Rather, we contribute strategies whereby occupational therapists working in educational settings can address play and leisure as a means, as well as an end, of occupational therapy in educational settings. Emphasis is on effectively using the skills and expertise of the occupational therapist as part of the educational team to ensure the best outcomes for the students served. In addition, the occupation of social participation is addressed, since this skill is often developed and reinforced through play and leisure activities.

BACKGROUND

Evolution, psychology, physiology, and sociology all present long-standing theoretical bases that note the existence and effects of play behavior. The early studies of evolution, which focused on animal behavior, have been joined by theories based in the study of human development. These theories include sociological views that address issues of roles (Reilly, 1974) and social participation (Parten, 1932) and psychological perspectives that identify play in terms of cognitive development (Piaget, 1962; Vygotsky, 1976). Play has also been studied from a physiological viewpoint by the examination of metabolic energy uses (Johnson, Christie, & Yawkey, 1987). Occupational therapy has drawn from these theories, and the role of play within occupational therapy practice has emerged from these foundations (Bundy, 1991; Daub, 1988; Florey, 1981; Kielhofner & Miyake, 1981; Llorens, 1974; Pratt, 1989; Reilly, 1974). Bundy (1993) suggested that play is a paradox: "play is also different from other occupations because it is not considered serious or real; it is not thought of as productive" (p. 218). This paradox seems to be most prevalent when occupational therapy services are provided in educational settings. Despite a wealth of research and other publications articulating the importance of play and leisure as occupations, evidence suggests that in educational settings play and leisure skills are seldom assessed or addressed through goals and objectives. Either play and leisure skill development is undervalued and underutilized, or interventions are casual and undocumented (this may be referred to as "underground practice [Fleming & Mattingly, 1994, p. 295]") rather than being an explicit part of a student's program (Neville-Jan, Fazio, Kennedy, & Snyder, 1997; Swinth, 2004; Swinth & Tanta, 2003; Tanta, Deitz, White, & Billingsly, 2005).

For infants, toddlers, and preschool children, play is the primary occupation and can be complex to evaluate. In addition, depending on the needs of the child, successful intervention requires a conscious team effort. Several researchers (e.g., Greenspan & Wieder, 1998) have recog-

nized the importance of play and have developed specific intervention strategies that will enhance a child's ability to participate in this occupation. For older children and adolescents, leisure skills have received less attention. Play and leisure activities, however, may be some of the "purest expressions of who we are as persons" and should be given emphasis equal to other areas of occupational performance during the occupational therapy process (Bundy, 1993, p. 217).

Recognition of the importance of play and leisure skills by occupational therapists does not appear to be an issue. Developing strategies for teaching specific play and leisure skills as part of occupational therapy intervention and articulating the importance of such intervention to team members seem to be challenges for therapists working in educational settings.

SCHOOLS AND PLAY, LEISURE, AND SOCIAL PARTICIPATION

School systems are the largest employer of occupational therapists, with approximately 30% of therapists working in educational settings (American Occupational Therapy Association [AOTA], 2003). Continued employment growth for school-based occupational therapists is anticipated because of an increase in both numbers of school-aged children and extended services for children with disabilities in school settings (U.S. Department of Labor and Statistics, 2001). Often occupational therapists who work in school settings address the occupation of student by emphasizing such skills as fine motor, visual-perceptual, and visual-motor abilities. In addition, however, school-based occupational therapists need to address and educate fellow team members about the importance of play and leisure skill development (Daub, 1988; Kielhofner, 1995) as an end, as well as a means of supporting foundational skills such as social participation, psychosocial health, and vocational skills.

Interestingly, an ongoing discussion in the education literature regards the use of play to support cognitive, emotional, and social development in young children (Farran & Son-Yarbrough, 2001; Guralnik & Hammond, 1999; Hestenes & Carroll, 2000; Rubin & Coplan, 1998). Even though the research indicates that play activities support learning in younger children, the current emphasis on accountability and high-stake testing (use of test scores to make critical decisions about education), which has resulted from recent education reform, has led to a decrease in play activities and playtime in early childhood curricula (Bergen, 2001). For elementary age children, with and without disabilities, the consequence is a decline in the number and the length of recess opportunities and a reduction in class "free choice" time. For junior high and high school students the academic demands continue to increase, often at the expense of elective classes (e.g., pottery, drafting, art, drama) that may support future leisure activities. Furthermore, because of these academic demands, students are spending more time after school completing homework rather than engaging in other leisure time activities such as socializing with peers. The potentially negative consequences of this trend are being studied, and current brain research repudiates such practices (Jensen, 1998).

Brink (1995) found that novel motor activities, such as those that occur during play and active leisure activities, increase brain growth and cognitive functions throughout a student's life. Several researchers have shown that a "constant interplay" (Jensen, 1998, p. 84) occurs between movement and learning, since both are processed in the same parts of the brain (Figure 11-1). Several studies have actually demonstrated an increase in test scores when movement and sensorimotor integration activities were part of the academic curriculum (Gilbert, 1977; Hannaford, 1995; Houston, 1982; Kearney, 1996). In many educational settings, movement activities most often occur during play and leisure opportunities such as recess and gym class. Such times for engagement in movement enhance academic learning and foster growth in other areas as well.

During play and leisure time children are afforded chances to develop social skills and emotional competence (Figure 11-2). These skills are critical to roles in adulthood (Jensen, 1998). For adults, social (or emotional) maturity may make the difference between success and failure in many employment, volunteer, or recreational activities (Goleman, 1995). Furthermore, lack of social (or emotional) competence may have negative effects on an individual's ability to develop and sustain relationships with others. Engagement in play and leisure activities crosses developmental domains and is essential for success both inside and outside the educational system.

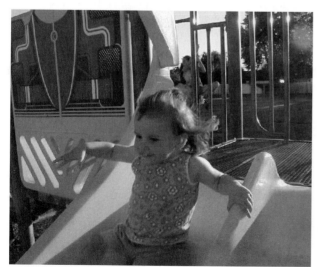

Figure 11-1
Slides can help support sensorimotor skill development.

WHY PLAY?

Play is considered to be developmentally and culturally relevant for all children (Reynolds & Jones, 1997). Few would dispute that children spend the majority of their time in play (Neville-Jan et al., 1997). Play (including but not limited to social interaction, pretend play, and physical activity) is an essential element in the development of a child and an educationally relevant domain for instruction (Bergen, 2001; Jensen, 1998). Reynolds and Jones (1997) proposed that mastering play skills is as important as mastering language and other academic skills. Hartley and Goldenson (as cited in Florey, 1981) indicated that professionals should be as concerned when a child cannot play as they are when a child does not eat or sleep.

As the "work" of children (Burke, 1993; Cherry, 1976; Simon & Daub, 1993) and one of the most elaborate occupations of humans (Royeen, 1997), play stimulates growth and learning (Illinois State Board of Education, 1994; Klugman, 1997; Reynolds & Jones, 1997) and prepares children for future engagement in adult role behaviors. Play is both skill and attitude (Ferland, 1997) and can be an influential medium for learning. Play should be included in the public school curriculum, yet its place within such institutions is far from being defined.

THE PROBLEM

Educators and other professionals have long recognized the importance of play and attempted to integrate play and leisure skills into educational settings. Froebel developed the German Kindergarten based on the philosophy of play, and Montessori also based an educational program on the importance of child-directed activities and play. More recently, however, many educators have come to perceive play as educationally irrelevant and developmentally trivial (Elkind, 1990; Robinson, 1977; Rubin, 1980; Scales, Almy, Nicolopoulou, & Ervin-Tripp, 1991). With the recent trends toward high-stake testing within the U.S. school system, as well as budget cuts in schools, play and leisure development has been removed even further from the school day. Many schools have decreased the number of elementary school recesses from two or three per day to one. Even in the early school years, when play is most likely to be prevalent in classrooms, instructional priority is given to goals and objectives that are drawn from developmental assessments primarily emphasizing skills other than play (Fewell & Kaminski, 1988). In the past, few educational researchers would have disagreed that play has a valued role in the educational process (Krasnor & Pepler, 1980), but currently play appears to be nonexistent in more academically oriented classrooms and curricula (Genishi, 1991; Reynolds & Jones, 1997) and opportunities for active engagement are few.

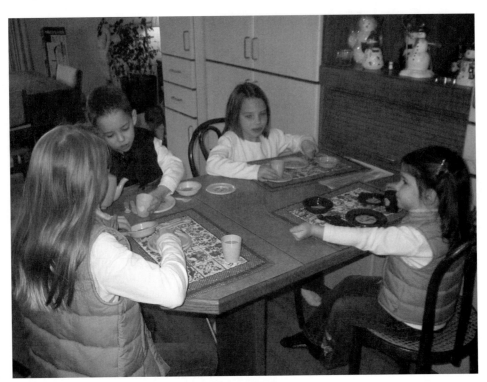

Figure 11-2
Children playing together.

Children often learn best through active play, yet they are frequently required to learn through passive activities (Humphrey & Humphrey, 1980; Jensen, 1998) under the assumption that learning takes place only through adult-directed teaching (Klugman, 1997). Reynolds and Jones (1997) suggested that this assumption may be wrong, since adult-directed teaching methods may not provide children with adequate opportunities to develop other important abilities such as initiative, problem solving, and innovation. All children need to develop play behaviors so that they may realize these higher order thinking skills, and efforts to promote the inclusion of these elements in the curriculum are needed.

Changes in public school curricula at the state and national levels may also be contributing to the disparities between historical and current views of play as parents and legislators push for reform and teaching the "basics" (Beardsly, 1991; Grubb, 1991; Scales et al., 1991; Smith, 1991; Washington State Commission on Student Learning, 1997). Research conducted by Rothlein and Brett (1987) indicated that many parents and teachers view play as having little value and believe that children do not need much playtime. In addition, teachers were noted to describe play and learning as distinctly separate activities. The evolution of kindergarten from a predominantly play-based learning experience toward structured academics is a prime illustration of such trends. These findings are of concern considering the evidence that play is an essential component of human development and is linked to, not separate from, learning new skills and behaviors.

Prominent educational philosopher John Dewey (1928) saw no antagonism between play and learning. His writings are still widely used in the preparation of educational personnel and are considered applicable today. Sociologists have argued that play, along with education, is a critical vehicle for social transformation and that it is imperative for all to learn to play (Reilly, 1974). Considering the rapid changes in the world and demands for knowledge and skills that are sensitive to the human condition, it is apparent that play and learning must be addressed together within the educational curriculum.

SCHOOL PROGRAMS: CONTENT, PROGRAM PLANNING, AND TRANSITION PLANNING

What role should play have within educational curricula? Smith (1991) quoted California School Superintendent Bill Honig (before the 1988 release of the California School Readiness Task Force Reports): "While it is important for children to learn basic skills, the teaching techniques and the curriculum must be balanced between child-centered activities and content-centered approaches that are appropriate for each child." Indeed we need a holistic approach to education, realistic goals for practice that value play, and educational contexts that support the development of play and leisure skills (Genishi, 1991; Reynolds & Jones, 1997).

One example of a school system model that has embraced play is that of the State of Illinois. The Illinois State Board of Education (1994) stated that school programs should aspire to assist children to acquire greater independence; learn to generalize skills across environments; gain social competence; and develop language, cognitive, motor, and self-help skills. In addition, the curriculum should be based in play and a successful school program must adopt a "child-centered" focus in the following ways:

1. A focus on developmental, not academic, goals
2. An emphasis on conceptual, not rote, learning to allow generalization
3. The use of natural, *play-based* settings
4. A view of children as active participants in the learning process
5. The promotion of *social interaction* through an emphasis on cooperation, rather than competition
6. A regard for the importance of stimulating growth in all developmental areas: intellectual, physical, emotional, *social and play*, self-help, language, and motor

Integral to these proposed elements, curricula should include the development of higher order skills, as discussed by Reynolds and Jones (1997). Initiative, problem solving, and innovation are skills possessed by skilled players. Children with these abilities are able to manage their own behaviors within social boundaries, recognize trends in information and experience, apply order to unstructured situations, and relate acquired knowledge and experiences to new situations. These are the skills required of successful, contributing members of society.

WHAT HAPPENS WHEN A STUDENT CANNOT PLAY?

The ease with which a child may learn to play and subsequently learn from play may be influenced by a variety of factors. When considering play, leisure, and social participation as aspects of occupation, the therapist can first identify factors that may be inhibiting a child's success and then design an appropriate intervention plan. Careful attention should be paid to the diversity of student learning styles and educational needs as they relate to play or leisure. To address play and leisure in relation to occupational therapy involvement in curriculum planning and implementation, we highlight four main issues: disability, social context, life skills, and transition planning.

Children with Disabilities

Children with disabilities have commonly been depicted as having types of play similar to their peers without disabilities, but with play repertoires and proficiencies that are often described as less well developed, less organized, and less varied (Bundy, 1989; Desha, Ziviani, & Rodger, 2003; Fewell & Kaminski, 1988; Harrison & Kielhofner, 1986; Howard, 1996; Linder, 1993; Restall & Magill-Evans, 1994). Their play skills may be limited by features or barriers related to their disabilities.

Barriers to the development of play behaviors in children with disabilities may occur in multiple ways: overdependence on caregiver; physical, psychological, or sensory limitations; environmental restrictions; or decreased social interactions (Missiuna & Pollock, 1991; Royeen, 1997). These obstacles to engagement in play activities may result in secondary disabilities such as increased dependence, decreased imagination, poor social skills, and lack of motivation (Missiuna & Pollock, 1991).

Barriers to play can result in learned helplessness. Learned helplessness is a secondary disability that can affect the functional skills and interactions of children with developmental delays. Learned helplessness is the individual's belief that he or she cannot exert control over outcomes experienced when interacting with the environment (Abramson, Seligman, & Teasdale, 1978; Gargiulo & O'Sullivan, 1986; Maier & Seligman, 1976; Weisz, 1979). When children perceive that they have little control over outcomes, motivational, cognitive, and emotional deficits result. They may develop low self-esteem, directly affecting how they interact and perform in the environment. They usually demonstrate a lack of initiation and an inability to cope with the events around them. In these instances educational interventions are needed to help children circumvent the aspects of their disabilities and environments that limit meaningful engagement in play, so that they may avoid secondary disabilities resulting from play deprivation (Missiuna & Pollock, 1991).

Research has shown that children with disabilities can be taught play skills that will be generalized across play situations (Ballard & Medland, 1986; Eason, White, & Newsom, 1982; Goldstein & Cisar, 1992; LeGoff, 2004; Lifter, Sulzer-Azaroff, Anderson, & Cowdery, 1993; Rogers, 2000). Such data lend support to instructional programs and objectives that address the development of play skills. In this manner the inclusion of play throughout the curriculum, for all students, is a realistic and necessary goal of curriculum planning.

Social Context

A deficit in play skill does not necessarily indicate a deficit in playfulness and vice versa. A child with a disability may have difficulty physically engaging in play or leisure activities and yet have a playful attitude toward life. Moreover, an activity that is play for one child may not be play for another. In addition, not all children and families value particular school-based play or leisure activities to the same extent. For some families it may be important that their child participate in school clubs, dances, sports, and other extracurricular activities. For others it may not. The occupational therapist must consider what is important to the child, family, and school when planning intervention.

Over the years, anthropologists and researchers have recognized that play and leisure are "genetically based and culturally modifiable" (Mohr-Modes, 2003, p. 1). Since play and leisure exploration and participation have a strong cultural component, the occupational therapist should take the time to hear from those in the child's or youth's environment who can provide insight into what is appropriate and culturally acceptable. This includes input from the teacher and other individuals within the educational setting.

Not all cultures value play in the same way, and the play of children may vary widely depending on their cultural context (Stahl, 1995). Cultural beliefs significantly influence play, so curriculum planning must begin with an understanding of the cultural background of the students to be served (Polk, 1994). To ascertain if a student is really deficient in play skills, educators need to know how play is viewed by the student and the community, taking the initiative to put play into the appropriate cultural context.

A qualitative study found that the social environment appeared to be one of the critical factors supporting play participation for adolescents with developmental disabilities (Pollock, Stewart, Law, Harvey, Sahagian, & Toal, 1997). This underscores the point that occupational therapists should ensure that an adequate assessment of the social environment (community and school) is part of the evaluation process and intervention.

Life Skills

The prevalence of play within the school environment typically decreases dramatically after the elementary years. The importance of knowledge learned through early play experiences, however, influences success in later school years as well as in life beyond the school years. Some advantages to the early acquisition of play skills that extend beyond school have been identified. These include improved social skills (Chadsey-Rusch & Heal, 1995), positive self-esteem (Whitney-Thomas & Hanley-Maxwell, 1996), and the development of higher order cognitive skills (Wilson & Sindelar, 1991). Higher order cognitive skills include the ability to take initiative, solve complex problems, and think critically. Employers typically seek individuals who are creative, culturally sensitive team players. Play offers a venue for the development of these skills. The need to address such skills throughout the school curriculum means the inclusion of play within life skills courses and job training opportunities for older students.

Transition Planning

The Individuals with Disabilities Education Improvement Act (IDEA, 2004) emphasizes the importance of developing a comprehensive transition plan for students with disabilities by the age of 16. One aspect of this plan should address the students' leisure skills in both current and future environments. The purpose of transition planning is to ensure that when students with disabilities graduate from high school, they are prepared for all aspects of life beyond the educational setting. As noted earlier, leisure skills not only support what a student does during free time, but also help a student develop important social skills that support occupational performance in other contextual settings such as community and work.

OCCUPATIONAL THERAPY PROCESS IN THE EDUCATIONAL SETTING

Within the educational setting, occupational therapists should use the occupational therapy process outlined in the Occupational Therapy Practice Framework (AOTA, 2002) to guide decision making in evaluation, intervention, and outcome determination when addressing play and leisure skills, as well as broader issues surrounding social participation. Although this process is frequently presented as linear, in reality each step often overlaps with one or more subsequent steps. It should also be noted that this process closely parallels the special education process as outlined in the IDEA (2004). That is, each process includes the need to gather qualitative information regarding the client, complete an evaluation, design intervention, and evaluate outcomes. The following sections briefly summarize the occupational therapy process, specific to play, leisure pursuits, and social participation as related to the educational setting.

Occupational Profile

According to the Framework (AOTA, 2002), the first step in the occupational therapy process is the development of the *occupational profile*. Through this step the therapist determines the need(s) of the client (e.g., parent, child, teacher, educational system), the reason that service is being sought, the occupations or activities that are successful and problematic, and the client's hopes, priorities, and targeted outcomes. The development of the occupational profile is a collaborative process that includes the child or youth (when appropriate), the family, and other individuals (e.g., teachers, caregivers, and community providers) who are part of the student's school, home, and possibly community environment. The occupational therapist needs to identify any history and experiences with play and leisure activities, as well as hopes, interests, values, and needs in this area. This is particularly critical when working with the educational team serving high school students and in preparing to develop the transition plan. As mentioned earlier, according to the IDEA (2004), the transition plan should include current and future leisure pursuits.

Box 11-1 summarizes some questions the occupational therapist who is developing an occupational profile with a focus on play or leisure might ask the child or youth, the family, and other professionals who are part of the environment. Gathering these data supports the development of a comprehensive analysis of occupational performance. It also enables the occupational therapy practitioner to address the "whole" child or youth.

Analysis of Occupational Performance

To complete the analysis of occupational performance, the occupational therapist must build on the information from the occupational profile by gathering additional data collected through a variety of assessment strategies. These may include methods (e.g., observations, review of records, interviews) or measures (e.g., standardized tests, range of motion measurements). The therapist interprets these data to identify the supports for and barriers to performance in play, leisure, and social participation. Within the educational environment it is often difficult to complete an occupational profile independent of the analysis of occupational performance. Thus these two steps in the process commonly occur concurrently.

The IDEA (2004) does not require standardized testing as part of the analysis of occupational performance. More often, assessment strategies such as skilled observation,

interviews, and record reviews are used. Ideally, to gain an accurate view of a student's play or leisure proficiency and social participation skills, performance should be observed in a variety of settings and activities, including indoor and outdoor play with adults and peers. Also important are observing the student during independent play and looking at play environments, the student's playfulness, the variety of opportunities available for play, the availability of playmates, and the frequency of opportunities for play activities. For older children the therapist should address performance skills (e.g., coordination of motor movements, ability to follow directions, self-regulation and level of arousal, ability to respond to environmental cues appropriately, social interactions) and patterns (e.g., specific habits, routines that are supporting or interfering with performance) related to play and adult leisure skills that will influence social functioning and employment.

In addition to skilled observation and other nonstandardized assessment tools, a comprehensive look at performance may require a more formal approach to assessment through the use of specific tools. As discussed in Chapters 2 through 6 in this book, numerous tools and taxonomies are available. Couch, Deitz, and Kanny (1998) found that if therapists did not explicitly assess a child's play skills, they were less likely to provide intervention in that area. Thus effective assessment is a key part of the evaluation process in these areas and should not be neglected.

If observation is the primary method for assessing play or leisure exploration and participation, therapists should be systematic regarding the data gathered. In a school environment many of the same skills are assessed as in other environments such as home and community. These may include the following:

How does the child or youth address social problem-solving skills such as sharing, taking turns, negotiating, and setting goals?

Can the child or youth access play or leisure toys or tools?

Can the child or youth access play or leisure environments of interest?

How does the child or youth react to being bullied?

Can the child or youth self-regulate to appropriately explore and participate in play or leisure activities?

Assessment tools that are specific to the educational setting and can address curriculum, environment, and student progress are available. The School Function Assessment (SFA) (Coster, Deeney, Haltiwanger, & Haley, 1998) and the Sensory Processing Measure (SPM) school forms (Miller-Kuhaneck, Henry, & Glennon, 2007) are examples of these. A portion of the SFA centers on playground and recess activities, looking at cooperation, game play, support for play, and social interactions. Box 11-2 is one occupational therapist's reflections on the SPM school forms (Parham, Ecker, Miller-Kuhaneck, Henry, & Glennoa, 2007) and on play and leisure in the schools.

Box 11-1 *Occupational Profile Questions*

1. What are the concerns relative to the child's or youth's ability to explore and participate in appropriate play, leisure, and social participation activities?
2. What are the child's, youth's, family's, or others' hopes regarding play, leisure, and social participation?
3. What are the strengths and weaknesses during play, leisure, and social participation activities?
4. What contexts support the engagement in exploration and participation in appropriate play, leisure, and social participation, and what contexts inhibit engagement?
5. What is the occupational history specific to exploration and participation in appropriate play, leisure, and social participation activities?
6. What are priorities and desired outcomes?

Modified from Swinth, Y. L., & Tanta, K. (2003). Play and leisure skill development in school-based practice. In Swinth, Y.L. (Ed.), *AOTA online course: Occupational therapy in school-based practice: Contemporary issues and trends.* Bethesda, MD: American Occupational Therapy Association.

Box 11-2 *Reflections Regarding the SPM School Form*

As an OT, I have a more complete understanding of the student's occupation...not only from a sensory motor and sensory processing perspective but also in social participation. This is why we included recess and playground as one of the environments rated by school staff in the Sensory Processing Measure (SPM). One student who was under responsive and a sensory seeker, was always getting into trouble on the playground because he would crash into others while playing ball (could not grade his movements). The school staff, including the playground assistant, decided to include heavy work activities into all their "ecological niches" and curricular activities for this student...including carrying the big box of heavy playground equipment for recess. Another student was referred because of social participation issues related to aggression and self isolation including on the playground. Using the SPM, we found her to have praxis issues, especially ideation difficulties as well as sensory over-responsivity. This caused her to be "lost" and overwhelmed during recess, not knowing how to join in play with her peers. The OT and school staff joined in to help her in recess by developing a circle of friends to play with her, initially designating a smaller quieter space to play. The same strategies were then used by the rest of the staff resulting in the student's improvement in her ability to function throughout the educational program.

Intervention

Development of sensorimotor, language, and social skills is considered a prerequisite to the acquisition of "master" play and leisure skills (Reynolds & Jones, 1997). The inclusion of adults and peers is an important component in the promotion of skill development. Ongoing teacher training, parent education, community networking, and interdisciplinary collaboration are needed to successfully incorporate play and leisure into the curriculum and to ensure the generalization of such skills beyond the classroom. Occupational therapists are not the only members of the team who may address play and leisure skills. The teacher, psychologist, or counselor may also promote skill acquisition in these areas. Furthermore, other professionals such as the speech language pathologist or physical therapist may use play in their interventions (Swinth & Tanta, 2003). Thus the occupational therapist works closely with other appropriate team members to design, implement, and evaluate intervention.

After the evaluation has been completed, the data are interpreted and information is shared with the team and incorporated into the Individual Family Service Plan (IFSP) or the Individualized Education Program (IEP). The occupational therapist and team should determine whether play or leisure will be used as a means or an end (Bundy, 1993). If the therapist is addressing play and leisure as an end, specific play-oriented goals and objectives should be developed. If these skills are addressed as a means, they are included in the occupational therapy intervention plan but may not have play-specific goals and objectives on the IFSP or IEP (Swinth & Tanta, 2003).

When other team members will also be addressing play and leisure skills, the occupational therapist collaborates with the team to determine if and how the unique skills and expertise of the occupational therapist can be used to support student outcomes. The occupational therapist may or may not provide direct intervention. If the therapist is not providing direct intervention, he or she may work more in a collaborative or facilitative role. This may include gathering and implementing appropriate adaptive equipment or environmental design to support play or leisure participation. It may also include helping with curriculum adaptations that support both play or leisure and social participation. For example, an occupational therapist may collaborate with a school counselor or a school psychologist to design and run a social group for third-grade girls, including girls with disabilities. Table 11-1 summarizes intervention considerations based on a student's developmental age and play characteristics.

The role of an adult in the process of facilitating play skills and establishing social play sequences is critical for modeling, questioning, introducing, and maintaining skills (Blanche, 1997; Krasnor & Pepler, 1980). A playful therapist is needed to foster playfulness in a child. A skillful therapist creates "just right challenges" (Koomar & Bundy, 1991) and provides learning opportunities for children within an enriching environment (Reynolds & Jones, 1997). Such occasions set the stage for the attainment or enhancement of play skills, which in turn provide the base for the acquisition of other skills, such as problem solving, conceptualization, independence, and creativity, that are required in the typical academic curriculum. Such academic gains will provide further validation for the inclusion of play as an instructional target in school programs.

Peers can be included in the intervention to serve as models of basic skills and partners for cooperative play experiences. Methods for promoting play behaviors through peer involvement can include the use of sociodramatic play scripts (Goldstein & Cisar, 1992), social skills training groups (Kamps et al., 1992), affection activities (McEvoy et al., 1988), peer monitoring of interaction skills (Dougherty, Fowler, & Paine, 1985), and vocational skills training activities.

When basic play skills are taught to a child with disabilities, the child's developmental level is an important consideration, regardless of the method of intervention. Lifter et al. (1993) described one such developmentally

Table 11-1
Intervention Considerations

Age Range	Play Characteristics	Intervention Considerations
Birth to 3 years	Shift from sensorimotor play behaviors of infancy to locomotor play (large muscle groups, e.g., running and jumping) Object play Social play Fantasy, symbolic, and pretend play Increased complexity in the second year	Parent, child, and environment (home, school center, playground) Parent-child-therapist interactions Lots of consultation, parent education Appropriate toys and tools available
Preschool	Practice and exploratory play Increased coordination Longer attention span More complex dramatization Social and peer play more prevalent Move from associative (parallel) to cooperative play Increased role playing Construction play predominates Props for play important	Interactions with other students Play groups School and playground accessibility Child-therapist-peer play Consultation with parents and teachers Recess Appropriate toys and tools available
Elementary school (middle childhood)	Recess is games period Games with rules predominate Constructive play more focused on end product Cooperation and competition Friends (making and keeping) Wanting to be liked Dramatic play (school plays)	Interactions with other students Transition to and from recess Direct therapy in groups Consult with child, teacher, and family Appropriate toys and tools available Environmental supports
Junior high	Success in peer groups Conformance to group norms "Best friends" Good understanding of group rules and increased flexibility Clubs—after-school cafeteria Socially competent player Peers important Achievement	Transition Peers Groups Consultation or direct collaboration with teacher Other students Appropriate tools available Environmental supports
High school	Achievement Socially competent player Sports and clubs Move to adulthood and adult leisure skills Activities more for amusement, spontaneous enjoyment, and self-expression Dating Work toward independent groups and leisure Leisure occupations selected now may become permanent part of a person's life	Transition Peers Groups Consultation Leisure counseling Appropriate tools available Environmental supports

Modified from Swinth, Y. L., & Tanta, K. (2003). Play and leisure skill development in school-based practice. In Swinth, Y. L (Ed.), *AOTA online course: Occupational therapy in school-based practice: Contemporary issues and trends*. Bethesda, MD: American Occupational Therapy Association.

appropriate strategy to successfully teach "doll as agent" play skills to preschool children with autism. In this method the child receives instruction and modeling in using a doll as an agent to complete an activity. The teaching is conducted primarily when the child is looking at or in physical contact with the doll. The adult scaffolds the prompts as follows:

1. Wait a few seconds to see if the child responds without a prompt.
2. Bring a second, complementary doll and materials (such as a cup, brush, or tissue) into view, and again wait for a response.
3. Guide the child through the desired action in a hand-over-hand manner.
4. Gradually fade any prompts until independence and generalization have been achieved.

This scaffold allows teaching to occur at the individual child's developmental stage. Within the school setting, similar scaffolding should occur. For example, when working with a child during recess, the therapist may need to use scaffolding such as the following:

1. Observe and wait a few seconds to see if the child responds without a prompt.
2. Bring the child over to a piece of playground equipment or near a group of peers, and again wait for a response.
3. Guide the child through the desired action through verbal cues or a hand-over-hand manner (e.g., help the child climb on the jungle gym).

4. Gradually fade any prompts until independence and generalization have been achieved.

Intervention Considerations

A variety of factors must be considered in the design and implementation of an occupational therapy intervention plan. The following sections address some of these considerations specific to the educational setting. Other chapters in this book discuss intervention in greater detail. Many of these discussions can be generalized to the educational setting as well. This chapter briefly describes occupational therapy service delivery models, intervention on the playground and during recess, assistive technology and toys and other equipment, and extracurricular activities.

Service Delivery

Although hands-on, direct therapy activities are commonly used to address play or leisure as an end, this service delivery model is not always the most effective. Occupational therapists may better use their skills and expertise to support identified student outcomes by working with others on the team or addressing issues within the system (Figure 11-3). Thus, when addressing play or leisure skills in an educational setting, the occupational therapist may have the teacher (or some other professional or parent) or the system as his or her "client," while providing services "on behalf of the child" (AOTA, 2002; IDEA, 2004). Table 11-2

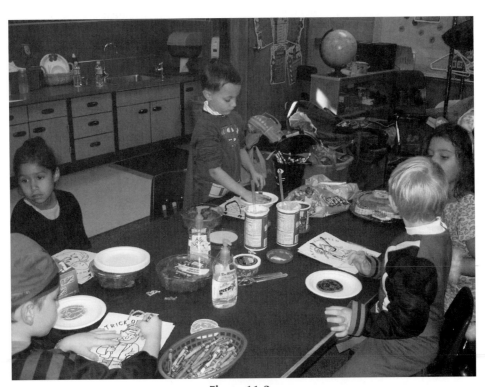

Figure 11-3
Helping a teacher set up a Halloween play activity can support motor and cognitive skill development.

Table 11-2
Play and Leisure Intervention: Who Is the Client?

Performance Skill	Student	Teacher, Parent, Other School Professionals	System
Motor skills	Does the child or youth have the postural, mobility, strength, and coordination skills needed for the task? Can he or she access toys or leisure tools and the environment? If not, see Considerations for Occupational Therapy below.	Do the environments (community, playground, and classroom), task, and expectations need to be adapted or modified to meet the child's or youth's needs? Are teachers, parents, and other professionals aware of appropriate play or leisure tools? Are teachers, parents, and other professionals aware of community linkages to support play and leisure participation? If so, see Considerations for Occupational Therapy below.	Does the center or district have a curriculum to address the child's or youth's needs? Is the environment (e.g., playground) accessible? Are there appropriate and accessible toys or leisure tools? If no, see Considerations for Occupational Therapy below.
Process skills	Does the child or youth have the skills to manage and modify his or her play or leisure exploration and participation? If not, see Considerations for Occupational Therapy below.	Do teaching methods and expectations need to be modified or adapted to meet the child's or youth's needs? Are there aspects within the environment that interfere with the child's ability to explore and participate in play or leisure activities? If so, see Considerations for Occupational Therapy below.	Is the curriculum accessible to the child? Are there appropriate and accessible toys or leisure tools? If not, see Considerations for Occupational Therapy below.
Communication and interaction skills	Does the child have the skills to communicate intentions and needs and interact with others? If not, see Considerations for Occupational Therapy below.	Do home or classroom rules, expectations, and routines need to be modified to meet the child's needs? If so, see Considerations for Occupational Therapy below.	Is there a school-wide or district-wide discipline program that supports student performance, teaches appropriate behavior, and creates a positive school climate? If not, see Considerations for Occupational Therapy below.
Considerations for Occupational Therapy	Consider direct services to support skill acquisition and performance.	Consider working with the teacher, parent, and other school professionals to solve problems and establish appropriate adaptations, accommodations, and modifications.	Consider working with the system to address environmental adaptations, acquisition of appropriate toys and tools, or curriculum needs.

This is not meant to be an exhaustive list of interventions. There will be variations depending on the unique needs of the system, classroom, and student.
Modified from Swinth, Y. L, & Handley-More, D. (2004). Elective Session 8: Handwriting, keyboarding, and literacy: What is the role of occupational therapy? In Y. L. Swinth (Ed.), *AOTA online course: Occupational therapy in school-based practice: Contemporary issues and trends.* Bethesda, MD: American Occupational Therapy Association.

lists questions the therapist can ask when making decisions about intervention with the various possible clients.

Playgrounds and Recess

As discussed earlier in this chapter, the amount of time that recess is available to children in schools has decreased markedly. In fact, according to the American Association for the Child's Right to Play, since 1989 many schools have abolished recess. This may be a result of safety and liability concerns as well as curricular demands and increased instructional accountability (Jarrett, 2003; Pellegrini, 1985). On the playground children are able to experiment with motor skills and sensory experiences and practice social play with peers through games. Recess is an important time for children to practice developmental skills and to "let off steam" so that they can return to schoolwork with increased concentration. Many social skills, such as taking turns and negotiating, are learned on the playground. Occupational therapists can promote playground and recess skills by collaborating with school staff about playground design and the benefits of recess (Figure 11-4). An accessible playground offers opportunities for skill acquisition, sensory exploration, social interaction, and physical exercise. For children with attention and sensory issues, recess and the playground are two of the most powerful sensory tools available at school.

Results of a recent study indicated that only about 50% of therapists working in schools provide intervention on the playground. Reasons given for not doing so included the time needed to get ready to go outside, weather, pressure to meet goals in other areas, and safety and liability concerns. The respondents in this study, however, recognized the value of working on the playground to address sensory and psychosocial needs (Knight, 2003).

Occupational therapists can work with school administrators to ensure that playgrounds are accessible, safe, and responsive to the sensorimotor needs of students. This may result in improved academic performance and classroom behavior. Box 11-3 gives one principal's thoughts regarding an accessible playground for all students. Box 11-4 addresses playground safety considerations, and Box 11-5 lists Internet resources addressing accessible playgrounds.

Assistive Technology, Toys, and Other Equipment

Other chapters in this book discuss the importance of assistive technology (Chapter 16) and equipment that supports play and leisure skills (Chapter 17). Each of these discussions is important and applicable to the educational setting. For some students assistive technology may be the only venue through which they can participate in play and leisure activities. In addition, the use of technological devices such as the Game Boy and iPOD is part of the play and leisure repertoire of students without disabilities. Occupational therapists may need to collaborate with teachers, parents, and others regarding the selection of appropriate toys and

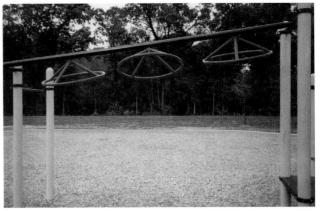

Figure 11-4
Adding specialized play equipment such as these spinning monkey bars helps to support sensory development, as well as play and social participation.

Box 11-3   *One Principal's Thoughts*

I worked with the occupational therapist at my school to redesign our playground. We added different equipment that supported the sensory needs of different students, such as spinning, climbing, and swinging. There was concern regarding falling and safety, but we put down a new surface. After updating our playground, we provided inservice training for our teachers and staff regarding safe use of the equipment and the importance of play and movement to support behavior, learning, and social skills. Many of our teachers reported a decrease in behavior problems such as distractibility.

Box 11-4   *Playground Safety Considerations*

Check to ensure that the equipment is a safe height.
Ensure that there are guard rails where needed (e.g., suspension bridges, decks on climbing toys).
Check for protrusions and sharp edges.
Avoid hard swing seats.
Make sure there are no areas where heads could get stuck or where fingers or extremities could be pinched or crushed.
Use a safe surface under playground equipment, such as organic mulch, wood chips, shredded rubber tires, or a commercially prepared surface.

Box 11-5   *Resources on the Web for Accessible Playgrounds*

www.gametime.com
www.playgroundgallery.com
www.playdesigns.com
www.access-board.gov/play/guide/intro.htm
www.insideoutplayground.org

Table 11-3
Outcomes for Play and Leisure Exploration and Participation

Types of Outcomes	Examples
Occupational performance	Student has improved ability to play. Student is able to participate in leisure activities with peers. Student is able to explore new play or leisure activities. Student is able to access play or leisure toys and tools. Student is able to access play or leisure environments.
Client satisfaction	Student is excited about new skill. Parents are pleased with student's progress. Student is motivated to play or participate in leisure activities.
Role competence	Student is able to meet the demands required of a preschooler. Student is able to participate as a fourth grader. Student is able to complete leisure activities.
Adaptation	Family knows how to adapt toys and tools for play or leisure activities. Teacher is able to adapt the classroom environment for play activities. School has adapted the playground for student access. Student is able to adapt a new play activity independently.
Health and wellness	Student is able to maintain psychosocial health in school.
Prevention	School develops a curriculum to address play or leisure skills for students with disabilities.
Quality of life	Student demonstrates self-determination skills across all environments and with unfamiliar adults. Student does not demonstrate play deprivation. Student is able to participate with peers across school and community environments.

Modified from Swinth, Y. L., & Frolek Clark, G. (2003). Overview of the *Occupational Therapy Practice Framework: Domain and Process* in school-based practice and other considerations. In Y. L. Swinth (Ed.), *AOTA online course: Occupational therapy in school-based practice: Contemporary issues and trends.* Bethesda, MD: American Occupational Therapy Association.

equipment to support the development of play and leisure skills. Such occupational therapy services may be more effectively provided through collaborative activities than by the traditional direct hands-on approach.

Extracurricular Activities
IDEA (2004) calls for supporting a student's involvement in extracurricular activities. This is another area in which an occupational therapist can promote the development of play or leisure skills. For example, a student with severe athetoid cerebral palsy lettered in football throughout his 4 years in high school. Although he could not play football, he wrote a majority of the plays for his team. This was possible because his occupational therapist worked with him in setting up the appropriate assistive technology on which to write the plays and addressing accessibility issues in his school stadium. The student's occupational therapist and physical therapist also collaborated with him, the coaches, and the administrators to devise strategies so that he could attend road trips. His long-term goal was to secure a job writing plays for a professional football team.

Outcomes

A variety of outcomes can result from addressing play or leisure within the educational setting. Using the Occupational Therapy Practice Framework as a guide, Table 11-3 provides some examples.

SUMMARY

As occupational therapists begin to address the occupational role behavior of play and leisure skills in the educational setting, they may be met with some reluctance and questions from teachers, administrators, parents, and other professionals on the educational team. It is important that they be able to articulate the critical roles of play and leisure skills in the overall development of a child. In addition, therapists need to be aware of evidence from the education and psychology literature to discuss the development of play with others on the collaborative team. Demonstrating that play and leisure participation may help a child learn self-determination skills, fine and gross motor skills, cognitive skills, and social skills will help others understand the critical need to address this type of occupation throughout a child's educational career. It is important that therapists assess play and leisure skills and develop play and leisure goals and objectives that reflect relevant outcomes. The goals and objectives should specifically address the long-term implications of play and leisure skill development, not simply the components of play and leisure skills.

The provision of occupational therapy in school settings should not be limited to interventions focused on remediation or attainment of motor or self-help skills. As a profession, occupational therapy looks holistically at an individual and at the rhythm of work, self-help, and play and leisure, and this approach should be evident in occupational therapy practice across all venues. Because successful play skills are essential for development and future successes as an adult member of society, school-based occupational therapists need to share their skills related to play as human occupation with the educational team to ensure that play is addressed in educational programs for children with special needs. Play and learning are not distinct entities, but rather companions for the successful education of children. The presence of one without the other would sacrifice learning opportunities for students. If occupational therapists are to continue to herald play as the work of children, an essential component of development, and a key element in the evolution of society, it must be addressed as such in the school curriculum.

That said, what became of Tyler, Rebekah, Reagan, Henry, and Greg as a result of school-based occupational therapy that addressed issues related to play, leisure, and social participation?

■ *Clinical Vignettes* ■

Tyler, the 3-year-old in a developmental program, no longer sits by himself during free choice. He is beginning to initiate interactions with his peers and responds when they initiate play with him. This has occurred in part because of a play group the occupational therapist developed and implemented in his preschool classroom twice a week during free play time. The classroom paraprofessional carried out the program on the other days of the week.

Rebekah, the first grader who loves to swing, has her climbing equipment back and is able to better attend to classroom activities. Her school occupational therapist facilitated a playground remodeling project that addressed both the sensorimotor play needs of the children and the safety and liability concerns of the school district.

Reagan, the fourth grader, now plays with other girls during recess. Social skills groups and a peer modeling program, developed and implemented through collaboration of the school occupational therapist and school counselor,

helped her to overcome her reluctance to interact with others. The occupational therapist and school counselor are collaboratively planning to implement a social skills curriculum with a sensory basis for all fourth-grade classrooms.

Henry, the junior high student, is no longer wandering and committing thefts during his free time. The school team had requested an occupational therapy evaluation, which included a leisure skills interest assessment. As a result, he spends his lunch hours in the music room practicing his drums with others interested in starting a band.

Greg, the 20-year-old high school student, has in place a transition plan (developed by his team, including the occupational therapist) that includes leisure skill development. He has completed an interest inventory, and whenever he sits in front of the television, he is encouraged to look at his list of interests and choose an alternative activity.

Review Questions

1. Are play and leisure included in the domain of occupational therapy as defined in the Framework?
2. What might intervention for play and leisure exploration and participation include?

REFERENCES

Abramson, L. Y., Seligman, M. E. P., & Teasdale, J. D. (1978). Learned helplessness in humans: Critique and reformation. *Journal of Abnormal Psychology, 87,* 49-74.

American Occupational Therapy Association. (2002). Occupational therapy practice framework: Domain and process. *American Journal of Occupational Therapy, 56,* 609-639.

American Occupational Therapy Association. (2003). American Occupational Therapy Association 2003 AOTA member compensation survey. Bethesda, MD: Author.

Ballard, K. D., & Medland, J. L. (1986). Collateral effects from teaching attention, imitation and toy interaction behaviors to a developmentally handicapped child. *Child and Family Behavior Therapy, 7,* 47-50.

Beardsly, L. (1991). Perspectives from the field: Teachers and parents respond to the call for developmentally appropriate practice in the primary grades. In B. Scales, M. Almy, A. Nicolopoulou, & S. Ervin-Tripp (Eds.), *Play and the social context of development in early care and education* (pp. 62-74). New York: Teachers College Press.

Bergen, D., (2001). Pretend play and young children's development? ERIC/EECE *publications-digests* (Report No. ED458045). Available http://www.ericdigests.org/2002-2/play.html.

Blanche, E. I. (1997). Doing with—not doing to: Play and the child with cerebral palsy. In L. D. Parham & L. S. Fazio (Eds.), *Play in occupational therapy for children* (pp. 202-218). St. Louis: Mosby.

Brink, S. (May 15, 1995). Smart moves. *U.S. News & World Report.*

Bundy, A. C. (1989). A comparison of the play skills of normal boys and boys with sensory integrative dysfunction. *Occupational Therapy Journal of Research, 9,* 84-100.

Bundy, A. C. (1991). Play theory and sensory integration. In A. G. Fisher, E. A. Murray, & A. C. Bundy (Eds.), *Sensory integration: Theory and practice* (pp. 46-68). Philadelphia: F.A. Davis.

Bundy, A. C. (1993). Assessment of play and leisure: Delineation of the problem. *American Journal of Occupational Therapy, 47,* 217-222.

Burke, J. P. (1993). Play: The life role of the infant and young child. In J. Case-Smith (Ed.), *Pediatric occupational therapy and early intervention.* Boston: Andover Medical Publishers.

Chadsey-Rusch, J., & Heal, L. (1995). Building consensus from transition experts on social integration outcomes and interventions. *Exceptional Children, 62,* 165-184.

Cherry, C. (1976). *Creative play for the developing child: Early lifehood education through play.* Carthage, IL: Fearon Teacher Aids.

Coster, W., Deeney, T., Haltiwanger, J., & Haley, S. (1998). *School function assessment.* San Antonio: The Psychological Corporation/Therapy Skill Builders.

Couch, K. J., Deitz, J. C., & Kanny, E. M. (1998). The role of play in pediatric occupational therapy. *American Journal of Occupational Therapy, 52,* 111-117.

Daub, M. M. (1988). Prenatal development through mid-adulthood. In H. L. Hopkins & H. D. Smith (Eds.), *Willard and Spackman's occupational therapy* (7th ed., pp. 50-74). Philadelphia: J.B. Lippincott.

Desha, L., Ziviani, J., & Rodger, S. (2003). Play preferences and behavior of preschool children with autistic spectrum disorder in the clinical environment. *Physical and Occupational Therapy in Pediatrics, 23*(1), 21-42.

Dewey, J. (1928). *Democracy and education.* New York: Macmillan.

Dougherty, B. S., Fowler, S. A., & Paine, S. C. (1985). The use of peer monitors to reduce negative interaction during recess. *Journal of Applied Behavior Analysis, 18,* 141-153.

Eason, L. J., White, M. J., & Newsom, C. (1982). Generalized reduction of self-stimulatory behavior: An effect of teaching appropriate play to autistic children. *Analysis and Intervention in Developmental Disabilities, 2,* 157-169.

Elkind, D. (1990). Academic pressures-too much, too soon: The demise of play. In E. Klugman & S. Smilansky (Eds.), *Children's play and learning: Perspectives and policy implications* (pp. 3-17). New York: Teachers College Press.

Farran, D. C., & Yon-Yarbrough, W. (2001). Title I funded preschools as a developmental context for children's play and verbal behaviors. *Early Childhood Research Quarterly, 16*(2), 245-262.

Ferland, F. (1997). *Play, children with physical disabilities, and occupational therapy: The ludic model.* Ottawa, Ontario, Canada: University of Ottawa Press.

Fewell, R. R., & Kaminski, R. (1988). Play skills development and instruction for young children with handicaps. In S. L. Odom & M. B. Karnes (Eds.), *Early intervention for infants and children with handicaps: An empirical base* (pp. 145-158). Baltimore: Paul H. Brookes.

Fleming, M. H., & Mattingly, C. (2003). The underground practice. In C. Mattingly & M. Fleming (Eds.), *Clinical reasoning: Forms of inquiry in a therapeutic practice* (pp. 295-315). Philadelphia: F.A. Davis.

Florey, L. L. (1981). Studies of play: Implications for growth, development, and for clinical practice. *American Journal of Occupational Therapy, 35,* 519-524.

Gargiulo, R. M., & O'Sullivan, P. S. (1986). Mildly mentally retarded and nonretarded children's learned helplessness. *American Journal of Mental Deficiency, 91,* 203-206.

Genishi, C. (1991). The research perspective: Looking at play through case studies. In B. Scales, M. Almy, A. Nicolopoulou, & S. Ervin-Tripp (Eds.), *Play and the social context of development in early care and education* (pp. 74-83). New York: Teachers College Press.

Gilbert, A. G. (1977). *Teaching the three R's through movement experiences.* New York: Prentice Hall.

Goldstein, H., & Cisar, C. L. (1992). Promoting interaction during sociodramatic play: Teaching scripts to typical preschoolers and classmates with disabilities. *Journal of Applied Behavior Analysis, 25,* 265-280.

Goleman, D. (1995). *Emotional intelligence.* New York: Bantam Books.

Greenspan, S. I., & Wieder, S. (1998). *The child with special needs: Encouraging intellectual and emotional growth.* Reading, MA: Addison-Wesley.

Grubb, W. N. (1991). Policy issues surrounding quality and content in early care and education. In B. Scales, M. Almy, A. Nicolopoulou, & S. Ervin-Tripp (Eds.), *Play and the social context of development in early care and education* (pp. 32-50). New York: Teachers College Press.

Guralnik, M. J., & Hammond, M. A. (1999). Sequential analysis of the social play of young children with mild developmental delays. *Journal of Early Intervention, 22*(3), 243-256.

Hannaford, C. (1995). *Smart moves: Why learning is not all in your head.* Arlington, VA: Great Ocean Publishing.

Harrison, H., & Kielhofner, G. (1986). Examining the reliability and validity of the Preschool Play Scale with handicapped children. *American Journal of Occupational Therapy, 40,* 167-173.

Hestenes, L. L., & Carroll, D. E. (2000). The play interactions of young children with and without disabilities: Individual and environmental influences. *Early Childhood Research Quarterly, 15*(2), 229-246.

Houston, J. (1982). *The possible human: A course in enhancing your physical, mental and creative abilities.* Los Angeles: Jeremy Tarcher.

Howard, L. (1996). A comparison of leisure-time activities between able-bodied children and children with physical disabilities. *British Journal of Occupational Therapy, 59,* 12.

Humphrey, J. H., & Humphrey, J. N. (1980). *Help your child learn the 3R's through active play.* Springfield, IL: Charles C Thomas.

Illinois State Board of Education (1994). *Special children, special care: Early childhood education for children with disabilities.* Springfield, IL: Author.

Individuals with Disabilities Education Improvement Act of 2004. DOCID: f:publ446.108, 20 USC 1400. Public Law 108-446.

Jarrett, O.S. (2003). Recess in elementary school: What does the research say? ERIC/EECE *publications-digests* (Report No. EDO-PS-02-5). Available at http://ericeece.org/pubs/digests/2003-2/jarrett02.html.

Jensen, E. (1998). *Teaching with the brain in mind.* Alexandria, VA: Association for Supervision and Curriculum Development.

Johnson, J. E., Christie, J. F., & Yawkey, T. D. (1987). *Play and early childhood development.* Glenview, IL: Scott, Foresman.

Kamps, D. M., Leonard, B. R., Vernon, S., Dugan, E. P., Delquadri, J. C., Gershon, B., et al. (1992). Teaching social skills to students with autism to increase peer interactions in an integrated first-grade classroom. *Journal of Applied Behavior Analysis, 25,* 281-288.

Kearney, P. (Aug. 3, 1996). Brain research shows importance of arts in education. *Star Tribune,* p. 19A.

Kielhofner, G. (1995). *A model of human occupation: Theory and application* (2nd ed.). Baltimore: Williams & Wilkins.

Kielhofner, G., & Miyake, S. (1981). The therapeutic use of games with mentally retarded adults. *American Journal of Occupational Therapy, 35,* 375-382.

Klugman, E. (1997). Foreword. In G. Reynolds & E. Jones. *Master players: Learning from children at play* (pp. vii-ix). New York: Teachers College Press.

Knight, M. (2003). *The use of playgrounds as a site for occupational therapy intervention* (Unpublished master's thesis, University of Puget Sound, Tacoma, WA).

Koomar, J. A., & Bundy, A. C. (1991). The art and science of creating direct intervention from theory. In A. G. Fisher, E. A. Murray, & A. C. Bundy (Eds.), *Sensory integration: Theory and practice* (pp. 251-314). Philadelphia: F.A. Davis.

Krasnor, L. R., & Pepler, D. J. (1980). The study of children's play: Some suggested future directions. In K. H. Rubin (Ed.), *New directions for child development* (pp. 85-94). San Francisco: Jossey-Bass.

LeGoff, D. B. (2004). Use of LEGO © as a therapeutic medium for improving social competence. *Journal of Autism and Developmental Disorders, 34*(5), 557-571.

Lifter, K., Sulzer-Azaroff, B., Anderson, S. R., & Cowdery, G. E. (1993). Teaching play activities to preschool children with disabilities: The importance of developmental considerations. *Journal of Early Intervention, 17,* 139-159.

Linder, T. W. (1993). *Transdisciplinary play-based assessment.* Baltimore: Paul H. Brookes.

Llorens, L. A. (1974). The effects of stress on growth and development. *American Journal of Occupational Therapy, 28,* 82-86.

Maier, S. F., & Seligman, M. E. (1976). Learned helplessness: Theory and evidence. *Journal of Experimental Psychology: General, 105,* 3-46.

McEvoy, M. A., Nordquist, V. M., Twardosz, S., Heckaman, K. A., Wehby, J. H., & Denny, R. K. (1988). Promoting autistic children's peer interaction in an integrated early childhood setting using affection activities. *Journal of Applied Behavior Analysis, 21,* 193-200.

Miller-Kuhaneck, H., Henry, D. A., & Glennon, T. J. (2007). *Sensory Processing Measure* (SPM)—Main classroom form and school forms. Los Angeles: Western Psychological Services.

Missiuna, C., & Pollock, N. (1991). Play deprivation in children with physical disabilities: The role of the occupational therapist in preventing secondary disability. *American Journal of Occupational Therapy, 45,* 882-888.

Mohr-Modes, B. (2003). *The power of play in the lives of preschool children within changing European and U.S. societies* (Unpublished master's thesis, University of Puget Sound, Tacoma, WA).

Neville-Jan, A., Fazio, L. S., Kennedy, B., & Snyder, C. (1997). Elementary to middle school transition: Using multicultural play activities to develop life skills. In L. D. Parham & L. S. Fazio (Eds.), *Play in occupational therapy for children* (pp. 35-51). St. Louis: Mosby.

Parham, L. D., Ecker, C., Miller-Kuhaneck, H., Henry, D. A., & Glennon, T. J. (2007). *Sensory Processing Measure (SPM) manual.* Los Angeles: Western Psychological Services.

Parten, M. B. (1932). Social participation among preschool children. *Journal of Abnormal and Social Psychology, 27,* 243-269.

Pellegrini, A. D. (1985). Social-cognitive aspects of children's play: The effects of age, gender and activity centers. *Journal of Applied Developmental Psychology, 6,* 129-140.

Piaget, J. (1962). *Play, dreams and imitation in childhood.* New York: W.W. Norton.

Polk, C. (1994, November 2). Therapeutic work with African-American families: Using knowledge of culture. *Zero to Three, 15,* 9-11.

Pollock, N., Stewart, D., Law, M., Harvey, S., Sahagian, S., & Toal, C. (1996). The meaning of play and work for adolescents with physical disabilities. *Canadian Journal of Occupational Therapy, 64,* 25-31.

Pratt, P. N. (1989). Play and recreational activities. In P. N. Pratt & A. S. Allen (Eds.), *Occupational therapy for children.* (4th ed., pp. 295-310). St. Louis: Mosby.

Reilly, M. (1974). An explanation of play. In M. Reilly (Ed.), *Play as exploratory learning* (pp. 117-150). Beverly Hills, CA: Sage Publications.

Restall, G., & Magill-Evans, J. (1994). Play and preschool children with autism. *American Journal of Occupational Therapy, 48,* 113-120.

Reynolds, G., & Jones, E. (1997). *Master players: Learning from children at play.* New York: Teachers College Press.

Robinson, A. L. (1977). Play: The arena for acquisition of rules for competent behavior. *American Journal of Occupational Therapy, 31,* 248-253.

Rogers, S. J. (2000). Interventions that facilitate socialization in children with autism. *Journal of Autism and Developmental Disorders, 30,* 339-409.

Rothlein, L., & Brett, A. (1987). Children's, teachers', and parents' perceptions of play. *Early Childhood Research Quarterly, 2,* 45-53.

Royeen, C. B. (1997). Play as occupation and as an indicator of health. In B. E. Chandler (Ed.), *The essence of play: A child's occupation* (pp. 1-14). Bethesda, MD: American Occupational Therapy Association.

Rubin, K. H., & Coplan, R. J. (1998). Social and nonsocial play in childhood: An individual differences perspective. In O. N. Saracho & B. Spodek (Eds.), *Multiple perspectives on play in early childhood* (pp. 144-170). Albany, NY: State University of New York Press.

Rubin, K. (1980). Foreword. In Rubin, K. *New directions for child development,* San Francisco: Jossey-Bass.

Scales, B., Almy, M., Nicolopoulou, A., & Ervin-Tripp, S. (1991). Defending play in the lives of children (pp. 15-31). In B. Scales, M. Almy, A. Nicolopoulou, & S. Ervin-Tripp (Eds.), *Play and the social context of development in early care and education.* New York: Teachers College Press.

Simon, C. J., & Daub, M. M. (1993). Human development across the life span. In H. L. Hopkins & H. D. Smith (Eds.), *Willard and Spackman's occupational therapy* (pp. 95-129). Philadelphia: J.B. Lippincott.

Smith, D. O. (1991). Here they come: Ready or not! Report of the California School Readiness Task Force. In B. Scales, M. Almy, A. Nicolopoulou, & S. Ervin-Tripp (Eds.), *Play and the social context of development in early care and education* (pp. 51-61). New York: Teachers College Press.

Stahl, C. (1995, January 30). The Navajo perspective: Not every culture values play. *Advance for Occupational Therapists, 17.*

Swinth, Y. L. (2004). *Current issues and trends in school-based occupational therapy.* Unpublished survey.

Swinth, Y. L., & Tanta, K. (2003). Play and leisure skill development in school-based practice. In Y. L. Swinth (Ed.), *AOTA online course: Occupational therapy in school-based practice: Contemporary issues and trends.* Bethesda, MD: American Occupational Therapy Association.

Tanta, K. J., Deitz, J., White, O., & Billingsly, F. (2005). The effects of peer-play level on initiations and responses of preschool children with delayed play skills. *American Journal of Occupational Therapy, 59,* 437-445.

U.S. Bureau of Labor and Statistics.(2001). *Occupational outlook handbook.* Washington, DC: Author.

Vygotsky, L. S. (1976). Play and its role in the mental development of the child. In J. Bruner, A. Jolly, & K. Sylva (Eds.), *Play: Its role in development and evolution* (pp. 537-554). New York: Basic Books.

Washington State Commission on Student Learning (February 22, 1997). *Essential academic learning requirements.* Olympia, WA: Author.

Weisz, J. R. (1979). Perceived control and learned helplessness among mentally retarded and nonretarded children: A developmental analysis. *Developmental Psychology, 15*(3), 311-319.

Whitney-Thomas, J., & Hanley-Maxwell, C. (1996). Packing the parachute: Parents' experiences as their children prepare to leave high school. *Exceptional Children, 63,* 75-88.

Wilson, C., & Sindelar, P. (1991). Direct instruction in math word problems: Students with learning disabilities. *Exceptional Children, 57,* 512-519.

IV

Play as a Goal of Intervention

12

Integrating Children with Disabilities into Family Play

JIM HINOJOSA AND PAULA KRAMER

KEY TERMS

family
play as a therapeutic medium
family play
family adaptations
Family Observation Guide

Several issues arose in the conceptualizing and writing of this chapter. The first is that play differs greatly among individual children and different cultures, whether the child has a disability or not. Play is strongly affected by the child's context, including family and peers, socioeconomic influences, and availability of time. What is considered play by one child may seem totally inappropriate and even distasteful to another child based on his or her prior experiences and personal preferences. Play is viewed as child-initiated activity that is not structured by an adult and does not have skill acquisition as a goal (Olson & O'Herron, 2004). The second issue is defining "family" in a manner that reflects the diversity of families as they exist in society today, without introducing overtones of discrimination or bias. Family is a complex concept that has to be defined broadly to include the many variations that occur. The values of the identified family affect the concept of play within that family. The third issue relates to the occupational therapist's perspective on the use of play as a therapeutic modality as opposed to play purely for the sake of pleasure. The therapist has a responsibility to work with the family to identify their valued occupations and routines related to play and then ensure the inclusion of the child with disabilities into the family play routines.

In this chapter play is any activity that is engaged in for its own sake. It may involve action on or with nonhuman objects or interaction with other people.

Play entails a freedom of choice in the activity, as well as a sense of enjoyment (Harkness & Bundy, 2001; Luebben, Hinojosa, & Kramer, 1999). Children play because it is fun and because they have an innate desire to play. When engaged in play activities, children often develop life skills without even realizing it. They are free to participate independently or to negotiate sharing of the activity with others (Olson & O'Herron, 2004). Thus play facilitates life skills and children's ability to function effectively within their environment. Depending on the disability, some children may not have the same access to play as children without disabilities. Therefore their play may be more contrived and have less inner direction than the play of other children. Children with more severe disabilities may have increased limitations, resulting in less access to play and less ability for play (Hackett, 2003; Harkness & Bundy, 2001). This affects skill acquisition and potential for developing play skills through experience and interaction with other children. Some children who have disabilities spend much of their formative time in medical and therapeutic environments and not in playgrounds or play groups. In addition, physical, cognitive, or behavioral disabilities can be restrictive in play situations, and other children frequently reject or avoid those who seem different from themselves.

The primary function of the family is to provide a supportive and nurturing environment for the child's development while meeting and recognizing the needs of all family members (Muhlenhaupt, Hinojosa, & Kramer, 1999). Families may include parents and children, grandparents, and other significant people. Nuclear, blended, extended, and single-parent households are all configurations of the family in current American society. Most families play and devote time to leisure activities. The range of activities and the level of participation of the individual members may vary. Families and individual members

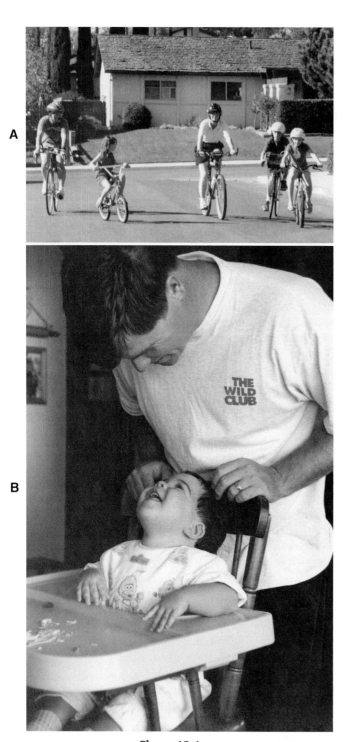

Figure 12-1
Play in the family context, **A,** *may be preplanned and organized or,* **B,** *may arise spontaneously in the course of daily routines. (Courtesy Shay McAtee.)*

operate in their own unique ways (Muhlenhaupt, Hinojosa, & Kramer, 1999). The presence of a child with a disability within the family may have a strong influence on the family's play styles and practices, especially if the family values inclusion of the child.

Play is a major modality for pediatric occupational therapists. Occupational therapists traditionally use play as a therapeutic modality, with a specific goal in mind. Therapists are highly skilled in the analysis, adaptation, and synthesis of play activities. The art of using therapeutic play in occupational therapy is that it allows the child to engage in and enjoy the activity as pure play, but simultaneously the therapist has a distinct goal in mind to achieve through the use of that play. Another key role of the therapist is to offer guidance and suggestions to parents in the family's use of play, both as an enhancement to therapy and as a means of strengthening their interaction with their child to provide an enjoyable childhood experience. The latter therapeutic role—to assist family members to engage in play with the child who has a disability—is one to which therapists are less accustomed; it is the focus of this chapter.

DEFINING PLAY AS IT RELATES TO THE FAMILY

Play within the context of the family is different from typical childhood play that takes place in a playground or in school. Whether family play is organized, such as a family football game, or spontaneous, such as tickling a child during dressing, it is always influenced by the family's values, culture, and setting (Figure 12-1). For example, building a dollhouse may be considered a play activity within one family, whereas it is considered work within another family. Play differs based on the child and the context surrounding the child.

No one set of characteristics defines play, but Tamis-LeMonda, Užgiris, and Bornstein (2002) have identified some common traits that frequently emerge from theories about play: a desire to play for the sake of playing; the intrinsic motivation of play; the laughter, smiles, and general good feeling when playing; the imaginative quality of play, allowing fantasy rather than focusing on reality pretense; and the redefinition of occurrences freely based on reality rather than the development of new meanings through play. Family child play is somewhat different in that it is viewed as supporting child development by providing varied experiences with emotional, social, and cultural issues and as enhancing communication between parent and child and between child and environment (Tamis-LeMonda et al., 2002).

The nature of play within a family is strongly influenced by the family's collective values. If the family values activity and physical fitness, the play may be more physically oriented. If the values are more intellectually oriented, activities involving learning may be more prevalent (Figure 12-2). Moreover, because children tend to emulate their adult role models, their family play may be geared toward the values and preferences of the adult participants. If play is a valued part of the adult routine, it will be included as part of the child's routine. Daily routines and arrangements will be adjusted to make time for the incorporation of play. It is not possible to impose play on a family because play arises out of the context of that particular family. If particular play activities are imposed from the outside, those activities may not be relevant to that family and may no longer be considered play. Children's concepts of what constitutes play are also influenced by their physical environment, their experiences individually and with other children, their culture and the cultures to which they are exposed, and their personality, age, and gender. They are also influenced by their experiences with the families of their peers, although often the families that interact together are fairly homogeneous. With the time constraints that occur in society today, the family has to value play in order to make time for it.

The family with a child who has a disability is a family first. Parents have the same values and responsibilities as other parents, but they now also have increased responsibilities toward this particular child. Sometimes these responsibilities cause play and pleasure-oriented activities to be placed on hold or to fall toward the bottom of a list of priorities. There is also a tendency for the family to become child centered. When the parents' primary focus is on the child with special needs, this may dominate the family activities.

The presence of a child with disabilities influences all family routines and practices, which has implications for the recreational and play needs of all family members. Current practice tends to support a family-centered philosophy that looks at the needs of the entire family. A typical family is fluid, with the needs of individual family members changing over time and the focus on different family members being adjusted as the needs arise. When a family has a child with special needs, that child's needs never fade into the background. Although other family members may become the focus of attention, the special needs of the child do not disappear. Family roles and routines always have to allow for the needs of the child. Recreational needs of families may be revised because of this, such as parents not taking time to go out by themselves without having a skilled babysitter for the child, siblings not going to a sports event that is not fully accessible, and grandparents not taking the children out camping. Because recreation and play are important needs for all families, they should be a priority both on an individual level and for the family group as a whole (Mactavish & Schleien, 2004; Tamm & Prellwitz, 2001).

For all families, developing and enjoying activities together encourages family cohesion. A family planning a trip to visit Grandma out of town can start with a discussion of how they will get there, what routes will they take, and what each family member wants to do when they arrive. When all members of the family have an opportunity to contribute

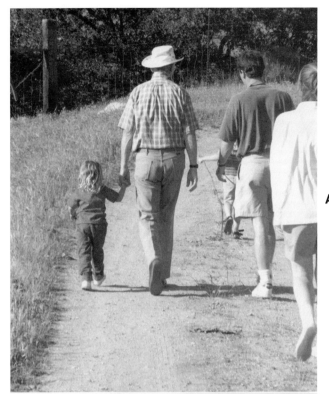

A

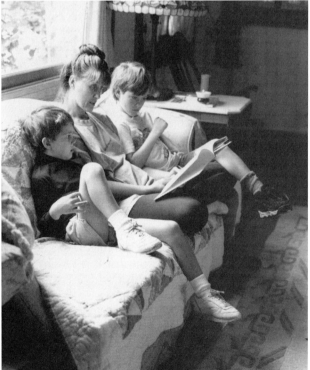

B

Figure 12-2

The collective values of a family influence their choices of play activities. **A,** *Physical and outdoor activities are prominent among families that value physical activity and fitness, whereas,* **B,** *literacy-oriented activities are emphasized among families that value intellectual and verbal pursuits. (Courtesy Shay McAtee.)*

ideas for the activities and feel that their personal desires are included, they can become invested in the activities. This breeds a sense of consideration and respect for other family members and inclusion of all members, and the task then truly becomes a group project. Through processes of this type, the family matures and functions as a unit.

CASE EXAMPLE 1
The Casey Family

The Casey family made a tradition of Sunday dinner. They viewed this Sunday dinner as part of their family recreational time. They enjoyed having a meal together and interacting with all the children and extended family around. Everyone was able to have fun together and talk about the things that had happened to each of them during the week. The table was always set with china and crystal because the family liked this time to be special. They needed to rethink this when they realized that Billy, age 6, who had cerebral palsy, might break the china and crystal accidentally because of his poor coordination when eating. The choice became whether to abandon the family tradition of Sunday dinner, modify the type of plates and glasses used, or continue in the same manner and accept the consequence of broken tableware. Their decision was to carry on the tradition by simply changing the type of dishes and glassware that everyone used. Maintaining a long-standing family tradition while including Billy became the important issue rather than the table service used. The family's time together could still be special without particular dishes and glassware. Everyone continued to enjoy Sunday dinner, with no one excluded or made to feel different. This family found a way to continue their tradition and develop family cohesion with the inclusion of Billy.

A child with a disability may influence the types of activity in which the family participates. The child with a disability should be included to the extent that it is possible; however, the family needs to realize that activities may have to be modified or that the child cannot be actively involved in some activities. Whatever the family situation, the child with disabilities should not preclude the development of family cohesion. By nature, families do things together and the child with a disability needs to be included, whether actively or passively. Although the child with special needs may require additional time and attention, the family's leisure activities can provide opportunities for focusing on the needs of the group rather than allowing the child's needs to take precedence.

Obviously, the degree and type of disability that the child has will affect his or her ability to engage in specific recreational or play activity. In other words, the disability affects the types of activity in which the child can participate and the degree to which the child can participate. The disability may also determine the satisfaction that a child receives from an activity. Congruent with this perspective, a child does not need to engage in an activity physically to enjoy it; he or she may be able to participate as a spectator (Figure 12-3). Although the potential exists for the child to feel like an outsider in this situation, the inclusion of the child in the activity to the extent that it is possible should be the focus rather than the child's inability to participate fully. Enjoyment happens in varying degrees of participation. Sometimes simply being part of the family experience brings its own pleasure.

PLAY AS A THERAPEUTIC MEDIUM

Therapists frequently use play as a means to achieve therapeutic goals for a child. These goals are related to creating an environment where the child can develop skills and successful behaviors. When play is used as a therapeutic medium, the therapist designs the play in a way that will promote positive changes in the child. In these situations play is the primary therapeutic medium to address occupational performance deficits, skill development, and the ability to interact with others.

Play is a useful vehicle for the development of imagination and higher level cognitive functioning. As distinct from purposefully therapeutic activities, therapeutic play requires some degree of self-selection and choice of activity on the part of the child. Play provides a safe venue for practicing skills and refining abilities where the child has control through choice. Guided by the theoretical approach, the therapist participates in the child's play. Thus the therapist creates an environment where the child with disabilities interacts around the play activity without focusing on the development of specific skills (Kramer & Hinojosa, 1999).

To introduce choice into therapeutic play, the therapist presents a number of options to the child. For example, a therapist gives a 3-year-old boy who lacks fine motor skills a choice of building a block tower or coloring a picture. Whichever activity the child selects, the therapist focuses on the development of fine motor skills while the child plays. The activity has been selected because it is age appropriate and has a therapeutic value for skill development. It attracts the child because it is fun, but that is not the primary reason that it was chosen by the therapist. Playing with blocks can be done within the home, where everyone takes part in constructing a group project. This is an activity that not only is therapeutic but can become part of family play. Similarly, a therapist may offer a card game, word game, or board game to help a 7-year-old with spina bifida who is in a wheelchair to develop cognitive skills of game rules, attention span, and interactive play. Whichever game is chosen, the child enjoys it. The therapist, meanwhile, has distinct goals for the child to achieve through playing the game; it will help the child develop cognitive skills of game rules, attention span, and

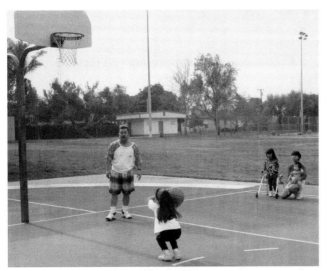

Figure 12-3

Being a spectator is a legitimate way that a child can participate in a family play experience, even if the presence of a disability precludes physical engagement. (Courtesy Shay McAtee.)

interactive play. Games of this type can easily be translated to an activity done in the home.

Using play as a medium appears simple but is really quite challenging because the therapist must be concerned with multiple contexts at one time. On one level the therapist must select an appropriate activity. This activity must be something that the child will enjoy and would typically want to do and must also be age appropriate. On another level the therapist considers the therapeutic goals for the child and how the play activity can be used to meet those goals, based on the theoretical approach to intervention (Kramer & Hinojosa, 2004, 2005). At the same time the therapist must look beyond specific deficits that require intervention and consider the play activity in the context of the child's life as a whole being. This requires a broader perspective than using play as a therapeutic tool to achieve change in one specific aspect of performance. Concerning the previous example of the 3-year-old child, in this broader perspective the therapist would provide the child with blocks without working specifically on the development of fine motor skills and the expectation of building a tower. Instead, the therapist would allow the child to be self-directed in the activity. Whether the child builds a tower, hits the blocks together, handles the blocks, or throws them, he is using the blocks to derive pleasure and simultaneously is developing creativity and spontaneity in play. In time, depending on the theoretical perspective being employed, the therapist might use a hand-over-hand approach or role modeling to demonstrate to the child how to build a tower. While still playing with the blocks, the child is now building fine motor skills at the same time.

The most complex level to be considered by the therapist is play within the family and how the child with a disability fits into that play structure. The therapist must gain an understanding of the types of play that are valued by the family, the types of play that are available to them, and the environment of family play. This includes the time spent on play, the environment of play, and any routines and habits that contribute to family play. Information is needed about the individual values of all family members and what each enjoys. The therapist also needs to understand the nature of family members' interactions with one another and with the child with disabilities.

To use play as a therapeutic medium within the context of a family, the therapist must understand play within the unique family structure. The Family Observation Guide (Box 12-1) has been developed to assist therapists in obtaining pertinent information related to family play. First, the therapist needs to become familiar with the family. The therapist may reflect on a number of questions: Who are the family members? What are each family member's roles within the family structure? What are each family member's values? What do they enjoy doing alone or as a family? Which family members tend to interact with each other? How does the family culture influence its choice of activities? What are the occupations of each family member and of the family as a whole? What are the family's habits and routines relating to play? How much time is devoted to play? Does time constrain play? What are the family's resources? Does the family have any limitations that should be considered? How does the family react to the child's disabilities, impairments, or handicaps? When the family is considered as a whole, is there anything that makes family recreation difficult? Because the family is the essential unit, it is the initial focus.

Following the focus on the family, the therapist is concerned with observing the child with a disability within the family context. What role does that child take in the family? What is the child capable of doing? What does the child enjoy doing? How much unstructured time is available to the child? What does the child generally do during this unstructured time? What does the child do spontaneously, without prompting from others? With which family members does the child interact, and how does he or she interact with them? With whom does the child interact in the daily life context, and whom does he or she seek out for interaction? What are the child's specific limitations in play and in activities in general? This information provides the basis for considering how the therapist can best facilitate play as occupational performance within the family (Figure 12-4).

Another important aspect for the therapist is information about the environment of the family. Where does play take place for this family? What objects, such as games,

---

Box 12-1   *Family Observation Guide*

Becoming Familiar with the Family
Who are the family members?
What are each family member's roles within the family structure?
What are each family member's values?
What do they enjoy doing alone or as a family?
Which family members tend to interact with each other?
How does the family culture influence its choice of activities?
What are the occupations of each family member and of the family as a whole?
What are the family's habits and routines relating to play?
How much time is devoted to play?
Does time constrain play?
What are the family's resources?
Does the family have any limitations that should be considered?
How does the family react to the child's disabilities, impairments, or handicaps?
Thinking about the family as a whole, is there anything that makes family recreation difficult?

Observing the Child with a Disability Within the Family Context
What role does that child take in the family?
What is the child capable of doing?
What does the child enjoy doing?
How much unstructured time is available to the child?
What does the child generally do during this unstructured time?
What does the child do spontaneously, without prompting from others?

With which family members does the child interact, and how does he or she interact with them?
With whom does the child interact in the context of daily life, and whom does he or she seek out for interaction?
What are the child's specific limitations in play and in activities in general?

Information About the Environment of the Family
Where does play take place for this family?
What objects, such as games, toys, and other materials, are available in the environment?
Are there space limitations?
Does the environment fit the activity (atmospheric elements, such as safety, sound level, lighting, temperature)?
Does the majority of family play take place within the home or outside of the home?
Are there other environments where family play takes place that the therapist should learn more about?

Matching the Information About the Family and the Child with Disabilities
Based on the activities the family enjoys, how can the child with his or her abilities, limitations, and interests be incorporated into these activities?
What does the family do to actively include the child?
Do the child's limitations preclude involvement in any of these activities?
If the child is unable to participate in these activities, is he or she able to observe them and still feel included as part of the family?
What environmental barriers may affect the child's ability to be involved with family play?

---

toys, and other materials, are available in the environment? Are there space limitations? Does the environment fit the activity (atmospheric elements, such as safety, sound level, lighting, temperature)? Does the majority of family play take place within the home or outside of the home? Does family play take place in other environments that the therapist should learn more about? By knowing the circumstances and settings where play takes place, the therapist can obtain a full picture of play for this family within its context.

After the information about play within the context of the family has been gathered, the next step involves matching the information about the family with information about the child with disabilities so that the child can be integrated into the routine play of the family. How can the child with his or her abilities, limitations, and interests

be incorporated into the activities that the family enjoys? What does the family do to actively include the child? Do the child's limitations preclude involvement in any of these activities? If the child is unable to participate in these activities, is he or she able to observe them and still feel included as part of the family? What environmental barriers may affect the child's ability to be involved with family play?

A comprehensive assessment of a child with a disability should include obtaining information about the child's play and the family's play. Data from assessment should allow the therapist to construct a total picture of the family leisure activities configuration. This will include what the family values, how they choose to spend their time, and what role each of the children has within the family.

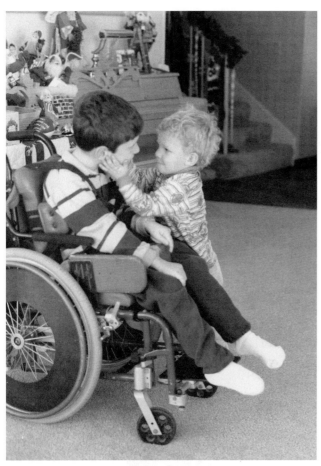

Figure 12-4
Sibling relationships are an important consideration in the evaluation of a child within the family context. Such relationships may be an important resource for facilitating play within the family. (Courtesy Shay McAtee.)

Therapists may find it hard to get a complete picture through an interview. If family members see therapists in their traditional roles of therapists, the family may think and talk in terms of what is therapeutic and therefore "good" for the child with disabilities. Because of this tendency for the family to give what they perceive as therapeutically acceptable answers, therapists need to give family members permission to talk about activities that are fun for each of them, activities that they like to do by themselves and with the child with a disability, and activities that the child enjoys doing alone or with each family member, without the burden of thinking about whether these activities are therapeutic. Therapists need to convey to the family that just by being fun, some activities can be beneficial to the child with disabilities and to the family as a whole.

One way that therapists augment information from an interview is through observation of the child and family within the natural environment. This might include the home, playground, community social events, or family celebrations. Observations such as this may not give a true picture of the "natural" event, however, because the inclusion of an outsider tends to change the event and the interactions. In addition, because play is typically spontaneous, fun, and at times fleeting, it may be difficult to observe.

Evaluation and possible intervention related to family play must be handled with skill and delicacy. Families require a balance of play that addresses the interests of all parties involved. The family may view the questions and observations of the therapist as intrusive, and if they are already actively involved in playing with their children, this focus may upset their natural balance of family play. Conversely, however, the therapist's line of questioning may facilitate the development of play within a family.

When guiding families to think of activities in terms of their play benefit, occupational therapists need to take into consideration the family's values, needs, and resources. Attention should be given to each family member's age, interests, and desires. Possible suggestions are activities the family may enjoy doing together, such as going to the beach, visiting the zoo, camping, or having a picnic. Although the therapist may make activity suggestions, strategies for doing the activities should come from the family. They need to individualize the suggestions, taking into account the physical and emotional setting in which the activity will take place. This perspective views the child as part of the family and not as an isolated person within the family. If the therapist devises the strategies instead of encouraging the family to develop their own strategies, the suggestions and strategies may become burdens on the family, who may feel compelled to comply with the suggestions for therapeutic reasons rather than enjoying the natural play that had been intended (Figure 12-5).

The following case study demonstrates how a family has developed an appreciation of its own balance of play, almost by accident, without intervention.

CASE EXAMPLE 2

The Jones Family

The Jones family consists of a single mother, her 15-year-old son, Tom, and her 12-year-old daughter, Valerie, who has athetoid-type cerebral palsy. They live in a two-bedroom apartment in New York City. Tom is a typical adolescent boy who enjoys riding his bike and playing with other children. Valerie has significantly delayed developmental milestones.

Valerie currently attends a center-based program where she receives occupational therapy, physical therapy, and speech therapy. Progress is slow because she is wheelchair bound and dependent in all aspects of activities of daily living. Psychological testing before she entered kindergarten revealed that she appeared to be mentally retarded, but the psychologist was unable to determine a specific score because of Valerie's extensive motor impairment and limited speech. Valerie was found to have a significant bilateral hearing loss and was fitted with hearing aids.

Tom attends high school. He is an average student who enjoys team sports and is on the school basketball team. He is protective of his sister and, with the exception of close friends, does not often bring friends home because he is concerned about how they may react to her. In general, he is social and outgoing.

The family is warm and loving. Mrs. Jones and Tom are actively involved in Valerie's intervention programs. Mrs. Jones attends most of Valerie's treatment sessions. She initially educated herself about Valerie's disability and took the initiative to obtain proper medical and therapeutic services for her daughter. She then explained Valerie's disability to Tom, who has become more concerned about Valerie, especially in social situations.

Until recently, family life revolved around Valerie and the various interventions she needed. They tried to follow home programs and were involved in outings with other families who had children with disabilities. Mrs. Jones described how the home program activities often resulted in frustration for both her and Valerie when a goal seemed difficult to reach or when Valerie did not want to cooperate. Gradually these sessions developed into playtime, using materials for having fun together that the therapists suggested. For example, while using playing cards to teach Valerie about sorting colors and shapes, Mrs. Jones tried to teach her how to play Go-Fish and War. After a while, she found that Valerie was able to understand these games and she started spending time playing the games with Valerie rather than doing the prescribed home activities. Whereas Mrs. Jones was very attached to Valerie's therapists, she felt that the therapists generally did not understand the need for a typical home life.

Mrs. Jones describes an incident during one summer when Valerie was a toddler that helped to change her perspective on her family life. It was a hot day, and her apartment had no air conditioning. Her automatic response was to take the children to the beach, but she wondered whether this was appropriate for Valerie. Tom, who was 7 years old at the time, and his best friend really wanted to go to the beach, where Mrs. Jones knew that they would play together. Despite her hesitancy, she decided to go, planning to place Valerie on a blanket under an umbrella. Once the family got to the beach, she found that her daughter had other ideas. Valerie rolled off the blanket toward the water and spontaneously began playing in the sand. Mrs. Jones talked about this as an enlightening experience: when she first realized that Valerie had the ability to adapt to her environment and had the natural capacity to find her own way to play like any other child.

Mrs. Jones recalls that she then began thinking that their family life was not typical and that she became concerned about whether the focus on Valerie was fair to Tom. After this incident she got him involved with Little League and outings became more family centered, rather than "Valerie centered."

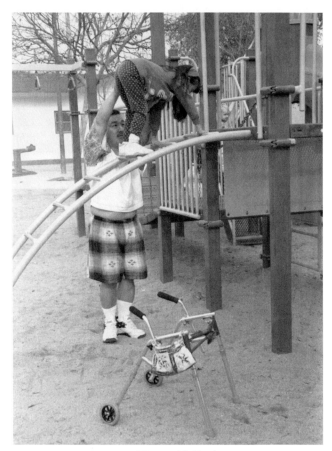

Figure 12-5
Strategies for involving the child with a disability in a family activity, such as going to the park, should be generated by the family rather than the therapist. Otherwise, the activity may be transformed into a chore that is done solely for therapeutic reasons rather than for fun. (Courtesy Shay McAtee.)

This case example illustrates the natural process that takes place in some families. This mother followed her instincts, considered the needs of the whole family, and was able to integrate the child with a disability into family play activities. Mrs. Jones did not feel supported by the occupational therapist in developing family play because the therapeutic focus was on Valerie's skill development. This occupational therapist did not facilitate family play and missed the potential to address an important occupational performance area. The next section illustrates the role of a therapist in facilitating the development of family play as part of the therapeutic process.

FAMILY PLAY AS PART OF THE THERAPEUTIC PROCESS

Some families naturally develop in a manner that allows them to integrate children with disabilities into their play, but other families may need assistance to achieve this. Occupational therapists can help families to develop their own strategies for integrating play into the life of the whole family so that the needs of all members can be met. Consistent with the family-centered philosophy, intervention plans may suggest changes in the family activity to promote enjoyment for its own sake within the family group, instead of providing direct treatment to the child. Intervention is intended to support play or leisure for the child and family and is not directly aimed at meeting specific treatment goals for the child. The interventions that occupational therapists may suggest fall into eight major categories: (1) the process of play, (2) the people engaging in play, (3) the environment where play takes place, (4) the psychosocial nature of play, (5) the materials used in play, (6) the imaginary and symbolic nature of play, (7) the cognitive and physical aspects of play, and (8) the balance of time in the family. A highly recommended approach is for the therapist to suggest natural ways that parents can interact with their child and find mutually enjoyable activities, rather than for the therapist to present these suggestions as a home treatment program. A home program may be perceived as an additional burden on the family, whereas suggested activities may promote comfortable patterns of interaction.

Process of Play

The process of play starts with an activity that spontaneously elicits pleasurable reactions. The process of play then follows a natural sequence of play development. The play sequence begins with mutual and reciprocal interactions between infant and parent. As development proceeds, solitary play becomes important and children are able to play alone and amuse themselves. Next, children tend to become involved in parallel play, playing side by side with other children without interacting. Later, they begin to take toys from each other while playing in a parallel manner, which signifies the beginning of cooperative play, when children actually begin to play together. Older children subsequently get pleasure from formal game play, whereas group play involves formalized rules and patterns (Olson, 1999; Pratt, 1989).

An example is a 4-year-old child who has severe cognitive impairment and is playing with blocks by banging them together. The child is using spontaneous sensorimotor play, banging the blocks together for fun. This is solitary play, which is typical of younger children; however, children with cognitive impairment often engage in play behaviors typical of younger children (Hellendoorn & Hoekman, 1992). Frequently, when parents realize that such behaviors are typical of younger children, they attempt to prevent the immature play from occurring. In the case of the 4-year-old child banging blocks, the parents may react by taking the blocks away, interrupting their child's play process. Therapists may intervene by educating the parents about the value of such play and by guiding the parents to become involved in the child's play. For example, therapists may suggest that the parents of the 4-year-old respond by encouraging the child with a smile as they imitate the banging or that they interact with the child in experimenting with different types of block play. In this manner the parents are becoming involved in the play process starting from the level at which the child is functioning, in an activity that the child has initiated, to increase the child's repertoires of behavior to include social interaction and imitation. If the parents were to move to a level of play complexity that was beyond the child's capability, such as stacking the blocks to build a tower, this might distort the activity or interactions in such a way that it would no longer be play or fun.

People Engaging in Play

The social dimension of play ranges from solitary activities to interaction with one or more individuals. Usually, children spontaneously interact with people around them, finding or creating play experiences wherever they are. Children with disabilities, however, are often limited in their opportunities to interact freely with other children or adults, and their lives tend to be more controlled by what they are unable to do or by what they are not expected to do because of their disabilities. Activities of daily living may take them longer, and they need to spend time in therapy sessions and at medical appointments. Therefore their time is often limited to interacting with adults instead of playing freely with other children (Mulderij, 1996, 1997). In addition, children tend to develop relationships with peers who are physically similar, further placing children with handicapping conditions at a disadvantage. This potentially limits the child's experience with children who do not have disabilities (Short-DeGraff, 1988).

Because the adults who surround a child with disabilities are often concerned with stimulating the child's development, they tend to be directive in their play with the child instead of encouraging spontaneous play. Adults generally want to assist the child to reach optimal performance, and this focus tends to preclude their attention to play and having fun with the child. In some cases this may be the result of a therapeutic recommendation, wherein the therapist has suggested particular activities or toys to parents or caretakers and they follow through in a contrived or artificial manner, concentrating on these activities rather than interacting spontaneously with the child as they would with any other child. Children with disabilities often have difficulty making friends and seldom have an opportunity to engage in sports or formalized recreational activities (Hackett, 2003; Tamm & Prellwitz, 2001).

An example is a 5-year-old girl, Ginny, who has spina bifida and is mobile only with a wheelchair. Although Ginny is mainstreamed in school, her opportunities to interact freely with children are limited because the wheelchair acts as a barrier to other children. Ginny is restricted in playground activities and cannot freely engage in imaginative play activities such as playing house or dress-up games. To intervene, an occupational therapist may show Ginny ways in which she can engage in some of these activities. She may engage Ginny in pretend cooking followed by cleanup. Although this would help to serve a therapeutic goal of developing a positive self-concept, it would also demonstrate that Ginny can engage in imaginative play and see herself in different roles. In addition, the occupational therapist may suggest to the family that Ginny invite other children with whom she feels comfortable to their house for a tea party.

Environment Where Play Takes Place

The environment is complex because it includes both the physical and the psychological contexts of the activity. The characteristics of both of these contexts equally affect play behavior. The physical environment has a strong influence on the types of activities that a person does. Children are active on a playground and sedentary in a movie theater. Children typically have experiences in many types of environments, and they tend to be creative in play within those environments. A revolving door may suddenly become a time capsule or part of an obstacle course. These spontaneous experiences in the physical environment, however, may not be possible for some children with disabilities. Children with disabilities tend to spend most of their time at home, at school, and in the places where they receive therapy.

Occupational therapists may explore with parents the various physical environments where their child spends time, suggesting how play can be incorporated into these physical environments and how the environments may be modified. Alternative environments may also be suggested.

Psychosocial Nature of Play

Play is an emotional experience for children. It allows them to express their emotions, feeling fun, excitement, pleasure, and the freedom to express sadness, anger, and fear. They learn to handle real issues of life in the context of a play experience. Interpersonal play helps to develop social and interpersonal skills, through an understanding of personal boundaries, rules, and acceptable and unacceptable behaviors. It also allows to children to learn and practice cultural experience and perceive their acceptance in a broader social world. Unfortunately, children with disabilities do not always have these opportunities. All professionals need to work together to support the family in understanding the importance of social interaction for the development of psychosocial skills. This must be done in a way that helps the child but supports the needs and values of the entire family (Tamis-Lemonda et al., 2002).

Materials Used in Play

Play materials vary depending on the activity, environment, and resources of the family. Any person, object, or material may become part of play. Children typically play with toys and household objects, but when family play is considered, objects may be less important than the interaction or the activity. For example, infants often begin to babble to crib toys. Parents who interact with the child by imitating the babbling sounds and picking up and tickling the child augment this spontaneous play. The play materials in this example are the crib toys, the parent, and the bodies of the parent and child. When the child is younger, the interaction between the people involved is important, but as the child gets older, the nature of play tends to focus more on the activity, the game, or the setting for enjoyment.

As noted earlier, an aspect of the therapeutic process is adaptation of the materials in the environment or the provision of alternative strategies for incorporating play into the family. Although therapists typically focus on adapting materials for the child, in family play situations the adaptations or alternative strategies are needed so that the family as a whole can become involved in play (Figure 12-6). The focus is not on simple adaptations of a specific toy but rather on complex strategies that take into account the players, their personalities, and the activities they enjoy. When therapists work with children who have motor impairments, they frequently adapt equipment to best meet a child's physical needs from a therapeutic perspective. In play situations the therapist may need to concentrate on removing materials that interfere with play rather than attending solely to proper positioning and adaptive devices. Recent innovations in technology can be used to enhance many aspects of play.

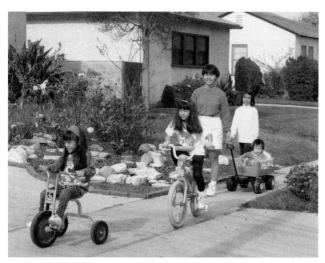

Figure 12-6

Families may have to make accommodations in their play routines, materials, or equipment to include a child with a disability while at the same time retaining the valued family activity so that all parties can enjoy it. (Courtesy Shay McAtee.)

Imaginary and Symbolic Nature of Play

Children become more sophisticated through the use of imaginary and creative play. The emphasis is on enjoyment and not on real-life situations. In imaginary play the child focuses on creativity and not reality. Objects are employed symbolically, which allows the child to use them in new and different ways. For the young child with a disability, imaginary play may allow the suspension of reality, if only briefly. The child can see the world from a different perspective. Play has a symbolic nature for all people, whether or not they have disabilities. As a person matures, imaginary play evolves into creative play that can continue through adulthood. Creative play may have to be role modeled for the child to imitate so that it can become spontaneous, since the child with a disability may have been guided into structured therapeutic activities without having the opportunity to develop a natural childhood sense of fun.

When dealing with creative play, the occupational therapist needs to understand the child and the family well enough to know the meanings of play activities to them—whether activities are specific to the culture, to the region, or to the individuals involved. The therapist cannot change the personal meanings of play to the participants or impose his or her creative sense on the family but must work with their preferences. The creativity should emerge from the family group, incorporating their meaning and values. Gender, roles, ethnicity, and related beliefs may be part of the scenarios, even in creative play. Furthermore, therapists need to be sensitive to the family's concerns about gender and cultural issues in play and not impose their views on the family.

Cognitive and Physical Aspects of Play

Play is widely recognized to be an enhancer of physical and cognitive development in children (Fjortoft, 2001; Goldberg, 2002; Johnson, Christie, & Yawkey, 1999; Rosenbaum, 1998). When parents or therapists choose toys or activities, it is important that they be at an appropriate cognitive and physical level for the child so that he or she can play and gain enjoyment without feeling frustrated. Therapists usually look at the child's cognitive and physical developmental levels when choosing toys. This often leads to a focus on the therapeutic properties of the toy rather than on its play properties. When the activity centers exclusively on the enhancement of learning or development, the fun aspects of play can be lost. Highlighting the therapeutic goal of the activity may interfere with the enjoyment or the play aspect of the activity (Procter, 1989).

The following example highlights the difficulties in balancing the suitability of a toy for play vis-à-vis therapeutic purposes. Daniel is an 8-year-old boy with mild cerebral palsy, spastic diplegia type. He frequently engages in independent play and has told his mother that for his birthday he wants a building set. His mother is concerned about his choice of this toy because, although this might be helpful in developing his fine motor coordination, it would not necessarily enhance his social interactive skills and foster play with other children, a goal suggested by his therapist. She finally decides to buy it for him because it is what he wants and is something he would enjoy.

Balance of Time in the Family

Time has become a precious commodity in family life. Families have difficulty coordinating the schedules of the parents, who have multiple responsibilities, and the children, who have multiple interests and skill levels. Family activities require considerable advance planning and preparation. This places constraints on family play and leisure activities (Mactavish & Schleien, 2004; Shaw & Dawson, 1998).

When intervening in the area of family play and leisure, therapists need to be aware of the time issue and sensitive to the needs and situations of the family. Time constraints complicate the goals of family-centered play, especially in the situation of a child with a disability. The parents may be juggling therapy schedules with cooking dinner for the family. A simple trip to the park may take much more time when a wheelchair is involved. It is hoped that time limitations would not prevent family play, but the therapist should be cognizant of this issue and understanding of the family's needs.

THERAPEUTIC INTERVENTION TO FACILITATE ADAPTATION

Although some families adapt naturally, as in the case example of the Jones family, others need intervention to facilitate adaptations to develop family play. The following case example describes the Wayne family, who required intervention to develop play activities that would include the whole family.

CASE EXAMPLE 3

The Wayne Family

Andrew Wayne, a 10-year-old boy, experienced anoxia following surgery when he was an infant, resulting in brain damage. He walks independently but has cognitive and motoric delays. Andrew comes from an upper middle class background. He lives in a large house with his parents, older sister Janet, and younger sister Carey.

Andrew's mother has taken most of the responsibility for his medical care and treatment because his father works long hours as a partner in a law firm. Andrew went to a therapeutic nursery school program, followed by special education in private schools. He has received occupational therapy and speech therapy, both inside and outside school. Progress has been slow, with periodic plateaus.

Currently Andrew is independent in most tasks, including activities of daily living with supervision, but does not have good social skills. He is still very dependent on his mother. He has few friends. Andrew has many toys but plays alone in his room most of the time. When family members are playing with Andrew, they let him choose the activity and frequently allow him to win games. Going to the zoo with his mother is a favorite activity, and she also takes him to movies and shows that she thinks he will enjoy. His sisters join them occasionally. They are very loving toward Andrew. Janet also takes him to the playground periodically. The family tries to eat together most nights, but Mr. Wayne frequently comes home late. Sunday dinner is a time for the whole family to get together.

The Wayne family lives near the city and enjoys going to many cultural events, such as museums and the theater. Often Andrew is not included in these outings because the family believes that he would not enjoy them.

The occupational therapist who is working with Andrew at home is concerned about his poor play and social skills. Using the Family Observation Guide, the therapist gains some insight into the family situation. Information about how the family interacts and plays with Andrew gives her the basis for an appropriate intervention plan. She encourages the family to spend more time playing with Andrew but suggests that they be involved in choosing the activities rather than always letting Andrew control the play situation. It is a gradual process to get the family accustomed to playing with Andrew and include him without focusing on him and treating him specially. Family members are included in some intervention sessions so that the therapist can role model play with Andrew without focusing on the skill-building aspects of intervention activities.

The therapist also suggests that Andrew be included in the family's cultural activities. Although some initial resistance is apparent, the family tries taking Andrew to a museum. He enjoys being included, although he needs some limits set on his behavior. The therapist reminds the family that all children need to learn how to behave in different situations and that in this regard Andrew is no different from other children. The therapist also suggests that other family members become involved in Andrew's chosen activities. Everyone can enjoy going to the zoo and the playground. The family members find that they enjoy watching Andrew's delight in these trips and soon became involved in the activities themselves.

Facilitating these changes in the family activities takes time and effort for all involved. It requires them to look at their styles of play and how they function as a family unit. The family loves Andrew but has viewed his care as part of Mrs. Wayne's role. He has been treated differently from other family members because of his limitations. The Waynes have had "Andrew activities" and "family activities," which they enjoyed but which often did not include Andrew. Through suggestions and gentle guidance from the occupational therapist, they are able to develop an awareness of family play and incorporate it into their lifestyle.

The intervention designed by the therapist facilitated several family adaptations. The process of play for this family included trips to the city and going to museums and plays, but Andrew was excluded from many of these activities. In addition, Mrs. Wayne took Andrew to the playground and the zoo but did not include Janet and Carey in these trips. The only time the family was consistently together was during Sunday dinner. Based on this information the therapist realized that she needed to suggest strategies to get the family to include Andrew in their activities. When the whole family was included in the trips to the museum or plays, all of them could gain new experiences and enjoy these activities together.

The people involved in play were the whole family as well as the dyadic groups of Andrew and his mother and Andrew and Janet. The therapist reinforced the aspect that Andrew's special times with his mother and sister were an important part of his playtime but suggested that it would help Andrew to see himself as a member of the family if he were also included in family outings. Whereas all family members needed time to pursue their own activities, the exclusion of Andrew alone from some family activities was not sensitive to Andrew's needs. The therapist guided the family to understand that each family member needs to have his or her own activities, as well as family activities, and that each family member should play a role in choosing activities that are done as a family group.

The family was initially resistant to including Andrew because the family members seemed to feel that a museum environment was not suitable for him. The therapist helped them to understand that all children need to learn how to act in different settings and that Andrew would not develop appropriate museum or theater behaviors unless he was given the opportunities or the experiences. Similarly, trips to the zoo or playground could be viewed as family outings instead of something just for Andrew to enjoy. As the family tried new activities as a group, its members became more comfortable with each other and in trying new things with Andrew. This also resulted in a change in the parents' attitude toward trying new things with their daughters.

The materials of play were not as relevant to this family, since they had many resources and preferred family outings to games or toys. The therapist was sensitive to the family's culture in choosing to stay with activities in which they were already involved and that suited their upper middle class stature. Andrew's inclusion in the family trips contributed to his understanding of himself as a family member.

This family's priorities focused on the cognitive nature of the activities they did together. The therapist helped them to understand that Andrew would enjoy some aspects of these trips and that, as with any child of this age, an interactive museum might be more enjoyable to him and his sisters. In suggesting family outings to the playground, the therapist pointed out that all of the children would enjoy the physical activities inherent in that setting.

SUMMARY

Play is an activity that people engage in for the sake of pleasure. Family play is the involvement of the various members in pleasurable activities individually and in groups. The family who has a child with a disability has to deal with many priorities because of the child's special needs and may not view family play as important in their daily activities. Attention should be given to the essential role of play in family life.

Occupational therapists have a unique contribution to the role of play in the family of a child with a handicapping condition. Although play is used as a modality for intervention to facilitate the child's development of functional skills, play or leisure is also an occupational performance area. The role of the therapist in facilitating this performance area is subtle and often overlooked. It requires the therapist to have a broader perspective in viewing the child within the context of the family rather than focusing on the child in isolation.

The Family Observation Guide is suggested as a format for gaining information about the family and play preferences. This approach includes the child as a member of the family and not as a focal point with more importance than any other member. Based on the information obtained, the occupational therapist can guide the family to develop activities in terms of their play benefit to the family and within the context of the family's culture and values. The therapist's role is to introduce strategies so that the needs of all family members are met. Intervention in this area is directly aimed at the play needs of the family as a whole and not at treatment goals for the child. The occupational therapist addresses eight major categories of concern: (1) the process of play, (2) the people engaging in play, (3) the environment where play takes place, (4) the psychosocial nature of play, (5) the materials used in play, (6) the imaginary and symbolic nature of play, (7) the cognitive and physical aspects of play, and (8) the balance of time in the family. Intervention is not focused on the child's developmental issues but involves suggesting changes to promote the integration of the child with a disability into family play as activity for its own pleasurable sake.

Review Questions

1. Consider how play may be viewed as an aspect of the performance area of play or leisure.
2. How is family play influenced by values, culture, and setting? Provide specific examples of each.
3. How do play and leisure activities contribute to family cohesion?
4. How may the presence of a child with a disability affect family play? When a member of the family is a child with a disability, what are the strategies a family can use to maintain a satisfying family play life? How can the therapist facilitate family adaptation using play?
5. How may "overfocusing" on the child with a disability have a negative effect on family play?
6. What are the four domains in the Family Observation Guide? Provide examples of the kinds of questions you might ask within each domain.
7. Describe how play may be viewed as a process and how this view may be incorporated into family play.
8. Discuss how the presence of a disability may affect the social dimension of a child's play.
9. Describe how physical and psychological contexts integrate to form the environment where play takes place.

REFERENCES

Fjortoft, I. (2001). The natural environment as a playground for children: The impact of outdoor play activities in pre-primary school children. *Early Childhood Education Journal, 29*(2), 111-117.

Goldberg, S. (2002). *Constructive parenting*. Des Moines, IA: Allyn & Bacon.

Hackett, J. (2003). Perceptions of play and leisure in junior school aged children with juvenile idiopathic arthritis: What are the implications for occupational therapy? *British Journal of Occupational Therapy, 66*(7), 303-310.

Harkness, L., & Bundy, A. C. (2001). The Test of Playfulness and children with physical disabilities. *Occupational Therapy Journal of Research, 21*(2), 73-89.

Hellendoorn, J., & Hoekman, J. (1992). Imaginative play in children with mental retardation. *Mental Retardation, 30,* 255-263.

Johnson, J., Christie, J., & Yawkey, T. (1999). *Play and early childhood development*. New York: Longman.

Kramer, P., & Hinojosa, J. (1999). Domain of concern of occupational therapy: Relevance to pediatric practice. In P. Kramer & J. Hinojosa (Eds.), *Frames of reference for pediatric occupational therapy* (2nd ed., pp. 9-26). Baltimore: Lippincott Williams & Wilkins.

Kramer, P., & Hinojosa, J. (2004). Activity synthesis as a means to occupation. In J. Hinojosa & M.-L. Blount (Eds.), *The texture of life* (2nd ed., pp. 136-158). Bethesda, MD: American Occupational Therapy Association.

Kramer, P., & Hinojosa, J. (2005). Philosophical and theoretical influences on evaluation. In J. Hinojosa, P. Kramer, & P. Crist (Eds.), *Occupational therapy evaluation: Obtaining and interpreting data* (2nd ed., pp. 19-36). Bethesda, MD: American Occupational Therapy Association.

Luebben, A. J., Hinojosa, J., & Kramer, P. (1999). Legitimate tools of pediatric occupational therapy. In P. Kramer & J. Hinojosa (Eds.), *Frames of reference for pediatric occupational therapy* (2nd ed., pp. 27-40). Baltimore: Lippincott Williams & Wilkins.

Mactavish, J. B., & Schleien, S. J. (2004). Re-injecting spontaneity and balance in family life: Parents' perspectives on recreation in families that include children with developmental disability. *Journal of Intellectual Disability Research, 48*(Part 2), 123-141.

Muhlenhaupt, M., Hinojosa, J., & Kramer, P. (1999). Perspective of context as related to frame of reference. In P. Kramer & J. Hinojosa (Eds.), *Frames of reference for pediatric occupational therapy* (2nd ed., pp. 41-66). Baltimore: Lippincott Williams & Wilkins.

Mulderij, K. J. (1996). Research into the lifeworld of physically disabled children. *Child: Care, Health & Development, 22*(5), 311-322.

Mulderij, K. J. (1997). Peer relations and friendship in physically disabled children. *Child: Care, Health & Development, 23*(5), 379-389.

Olson, L. (1999). Psychosocial frame of reference. In P. Kramer & J. Hinojosa (Eds.), *Frames of reference for pediatric occupational therapy* (2nd ed., pp. 323-376). Baltimore: Williams & Wilkins.

Olson, L., & O'Herron, E. R. (2004). Range of human activity: Leisure. In J. Hinojosa, & M.-L. Blount (Eds.), *The texture of life* (2nd ed., pp. 355-366). Bethesda, MD: American Occupational Therapy Association.

Pratt, P. N. (1989). Play and recreational activities. In P. N. Pratt & A. S. Allen (Eds.), *Occupational therapy for children* (2nd ed.). St. Louis: Mosby.

Procter, S. A. (1989). Play and recreational activities. In P. N. Pratt & A. S. Allen (Eds.), *Occupational therapy for children* (2nd ed.). St. Louis: Mosby.

Rosenbaum, P. (1998). Physical activity play in children with disabilities: A neglected opportunity for research? *Child Development, 69*(3), 607-608.

Shaw, S., & Dawson, D. (1998). *Active family lifestyles: Motivations, benefits, constraints and participation*. Ottawa, Ontario, Canada: Canadian Fitness and Lifestyle Research Association.

Short-DeGraff, M. A. (1988). *Human development for occupational and physical therapists*. Baltimore: Williams & Wilkins.

Tamis-LeMonda, C. S., Užgiris, I. C., & Bornstein, M. H. (2002). Play in parent-child interaction. In M. H. Bornstein (Ed.), *Handbook of parenting. Vol. 5. Practical issues in parenting* (2nd ed., pp. 221-241). Mahwah, NJ: Lawrence Erlbaum.

Tamm, M., & Prellwitz, M. (2001). 'If I had a friend in a wheelchair': Children's thoughts on disabilities. *Child: Care, Health and Development, 27*(3), 223-240.

13

Fostering Early Parent-Infant Playfulness in the Neonatal Intensive Care Unit

ELISE HOLLOWAY

KEY TERMS

parent-infant play
social-emotional context of infancy
neonatal intensive care unit
neurobehavioral organization
neuroregulatory abilities
nonprescriptive stance

The neonatal intensive care unit (NICU) is an acute care environment that focuses primarily on the medical needs rather than the social-emotional and developmental needs of its patients. The NICU staff is highly trained to care for preterm and sick full-term newborns during the most critical phases of their hospital care. In fact, neonatology and neonatal nursing have been called emergency medicine specialties because of the critical nature of the care they give (Gilkerson, Gorski, & Panitz, 1990). Advances in the care of these immature and critically ill newborns have resulted in improved survival rates and an ongoing interest in optimizing their cognitive, neuromotor, and social-emotional outcomes (Als, Duffy, McAnulty, & Badian, 1989; Hack et al., 1991; Symington & Pinelli, 2003). Occupational therapy is one of many health and development disciplines to show this interest (American Occupational Therapy Association [AOTA], 2000; Gorga, 1994; Hunter, 2005; Vergara & Bigsby, 2004).

This chapter addresses parent-infant playfulness within the context of the NICU. Before this is discussed, however, an overview of relevant play theories and concepts of neonatal developmental care is presented. This information can help set the stage for a consideration of parent-infant playfulness within the NICU environment.

APPROACHES TO PLAY

As is apparent from the various chapters in this book alone, there are many theories and perspectives regarding the purposes of play. Solnit and Cohen (1993) viewed play from a child-centered psychotherapeutic perspective in describing the multiple roles that play has for children: Play expresses and represents to the child and others the child's life experiences. Children may use play to learn about and cope with unhappiness, conflict, and trauma. In this view, play becomes a window into the child's cognitive and emotional functioning. Psychotherapists suggest that play can be an intermediary process between acting and thinking and between acting and emoting and so can help therapists to understand the child's internal processes (Solnit, 1993).

The evolutionary perspective on parent-child play suggests that behavior as common as play must have an evolutionary function and that it represents an important adaptation. Play is conceptualized as an "environment-engagement device" (MacDonald, 1993, p. 117) with the purpose of providing stimulation for the child, which will assist in the development of neural structures that help the child adapt to his or her environment. Play and neurological development are thus viewed as intimately connected to each other.

Cultural-ecological theories suggest that children's play varies depending on the ecological characteristics of the play setting. Whereas parent-infant play has a unique, species-typical character of rhythm, tempo, synchrony, and body and eye contact, broader cultural norms, values, and beliefs define children's play contexts and the type of play activity. This type of sociocultural interaction theory recognizes that social interaction is embedded within family routines and that culture is transmitted via active participation in daily activities. Children are assumed to have an intrinsic interest in their world and to have the skills to participate in it. They are viewed as active and motivated participants because they have internalized species-specific and culture-specific behavior; this behavior is elaborated on by experience (Bloch & Pellegrini, 1989; Fogel, Nwokah, & Karns, 1993).

It has been suggested that even though parent-child play is species and culture specific, it cannot be explained solely by genetics or infant maturation and learning. Fogel et al. (1993) suggested that "parent-child play is a creative process, emergent from the dynamics of social discourse between two different individuals in a particular cultural and physical context" (p. 45). In the view of these authors, other theories that rely on internal schemes to account for play and interactive behavior are inadequate to account for the spontaneity, variability, and creativity that are seen within an interaction. Instead, these interactive rules may result from the dynamics of interaction between parent and infant. This two-person system is thought to be self-organizing and process oriented. Consequently, a wide variability is seen in parent-infant play even within one cultural setting. Furthermore, a change in the dynamics of the interaction results in a change in patterns of parent-infant social play. An example of this process is provided by Tronick and Cohn's still-face paradigm (Cohn, 1993; Cohn & Tronick, 1983). During face-to-face play, mothers were asked to simulate depression with a flattened affect while continuing to look at their babies. Initially the infants attempted to sustain play, but after just a few minutes they reduced their smiling and gazing.

Occupational therapists have various perspectives on play as well. The Occupational Therapy Practice Framework definition of play is "any spontaneous or organized activity that provides enjoyment, entertainment, amusement, or diversion" (AOTA, 2002, p. 633). Play is considered to be an occupation. To many occupational therapists, however, play is a tool, much in the same way that neurofacilitation techniques and assistive technology are tools. For example, play has been used to motivate a child to accomplish a specific motor act or to "learn" spatial relationships. It also has been used by therapists to engage children in environmental exploration (Bundy, 1991; Burke, 1993). Although occupational therapists may emphasize the role of intrinsic motivation in play behavior, they usually tie it to the rationale of using play to support the development of skills. Less frequently, an outcome of occupational therapy treatment is play for its own sake, that is, for the process as described by Fogel rather than the outcome of skill development (Burke, 1993; Fogel et al., 1993). Play has been defined as self-initiated, self-directed, and flexible, yet occupational therapists frequently choose to direct a child's play activity to achieve a therapist-driven goal.

Bundy (1997) suggested that because play is more process oriented than the product-driven occupations of work and self-care, occupational therapists find play difficult to assess and measure as an outcome. She and others (Bazyk, Stalnaker, Llerena, Ekelman, & Bazyk, 2003) posited that instead of defining and measuring play, it may be more useful to address playfulness in a variety of contexts. That is, it may be more meaningful for the therapist and the client to examine *how* an individual engages in an activity rather than *whether* a specific activity is play.

Sutton-Smith (1993) warned that play has become more supervised and controlled by adult interests as it has been shown to be a means of improving academic competence. He suggested that influencing play to improve developmental outcomes can be a device to justify the socialization of one cultural group according to the standards of another group. One occupational therapy view of play is that if the child is successful as a player, he or she experiences feelings associated with productivity, satisfactory quality of life, meaningfulness, and value (Burke, 1993). Although these are qualities that the dominant culture of the United States generally values, occupational therapists must be careful not to project them onto families whose own cultures may not value play activities per se or these types of value-driven outcomes (Bazyk et al., 2003; MacDonald, 1993). When therapists overgeneralize the values of the dominant culture, they themselves fall into the trap to which Sutton-Smith (1993) referred.

SOCIAL-EMOTIONAL CONTEXT OF INFANCY

Infants develop in a social-emotional context. From the moment of birth they are involved in social interactions with adults, primarily their family members, in their environment. Infants have been shown to respond differently to adults, with slower movements of the extremities and more alert facial expressions, than they do to objects. Some interactions meet infants' daily care needs, but other interchanges are more playful, with mutual engagement and synchronized exchanges of smiles, sounds, and gazes; enjoyment and connectedness are the only purpose (Brazelton, Koslowski, & Main, 1979; Whaley, 1990). Infants need adequate support from the caregiving environment to master their social, interactive, and exploratory skills. How parents engage with their newborn plays a critical role in facilitating or interfering with the infant's ability to master these skills and to experience pleasure in the process (Beeghly, 1993; Greenspan, 1990).

Beeghly (1993) described the perspective of organizational developmental psychopathology on early infant development and parent-infant play. In her view, behavioral systems such as cognition, social-communicative behavior, affect, and self-regulation are organized hierarchically and are all interrelated. In each stage of development a child must negotiate a series of cognitive, social, and affective tasks. Accomplishing a certain developmental task helps the child adapt to the environment and readies him or her to develop competence in a more complex task. Establishing competence via play promotes age-appropriate adaptation later on by integrating earlier competencies in the social, emotional, and cognitive realms into later function. This organizational perspective, when applied to parent-infant play, implies a multidimensional approach that takes into consideration the child's unique characteristics, his or her age and developmental level, the interrelationships among the various developmental realms, and the unique characteristics of the caregiving and sociocultural environment provided by the parent (Beeghly, 1993).

The organizational approach describes major tasks of infancy that occur and must be mastered in a developmental sequence for the individual to function adaptively. For each task infants must use their full range of social, affective, cognitive, and self-regulatory capacities, enabling their current level of behavioral competence to be observed. The major tasks for the birth to 3-month period are regulatory ones. These are to stabilize sleep-wake cycling, patterns of feeding and elimination, and state organization. If the tasks are achieved, the infant is able to interact more consistently with the caregiver within the infant's environment and begin to establish a reliable early signaling system. How well infants accomplish one task has an impact on their accomplishment of future tasks. For example, a newborn's difficulty regulating his or her state of arousal may interfere with the infant's ability to engage in a social task such as face-to-face interaction with a parent. Infants who are biologically at risk may have difficulty with state organization or regulation and mastery of social-interactive and exploratory skills that are crucial for negotiating the next developmental task successfully (Als, Lester, Tronick, & Brazelton, 1982).

One significant task of parenting in the newborn period is establishing parent-infant interaction and patterns of communication. These interactions are often embedded within other aspects of parenting such as child-care activities and nurturance (Patteson & Barnard, 1990). Newborns are viewed as active participants in any interchange; they are social organisms that are innately predisposed to interact with their environment. These interactions have been noted to be bidirectional, that is, involving communication from parent to infant and from infant to parent (Gianino & Tronick, 1988). Because of both external and internal feedback processes, this interchange cannot be predicted solely by a linear model but must include the dynamic process between parent and child (Nugent & Brazelton, 1989; Nugent et al., 1993). The infant's development takes place in a particular cultural context or niche: his or her family. The family structure provides the social resources to help organize the infant's niche so as to provide nurturance and stimulation to

engage in this parent-infant dance of interaction (Nugent et al., 1993).

Parents attribute intention and motives to infants. Frequently infants are viewed as individuals with subjective experiences, social awareness, and a sense of self from birth (Brazelton & Cramer, 1990). Meanings that parents attribute to their infant's behavior may arise from the parents' personal histories and memories, as well as from their infant's unique characteristics. This provides parents with a set of internal rules for interpreting their infant's behaviors. Parental perceptions of their newborn's interactive behaviors guide their interactions with the baby (Brazelton & Cramer, 1990; Cardone & Gilkerson, 1990, 1992).

Cross-cultural research has shown significant variability in parent-infant interaction patterns, with the range and form of adaptations shaped by both the demands of culture and the dynamics occurring between parent and infant. Patterns of feeding, diapering, swaddling, holding, touching, and looking are all mediated by these processes (Finn, 2003). It is important, then, to focus not on the "*what* of behavior but the *how* of behavioral responsivity" (Nugent & Brazelton, 1989, p. 94) of both partners in understanding early parent-infant play.

During the newborn period, both the parents and the infant are in a state of heightened readiness for exploratory interaction to assist in reorganizing the family niche (Nugent & Brazelton, 1989). In addition to the cultural context, the infant's social responsivity and communication cues may determine the amount of caregiving that he or she elicits from parents. Research has shown that a certain degree of unpredictability or variability in the infant's state behavior may elicit more parental caregiving involvement (Nugent et al., 1993).

The variability in infant behavior, parent attributes, and cultural values about the nature of infant care and development necessitates that therapists take a "nonprescriptive stance" (Nugent & Brazelton, 1989, p. 93) when engaging therapeutically with parents and newborns. This nonprescriptive stance is one that sensitizes parents to their infant's unique adaptive abilities and communication cues without adding a label or value to those capacities. In this way the therapist may initiate a positive cycle of mutually rewarding social and emotional interactions, essentially defined by the parent-infant dyad itself, which may result in positive long-term influences on parent-infant relations and infant developmental outcomes (Brazelton & Cramer, 1990; Nugent & Brazelton, 1989; Patteson & Barnard, 1990).

Parent-infant research and clinical experience, such as those just described, have resulted in a growing realization by many health and development disciplines that the infant's experience of his or her primary relationships influences future development. The multidisciplinary field of infant mental health, composed of health, education, and social service disciplines, embraces the philosophy that each infant's optimal growth and development occur within nurturing relationships and that a "therapeutic presence" (Weatherston, 2002, p. 2) with high-risk infants and at-risk families may reduce the chance that their relationship will fail. The field of infant mental health focuses on the biological, psychological, and social aspects of risk; protective factors, resilience, developmental processes, and psychopathology in the infant and parent; and most important, their relationship. The emphasis of study, assessment, and intervention is this relationship and the central role it plays in the infant's development (Schultz-Krohn & Cara, 2000; Weatherston, 2002; Zeanah & Zeanah, 2001). Occupational therapy is an acknowledged player within the infant mental health arena, especially for its unique contributions related to emerging occupations and sensory processing when applied to parent-child relationships.

The infant mental health perspective is an important consideration for therapists working with high-risk populations, such as infants who are biologically at risk. However, definitions of risk are cultural constructions, so what constitutes risk status in one setting, such as the hospital, may not in another, such as the community (Nugent et al., 1993). Thus it is even more important that the therapist integrate the "nonprescriptive stance" into her or his work with infants and families in the NICU. This strategy is discussed further in the following sections.

DEVELOPMENTAL CARE IN THE NEONATAL INTENSIVE CARE UNIT

With the advent of specialized neonatal intensive care units in the late 1960s and early 1970s, survival rates of preterm and critically ill newborns improved significantly. Research emphasis in the new field of neonatology began to shift from mortality to neurodevelopmental morbidity. Outcome studies indicated that many infants had cognitive and neuromotor deficits (Browne, 2003; Gottfried & Gaiter, 1985). During that time researchers in development postulated that the isolating and sensorially depriving hospital environment contributed to these poor outcomes. Accordingly, intervention studies looking at various combinations of sensory stimulation, most frequently tactile, vestibular, and kinesthetic-proprioceptive, were initiated (Gregg, Haffner, & Korner, 1976; Leib, Benfield, & Guidubaldi, 1980; Powell, 1974; Rice, 1977; Scarr-Salapatek & Williams, 1973; Solkoff & Matuszak, 1975; Solkoff, Yaffe, Weintraub, & Blase, 1969; White & LaBarba, 1976). Although almost all of these studies reported positive outcomes in terms of improved weight gain, feeding abilities, state regulation, motor development, and visual attention, there were clear methodological problems that limited their applicability.

The intervention programs varied in timing, type, and intensity of stimulation. Some were applied to infants of one gestational age, whereas others were used with infants of varying ages. In general, these studies did not report baseline environmental conditions before, during, or after their intervention, complicating even further the analysis of the effects of these supplemental stimulation programs (Cornell & Gottfried, 1976; Pressler, Turnage-Carrier, & Kenner, 2004). Another significant limitation was the lack of understanding of the preterm infant's central nervous system (CNS) organization; there was little knowledge about CNS regulation of heart rate, respiration, or arousal (Gilkerson et al., 1990). Furthermore, these studies were carried out with a relatively low-risk, stable infant population. Today's NICU sees a much more fragile, gestationally immature infant, whose nervous system is more vulnerable to environmental demands and who may indeed be compromised physiologically by caregiving activities that are appropriate for robust full-term infants and even for more stable preterm infants (Als et al., 2003; AOTA, 2000; Gilkerson et al., 1990).

When the NICU sensory environment was examined in research, it was not found to be consistently sensorially depriving. In fact, at times it was noted to be overwhelming to some infants. In general, stimulation levels did not seem to match the states of arousal or behavioral readiness of the infants and appeared to affect them physiologically. For example, ambient noise levels were often quite high and correlated with decreases in infants' blood oxygen levels and increases in intracranial pressure (Bess, Peck, & Chapman, 1979; Long, Lucey, & Philip, 1980; Speidel, 1978). Routine caregiving procedures that were standard for all infants were also found to result in physiological changes (Long, Philip, & Lucey, 1980). Little diurnal variation in activity or lighting levels was noted; the nursery's schedule was based on caregiver needs rather than infant needs. Handling or talking usually was not related to the infant's state of arousal. Infants showed both immediate and delayed, subtle and gross signs of distress related to caregiving and other environmental events (Bozzette & Kenner, 2004; Gaiter, 1985; Gottfried et al., 1981; Linn, Horowitz, & Fox, 1985; Newman, 1981).

The current trend in NICU developmental intervention research is directed toward understanding the immature and sick infant's neuroregulatory abilities and then letting this guide developmentally supportive interventions (Ballweg, 2004). This approach began with the characterization of the healthy full-term newborn as competent, capable of responding to the environment, and able to elicit responsive behaviors from the caretaker in order to receive the kind of interaction and caregiving he or she needs (Nugent & Brazelton, 1989). The infant was viewed as effectively communicating via behavioral cues to indicate his or her readiness for stimulation, stress, and need for rest. With this perspective in mind, researchers such as Als, Gorski, and Barnard began to describe behaviors of sick and immature newborns in attempts to understand these infants' thresholds of stress and stability and then to design supportive intervention programs in which the infant's behavior guided the caregivers' actions. This approach recognizes and treats infants as individuals and consequently individualizes each infant's intervention program (Als, 1986; Barnard & Bee, 1984; Gorski, Leonard, Sweet, Martin, & Sehring, 1990; Symington & Pinelli, 2003).

The work of Als and her associates is one example of the developmental intervention trend. Als conceptualized a model termed the Synactive Theory of Newborn Neurobehavioral Organization. This model describes the newborn's emerging behavioral organization and how development proceeds via a continuous balancing of infant-environment interactions and the continuous interplay among the following five neurobehavioral subsystems within the infant (Als, 1983, 1986; Als et al., 1982, 1986, 1989):

1. *Autonomic system.* The newborn's primary task is to stabilize and integrate autonomic functions such as heart rate, respiration, thermoregulation, and digestion.
2. *Motor system.* The newborn demonstrates varying degrees of postural adjustments and modulation of muscle tone.
3. *State organizational system.* The newborn demonstrates differentiation of states of arousal with emerging sleep, wake, and crying states; distinctness versus diffuseness of states and patterns of state transition are observed.
4. *Attention-interaction system.* The infant shows ability to modulate arousal and attention to interact with and elicit input from the world.
5. *Regulatory system.* The infant demonstrates ability to maintain or regain a stable, well-modulated subsystem balance. This includes the facilitation that the infant requires from his or her environment to achieve and sustain this balance.

Each of these subsystems matures sequentially, and all are interdependent. Autonomic system instability can be observed in changes in respiratory patterns, skin color, and various visceral signs. Motoric organization is seen via muscle tone, posture, and movement. The range of availability of the infant's states of arousal and transitions between states, that is, sleep to drowsy to alert, influences both motoric stability and the infant's attentional-interactional system. Once the infant is able to achieve and maintain an alert state, interactive responses demonstrate his or her ability to orient and attend to visual and auditory stimuli without becoming fatigued. In the healthy, term newborn, these subsystems function smoothly and in synchrony via the regulatory system. The less mature or ill newborn shows a less organized interplay of subsystems, with lower thresholds for stimulation and relatively fewer self-regulatory abilities. Therefore routine caregiving and interactive demands can be stressful and cause physiological instability in such an infant.

The work examining neuroregulatory abilities emphasizes the individualized caregiving needs of preterm and sick newborns. The infant's readiness for environmental demands and ability to cope with the potential mismatch between the infant's capabilities and the environment continues to be at the heart of developmental intervention research. This model is one that "focuses on the way individual infants handle the experience of the world around them rather than on skills" (Als et al., 1989, p. 6).

Gilkerson et al. (1990) appropriately pointed out that understanding of infant regulatory functions is still very limited. They questioned whether intervention efforts should be focused on changing or shaping behaviors that are not well understood. For example, they asked whether it is appropriate at any given point in an infant's neuromaturation to attempt to change the amount of time that an infant is in awake states, possibly at the expense of other states; they suggested that losing time in other arousal states that "might serve some less obvious but equally vital purpose during a particular stage of maturation" (Gilkerson et al., 1990, p. 460) could have as yet unknown consequences. This perspective regarding the current limited knowledge of the neuroregulatory abilities of newborn infants, along with the better understood organ system fragility of these infants, must underlie any discussion of occupational therapy intervention in the NICU.

PARENTAL EXPERIENCE IN THE NEONATAL INTENSIVE CARE UNIT

Parents' assumptions' about themselves, the world, and how their family will function can be violated by having a preterm or critically ill newborn hospitalized in the NICU (Affleck & Tennen, 1991). This experience can pose a significant threat to the parents' psychological well-being; emotional distress is common. Throughout the infant's hospitalization, parents show a range of emotional reactions in a "rollercoaster ride" (Hughes & McCollum, 1993, p. 57; Price, 2003) that follows the ups and downs of their infant's hospital course. Emotional stressors reported by parents include separation from the infant, concern regarding the infant's health, disruption in family routines, not feeling like a parent, ambivalence about their emotional investment in the infant, and anxiety concerning the infant's future development (Hughes & McCollum, 1993; McGrath & Myer, 1992; Talmi & Harmon, 2003). Coping strategies are linked to each individual's perception of personal stressors. To cope, parents report that they have sought out social support, information regarding their child's problem, a meaning to the whole perinatal-neonatal experience, and escape (Able-Boone & Stevens, 1994; Affleck & Tennen, 1991; Affleck, Tennen, & Rowe, 1990;

Hughes, McCollum, Sheftel, & Sanchez, 1994). Parental coping efforts could influence the nature of their current and future interactions with their infant and must be considered in attempts to foster a mutual interchange between parent and infant.

PLAYFULNESS IN THE NEONATAL INTENSIVE CARE UNIT

As mentioned earlier, infants develop in a social-emotional context. They are born adapted to their family niche. They have innate abilities to organize their physiological, motoric, state, and interactional systems to elicit caregiving and nurturance from their parents. Parents, for their part, bring their own contributions to the dynamic interchange that forms the basis of parent-infant playfulness and play. Their values, beliefs, and memories assist them in reading and interpreting their infant's communications. This process supports the infant in achieving an early primary task: feeling calm and alert and ready to develop a consistent, refined signaling system by which to engage with the parent. This signaling system facilitates the emergence of the infant's occupational being through enabling the infant's participation in a relationship with the parents and in family life.

With the preceding perspective in mind, the occupational therapist may use the Occupational Therapy Practice Framework to address the emerging infant-parent occupational performance within the context of the NICU. To develop an intervention process that supports both current and emerging parent-infant co-occupations, including playfulness, the therapist may assess client factors, activity demands, context, and performance skills (AOTA, 2002). These areas for assessment are indicated in italics in the following discussion.

Because of their immaturity or illness, infants in the NICU are not necessarily adapted to extrauterine life and its demands. They may be inconsistently able to organize smooth functioning of their neurobehavioral subsystems. Their efforts to do so, especially in the face of the environment's social and physical demands, may be physiologically destabilizing, causing apnea, bradycardia, and hypoxia. As preterm infants mature, they begin to achieve a balance in these subsystems. Any extra demand, however, can threaten that fragile balance (*client factors*).

The fragility of the hospitalized infant creates stress for parents (*client factors*). In addition, the NICU experience may impose additional stress on parents as they attempt to establish a relationship with their infant (Talmi & Harmon, 2003). When a parent enters the NICU, she or he sees a high-tech, unfamiliar environment with monitors and equipment evident both visually and auditorially (*context*). Even the location of the infant in that environment may not be obvious at first (Figure 13-1). The sense of being overwhelmed may grow as the parent draws near

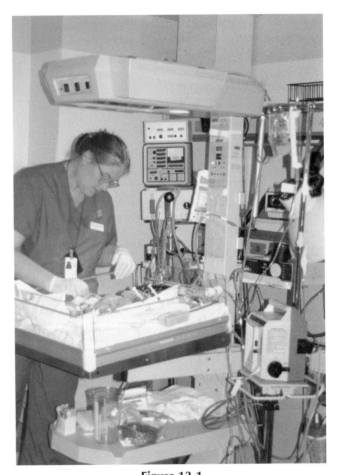

Figure 13-1
The overwhelming environment of the neonatal intensive care unit.

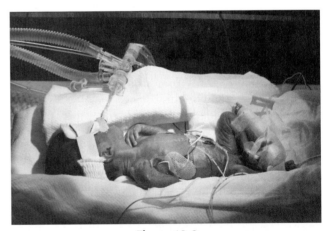

Figure 13-2
Initially the fragile infant struggles with physiological stability.

to the infant's bed and sees the baby (Figure 13-2). Parents have reported that it can take weeks or even months, watching their infant grow and recover, before they are comfortable touching or holding their infant (Holloway, 1994). With an understanding that infants engage in co-created occupations with parents (Lawlor, 2003) and an appreciation of the infant's fragility and parents' emotional status, the occupational therapist must seek to determine what therapeutic processes will assist them in beginning to co-create their family occupations, whether these are feeding, diapering, or playing together.

Als and her associates suggested that preterm and sick infants communicate their needs via their behaviors (Als, 1997; Als et al., 1982, 2003). They can be overstimulated easily but may be able to indicate this, as well as their readiness for interaction, to their caregivers. These behavioral cues become more evident as an infant grows and matures, becoming more physiologically stable. The infant in this process is working on the first major developmental task of infancy, according to the organizational perspective (*performance skills*). However, the developing signaling system may be inconsistent or difficult to read at first. If a young infant is struggling to establish his or her neurobehavioral balance within the environment and has just begun signaling, the infant is not yet ready to participate in a playful moment. The nature of play (*activity demands*) and the attributes and skills needed by both partners for a successful, playful interchange suggest that these infants, and often their parents, are not ready for playful interchanges during most of their hospitalization (*client factors*).

Occupational therapists practicing in the NICU can support the precursors of playfulness by helping the parents read their infant's communication signals, assign their own meaning to these signals, and feel comfortable with the actions that they do and do not take with their baby (*performance skills*). Infant signals can be subtle or very obvious to a parent (*performance skills*). For example, an infant who is overaroused (Figure 13-3, *A*) is as unavailable for a positive interchange at that moment as one who is underaroused (Figure 13-3, *B*). Similarly, an infant who is grimacing, splaying her or his fingers, or yawning may be signaling the need for a break in the interaction (Figure 13-4). Parents may learn that just sitting quietly, looking at their infant or possibly touching her or him, provides exactly the right amount of sensory information to match their infant's arousal threshold (Figure 13-5).

Occupational therapists may support parents in learning alternative ways of engaging with their infant. The father in Figure 13-6 discovered early on that his daughter Amanda loved to suck on his little finger, and he expressed great pleasure in this. Amanda's act of sucking on his finger symbolized to him her acceptance and responsiveness to him. This became the basis for their growing signaling and engagement system. The positive meaning that he attached to his infant's sucking encouraged him to try to engage with her in other ways and at other times, such as during dressing (Figure 13-7, *A*). Figure 13-7, *B*, shows another instance of parent-infant engagement

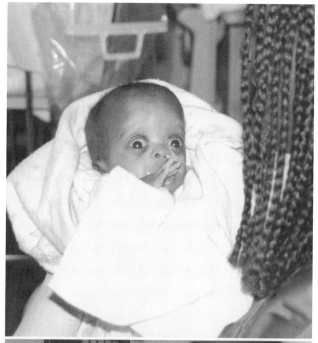

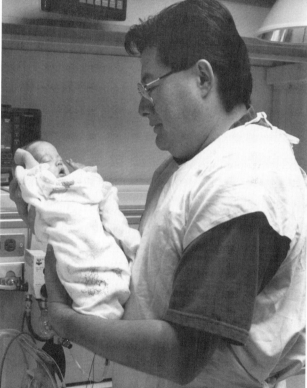

Figure 13-3

A, *An infant who is hyperalert may be overwhelmed by social interaction.* **B,** *Immature infants may have difficulty achieving and maintaining an alert state. (Courtesy Shay McAtee.)*

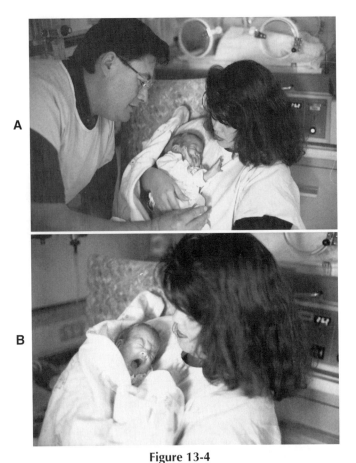

A

B

Figure 13-4

Parents may adjust their interaction styles based on infant communication signals. (Courtesy Shay McAtee.)

occurring spontaneously within the context of a daily care activity, bathtime. These moments cannot be taught via parent education but can be facilitated and supported by the occupational therapist as she or he seeks to understand what is meaningful to the parent and how that may relate to the infant's neurobehavioral capacities.

The therapist accomplishes such facilitation and support processes through his or her therapeutic use of self and "doing with" the parent-infant dyad. Price, in her research regarding occupation-centered practice in the NICU, observed that it is the "intra-personal aspects of the therapeutic process and the inter-subjective aspects of the therapeutic relationship" while therapist and parent are mutually engaged with the infant in therapy activities that "enable the creation of meaning, making the activities occupational" (Price, 2003, p. 301)

Parent-infant interchanges, which become more active and frequent as the infant becomes more medically stable, more mature, and closer to going home, can help to establish the beginning of playfulness between parent and infant. As the parent learns to read the infant's rhythms and subsequently adapts his or her behavioral tempo, and as the infant matures in self-regulation, their mutually positive experience is

prolonged. The short-term therapy goal is that both parent and infant experience satisfying interchanges, some of which are playful in nature. The long-term goal is to promote a nurturing relationship that supports development of the child as an occupational being with full participation in daily family life. Through the therapeutic use of self and a focus on the "how" of parent-infant responses and engagement, the occupational therapist can help to create an emotional space for a creative, playful process to emerge from the growing dynamic between parent and infant as they go home together.

Chronic health conditions sometimes develop in infants hospitalized in the NICU, necessitating more prolonged hospitalization (Browne, 2003; Gottfried & Gaiter, 1985). With these longer stays in the NICU, there may continue to be a mismatch between the infant's neurobehavioral capabilities and the environment's demands. Whether the occupational therapist's approach is based on the evolutionary perspective that the infant uses play to engage the environment so as to obtain the stimulation necessary for neural structure development, or on the contention of Fogel and occupational therapy theorists that play is important for its own sake, the therapist's challenge becomes threefold: facilitating the infant's ongoing development, learning the meaning of play for the parent, and adapting the environment to encourage both infant's and parent's readiness so as to provide opportunities for playful moments.

First, the occupational therapist must return not only to examining the infant's developmental skills, such as reaching for a toy, but also to the "how" of accomplishing those skills. How does the infant process the environment's sensory input? How and in what way does he or she engage? Does the infant behave differently when he or she is having difficulty with feedings or when having respiratory distress? Understanding all of the infant's interrelated physiological, sensory, neuromotor, and social-emotional processes provides the foundation for developing therapy interventions that promote playfulness (*client factors, performance skills*). This understanding comes about from direct interaction with the infant, in addition to observation of the infant during nursing care procedures and parent interactions.

In some instances one-to-one therapy with the infant, such as focusing on strengthening, may be appropriate. The reason for strengthening might be to improve head control in a supported sitting position, to promote postures that support the infant's engagement with the therapist, or ultimately to enable the infant to hold his or her head up during playtime with the mother. Other reasons for direct intervention might be to assist the infant to remain available for interaction in the face of environmental demands or to determine

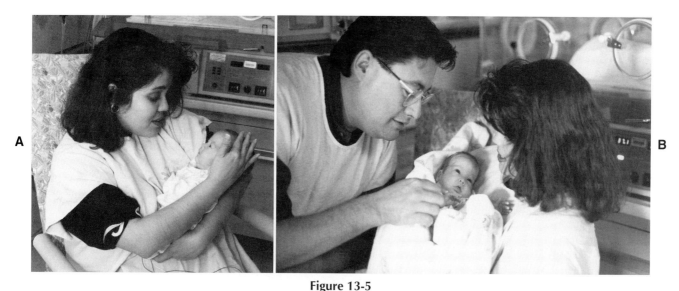

Figure 13-5
A, *Quietly looking at each other can be a mutually rewarding interchange.* **B,** *At other times the infant may be able to respond to her parents'*
voices. (**A,** *Courtesy Shay McAtee.*)

how the infant indicates his or her needs and what events interfere with the infant's signaling efforts (*performance skills, activity demands*).

Since parents and infants work toward a dance of give and take in interaction and play (Nugent et al., 1993), therapy time can be devoted to facilitating the infant's ability to participate in two-way communication and to string several behaviors together (*performance skills*). The occupational therapist can plan to wait and watch for infant responses and then act in a manner contingent on the infant's behavior to facilitate the infant's portion of the "dance." In addition, the therapist needs to be able to tap into a personal sense of playfulness and express that to the infant in a well-modulated way, matching the infant's own tempo and rhythms, to elicit the infant's playfulness.

Environmental adaptations (*context*) are not only physical in nature (e.g., turning down bright hospital lights), but also social. Since playful moments often occur within the context of daily activities, the older chronically ill infant may benefit from having a daily schedule with built-in routines. Consistency of caregivers and caregiving approaches promotes the infant's sense of predictability and assists the caregivers in getting to know the infant. This may allow the infant's subtle or fleeting efforts at signaling to emerge and to receive an appropriate response. Daily routines and schedules can be arranged so that an infant is "ready" for the parents, if possible. In this way the infant may be at his or her rested and responsive best for play with dad, even if it is at 10 pm after the father gets off work (*context*).

With the understanding that each individual family's cultural norms, values, and beliefs define where and how family members play, the therapist must seek to learn the parents' view of playfulness and play. The only

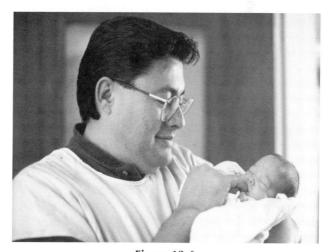

Figure 13-6
Touch can be as meaningful as looking and listening. (Courtesy Shay McAtee.)

assumption regarding this definition that the therapist may safely make is that few parents idealize the NICU as a play environment! The therapist should elicit the following information from parents: What needs to happen for the parent to feel comfortable in the NICU? How would the parent like to act with his or her baby if no one were around? Does the parent wish for one-on-one time or for the whole family to be together? If there were no rules, where would the parent like to be with his or her baby: in a chair, in bed, on the floor? When does the parent feel most at ease in the NICU? Is the parent a morning or night person? How does the parent characterize his or her current coping? Does the parent feel like playing?

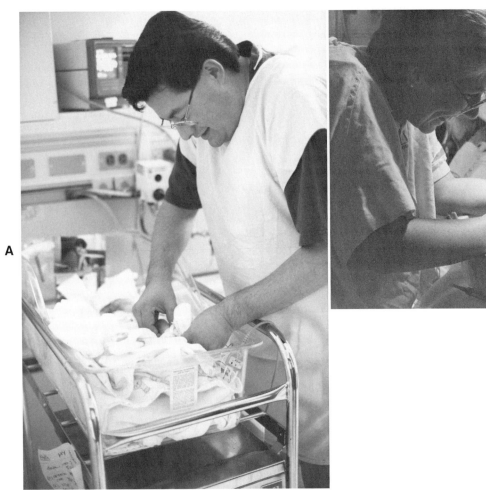
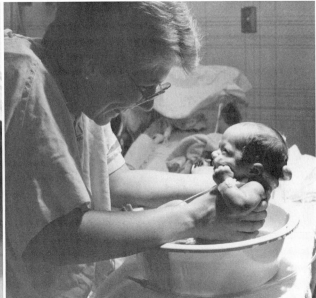

Figure 13-7
Parent-infant engagement occurs within the context of daily care activities. (**A,** *Courtesy Shay McAtee.*)

Information about a parent's views of play can assist the occupational therapist in facilitating a play dynamic between parent and infant. Together the therapist and parent can discover the types of activities and infant responses that have meaning to them, that may be perceived as fun or playful. Although sharing what has worked between the therapist and the infant during their therapy sessions may be helpful, the goal is to take a nonprescriptive stance by encouraging the parents' vision of play and nurturing (Nugent & Brazelton, 1989). For the parents, play may mean smiling face to face with the baby (Figure 13-8, *A*), feeling the baby holding onto a parent's shoulder as the parent "dances" (Figure 13-8, *B*), or something that baby, mother, and father create together (Figure 13-8, *C*).

CASE EXAMPLE 1
Amanda

Amanda was delivered at 23 weeks gestation with a birth weight of 510 grams. Her primary medical diagnoses during her rocky hospital course were respiratory distress syndrome, bronchopulmonary dysplasia, bilateral grade IV intraventricular hemorrhage, and posthemorrhagic hydrocephalus with a resultant ventriculoperitoneal shunt. Several times during the early days of her hospitalization, Amanda's parents met with the neonatologists to determine how aggressive her medical care should be, considering her poor prognosis for survival and neurodevelopmental outcome. Until she was 7 weeks old, occupational therapy intervention was indirect, through consultation with nursing to integrate developmental care strategies into her overall nursing care plan.

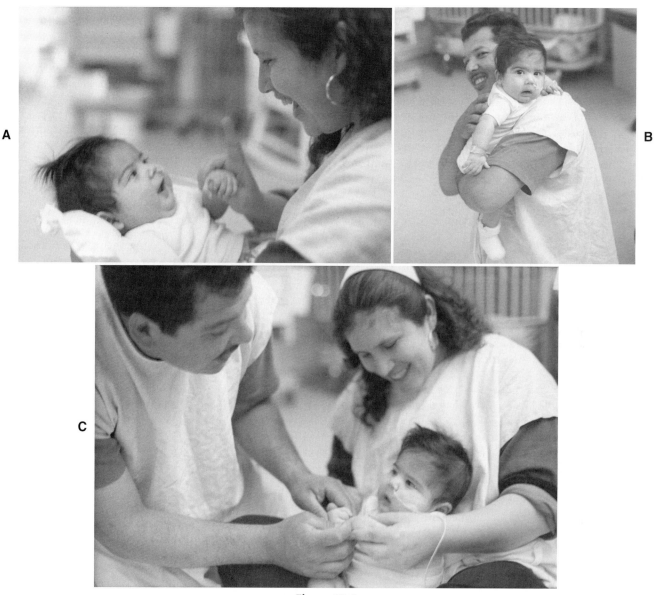

Figure 13-8
The parent-infant dyad or triad determines the nature of their play.

As Amanda's survival became more assured, more direct occupational therapy involvement was offered to her parents. At this time she was 30 weeks gestation, in an Isolette, and receiving assisted ventilation via continuous positive airway pressure and supplemental oxygen. Her parents indicated a reluctant interest in what occupational therapy had to offer. The course that the therapist took to establish a collaborative relationship was guided by Amanda's parents and by Amanda herself. First, the therapist encouraged Amanda's parents to describe their view of their precious little girl. They understood that she was still very fragile and yet saw strength in her because she had already come through so much. They clearly communicated that this was the manner in which they wanted everyone to view her. The therapist and parents watched Amanda together during her diaper changes, nasogastric tube feeding, and respiratory therapy treatments and then described her behaviors that indicated to them her strengths and her fragility. Her parents, however, always led the way in describing her. They attributed her various characteristics to one parent or the other, as well as to the current situation. The therapist added her observations regarding their own capable ways of knowing and responding to their baby. They discussed Amanda's rhythms during caregiving and the type of pacing that she needed. When Amanda showed fatigue or a sign of stress, they talked about it and tried different interventions that might help her to cope.

As Amanda matured and recovered, the parents and the therapist continued their partnership in supporting Amanda's development. As mutual trust grew, they were able to speak more openly about what happened when Amanda showed a response that was not what her parents wished. They discussed the meaning of her behaviors to them. For example, sucking her father's finger meant acceptance of him (Figure 13-6). To her mother, it meant that breastfeeding was still a possibility and that her husband was experiencing delight in being with their daughter. Parents and therapist interpreted her signaling behaviors together, respected her self-regulatory attempts, and brainstormed the types of neurobehaviorally supportive activities that they could do with Amanda so that she could be available to engage with her parents in their beginning family "dance."

CASE EXAMPLE 2

Alejandro

While Alejandro's mother was pregnant with him, a fetal ultrasound showed a congenital left diaphragmatic hernia. His mother was transported 200 miles away from home so that he could be born at a hospital with a tertiary-level NICU. Alejandro was delivered by cesarean section, intubated in the delivery room, and taken immediately to the NICU. He was placed on extracorporeal membrane oxygenation (ECMO), a type of heart-lung bypass, to ensure adequate oxygenation. On his fifth day of life, Alejandro underwent surgical repair of his congenital diaphragmatic hernia. After surgery ECMO was discontinued, but he continued to receive mechanical ventilation for the next 2 months because the right side of the diaphragm was paralyzed. Alejandro stayed in the hospital for 4 months because of right-sided diaphragmatic paralysis, hypoplasia in the left lung, feeding intolerance, gastroesophageal reflux, delayed stomach emptying, intestinal adhesions, and a dilated small bowel. The complexity of his medical problems required that he remain in the tertiary-level NICU rather than moving to another hospital closer to home.

Alejandro's parents stayed with friends near the hospital for the first month after he was born. They were at his bedside every day. His father, however, had to go back to work and to go home to care for Alejandro's two sisters. His mother was able to stay for another month, and then she also needed to return home to her family. For the next 2 months his parents traveled the 200 miles every weekend so that they could be with Alejandro.

When he was able to go home, Alejandro was receiving 1 liter of 100% oxygen by nasal cannula and continuous drip feedings via gastrostomy button. Because of his chronic respiratory and nutritional problems, Alejandro had limited endurance for activity. If he was pushed beyond his limit, he showed poor oxygenation and respiratory distress. His muscle tone and strength were well below expectations for his age, with subsequent delays in his development. His interactive abilities were his strength, however. Alejandro established eye contact, smiled, and kicked his legs to show his excitement. At hospital discharge he was a non-oral feeder because of his gastrointestinal problems. During his hospitalization the occupational therapist and nurses worked together to adapt his daily schedule and immediate environment so that it was developmentally supportive, provided direct treatment to address oral-motor and developmental issues, and collaborated with his parents to support their vision of parenting a hospitalized infant.

Alejandro was a big, full-term infant who grew well while he was in the hospital (Figure 13-8). When resting and with his nasal cannula in place, he often looked pink and in no distress. He looked like a "normal" baby, as if he could easily tolerate and participate in his daily care activities. There was a real mismatch, however, between the way he looked at rest, his physical status, and his parents' dreams for him.

Alejandro's parents and the therapist met frequently at his bedside. They talked about what Alejandro and his parents did together during their visits. The parents described how he showed them what he liked and disliked when they performed some of his nursing care or attempted to interact with him. At one meeting the therapist asked them to describe what they would like to be able to do with him.

His mother wanted to cuddle and to play social games but felt that he was uncomfortable and not able to breathe well in her arms. When questioned, she reported that she felt restricted by having to sit in a chair while holding him. She also felt that everyone else in the room was watching them during her special time with Alejandro. She was open to the idea of being down on the floor with him; in fact, that is where she had envisioned them playing together at home. The therapist brought her a small mat that could be placed on the floor between the wall and the crib. This gave the mother and infant a feeling of privacy and yet allowed the nurses to observe Alejandro's status via his monitors. His mother sat on the mat, leaning her back against the wall with her knees flexed while Alejandro sat in her lap, facing her. The support of her legs allowed his trunk to stay relatively more extended rather than collapsing into trunkal flexion, which compromised his respiratory status while he was in her arms. She continued to have full contact with him, and this position emphasized his interactive strengths. His mother's hands were free for any spontaneous movement or interaction (Figure 13-8, *A*).

Alejandro's father wanted him to hold his head up, grasp his father's finger, and be able to tolerate bouncing in the air. At the same time the father indicated that he actually did very little physical handling of Alejandro. Alejandro's mother and the therapist assisted his father in holding him. By smoothing transitions and giving frequent, well-supported rests, they adapted their rhythms to those of Alejandro. Although he could not yet tolerate bouncing or flying, Alejandro enjoyed being held well supported at his father's shoulder, and his father could gently and smoothly sway or rock (Figure 13-8, *B*). His mother and the therapist pointed out Alejandro's stable monitor readings and used a mirror so that his father could see Alejandro's face. This positive feedback helped the father to feel more relaxed while holding Alejandro and enabled him to try other ways of holding and playing with his baby. Through developmental guidance, mutual problem solving, and structuring of Alejandro's daily schedule, the parents discovered ways to meet his physiological and developmental needs while addressing their needs in the realm of nurturing their infant.

CASE EXAMPLE 3

Tamisha

Tamisha's "spa day" is an example of parents creating a playful moment with their infant. After Tamisha, a ventilator-dependent older infant, had been hospitalized for weeks, her parents were finally able to give her a tub bath, an activity they had longed to perform because it meant that she was starting to do more babylike things. Because of her fragility, neuromuscular status, and medical equipment, the family requested and received staff support. During the bath the occupational therapist specifically chose to comment that with so many people participating in the bath, Tamisha must be feeling quite pampered. Her mother than began to elaborate on a playful scenario, calling the bath "Tamisha's spa day." The nurse and respiratory therapist became facialist and manicurist. Mother was masseuse, and father had the all-important role of Jacuzzi jets! In this way a perfunctory, potentially stressful bath was elaborated on to become spalike activities. Over the next several days Tamisha began to collect an assortment of soaps and lotions, beauty aids her mother called them, in anticipation

of spa day's becoming a weekly event. This tub bath scenario was enjoyed and playful for its own sake, but it also encouraged the parents and caregivers to see Tamisha as an individual with likes and dislikes. Furthermore, it enabled her parents to begin to plan for Tamisha's future and real days at a spa.

SUMMARY

Infants thrive and develop within the context of their families. Unfortunately, some preterm and seriously ill newborns enter their families as they struggle for physiological stability in the NICU. Because of the nature of the infant's medical status and neuromaturational processes, as well as the parents' emotional distress in many cases, engaging and playing with one another are delayed. The task of the occupational therapist is to discern when both infant and parents are robust enough to begin this work together.

The therapist adapts the environment and activities to account for the infant's medical fragility and the parents' definition of play. Using Nugent's "nonprescriptive stance," therapist, infant, and parent elaborate on their current successful engagement and early playful experiences. At these times the infant's posture may not be optimal, the hand splints may need to be forgone temporarily, or the opportunity to teach a therapy technique may be postponed (Figure 13-9). The therapeutic process enables connectedness, attachment, and participation for both infant and parents (Price, 2003). Knowledge of each infant's physiology and neurobehavioral maturation, along with an understanding of the parents' dreams, fears, beliefs, and sense of playfulness, is necessary for the therapist to support the creative, dynamic process that most often occurs spontaneously for other families.

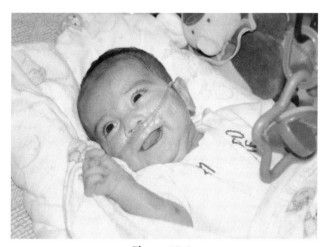

Figure 13-9
Regardless of posture, a playful interchange can take place.

Review Questions

1. Consider the relevant play theories discussed in this chapter. Describe how these relate to the infant in the NICU.
2. Describe the social-emotional context of the infant. How does the environment of the NICU alter this social-emotional context?
3. How does the infant's stay in the NICU alter the development of parent-infant communication and play?
4. What are neuroregulatory abilities, and how do they influence parent-infant interactions, including play?
5. Hospitalization of a preterm or critically ill newborn in the NICU can have a tremendous impact on the parents. Describe parental experiences in the NICU, and indicate how occupational therapy can intervene to enhance parental coping.
6. Describe some of the ways occupational therapists practicing in the NICU may assist parents in supporting the precursors of play.

REFERENCES

Able-Boone, H., & Stevens, E. (1994). After the intensive care nursery experience: Families' perceptions of their well-being. *Children's Health Care, 23*(2), 99-114.

Affleck, G., & Tennen, H. (1991). The effect of newborn intensive care on parents' psychological well-being. *Children's Health Care, 20*(1), 6-14.

Affleck, G., Tennen, H., & Rowe, J. (1990). Mothers, fathers and the crisis of newborn intensive care. *Infant Mental Health Journal, 11*(1), 12-25.

Als, H. (1983). Infant individuality: Assessing patterns of very early development. In J. Call, E. Galenson, & R. Tyson (Eds.), *Frontiers of infant psychiatry* (pp. 363-378). New York: Basic Books.

Als, H. (1986). A synactive model of neonatal behavioral organization: Framework for the assessment of neurobehavioral development in the premature infant and for the support of infants and parents in the neonatal intensive care environment. *Physical and Occupational Therapy in Pediatrics, 6*(3/4), 3-53.

Als, H. (1997). Relationship-based developmental NICU care. *Seminars in Perinatology, 21*(3), 178-189.

Als, H., Duffy, F. H., McAnulty, G. B., & Badian, N. (1989). Continuity of neurobehavioral functioning in pre-term and full-term newborns. In M. H. Bornstein & N. A. Krasnegor (Eds.), *Stability and continuity in mental development: Behavioral and biological perspectives* (pp. 3-28). Hillsdale, NJ: LEA Publishers.

Als, H., Gilkerson, L., Duffy, F. H., McAnulty, G. B., Buehler, D. M., Vandenberg, K., et al. (2003). A three-center, randomized, controlled trial of individualized developmental care for very low birthweight preterm infants: Medical, neurodevelopmental, parenting, and caregiving effects. *Journal of Developmental and Behavioral Pediatrics, 24*(6), 399-408.

Als, H., Lawhon, G., Brown, E., Jibes, R., Duffy, F. H., McAnulty, G., et al. (1986). Individualized behavioral and environmental care for the very low birth weight pre-term infant at risk for bronchopulmonary dysplasia: NICU and developmental outcome. *Pediatrics, 78*, 1123-1132.

Als, H., Lester, B. M., Tronick, E. Z., & Brazelton, T. B. (1982). Assessment of pre-term infant behavior (APIB). In H. E. Fitzgerald & M. Yogman (Eds.), *Theory and research in behavioral pediatrics* (pp. 64-133). New York: Plenum Press.

American Occupational Therapy Association (2000). Knowledge and skills for occupational therapy practice in the neonatal intensive care unit. *American Journal of Occupational Therapy, 47*(12), 1100-1105.

American Occupational Therapy Association (2002). Occupational therapy practice framework: Domain and process. *American Journal of Occupational Therapy, 56*, 609-639.

Ballweg, D. D. (2004). Individualized care: Actions for the individualized staff member. In C. Kenner & J. M. McGrath (Eds.), *Developmental care of newborns and infants.* St. Louis: Mosby.

Barnard, K. E., & Bee, H. L. (1984). The assessment of parent-infant interaction by observation of feeding and teaching. In T. B. Brazelton & B. Lester (Eds.), *New approaches to developmental screening in infants.* New York: Elsevier.

Bazyk, S., Stalnaker, D., Llerena, M., Ekelman, B., & Bazyk, J. (2003). Play in Mayan children. *American Journal of Occupational Therapy 57*(3), 273-283.

Beeghly, M. (1993). Parent-infant play as a window on infant competence: An organizational approach to assessment. In K. MacDonald (Ed.), *Parent-child play: Descriptions and implications* (pp. 71-111). Albany, NY: State University of New York Press.

Bess, F. H., Peck, B. F., & Chapman, J. J. (1979). Further observations on noise levels in infant incubators. *Pediatrics, 63*(1), 100-106.

Bloch, M. N., & Pellegrini, A. (1989). Introduction. In M. N. Bloch & A. Pellegrini (Eds.), *The ecological context of children's play* (pp. 1-5). Norwood, NJ: Ablex Publishing.

Bozzette, M., & Kenner, C. (2004) The neonatal intensive care unit environment. In C. Kenner & J. M. McGrath (Eds.), *Developmental care of newborns and infants.* St. Louis: Mosby.

Brazelton, T. B. & Cramer, B. G. (1990). *The earliest relationship.* Reading, MA: Addison-Wesley.

Brazelton, T. B., Koslowski, B., & Main, M. (1979). The origins of reciprocity: The early infant-mother interaction. In M. Lewis & L. A. Rosenblum (Eds.), *The effects of the infant on the caregiver.* New York: John Wiley & Sons.

Browne, J. V. (2003). New perspectives on premature infants and their parents. *Zero to Three 24*(2), 4-12.

Bundy, A. C. (1991). Play theory and sensory integration. In A. G. Fisher, E. A. Murray, & A. C. Bundy (Eds.), *Sensory integration: Theory and practice* (pp. 46-68). Philadelphia: F.A. Davis.

Bundy, A. C. (1997). Play and playfulness: What to look for. In L. D. Parham & L. S. Fazio (Eds.), *Play in occupational therapy for children.* St. Louis: Mosby.

Burke, J. P. (1993). Play: The life role of the infant and young child. In J. C. Smith (Ed.), *Pediatric occupational therapy and early intervention* (pp. 198-224). Andover, MA: Andover Medical Publishers.

Cardone, I. A., & Gilkerson, L. (1990). Family administered neonatal activities: An exploratory method for the integration of parental perceptions and newborn behavior. *Infant Mental Health Journal, 11*(2), 127-141.

Cardone, I. A., & Gilkerson, L. (1992). Family administered neonatal activities: An adaptation for parents of infants born with Down syndrome. *Infants and Young Children, 5*(1), 40-48.

Cohn, J. F. (1993). Mother-infant play and maternal depression. In K. MacDonald (Ed.), *Parent-child play: Descriptions and implications* (pp. 239-256). Albany, NY: State University of New York Press.

Cohn, J. F., & Tronick, E. Z. (1983). Three month-old infants' reaction to simulated maternal depression. *Child Development, 54*, 185-193.

Cornell, E. H., & Gottfried, A. W. (1976). Intervention with premature infants. *Child Development, 47*, 32-39.

Finn, C. D. (2003). Cultural models for early caregiving. *Zero to Three, 23*(5), 40-45.

Fogel, A., Nwokah, E., & Karns, J. (1993). Parent-infant games as dynamic social systems. In K. MacDonald (Ed.), *Parent-child play: Descriptions and implications* (pp. 43-69). Albany, NY: State University of New York Press.

Gaiter, J. L. (1985). Nursery environments. In A. W. Gottfried & J. L. Gaiter (Eds.), *Infant stress under intensive care* (pp. 55-82). University Park, MD: University Park Press.

Gianino, A., & Tronick, E. Z. (1988). The mutual regulation model: The infant's self regulation and coping and defensive capacities. In T. M. Field, P. M. McCabe, & R. Schneiderman (Eds.), *Stress and coping across development*. Hillsdale, NJ: Lawrence Erlbaum.

Gilkerson, L., Gorski, P., & Panitz, P. (1990). Hospital-based intervention for pre-term infants and their families. In S. J. Meisels & J. P. Shonkoff (Eds.), *Handbook of early childhood intervention*. New York: University of Cambridge.

Gorga, D. (1994). The evolution of occupational therapy practice for infants in the neonatal intensive care unit. *American Journal of Occupational Therapy, 48*(6), 487-489.

Gorski, P. A., Leonard, C. H., Sweet, D. M., Martin, J. A., & Sehring, S. A. (1990). Caregiver-infant interaction and the immature nervous system: A touchy subject. In K. E. Barnard & T. B. Brazelton (Eds.), *Touch: The foundation of experience* (pp. 229-251). Madison, WI: International Universities Press.

Gottfried, A. W., & Gaiter, J. (1985). *Infant stress under intensive care*. Baltimore: University Park Press.

Gottfried, A. W., Lande, P. W., Brown, S. S., King, J., Coen, C., & Hodgman, J. E. (1981). Physical and social environment of newborn infants in special care units. *Science, 214,* 673-675.

Greenspan, S. I. (1990). *Infancy and early childhood: The practice of clinical assessment and intervention with emotional and developmental challenges*. Madison, WI: International Universities Press.

Gregg, C. L., Haffner, M. E., & Korner, A. F. (1976). The relative efficacy of vestibular-proprioceptive stimulation and the upright position in enhancing visual pursuits in neonates. *Child Development, 47*, 309-314.

Hack, M., Horbar, J. D., Malloy, M. H., Tyson, J. E., Wright, E., & Wright, L. (1991). Very low-birth weight outcomes of the National Institute of Child Health and Human Development neonatal network. *Pediatrics, 87*, 587-597.

Holloway, E. (1994). Parent and occupational therapist collaboration in the neonatal intensive care unit. *American Journal of Occupational Therapy, 48*(6), 535-538.

Hughes, M., & McCollum, J. (1993). Maternal stress and coping in the NICU: An exploratory study. *ACCH Advocate, 1*(1), 57-61.

Hughes, M., McCollum, J., Sheftel, D., & Sanchez, G. (1994). How parents cope with the experience of neonatal intensive care. *Children's Health Care, 23*(1), 1-14.

Hunter, J. G. (2005). Neonatal intensive care unit. In J. Case-Smith (Ed.), *Occupational therapy for children* (5th ed.). St. Louis: Mosby.

Lawlor, M. C. (2003). The significance of being occupied: The social construction of childhood occupations. *American Journal of Occupational Therapy, 57*(4), 424-434.

Leib, S. A., Benfield, G., & Guidubaldi, J. (1980). Effects of early intervention and stimulation on the pre-term infant. *Pediatrics, 66*, 83-90.

Linn, L., Horowitz, F. D., & Fox, H. A. (1985). Stimulation in the NICU: Is more necessarily better? *Clinics in Perinatology, 12*(2), 407-422.

Long, J. G., Lucey, J. F., & Philip, A. G. (1980). Noise and hypoxemia in the intensive care nursery. *Pediatrics, 65*(1), 143-145.

Long, J. G., Philip, A. G., & Lucey, J. F. (1980). Excessive handling as a cause of hypoxemia. *Pediatrics, 65*, 203-207.

MacDonald, K. (1993). Parent-child play: An evolutionary perspective. In K. McDonald (Ed.), *Parent-child play: Descriptions and implications* (pp. 113-143). Albany, NY: State University of New York Press.

McGrath, M. M., & Myer, E. C. (1992). Maternal self-esteem: From theory to clinical practice in a special care nursery. *Children's Health Care, 21*(4), 199-205.

Newman, L. F. (1981). Social and sensory environment of low-birth weight infants in a special care nursery: An anthropological investigation. *Journal of Nerve and Mental Disability, 169*(4), 448-455.

Nugent, J. K., & Brazelton, T. B. (1989). Preventive intervention with infants and families: The NBAS model. *Infant Mental Health Journal, 10*(2), 84-99.

Nugent, J. K., Greene, S., Deering, D. W., Mazor, K. M., Hendler, J., & Bombardier, C. (1993). The cultural context of mother-infant play in the newborn. In K. McDonald (Ed.), *Parent-child play: Descriptions and implications* (pp. 367-386). Albany, NY: State University of New York Press.

Patteson, D. M., & Barnard, K. E. (1990). Parenting of low-birth weight infants: A review of issues and interventions. *Infant Mental Health Journal, 11*(11), 37-56.

Powell, L. F. (1974). The effect of extra stimulation and maternal involvement on the development of low-birth weight infants and on maternal behavior. *Child Development, 45*, 106-113.

Pressler, J. L., Turnage-Carrier, C. S., & Kenner, C. (2004). Developmental care: An overview. In C. Kenner & J. M. McGrath (Eds.), *Developmental care of newborns and infants*. St. Louis: Mosby.

Price, P. (2003). Occupation-centered practice: Providing opportunities for becoming and belonging. *Dissertation Abstracts International*, 65 (05), 2382B. (UMI No. 3133327).

Rice, R. D. (1977). Neurophysiological development in premature infants following stimulation. *Developmental Psychology, 13,* 69-76.

Scarr-Salapatek, S., & Williams, M. L. (1973). The effects of early stimulation on low-birth weight infants. *Child Development, 44,* 94-101.

Schultz-Krohn, W., & Cara, E. (2000). Occupational therapy in early intervention: Applying concepts from infant mental health. *American Journal of Occupational Therapy, 54*(5), 550-554.

Solkoff, N., & Matuszak, D. (1975). Tactile stimulation and behavioral development among low-birth weight infants. *Child Psychiatry and Human Development, 6,* 33-37.

Solkoff, N., Yaffe, S., Weintraub, D., & Blase, B. (1969). Effects of handling on the subsequent development of premature infants. *Developmental Psychology, 1,* 765-768.

Solnit, A. J. (1993). From play to playfulness in children and adults. In A. J. Solnit & D. J. Cohen (Eds.), *The many meanings of play: A psychoanalytic perspective* (pp. 27-53). New Haven, CT: Yale University Press.

Solnit, A. J., & Cohen, D. J. (1993). Introduction. In A. J. Solnit & D. J. Cohen (Eds.), *The many meanings of play: A psychoanalytic perspective.* New Haven, CT: Yale University Press.

Speidel, B. D. (1978). Adverse effects of routine procedures on pre-term infants. *Lancet, 1,* 864-865.

Sutton-Smith, B. (1993). Dilemmas in adult play with children. In K. MacDonald (Ed.), *Parent-child play: Descriptions and implications* (pp. 15-42). Albany, NY: State University of New York Press.

Symington, S., & Pinelli, J. (2003) Developmental care for promoting development and preventing morbidity in preterm infants. *Cochrane Database of Systematic Reviews*, Issue 4, Article No: CD001814.

Talmi, A., & Harmon, R. J. (2003). Relationships between preterm infants and their parents: Disruption and development. *Zero to Three, 24*(2), 13-20.

Vergara, E. R., & Bigsby, R. (2004). *Developmental and therapeutic interventions in the NICU.* Baltimore: Paul H. Brookes.

Weatherston, D. J. (2002). Introduction to the infant mental health program. In J. J. Shirilla & D. J. Weatherston (Eds.), *Case studies in infant mental health: Risk, resiliency, and relationships.* Washington, DC: Zero to Three.

Whaley, K. K. (1990). The emergence of social play in infancy: A proposed developmental sequence of infant-adult social play. *Early Childhood Research Quarterly, 5,* 347-358.

White, J. L., & LaBarba, R. C. (1976). The effects of tactile and kinesthetic stimulation on neonatal development in the premature infant. *Developmental Psychology, 9,* 569-577.

Zeanah, C. H., & Zeanah, P. D. (2001). Towards a definition of infant mental health. *Zero to Three, 22*(1), 13-20.

14

Play in Children with Autism: Structure and Experience

Susan L. Spitzer

KEY TERMS

autism
play experience
social play

What is play for children with autism? Do children with autism really play? How can we help children with autism play? The playfulness, spontaneity, and flexibility that seem to be essential qualities of play stand in contrast to the repetitive and inflexible behavior so often observed in children with autism. Many children with autism do not seem to want to *work* on the skills needed to support engagement in conventional forms of play and may prefer unconventional forms. A child with autism may have difficulty participating in common play forms and may miss out on the developmental benefits of play. What the child does experience as play may be difficult for an adult to understand. Reconciling and negotiating play's structural elements and personal meaning are essential for promoting play for the child with autism. This is reflected in occupational therapy's practice framework, which emphasizes addressing an individual's occupational performance and occupational profile (American Occupational Therapy Association [AOTA], 2002).

STRUCTURE OF PLAY

Play has structure as an activity, as action (Sutton-Smith, 1997). A child's observable occupational performance in play is a function of the child's skills, interests, and environmental opportunities and supports (Box 14-1). The structure of play is described most commonly in terms of how children use objects, pretend, and interact with other people. This typology clearly dominates the literature on play in children with autism. For most children the structure of play becomes increasingly complex as they develop. The structural elements of play are closely linked with social, cognitive, and adaptive functions of play. Play can be seen as reflecting and promoting the development of social and communication skills (Piaget, 1951/1962; Rubin, Fein, & Vandenberg, 1983); cognitive skills, including creativity and problem solving (Piaget, 1951/1962); and adaptive behavior, such as flexibility and an ability to adjust to novel situations (Rubin et al., 1983). It is the developmental functions of play through the use of objects and social interaction that may be very important to parents, teachers, and therapists, especially when looking at functional gains for children with autism.

Autism influences and is reflected in the child's play. Autism is a neurobiological disorder that is manifest within the first 3 years of a child's life. It includes (1) a qualitative impairment in social interaction, (2) a qualitative impairment in communication (atypical or reduced speech and nonverbal communication), and (3) restricted repetitive and stereotyped patterns of behavior, interests, and activities (American Psychiatric Association [APA], 1994). Although not part of the diagnostic criteria, atypical sensory processing, motor difficulties, and cognitive impairments are also common (Baranek, Parham, & Bodfish, 2005; Grandin, 1996; Ornitz, 1974; Rapin, 1991). Children may manifest these symptoms to varying degrees, resulting in an extremely heterogeneous population. Strengths have been noted in rote memory, mathematics, mechanical abilities, and visual perception (Happe, 1996; Kanner, 1943; Rapin, 1991; Ritvo & Freeman, 1978; Rutter, 1978; Schreibman & Charlop, 1989). Autism is a lifelong disorder, and the symptoms may change with development (Bristol et al., 1996).

Most descriptions of the play of children with autism are consistent with the clinical criteria of the diagnosis. For example, object play tends to reflect the child's restricted repetitive and stereotyped patterns of behavior, interests, and activities. Delays or abnormal symbolic play fulfills a criterion in the diagnosis of autism (APA,

Box 14-1   *Play in Children with Autism: Observation Guide*

Play Preferences and Interests
Self-initiated:
High frequency/duration:
Strong positive affect displayed
    during:

Object Play
Objects:
Self-initiated:
Suggested by Others:
Directed by Others:
Uses:
    Mouthing
    Holding
    Manipulating
    Pulling
    Dropping
    Banging
    Shaking
    Waving
    Fingering
    Other
Variety:
    Of objects
    Of uses

**Object Relational Play
(2+ Objects Together)**
Forms:
    Touching
    Banging
    Pouring
    Container play
    Pull apart

Constructing and building (put
    together)
Knocking against or into
Using tools (i.e., bat to hit ball,
    tongs, etc.)
Qualities:
    Degree of precision and control
    Variety
    Complexity
    Self-initiation

**Functional Play (Realistic Pretend
Object Use)**
Themes:
    Self-care (grooming, feeding,
        eating, sleeping)
    Play
    Work
    Mechanical actions (drive car,
        fly plane, etc.)
Directed toward:
    Self
    Other person
    Doll, character, or figure
Qualities:
    Number of steps or complexity
        of "story"
    Variety
    Self-initiation

Symbolic Play
Forms:
    Pretends objects are something
        else

When the object is very similar
    looking
When the object is dissimilar
Uses doll to act like person
Pretends roles
Uses story narrative (multistep;
    beginning, middle, end)
Themes and content
Qualities:
    Imitate
    Improvise
    Variety

Sensorimotor Play
Actions
Materials and objects
Social aspects
Variation
Self-initiation

Social Play
Adults:
Children:
Components:
    Tolerates others in close space
    Shares objects and materials
    Reciprocal interaction
    Joint attention
    Initiates with others
    Shares affect and emotion
        (expression and response)
    Responds to others
    Imitates others
    Tolerates and negotiates play
        structure with others

This guide is organized primarily according to categories of play structure. Within each category, identify the child's preferences to indicate what is internally important to the child.

To build play, incorporate these preferences to build the child's interest and self-direction. Expand on existing play by adding features that are somewhat similar to what the child currently does within and across categories. Play structure may be enhanced by the building of self-initiation, variation, and complexity within a category or by the use of elements from one category to cross into another category.

1994). Social play is greatly affected by impairments in social interaction and communication. Play skills are often cited as one of the major deficits for children with autism and can be a significant concern. Both independent and social play may be affected (Ritvo & Freeman, 1978). The bulk of the autism research and literature indicates that the play of children with autism is not simply delayed, but rather is qualitatively different from that of children who are typically developing and those

with developmental delays (Wulff, 1985). The research findings, however, are not consistent and probably reflect the heterogeneity of autism. This section provides a review of literature that may be helpful for occupational therapists in assessing potential structural differences in the play of individual children with autism, but it should not be seen as an absolute description of what the therapist will find, since this can vary dramatically from child to child.

Object Play

The use of objects starts in infancy, when children first manipulate objects. Object manipulation involves contact with the object. Typically the child uses an increasing variety and combination of "schemas" for acting on objects (Piaget as cited in Cole & Cole, 1993), such as mouthing, holding, pulling, dropping, banging, shaking, waving, or otherwise manipulating an object (Power, 2000). Such behaviors may be repeated as a child explores new materials. The child experiences the object's sensory properties and what the object can do. Gibson (1988) referred to this as perceiving the object's "affordances," the opportunities and possibilities that an object provides for use. Increasingly precise motor and perceptual skills correspond with the development of manipulating and relating objects. Although simple object exploration (banging, mouthing, fingering, and visual exploration) typically declines quickly after the first year (Largo & Howard, 1979), even adults may engage in playful object manipulation during leisure activities such as finding rocks and seashells or watching a sunset. Artists who work with various media may spend significant amounts of time in exploring objects and materials.

Children with autism differ in their object play from their developmentally matched peers, but these differences may not emerge until after the first year of age. In a retrospective study of children later identified as having autism, a developmental delay, or typical development, Baranek, Barnett, et al. (2005) found that the duration and level of object play in infants aged 9 to 12 months did not differ significantly among the groups.

The differences in object play for children with autism have been identified in children older than 1 year of age. This research has found that children with autism tend to spend more time manipulating objects than do other children their age, who have moved on to other types of play (Black, Freeman, & Montgomery, 1975; Ungerer & Sigman, 1981), and tend to manipulate objects in atypical ways (Williams, 2003; Williams, Costall, & Reddy, 1999). They may use the objects in limited ways, such as playing with only a few objects, having intense attachment to particular objects, and playing with objects in the same ways (Rapin, 1991; Rutter, 1978). Children with autism may also demonstrate more interest in the parts of objects (APA, 1994), such as the wheels on a toy car rather than the car itself. Sometimes object manipulation is focused on self-stimulatory toy use (Black et al., 1975; Charlop, Schreibman, & Kurtz, 1991; Ritvo & Freeman, 1978; Schreibman & Charlop, 1989; Wulff, 1985) rather than exploration of the properties of the objects. For example, a child might hold up a toy airplane close to his eyes and repetitively spin the propeller. Toy play may involve more negative interactions, such as throwing a toy across the room (Black et al., 1975). In sum, children with autism tend to retain an interest in objects that lasts longer and takes a different form from the object play of most children without autism.

Relational Play

Relational play with objects typically emerges by 9 months (Fensom, Kagan, Kearsley, & Zelazo, 1976). Initially, children combine objects in nonfunctional manners such as touching or banging two blocks together. In this way children extend their exploration of objects to learn how objects relate to each other (Piaget as cited in Cole & Cole, 1993; Robinson, 1977) and to gain competency in effectively using objects in their environment (Reilly, 1974). Praxis and fine motor skills can also be important for relating objects effectively. Increasingly complex relational play with objects develops as children relate objects in more precise ways, such as putting objects into a container, taking objects apart, placing rings on a pole, stacking blocks, using shape sorters and puzzles, and doing constructional activities (Knox, 1997) (Figure 14-1). Relational object play also moves from a trial and error approach to mental manipulation and memory of ways for relating objects. Collecting objects and construction continue to be typical play interests in middle childhood (Florey & Greene, 1997; Takata, 1974). Adolescent and adult hobbies such as building models may be seen as advanced relational object play. Fields such as engineering may be an outgrowth of such play and hobbies (Petroski, 1999).

Young children with autism tend to engage more in relational object play than typical children their developmental age, who have moved on to more functional play (Ungerer & Sigman, 1981). The relational play can also be more rigid and repetitive than in typical children. For example, a child with autism may tend to line up objects

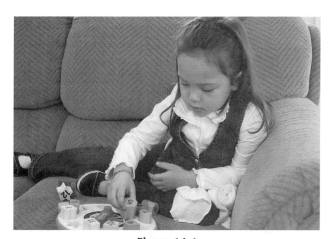

Figure 14-1

Children with autism often demonstrate a preference and skill for relating objects in construction activities and puzzles. (Courtesy Shay McAtee.)

in the same ways rather than explore other ways of relating the objects. Self-stimulatory behavior has been found to be a barrier to appropriate toy play (Koegel, Firestone, Kramme, & Dunlap, 1974). Children with autism often develop their greatest strengths and strong interests in relational object play, such as using puzzles and construction toys. Furthermore, many adults with autism excel in activities that rely on advanced skill and knowledge of object relations, such as engineering and art.

Functional Play

Functional play typically emerges at around 9 to 12 months and becomes dominant at 15 months (Largo & Howard, 1979). Functional play is sometimes called presymbolic play. It refers to the appropriate or conventional use of objects, such as a spoon to feed. Functional play involves the use of realistic objects (a real cup or a play phone) for their intended purpose (i.e., as a cup or a phone) (Figure 14-2). Initially, functional play is focused on the child (such as "drinking" from an empty cup), and then the action transfers to a doll (such as giving the doll a "drink" from an empty cup), which is often called representational play. The development of functional play also includes the sequencing of actions on more than one object, such as feeding self, then mother, then a doll.

Functional play adds a social element to object play in that children use objects in the ways that society conventionally uses them—a spoon is put up to the mouth, not to the leg. Although functional play is still a concrete, physical use of objects, it focuses on the socially ascribed use(s) rather than the full range of object affordances. Williams et al. (1999) asserted that the functional use of objects for children with autism is associated with basic social relations because children learn most functional play through other people, a social context.

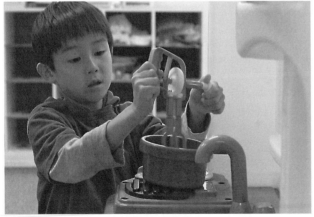

Figure 14-2

This boy's functional play of cooking involves the use of a hand-mixer for its socially accepted purpose. (Courtesy Shay McAtee.)

The research is inconsistent on the amount of functional play in which children with autism engage; however, studies do indicate significant qualitative differences in the functional play of children with and without autism. For example, in a study of 16 young children with autism with a mean mental age of 24.8 months, Ungerer and Sigman (1981) found that spontaneous doll-directed functional play was consistently less than or equal to self-directed functional play. In typical children of this developmental age, doll-directed functional play occurs more frequently. The ability to engage in doll-directed functional play is believed to be important for the later development of symbolic play as the child becomes able to separate his or her physical involvement in the play. Williams, Reddy, and Costall (2001) found that the functional play of young children with autism was less elaborated, less varied, and less integrated than that of developmentally matched children with Down syndrome and typically developing infants. In this study the functional play of the children with autism often consisted of a simple one-step act involving a single object. Williams et al. (1999) suggested that the children's repetitive and ritualistic object play may interfere with functional object play because objects often have unconventional meanings for children with autism. They called for more research in object use, which they asserted is a neglected and less well-understood area.

Symbolic Play

Symbolic play, which tends to replace functional play and involves the use of objects as symbols, emerges around 24 months of age (Piaget as cited in Cole & Cole, 1993). The object's use is not bound by its physical properties but still relates to the social-cultural environment. For example, a child may use a block like a phone or a ball as an apple. The child may also have a doll act like a person. The child is able to pretend—to have a representation of what the object symbolizes in his or her thoughts. As a child grows older, symbolic play becomes more elaborate with the involvement of more children, detailed roles to play out, and decreasing reliance on objects. Both imitation and drama are features of symbolic play (Knox, 1997). Symbolic play has an increasingly narrative quality of acting out a story, although it may not have a logical ending or outcome (Singer & Singer, 1990). A child may pretend to be a ballerina, firefighter, or superhero involved in a multipart plot. Singer and Singer (1990) argue that symbolic play moves "underground" into fantasy for adolescents and adults.

Most of the recent research on play in children with autism has focused on symbolic play. As in many areas of research on this population, methodological issues abound (Jarrold, Boucher, & Smith, 1993) and the current state of knowledge will surely evolve with future research. Most recent assessments of symbolic play in research studies compared their subjects' performance to that of other children with a similar mental age, especially verbal mental age because symbolic play has been associated with cognitive and communication development. In comparing the play of children who have other developmental disabilities with typically developing children of a similar mental age, scholars have described the pretend play of children with autism as occurring less frequently and, when it occurs, lacking symbolism, creativity, and complexity (Riguet, Taylor, Benaroya, & Klein, 1981; Rutherford & Rogers, 2003; Wulff, 1985). Based on their review of the literature on play and children with various disabilities, Rutherford and Rogers (2003) concluded that "pretend play is most severely affected by visual impairments and by autism" (p. 290).

Early research studies noted that spontaneous pretend play seemed to be most impaired in children with autism, whereas play that was elicited with cues, structure, or instruction seemed to be less impaired (Sigman & Ruskin, 1999). For example, Ungerer & Sigman (1981), in a study of 16 children with autism (mental age $M = 24.8$ months), found that the children engaged in less symbolic behavior, doll play, and diversity of play acts than would be expected for their developmental age. The number of different acts was higher, however, in a structured setting, where a single toy or a set of toys was provided at a time, with instructions and modeling as needed, than it was in the unstructured free-play setting. Differences among the children in play skills were associated with differences in language comprehension. Riguet et al. (1981) studied 10 autistic children (verbal mental age $M = 2.5$ years) and found that the children with autism, in comparison with matched samples of children with Down syndrome and children without disabilities, spent less time in symbolic play and more time in lower levels of symbolic play with fewer substitute symbolic uses of objects. The symbolic play of children with autism improved significantly after modeling, but it still did not reach the levels of the other groups. Furthermore, the children with autism engaged in significantly more off-task and nonplay behavior.

Although the early research indicated deficits in symbolic play, it also demonstrated that children with autism have the *capacity* for symbolic play (Jarrold, 2003; Jarrold et al., 1993). Under structured conditions, children with autism demonstrated more functional and symbolic play skills than in unstructured conditions.

Researchers in the last two decades have been trying to understand what factors influence or limit symbolic play in children with autism. A number of research studies have looked at imitation in general and have found that children with autism have deficits in imitation skills; deficits were greater in the imitation of body movements than in the imitation of object manipulation (Baranek, Parham, et al., 2005; Rogers, Hepburn, Stackhouse, & Wehner, 2003; Stone, Ousley, & Littleford, 1997). Libby, Powell,

Messer, and Jordan (1997) examined different aspects of imitation of pretend play. They studied 10 children with autism matched on verbal mental age ($M = 2½$ years) with typically developing children and children with Down syndrome. An adult modeled a pretend action(s), handed the object to the child, and instructed the child to do it. The experimenters used three different types of items: (1) a single act, (2) multiple acts presented in a common sequence, and (3) multiple acts presented in a scrambled order. They found that for single-action items the children with autism were significantly more likely to give a correct response than the typically developing children. The authors suggested that this finding may relate to the greater experience and educational influences of the children with autism because they were chronologically much older than the control groups (autism, $M = 126$ months; Down syndrome, $M = 55$ months; typically developing, $M = 28$ months). There were no significant differences among the groups in imitating multiple tasks, whether presented in correct sequence or in scrambled order. The children with autism, however, were less likely to correct the scrambled order items than were the other children, which the authors concluded may indicate that children with autism copy actions without the understanding that accompanies true imitation.

Whether or not children with autism can understand pretend play has been another area of research. In these studies a symbolic action is demonstrated for the child and then the child is asked to identify the correct outcome. Generally, one option is that the toy stays the same (what has been visually seen), another option is that the toy is changed as would be expected by the symbolic act observed, and sometimes a third option is available that does not relate to the concrete or symbolic aspects of the experiment (a distraction item). In the studies the children with autism responded with better than 50% correct (better than expected by chance alone) and rarely selected the distraction items (Jarrold, Smith, Boucher, & Harris, 1994; Kavanaugh & Harris, 1994). In the Jarrold et al. (1994) study, the children with autism (receptive verbal mental age $M = 54.5$ months) performed similar to children with moderate learning difficulties and without disabilities, matched on verbal mental age. Kavanaugh and Harris (1994) identified this as a skill that typical children can do by 3 years of age, although the children with autism were much older in both these studies (mean chronological age of 8 years, 8 months in Jarrold et al. [1994], and 6 years, 6 months in Kavanaugh & Harris [1994]). These studies suggest that children with autism may be able to understand pretend play beyond that which they themselves display (Jarrold, 2003); however, mental age must also be considered. If children with autism have the capacity to pretend, it may be that they have difficulty using this capacity or lack interest in pretend play (Jarrold, 2003).

Generativity is another factor being examined by researchers studying the symbolic play of children with autism. Generativity or generative ability refers to the ability to generate ideas for use, such as in play. It is similar to the concept of ideation in a sensory integration approach (Trecker & Miller-Kuhaneck, 2004). Lewis and Boucher (1995) asserted that individuals with autism may have difficulty accessing stored knowledge or information to generate creative and original ideas. The individual must be able to disengage partially from the current immediate context, inhibit behavior that is related to the concrete surroundings, and switch attention to internal mental structures (e.g., creativity, pretense, goals) to activate novel behavior (Lewis & Boucher, 1995; Rutherford & Rogers, 2003). In the Lewis and Boucher (1995) study, 15 children with autism, aged 6 years, 6 months to 15 years, 8 months (verbal mental age $M = 5$ years, 5 months) were matched on verbal mental age to a group of children with moderate learning difficulties and a group of younger normal children. Each child was presented with a car and then a doll in an elicited play condition (the child was directed to show what the toy could do) and an instructed play condition. The researchers found that the children with autism had more difficulty generating original play ideas in the elicited play condition than demonstrating symbolic and functional play acts in the instructed play condition. Specifically, in the instructed play condition no significant differences were found among the groups of children in amounts of functional and symbolic play with the two toys. In contrast, in the elicited play condition, the young people with autism had significantly more original ideas for the doll than the car, a pattern not found in other groups. Furthermore, the individuals with autism demonstrated significantly fewer original ideas with the car than did the other children in the elicited play condition. The authors attributed the difference in generating ideas for the two toys to the doll's flexible body and movable limbs, which provided cues for play actions. By physically manipulating the doll, the children with autism identified ideas for play actions.

Rutherford and Rogers (2003) examined the ability of different factors to predict pretend play in 28 young children with autism (overall mental age $M = 20.01$ months), 24 children with other developmental disorders, and 26 typically developing children matched on overall mental age. In their protocol each child was allowed to use an object, and if the child did not, he or she was prompted. The children with autism engaged in significantly less spontaneous pretend play than did the other children. When all the children were grouped together, generativity task scores (different ideas) accounted for 27% of variance in both spontaneous and overall pretend play even when mental age was factored out. Joint attention and set shifting (shifting of attention) measures were not associated with variance in pretend play. In addition, verbal mental age and nonverbal mental age were correlated with spontaneous pretend play in the control groups only, not in the children with autism. The authors concluded that both experience and developmental maturity play a role in early pretend play development and that in children with autism the general developmental level is not accounting for play skills. At this point the concept of generativity appears to explain some aspects of the impairment of symbolic play skills in children with autism.

Other hypotheses about the causes of deficits in symbolic play in children with autism include deficits in social impairment, motivation, metarepresentation, and executive functions (Jarrold et al., 1993). Certainly, more research is needed to explain and understand fully the symbolic play of children with autism and the various factors that may be involved. Only signs of the mental processes implicit in symbolic play can be observed, not the actual symbolism. "Without children's verbalizations it is difficult to determine how imaginative or creative they are in their play" (Singer & Singer, 1990, p. 62). Given the language deficits in children with autism, assessing and understanding their symbolic play are especially challenging.

Sensorimotor Play

Sensorimotor or physical play may or may not involve manipulating and relating actual or symbolic objects. It does involve physical interaction with the environment (Figure 14-3). Although object manipulation can be sensorimotor play, sensorimotor play is not necessarily limited to objects, especially not to objects that can be easily moved or manipulated. Sensorimotor play tends to involve a greater use of space. The actions are done purely for the pleasure of doing them. "Practice games" involve repeating physical actions (often gross motor actions) without pretending or attending to social rules (Piaget, 1962). Sensorimotor play is common in the first 2 years of life or when learning new skills (Piaget as cited in Cole & Cole, 1993; Takata, 1974). Rough-and-tumble play is a social form of sensorimotor play that is more common in boys and continues for several years (Pellegrini, 1995). Elements of sensorimotor play may continue for an individual who loves to do physical activities such as swim, dance, or run for the intrinsic "feeling" of it, rather than for symbolic or social reasons (e.g., competition, health, achievement).

Children with autism seem to prefer sensorimotor play to other forms of play, but little research has been reported. Rutherford and Rogers (2003) reported that the young children with autism in their study engaged in more sensorimotor play than pretend play. The children still engaged in significantly less spontaneous and

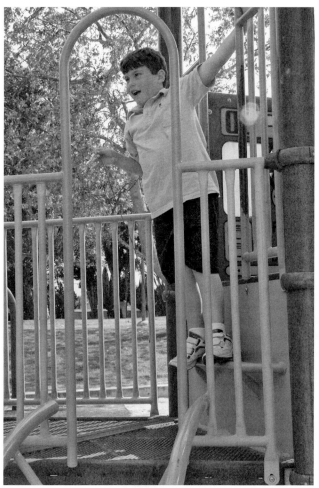

Figure 14-3

Children with autism may prefer the sensations of engaging in sensorimotor play to pretend play. (Courtesy Shay McAtee.)

prompted sensorimotor play than did matched samples of children with developmental disorders and children who were typically developing.

Social Play

Children's play develops socially first with adults (Figure 14-4, *A*) and then with peers (Figure 14-4, *B*). Social aspects of play are not necessarily distinct from the use of objects, the physical environment, or the world of make-believe. As children develop, they tend to increase in the amount and complexity of social participation in their play from independent to cooperative (Knox, 1997; Parten, 1932).

Early social interaction typically occurs with adults through a dialogue of actions and interactions. The adult and child engage in reciprocal early turn taking that becomes predictable, routine, and repeatable (Owens, 2001). They take turns making sounds and imitating in face-to-face play. Around 6 to 12 months, play becomes

more structured and defined through conventional games, such as peekaboo and pat-a-cake, and object-mediated dyadic play, such as sharing objects or pointing out objects (Field, 1979; Fraits-Hunt & Zemke, 1996; Williams, 2003). Toward the end of the first year, an infant typically begins to initiate an action to get a reaction from another person, such as teasingly offering and then withdrawing a toy, doing things in silly ways such as putting shoes on his or her head, or showing off gestures, actions, or sounds (Williams, 2003).

The social play of children with autism tends to be characterized by less social-interactive and cooperative play than occurs with typically developing or developmentally delayed children (Restall & Magill-Evans, 1994; Ritvo & Freeman, 1978). Like symbolic play, complexity of social interaction tends to be associated with cognitive and language abilities (Restall & Magill-Evans, 1994; Sigman & Ruskin, 1999; Tardif et al., 1995). Limited social interaction is a primary defining feature of autism. Deficits in social play commonly include withdrawal, isolation, and deficits in joint attention, affective sharing, empathetic responses, imitation, initiation of social interaction, and social responsiveness.

Many children with autism play in isolation from other people (Sigman & Ruskin, 1999). Initially their isolation was thought to indicate a difficulty with attachment to others, but this has not been supported by research (e.g., Buitelaar, 1995; Dissanayake & Crossley, 1996; Sigman & Ungerer, 1984). Children with autism do demonstrate attachment behaviors, for example, seeking proximity and closeness to a particular person such as a parent (Dissanayake & Crossley, 1996), and show an increase in attachment behaviors when reunited with their mothers (Sigman & Ungerer, 1984). Nonetheless, they tend to play alone more than other children do.

Joint attention involves nonverbal communication exchanges between the child and another person about an object or common interest. Often it involves looking back and forth between the person and the object, pointing, or gesturing to indicate a sharing of the object or event. It establishes a single focus of attention shared by the two people. Joint attention tends to emerge as object play develops (Kasari, Sigman, Mundy, & Yirmiya, 1990). It provides a foundation for social interaction through sharing an experience but is often compromised in children with autism (Charman et al., 1997; Kasari et al., 1990; Mundy & Crowson, 1997; Mundy, Sigman, & Kasari, 1990; Sigman & Ruskin, 1999). Children with autism are more likely than developmentally matched peers without autism to directly manipulate the examiner's hand to request or show objects (Stone, Ousley, Yoder, Hogan, & Hepburn, 1997). Joint attention deficits tend to emerge early in life for children with autism and are thought to be an early sign that distinguishes between individuals with and without autism (Mundy & Crowson, 1997;

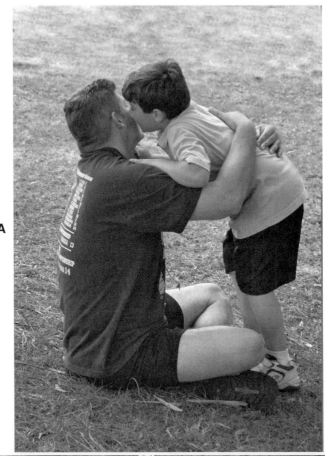

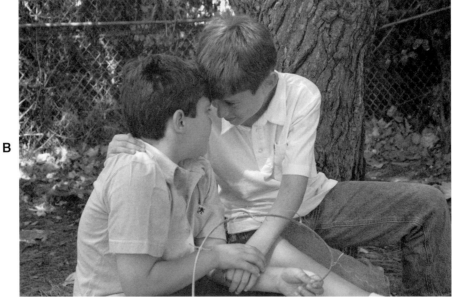

Figure 14-4
A, *The social play of children with autism may involve a physical closeness to particular person.* **B,** *Play with other children tends to occur less frequently than in typically developing children. (Courtesy Shay McAtee.)*

Sigman & Ruskin, 1999). Children with autism may avoid eye contact with other people, especially less familiar people (Miller, 1996), unless in close physical space (Pedersen, Livoir-Petersen, & Scheide, 1989). Features of social play in young children with autism that may enable joint attention include sharing sensorimotor features, sensory perception (visual and auditory), objects, or simple scripted action (Spitzer, 2001).

The ability to share an affective or emotional state with another person typically begins in the first years of life as infants exchange affective expressions with caregivers. Children with autism often do not demonstrate empathy when someone is injured (Charman et al., 1997). Dawson, Hill, Spencer, Galpert, and Watson (1990) found that young children with autism smile as often as normally developing children, matched on receptive age, but they are less likely to combine smiles with eye contact and are less likely to smile in response to their mothers, which implies an intention to communicate or share the emotion. Children with autism pay less attention to the faces of other people whatever their affect, but a strong expression of affect may draw their attention (Sigman & Ruskin, 1999). Greenspan (2001) asserted that a difficulty in connecting affect to motor planning, sequencing, and symbol formation is a core deficit in autism. Thus emotion needs to be connected to play actions.

Impairments of imitation skills also seem to affect social play. Imitation of facial movements is consistently more impaired in toddlers with autism, compared with control subjects who have fragile X syndrome, other developmental disorders, or no disability, and seems to distinguish autism from other disabilities (Rogers et al., 2003). Imitation is thought to be important for the early development of intersubjectivity (shared understandings with other people) and hence the emergence of communication and social interaction in children with autism (Gopnik & Meltzoff, 1993; Hobson & Lee, 1999; Rogers & Pennington, 1991).

Many researchers and experts contend that deficits in joint attention, affective sharing, and empathy are signs of deficits in social understanding (Pennington, 1991). Individuals with autism seem to have difficulty understanding other people, social interaction, and social norms. Even high-functioning individuals with autism find it hard to understand the nuances and subtleties of social interaction and thus determine appropriate social responses.

Sigman and Ruskin (1999) conducted a longitudinal study of several groups of children, including children with autism, developmentally matched typically developing children, and developmentally matched children with developmental delays. They found that school-age children with autism tended to play in isolation, initiated interaction less frequently, and accepted other children's overtures less frequently. The children with autism were no more likely to be rejected by their peers, since they received a similar number of approaches by others and had a similar number of their initiations accepted by others. Once an interaction was started, children with autism tended to maintain it as long as others. Nonverbal communication and representational play at young ages predicted social engagement in school-age children with autism.

EXPERIENCE OF PLAY

General descriptions of the experience of play contrast markedly with descriptions of the play of children with autism. In general, play is described as a pleasurable experience that provides meaning for living a person's life and is a means for children to shape individual identities. Such examinations of play in the autism literature are noticeably absent. The scarcity of research on play as an experience for children with autism makes this area of practice challenging but cannot be forgotten. Therapists must rely on the knowledge that is available and the state of research as it exists today. As a result, the general literature on play as experience is explored here in some depth, as well as the few studies of individuals with autism and similar developmental disabilities, as a knowledge base for informing practice.

The experience of play is central to a child's occupational profile (AOTA, 2002) as it occurs through participation in play (Bundy, 1991, 1993, 1997; Henricks, 1997). Play is "some quality of experience that is generated and sustained by certain actions" (Henricks, 1997, p. 8). This experience refers to the excitement, engagement, and emotional states generated by play. In occupational therapy, Anita Bundy (1991, 1993, 1997; see also Chapter 4) has pioneered the conceptual development of play as experience, which she labels "playfulness." Bundy (1993) has described playfulness as a style or approach for engaging in activities. Although research suggests that some children may be more disposed to play and possess what has been labeled a playful personality trait (Barnett, 1998; Rogers et al., 1998), playfulness cannot be limited to a personality trait and thereby be restricted to "playful" people. Rather, play is a complicated interaction between people and their environments (Henricks, 1997; Rubin et al., 1983).

A play experience is characterized by the presence of intrinsic motivation, internal control, and the freedom to suspend reality (Bundy, 1991, 1993, 1997). An activity that is intrinsically motivated is one in which the individual engages for its own sake (Bundy, 1997; Florey, 1969; Henricks, 1997; National Institute of Mental Health, 1995; Parham & Primeau, 1997; Rubin et al., 1983; Wing, 1995). In other words, people play for the sake of play. Internal control refers to the person's ability to direct his or her actions (Bundy, 1997; Henricks, 1997; Parham & Primeau, 1997; Wing, 1995). The individual is in a sense "free" to shape the form of his or her own play (Henricks, 1997). The freedom to suspend reality means that players act "as if" there were no external rules, seeking out challenges and exploring a range of alternative futures. For example, Barnett's (1998) research suggested that through play, children manage their environments to reduce anxiety from stressful situations. Although this aspect seems to emphasize a sort of imaginative or pretend play, it should not be confused with imaginative or pretend play per se. It may involve imaginative play, but the imagining may simply be a child's feeling that she or he can do more physically, such as climb to a higher bar on the jungle gym. In this way, play has a transformative quality (Henricks, 1997).

Play and Meaning

For years the meaning of play has been closely linked to pleasure (Freud, 1920/1955). Play is hypothesized to provide meaning for a person's life by making life livable, by giving the person a sense that life is worth living (Parham, 1996; Sutton-Smith, 1971, 1994). When people play, they enjoy living (Sutton-Smith, 1971). Most simply, play is fun. In addition to providing meaning for life, play engages people's sense of their potentiality (who they might become) and energizes them to further engage in ongoing daily activities of life. This hypothesis is perhaps best credited to the work of Brian Sutton-Smith, who after a lifetime of research on play has concluded, "So the function of play in my mind is to pretend that we exist in a life worth living" (1994, p. 20). Play is what makes life livable. Occupational therapists are especially committed to play for its own sake and as a valid treatment outcome (e.g., Blanche, 1997; Bundy, 1997; Deitz & Swinth, 1997; Hinojosa & Kramer, 1997; Holloway, 1997; Parham, 1996; Parham & Primeau, 1997). Play is "an active ingredient of a healthy, satisfying lifestyle" (Parham, 1996, p. 78). Such positive emotions have been linked with psychological well-being (National Institute of Mental Health, 1995), physical health (Fredrickson, 2003), and the development of other skills (Greenspan, 2001).

Play and the Self as an Occupational Being

Play is understood to contribute to and convey an individual's self-identity. The self is developed through the transformative aspect of play (Henricks, 1997; Mook, 1994). The player changes as he or she experiences play. Nonplay experiences may also be transformative and influence identity. What makes play unique in the development of the self is that the player is self-motivated and self-directing this process. "During play, the subject itself controls the models of how the self will develop in an open process" (Schafer, 1994, p. 84). In play, people challenge themselves, try different roles, and explore other possibilities for themselves.

Play as experience offers great potential for expressing the *individualized, complex,* and *meaningful* aspects of occupation, which are key concerns of occupational therapists (Clark et al., 1991; Yerxa et al., 1990). Because play is intrinsically motivated and self-directed, children express themselves by indicating what is important to them (Axline, 1947/1969; Barnett, 1998; Bundy, 1993; Holloway, 1997; Mook, 1994; Parham, 1996; Sutton-Smith, 1997). Children demonstrate their unique play styles (Knox, 1997; Singer & Singer, 1990). Bundy (1993) asserted that it is playfulness, rather than a "play" activity, that is at the essence of understanding play as occupation. Understanding the play experience and other occupational experiences is central to understanding people as occupational beings.

An example of a child's experience of play was provided by the research of Kelly-Byrne (1989). She presented a rich account of a single child's perspective and of an adult who played with the child intensively over an extended period. Her focus was to understand the 7-year-old child, Helen, as a person participating in intentional acts. Kelly-Byrne found Helen's play themes to be symbolic of her struggles over her personal, social, and sexual identity and her need to establish her own sense of power in daily activities. Helen's play consistently involved battle stories she developed, which seemed symbolic of her inner battle between what she was and what she wished to be.

Experience of Play for Children with Autism

In children with autism, as in other disabilities, play has been understood primarily in terms of their disabilities, deficits, and limitations. Few studies have attempted to understand play as an experience for children with developmental disabilities. The limited research suggests that researchers have felt that the experience of play for children with autism either does not exist or is not worthy of study. For example, Wulff (1985) noted that play seemed to lack pleasure for children with autism but did not question why. A more recent article by Ziviani, Boyle, and Rodger (2001) similarly dismissed the experience of play because "The term 'playful' is difficult to apply to children with ASD [autism spectrum disorders] because it involves spontaneity, a quality that these children have difficulty in displaying" (p. 20). Relatively little is known about the play of children with disabilities such as autism in terms of what they *can* do (Hellendoorn, van der Kooij, & Sutton-Smith, 1994). Children with developmental disabilities may have play strengths. They may, in fact, develop capabilities and competencies that are lacking in individuals without disabilities by virtue of their distinctive life experiences as persons with a disability (Hahn, 1989).

More recently, perhaps spurred on by the disabilities rights movement, there seems to be "a growing concern for these children's own identities and their own ways of playing" (Hellendoorn et al., 1994, p. 2). This is important because to equate a child's play with her or his disability is to obscure the child and the child's shared humanity. To understand a child's play only in terms of deficits or deviations from "normal" is to diminish both the diversities and the commonalities in children's play.

One of the first people to look at play in children with autism as an experience rather than just play skills was Pamela Wolfberg. Wolfberg (1999) conducted a longitudinal qualitative study of three children with autism as they participated in a play intervention program from ages 7 to 9 years. Although her focus was predominantly on the children's play skills and development, she also included the children's experiences. She found that the impulse to play was significantly subdued in the children with autism as compared with typically developing children. The children with autism had a tendency to stay with repetitive behaviors, actions, objects, people, and routines that were familiar to them. Often their subtle attempts to initiate play with others went unnoticed by typically developing play partners. Once the children with autism and their peers were given adult guidance and support to play with one another, they played together more often and in more flexible and novel ways, developing functional and symbolic play skills. As they did so, many of the children's unique interests were integrated into more conventional activities and appeared to be accepted as the new "norm." Many early interests continued in different forms in pretend play, games, and other activities.

Although she did not limit her study to play, Spitzer's (2001) study of the experience and interests of five 3- and 4-year-olds with autism in daily activities certainly overlaps with play. In this qualitative study she observed and participated in the children's daily activities in home, school, and community settings over several months. She found that by examining the details of how the children did and did not participate in activities, adults could identify what was meaningful and important to the individual child in that activity. For example, she described how Britany enjoyed repetitively hitting her dolls on the kitchen floor in such a way as to provide a steady rhythm that was soothing and restorative for her in a location where she could be near the social interactions of her family. With this information, adults could successfully join in and share the activity with the child in an interactive way. For example, Britany's mother would sit with her and provide sound effects in time (rhythm) with Britany's

banging her dolls. In this way Britany and her mother would monitor each other's actions to change the tempo or pitch and thus keep their sounds in alignment with each other as they composed their own "music" together. Such information about the child's occupations provides a sense of the child's identity as an occupational being and hints about what else the child might like to do or be. This knowledge about how such occupations may occur in daily life provides a foundation for occupational therapists to identify and use the interests of a child with autism to facilitate playful experiences for the child (Spitzer, 2004).

Desha, Ziviani, and Rodger (2003) specifically examined the play interests of 24 preschool-age children with autism. They studied the spontaneous play of the children in an occupational therapy clinic. These children demonstrated clear preferences for play objects in the form of popular characters (e.g., Thomas the Tank Engine) and those with sensorimotor properties.

In 2003, Jean-Paul Bovee, an individual in whom autism had been diagnosed, described his childhood play experiences from a different perspective than his mother (Donnelly & Bovee, 2003). Bovee recounted that his favorite play was making lists, especially of genealogical family trees and cities of the world, and making up genealogies for characters in books. He also made up ball games with players on baseball cards and watched drops of liquid "race" down a window. These fun activities were play for him. He found the conventional play activities his mother encouraged him to do, such as sports, to be challenging, frustrating, and not enjoyable. For Bovee, his play was a form of imagination based on an interest in finding and remembering information. Now his childhood play connects to his adult work as an information specialist.

Most young children delight in learning new skills, even in nonplay activities. Given the challenges that children with autism experience in so many activities, they are less likely than children without disabilities to have positive activity experiences and to experience the joy of play (Brockmeyer, 2001). A lack of positive experiences is a natural disincentive to engage and participate in the variety of daily activities available to these children. Thus, encouraging play as a full experience and playful moments is important for the overall well-being of the child and the promotion of a trajectory of occupational engagement. Children with autism need and deserve to play more.

INTERVENTION TO SUPPORT PLAY FOR CHILDREN WITH AUTISM

Occupational therapists are concerned with the structural performance and occupational profile of play (see Box 14-2 for examples of play goals). At times an

Box 14-2	*Common Goals for Promoting Play in Children with Autism*

Expand variety in the child's object play repertoire.
Enhance diversity, complexity, and creativity of play.
Develop participation in peer play.
Facilitate playful engagement with persons or objects.
Improve motivation to play.

From Baranek, G. T., Reinhartsen, D. B., & Wannamaker, S. W. (2001). Play: Engaging young children with autism. In R. A. Huebner (Ed.), *Autism: A sensorimotor approach to management* (p. 337). Gaithersburg, MD: Aspen Publishers.

occupational therapist may focus on pieces of play, but clinical reasoning should always be directed toward the potential for expanding to a full, rich play activity. Therefore intervention is described here in terms of both facilitating a playful experience and building structural components for play.

Promoting Play Experiences: Imagining and Realizing Possibilities

Play experiences are promoted by imagining possibilities for play to emerge, creating a play milieu, and providing support for play to emerge. This is a rather playful process for the occupational therapist. The therapist frees himself or herself to some degree from the child's clinical picture of diagnosis and deficits. Instead, the therapist plays with other possibilities of who the child is and might become. Using complex analysis and a creative individualized approach, the therapist imagines and explores "what if" the child did not have autism and constructs opportunities "as if" the child *might* play. These possibilities reach outside what the child typically does but are still possible within the realities of the child's abilities. The possibilities may not seem probable or likely, but this is the world of play, where players are transformed whether they are therapists or clients. "In play a child always behaves beyond his average age, above his daily behavior; in play it is as though he were a head taller than himself" (Vygotsky, 1978, p. 102).

Three strategies can be used to promote a play experience for children with autism. First, the therapist must have an advanced knowledge and understanding of play to offer and support possibilities that transcend the everyday "reality" of the diagnosis. Second, the therapist uses the knowledge of the child's specific interests and knowledge of the activities to reframe previously meaningless activities into personally meaningful, intrinsically motivating play. Third, the therapist is free to look for and support opportunities to infuse playfulness into diverse activities. In other words, the occupational therapist "plays," as well as works to support play.

Recognizing and Extending Hints of Play

To recognize hints of play possibilities and to extend those into play activities, the occupational therapist must become familiar with the complexity of typical play (described throughout this book and in play research). As the therapist works with a child with autism, he or she is always looking for hints of play. Hints of play may be moments when the child engages in more complicated object play, glances at another person, acts or comments on a piece of a narrative play story, or suggests a play theme. At the moment the therapist perceives a hint of a play possibility, he or she must support the child by helping to structure and elaborate this isolated playful moment into a play activity. For example, the therapist may show the child more ways to use a toy to accomplish what the child wants. Spitzer (2001) recounted an example of Emma, a preschooler with autism, who enjoyed incorporating adult interaction and change when it was play.

CASE EXAMPLE 1

Emma

Emma is a preschooler who enjoys the process of collecting and carefully placing various items such as toys, neckties, and scarves. She generally resists anyone's attempt to move aspects of her creations. One day, the occupational therapist remarks that her creation looks like roads. Emma's mother and the occupational therapist model using toy cars to go through "roads" in her creations and "park" the cars in a pattern at the other end. Emma begins to drive the cars as well, taking turns and waiting for additions to the roads. By honoring Emma's play of creating a project, her mother and the therapist are able to stretch her relational play to include functional play. Flexibility and tolerance for interaction with others are additional skills that are incorporated within the process (Spitzer, 2001, p. 263).

Playing the role of superheroes is a common theme in the make-believe world of typically developing children but often overlooked in children with autism. Adults tend to encourage more realistic forms of pretend play, for example, pretending to be a real entity such as a mother, father, pilot, or animal. Sometimes adults become concerned when children with autism want to pretend to be a fictional character because they may perseverate with a particular character, such as Thomas the Tank Engine. Adults may also be concerned about the ability of a child with autism to tell the difference between reality and make-believe or doubt the child's capability to participate in such elaborate pretend play. In contrast, the play research with typical children suggests that being a superhero can be a powerful form of play (Kelly-Byrne, 1989;

Singer & Singer, 1990). Consequently, children with autism, who might be able to experience this form of play too, are owed the opportunity to do so. The following two case examples illustrate how this occurred in boys with autism who seemed unlikely to engage in such symbolic play but had provided hints that the occupational therapist recognized and helped support.

CASE EXAMPLE 2

Christopher

Christopher is a 10-year-old with autism. He is big for his age and strong. He is able to use two-word phrases to communicate simple concrete needs and wants. During daily activities he breaks items and hurts other people constantly throughout the day because he is very dyspraxic and is unable to regulate force. He cries and says "Sorry" each time he sees the damage or when someone points it out to him. It is almost as if everyone and everything he touches is hurt by him. Often he resists or refuses engagement in activities. During his occupational therapy using a sensory integration approach, the therapist urges him to help arrange equipment. She knows this will be a good way to provide Christopher with the additional proprioceptive input his body needs, but Christopher refuses, saying, "You (do it)." So the therapist models trying to move the equipment, saying, "It's too heavy for me. I need help." Christopher is watching her carefully, smiling in response to her dramatic expressions, and comes rushing over to help. "Oh, you're so strong," she says, "just like Superman." "Superman," he repeats in an excited voice. This becomes the theme of many of their sessions. Whenever the therapist wants to encourage Christopher's more active involvement, she calls on "Superman" and "Super Chris." Christopher is transformed into "Superman," whose strength and force are positive, where he is able to help and "save" other people. He is able to experience in play a different sense of who he is, transformed from one who destroys with unregulated force into one who helps by virtue of his "superhero" strength. He begins to take on this helper role outside of occupational therapy as well.

Christopher's breakthrough started with the occupational therapist's recognition that his role in helping an adult move a "heavy" object was like being a superhero. Although no one was likely to suspect that Christopher could pretend to be a superhero, his occupational therapist was willing to suspend traditional notions of autism, explore "what if," and structure this opportunity, of which he took full advantage.

CASE EXAMPLE 3

William

William is a 7-year-old with autism and a generally low activity level. The general goal for occupational therapy is for William to initiate, carry out, and sustain engagement in multistep activities. He often echoes single words but seldom uses speech to communicate. One day, William is going through an obstacle course during his occupational therapy session. He lies down and stops in the middle of a cloth tunnel. The therapist encourages him to continue on, but he just lies there repeatedly saying something like "ler-cul-ees." The therapist looks quizzically at his mother, who explains, "Hercules." The occupational therapist then encourages him by saying, "Go Hercules! You're so strong! Go Hercules!" William laughs and begins crawling quickly through the tunnel. At the end of the tunnel the therapist lifts up a large weighted ball in the stance of Atlas and says, "Yeah, Hercules!" She then hands the ball to William, who copies her. His mother is excited to see William play in this way, since she has never observed it before. For months afterward, William asks to play "Hercules"—an obstacle course. As the therapist calls him "Hercules," he smiles and a surge of energy propels him forward.

It is not clear whether William came up with an idea to play Hercules or was simply echoing the word from one of his videos as he often did. Rather than focus on clinical diagnostic reasons for why he was saying the word, his occupational therapist seized the opportunity to structure it as play.

Often adults discourage children from certain play themes such as violence, death, sexuality, or other behavior that adults feel is "wrong" or "bad." Such themes are common in the play of typically developing children (Goldstein, 1995; Pellegrini, 1995; Singer & Singer, 1990). They seem to be helpful for children who are struggling to understand these issues (Singer & Singer, 1990). For children with autism, adults may be even more likely to stop this play because of the desire to see them learn socially appropriate behavior in real-life situations. If children learn to understand ideas by playing with them, however, perhaps children with autism should be allowed an opportunity to participate in such play as well. Caution must be exercised to ensure that the child understands the limits of any such play, and the occupational therapist must feel confident of having the ability to address potential social-cultural ramifications. At minimum, when the play emerges from the child, the occupational therapist must recognize it as play and evaluate his or her own abilities to venture into this area before automatically stopping the play. The following case provides an example of how this might occur.

CASE EXAMPLE 4

Peter

It is the last day of occupational therapy for Peter, a 7-year-old with autism. He was referred to occupational therapy for tactile defensiveness and difficulty with tool use. His occupational therapy sessions have been rich with imaginative play—acting out characters and scenes based on different children's videos. During this last session, Peter creates a scene involving jumping into a "cake" (a pile of cushions and an inner tube). At the end, Peter, his mother and sister, and the occupational therapist sit down to celebrate Peter's graduation by each having a piece of real cake. Peter looks at his and asks, "Can I put it in my face?" After glancing quickly at Peter's mother, who is smiling, the occupational therapist says, "Yes." With much drama, Peter proceeds to smash the cake in his own face. They all laugh together. As the therapist offers a towel to help clean up, she asks him, "It's funny, like on TV, huh?" "Yes," he replies. "But are you supposed to smash cake in people's faces?" she asks. "No," he responds. Follow-up later indicates that this is indeed a one-time play event.

Although it was clearly not appropriate mealtime behavior, Peter's interest in playing with food seemed related to trying to understand things he had seen and to conquering his own sensory challenges. The occupational therapist, with support from Peter's mother, recognized this as play, not the typical play of a child with autism, but the typical play of a typically developing boy.

Reframing Activities into Play

Occupational reframing involves modifying activities in such a way that they become transformed into individually meaningful occupations. Spitzer (2001, 2004) provided a detailed model for occupational reframing in children with autism. In the case of children, reframing activities into preferred occupations often has a playful quality. Spitzer (2003) suggested that occupational therapists carefully analyze a child's preferred occupations by examining the child's intentional actions. By observing the details of what a child does and how the child does it, the occupational therapist can make interpretations about the subjective meaning of the activity. These subjective meanings and the child's interests can provide the therapist with ways to reframe meaningless activities into occupations the child wants to do (Spitzer, 2001, 2004). By incorporating materials or themes of interest to the child, the occupational therapist can help transform an activity of little interest into a real play experience for that particular child. Spitzer (2004) recounted

the detailed cases of David, Austin, and Kenneth, who illustrate this point. David did not even hold a pencil or attempt to make marks on his own but found "drawing" the letters of car names to be a fun activity that he initiated. Austin, who preferred to bang toys, was delighted to put objects into a shape sorter once his occupational therapist showed him how items put inside the container could be shaken to create even more noise. Kenneth, who resisted most activities with his hands, joyfully put on and removed a container lid when the container was used as a garage for a favorite toy bus to go to "sleep" and "wake up."*

Embedding Play into Everyday Activities

Sometimes everyday activities present opportunities for play moments. When typically developing children do schoolwork, especially in younger grades, it is striking how playful moments and genuine interest are interspersed with the "work." Play and work are not always distinct categories. In contrast, when children with autism laugh, joke, or stop to manipulate an object during work tasks, they are usually chided for off-task behavior. It seems that children with autism might be more interested in "work" if it were more fun (Brockmeyer, 2001). While sometimes it is important to encourage a child with autism to use a particular defined behavior, sessions do not have to be serious all the time, especially if play is also important. During targeted opportunities, lifting the rules and restrictions to allow the child to direct his or her own actions can enable play experiences. The case of Jackie (Case Example 5) illustrates how an occupational therapist might take advantage of potentially playful moments to build a store of play experiences that will help balance out the continual challenges faced by a child with autism.

In sum, the occupational therapist promotes play as an occupational experience for children with autism by playing with the child. The occupational therapist must be prepared to suspend reality to see hints of play, to tap intrinsic motivation to reframe activities into play, and to suspend behavioral "rules" to be flexible and adaptive. In the process of participating in play, the child shapes a trajectory of occupational engagement and develops other skills for greater well-being.

Promoting the Structure and Skills for Play

Research suggests that the play skills in children with autism may respond to a variety of approaches (Jordan, 2003; Rogers, 2000) (Box 14-3). Some approaches have

---

*Geist and Kielhofner (1998) and Goode and Gaddy (1976) also provide good suggestions for identifying interests in children.

CASE EXAMPLE 5
Jackie

Jackie is a 4-year-old with autism. Her occupational therapist is working with her on tolerating adult structure so that she can participate in preacademic activities such as using a pencil to make different strokes on a page. To increase interest and sensory feedback, the occupational therapist decides to introduce a vibrating pencil. Because Jackie is so resistant to adult structure, the occupational therapist will initially have only one rule for the activity. Jackie can use the pencil in any way as long as she physically stays at the table. Jackie tolerates this structure by the therapist and explores the pencil by manipulating it in different ways in addition to making some marks with it. Jackie seems interested in the pencil, which is the occupational therapist's primary goal for the session. Suddenly within this exploration Jackie holds the vibrating pencil toward the therapist's face. The therapist remains still, and Jackie touches the tip to the therapist's nose. The therapist giggles in an exaggerated fashion and then moves the pencil toward Jackie's nose. Jackie laughs. The two go back and forth several times, embedding social play into a work-oriented activity.

Box 14-3 *Key Approaches for Promoting the Structure of Play in Children with Autism*

Use toys and themes that interest the child.
Modify the environment and activities.
Teach and guide the development of social, object, sensorimotor, and pretend play.
Cue, prompt, direct (emphasize a visual learning approach).
Model play actions and behavior.
Use visual strategies and cues.
Reinforce successes and attempts.
Target key play skills:
  Add new steps or materials.
  Share activities through physical interaction, perceptual play, objects, or repeatable sequences.
  Teach body language, how to stay on topic, share, help, take turns, initiate, respond.
  Explain social situations and contexts to build understanding (e.g., social stories).
  Include play partners, especially peers.
  Build foundational skills (e.g., sensory integration, motor skills, imitation).

---

received more research than others. Most have been studied only with small numbers of children. Seldom have strategies been researched on a large scale or compared with different strategies. As a result, little research is available on which strategies are most effective or for which children a particular strategy may be most effective. Therefore the selection of strategies for use with an individual child is a matter of clinical reasoning. The occupational therapist matches the child's needs and strengths with complementary strategies.

Incorporating the Child's Interests

Not only does incorporating the child's interests help promote a play experience for the child, but research suggests that it can also assist in building a child's play skills. Selecting toys and play activities that interest the child taps the child's intrinsic motivation, helping him or her to realize that the activity offers something enjoyable that makes it worth the effort (Arthur, Bochner, & Butterfield, 1999). The child becomes more likely to initiate and sustain participation in play (Figure 14-5). By participating, the child develops more play skills.

Drawing on the child's interests may start with joining the child in the activity she or he is doing, such as by imitating the child (Huebner & Kraemer, 2001). Tiegerman and Primavera (1981) found that the frequency and duration of object manipulation in children with autism was greatest when the adult imitated the child by using both the materials and methods of play that the child had chosen, rather than performing a different action on the same object or performing a different action on a different object.

Koegel, Dyer, and Bell (1987) found that when children with autism were engaged in their preferred activities, they avoided other people less and were more responsive to social initiations by others. Furthermore, prompting children with autism to engage in their preferred activities was more effective for decreasing social avoidance, increasing social responsiveness, and increasing and maintaining verbal interactions than was prompting them to engage in arbitrary activities. Baker, Koegel, and Koegel (1998) used the obsessive interests of three children with autism to create playground games that were intrinsically motivating for those children and appropriate for typical peers as well. The activities included tag games based on a map of the United States and on movie themes and a follow-the-Disney-character-leader game. With adult prompting and support the amount of social play at recess increased dramatically for each child and was maintained for 2 months without the adult's presence. Significant increases in affect (interest and happiness) were also noted in each child and their typical playmates and were maintained for 2 months. Further research on the use of a child's interest for building play skills can be found in the literature on particular intervention models such as

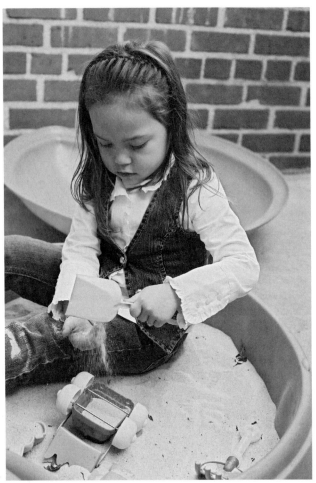

Figure 14-5
Incorporating the child's interests helps to promote both a play experience and motivate the child with autism to engage in play activities. (Courtesy Shay McAtee.)

Pivotal Response Training (e.g., Stahmer, 1995; Stahmer, Ingersoll, & Carter, 2003); the Developmental, Individual-difference, Relationship-based (DIR) model (e.g., Weider & Greenspan, 2003); and Integrated Play Groups (Wolfberg & Schuler, 1993).

Play that incorporates visual feedback, construction, sensory properties, sensorimotor engagement, favorite toys, and narratives from favorite stories or movies can be a good start to engage a child with autism. Given that children with autism tend to have strengths in visual processing, toys and activities that provide an observable effect of the child's actions can be more interesting (Brockmeyer, 2001). For example, throwing a beanbag at a stack of blocks that falls down when hit can be more interesting than throwing at a target. Spinning tops and wind-up or pop-up toys can also be intriguing activities. Since constructional skills tend to be stronger in children with autism, offering a variety of different objects that can be put together or fit together into a larger object, such as chain links, pop beads, puzzles, and blocks, may be more motivating. The toys selected should be easy enough for the child to manipulate given her or his motor skills. Sensory-rich play also motivates many children with autism (Baranek, Reinhartsen, & Wannamaker, 2001; Hayes, Rincover, & Volosin, 1980; Van Berckelaer-Onnes, 2003). For example, sensorimotor games can be a good context for working on social play (Black et al., 1975). Adding sensory elements such as sand can increase a child's interest, as the case of Greg illustrates. Play activities that "have an obvious, identifiable and prescribed process (story lines from Thomas the Tank Engine), and have easily repeatable acts (for example, blowing bubbles)" (Ziviani et al., 2001, p. 20) are highly engaging for children with autism. Even so-called obsessions can be used to support play (Brockmeyer, 2001). Chapter 7 provides suggestions on selecting interesting toys for children.

CASE EXAMPLE 6

Greg

Greg is a 2½-year-old whose autism was just diagnosed. He prefers sensorimotor play. His object play consists of a few seconds of rolling a toy vehicle around and dumping out bins of toys to kick them around. Whenever anyone offers him toy figures or models actions with toy figures, he knocks the toys away. Occupational therapy is focused on increasing his ability to tolerate structured activities and enlarging the repertoire of activities in which he will engage. One day the occupational therapist pulls out a small bin of damp sand, hoping to interest Greg in imitating various lines in it. Greg shows little interest in the lines but digs his hands into the sand, manipulating it and smiling at the therapist. His interest in the sand seems like a prime opportunity, so the therapist gives up the prewriting ideas and decides to explore other options. She makes a little "cookie" and holds it up to her mouth to "eat" it. Greg watches her carefully, and then she offers it to him. He holds his mouth still while she "feeds" him. They take turns eating. Then the occupational therapist wonders if the interest in sand and pretend eating can be extended. She gets out toy characters and "feeds" them. Before long, with the occupational therapist's narrative prompts, Greg is carrying out a simple play sequence of feeding the toys, putting them to bed covered by a paper towel, and waking them up to dance and kick around in the sand. He repeats this many times with great excitement. This is the first time he has played with toy characters in a functional way.

Modifying the Environment

Given the child's underlying deficits, grading the physical environment and play activities to match the child's abilities can be important in supporting play (Baranek et al., 2001; Black et al., 1975; Tanta, 2004). For example, too many objects or a noisy place may be overstimulating, making it difficult for the child to participate in the activity at hand. A game that requires refined precision of motor coordination may be too frustrating. On the other hand, reducing the number of objects, background sounds, and motor demands may enable a child to participate in a higher level of play. The properties of certain toys lend themselves more readily to different types of and ideas for play (Baranek et al., 2001; Lewis & Boucher, 1995; Wolfberg & Schuler, 1993). "For example, a brightly colored rattle with a bell invites manipulative exploration; whereas a drum and a drumstick or wooden spoon invite relational play; and a toy cup invites functional—or possibly symbolic—play" (Van Berckelaer-Onnes, 2003, p. 419). Objects can even be used to facilitate and bridge social interaction through such actions as sharing, taking turns, or modeling (Baranek et al., 2001; Williams et al., 1999)

Teaching and Guiding the Development of Play

Research suggests that providing interesting opportunities is often not enough to increase the level of play in children with autism. Spontaneous play is unlikely to emerge unless structured guidance is provided. Techniques and programs for explicitly addressing play abound. Instructing, prompting, modeling, and reinforcing are the most common researched techniques. Many recent studies and programs combine techniques and emphasize more natural settings.

An adult may instruct a child directly to perform a particular play act such as, "Feed the doll" (Jarrold, 2003; Lewis & Boucher, 1995; Pierce & Schreibman, 1995; Stahmer et al., 2003; Strain, 1980). The adult may provide the child with a verbal cue or hint of what to do or how to respond. For example, the therapist may say to the child, "Show me what you can do with the car" or "What can we do with this toy?" (Charman & Baron-Cohen, 1997; Jarrold, 2003; Stahmer et al., 2003) Visual prompts increase the visual stimuli to help the child identify what to do. For example, pointing to or tapping a toy or part of a toy may encourage the child to use that toy. Visual cues about what constitutes the child's personal space and cue cards about what to do are also frequently employed (Charlop-Christy, 2003; Densmore, 2004; Piantanida, 2004). Physically prompting the child may involve guiding his or her hand toward a toy to use or turning the child's body to face the person with whom he or she is to interact. With prompts, school-age children and adolescents with autism can produce functional play and symbolic play equal to that of children of the same mental age who do not have autism (Charman & Baron-Cohen, 1997). Generally the lowest level of direction should be used so that the child does not become dependent on high levels of elaborate support. Fading adult prompting, rather than stopping it, can help maintain play skills beyond the intervention period (Romanczyk, Diament, Goren, Trunell, & Harris, 1975). Using different cues and presenting instruction in different ways also help carryover because the child learns to respond to a variety of cues that may exist in the natural environment rather than one specific cue that may not always be present.

Modeling has been found to be an effective strategy for teaching object, pretend, and social play skills (e.g., Charlop-Christy, 2003; Mesibov, 1984; O'Connor, 1969; Pierce & Schreibman, 1995; Riguet et al. 1981; Stahmer, 1995; Stahmer et al., 2003; Tryon & Keane, 1986; Van Berckelaer-Onnes, 2003). Adult, peer, and video modeling has been used. A key to using models effectively may be to ensure that the child is attending to the model (Tryon & Keane, 1986). Modeling of play with objects helps a child understand that different possibilities exist for playing with the toys (Van Berckelaer-Onnes, 2003).

Reinforcement has been a feature of effective play skill programs but appears to be most successful when combined with other techniques (Stahmer et al., 2003). Usually naturalistic forms of reinforcement are emphasized, such as verbal praise and the ability to play with preferred toys (Stahmer, 1995). Some forms of play can be structured to be naturally reinforcing, such as taking turns to play with a preferred toy. Each time the child asks for a turn, he or she is naturally reinforced by getting to play with that toy. As they are learning a play skill, some children need more explicit reinforcement of attempts or approximations of the skill. To maintain the behavior, gradual fading of supplemental reinforcement is recommended (Romanczyk et al., 1975).

Several areas of play are commonly targeted in children with autism. Some programs teach types of play in developmental sequence: manipulative and relational play, then functional play, then symbolic play (Van Berckelaer-Onnes, 2003); however, it is not clear from the research whether this is necessary (Williams, 2003). Weider and Greenspan (2003) recommended targeting the ongoing elaboration of more complex symbolic play. Narrative play, a common symbolic play form in typically developing children, is often overlooked in children with autism (Schuler, 2003) and may require targeted intervention to develop (Densmore, 2004; Schuler, 2003). The case of Greg provides one example for promoting narrative play (see also Chapter 18 for additional strategies for using stories in treatment). Limited play routines can be expanded by modeling or prompting new steps or introducing new materials for the same play routine (Baranek et al., 2001). For social play it may be beneficial to first emphasize sharing an activity (Carpenter, Pennington,

& Rogers, 2002) through physical interaction, perceptual play, objects, or a series of repeatable and predictable actions (Spitzer, 2001). Joint attention can be enhanced by pointing to an object. Other specific social skills that are often targeted are body language, staying on topic, sharing and helping others, initiating interactions, responding to others' initiations, and taking turns (Densmore, 2004; Piantanida, 2004; Rogers, 2000; Sigman & Ruskin, 1999). Teaching children with autism to initiate play by offering a toy or object has been an effective technique in increasing cooperative play (Gaylord-Ross, Haring, Breen, & Pitts-Conway, 1984; Haring & Lovinger, 1989). Children with autism may also need help putting these skills together to build relationships and friendships (Arthur et al., 1999). (See also Chapter 10 for additional suggestions for building specific social skills.)

With more complex social interactions, the child may need concrete, explicit explanations of why people engage in the behavior that they do and why the child should engage in this behavior. For example, something as simple as understanding why people smile may not be recognized by a child with autism unless it has been explained explicitly. One of the most popular strategies for explaining social behavior so that a child with autism can understand the reasoning behind actions is the use of social stories (Gray, 1994/2000; Kuoch & Mirenda, 2003). Social stories are written by an adult or with the child to clearly explain detailed information about social situations, subtle cues, and people's expectations for social behavior. Verbal explanations, problem solving, and video reviews can also be helpful approaches in building a child's understanding of why the child should or should not engage in particular social behaviors (Densmore, 2004).

Some children with autism need similar explanations about what pretend play is so they can understand how it differs from "reality." Initially they may resist pretend play or want to pretend in very literal ways. Explicit explanations that this is "pretend" and encouragement to try different ways can help expand pretend play, as the example of Joe illustrates.

CASE EXAMPLE 7

Joe

Joe is a bright 3-year-old with autism who has a strict routine that he and his family follow. When anything deviates from this routine, Joe screams and throws himself to the ground, often injuring himself and requiring more than 30 minutes to calm. When the occupational therapist first introduces play ideas, such as suggesting that he looks like a snake wrapped around a post or that a red ball be an apple, Joe yells at her, "No! I'm not a snake! I'm a boy!" or "No! It's not an apple! It's a ball!"

Using sensory integration techniques to calm Joe, the occupational therapist gradually introduces these ideas with explicit explanations that this is "just pretend." The therapist first models the pretend play behavior. "This is a ball, but I am going to *pretend* it is an apple and pretend to eat it," says the occupational therapist, who then models actions of eating the apple. "Now I'm going to use it like a ball" and she throws it into a bin. Similar play actions are modeled and explained. As Joe is able to tolerate the therapist's actions, she begins to offer him opportunities to pretend as well. Gradually he starts to pretend, starting with copying the therapist and then coming up with his own ideas. His pretend play skills blossom, and he begins to comment on how certain materials put together look like something else (such as three rocks looking like a triangle). Nine months later, his preschool teacher in a regular education community class remarks that Joe is the most creative child in the class.

Including Play Partners

Research suggests that the best results in social play are found when the child actually plays with other people (Jordan, 2003; Rogers, 2000; Weider & Greenspan, 2003; Wolfberg, 1999) (Figure 14-6). This may be the therapist (Figure 14-7), the parents, or peers.

Peers are believed to be an essential component of interventions designed to build peer play (Wolfberg & Schuler, 1993). Most studies use typically developing children as peers, but children with mild disabilities have been used successfully as well (e.g., Ragland, Kerr, & Strain, 1978; Shafer, Egel, & Neef, 1984). The presence

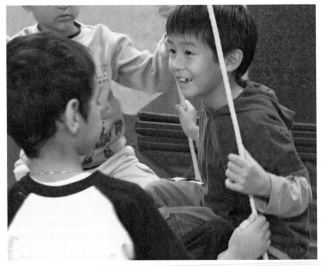

Figure 14-6

Including peers in occupational therapy treatment sessions can be an important element in building peer social play skills for children with autism. (Courtesy Shay McAtee.)

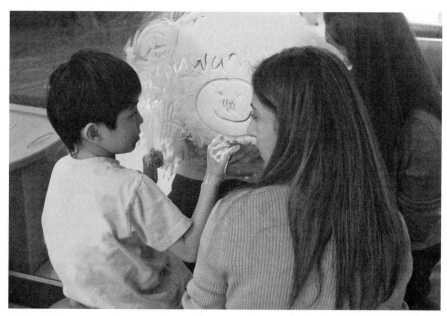

Figure 14-7

The occupational therapist can be a play partner to facilitate social play in a child with autism. (Courtesy Shay McAtee.)

of peers in integrated settings may be essential for generalization of skills (Strain, 1983) but is not adequate for building social skills (Odom & Strain, 1984). At a minimum, peers need to be explicit models (Tryon & Keane, 1986) or be given instructions for interacting with the children with autism (Strain, 1980). In McHale's (1983) study, general instructions to peers to teach the children to play resulted in increased social interaction in a sample of six children with autism; most programs, however, use more structured peer training. For example, in a pivotal response training program, peers are often trained in the following techniques to teach play to children with autism: ensure that the child is attending, give the child choices, vary the toys used, model appropriate social behavior, reinforce the child's attempts, encourage conversation, extend conversation by asking questions, take turns, narrate play such as "I'm going to cook the pizza," and use multiple cues (Pierce & Schreibman, 1995).

Wolfberg's (1999) Integrated Play Groups model provides another structure for including peers. Children with autism are considered to be "novice players," who participate in play with socially competent peers ("expert players") through guided participation of an adult. The adult guide's role is to monitor play and give temporary support only as needed. Support is provided to help the children with and without autism recognize and respond to each other's initiations. Wolfberg recommended choosing playmates who complement one another. This approach has been effective in increasing social, functional, and symbolic play (Wolfberg & Schuler, 1993; Yang, Wolfberg, Wu, & Hwu, 2003).

Building Foundational Skills

Additional gains in play skills may result from helping a child to build skills in sensory processing, motor coordination, and imitation, which are involved in play and lay a foundation for participation in play. For example, mulitsensory processing has been associated positively with participation in more mature play for children with autism (Gaines, 2002). A sensory integration approach may promote engagement in play by building efficient sensory processing and praxis, as well as incorporating opportunities to participate in play (Cross & Coster, 1997; Trecker & Miller-Kuhaneck, 2004) (see also Chapter 9). Improved motor skills may give a child access to a greater range of play activities. Learning to imitate others, first with objects and then with increasingly complex body actions, may help a child learn to imitate play more effectively.

Whatever skills are taught and whatever methods employed, the literature suggests that opportunities for ongoing supported practice are usually necessary to ensure maintenance and generalization of skills to a variety of people, settings, and materials.

SUMMARY

Children with autism have the potential to engage in a wider variety of play but often prefer less conventional forms of play. Their participation in traditional forms of play is both immature and qualitatively different from the play of developmental age–matched peers. Children with autism often lack interest and skills for engaging in the full realm of play activities. Without participating in the diversity of available play activities, they may miss out on the opportunities for further cognitive, social, fine motor, and adaptive skill development. Instead, children with autism tend to prefer play that goes unrecognized and unvalued by others.

Children with autism deserve to experience the joy and meaning of play and to maximize their potential to participate in the play activities of society. The child's interests must be respected by the incorporation of favorite materials, toys, themes, and even "obsessions" into play. At the same time, the child with autism often needs additional structure to maximize opportunities to play. Fusing the development of play skills and the experience of play is necessary to ensure that the child can experience an activity as true play and can develop the skills for greater participation in play activities. An increase in participation allows further practice and development of skills, greater opportunities for the child to maximize his or her potential for engagement in society, and cultivation of a meaningful, healthy life.

Review Questions

1. How does the play of children with autism differ from that of typically developing children in the six structural categories discussed?
2. Discuss the differences between the structure and the experience of play for children with autism.
3. What are specific observations that an occupational therapist can make to help determine what a child with autism experiences as play?
4. List general goals for promoting play in children with autism. Apply these specifically to the children in the case examples.
5. Describe three intervention methods an occupational therapist can use to promote play experiences for a child with autism.
6. Describe five intervention strategies an occupational therapist can use to promote the development of play skills in a child with autism.

REFERENCES

American Occupational Therapy Association (2002). Occupational therapy practice framework: Domain and process. *American Journal of Occupational Therapy, 56*, 609-639.

American Psychiatric Association (1994). *Diagnostic and statistical manual of mental disorders* (4th ed.). Washington, DC: Author.

Arthur, M., Bochner, S., & Butterfield, N. (1999). Enhancing peer interactions within the context of play. *International Journal of Disability, Development and Education, 46*(3), 367-381.

Axline, V. M. (1969). *Play therapy.* New York: Ballantine Books. (Original work published 1947).

Baker, M. J., Koegel, R. L., & Koegel, L. K. (1998). Increasing the social behavior of young children with autism using their obsessive behaviors. *Journal of the Association for Persons with Severe Handicaps, 23*(4), 300-308.

Baranek, G. T., Barnett, C. R., Adams, E. M., Wolcott, N. A., Watson, L. R., & Crais, E. R. (2005). Object play in infants with autism: Methodological issues in retrospective video analysis. *American Journal of Occupational Therapy, 59*(1), 20-30.

Baranek, G. T., Parham, L. D., & Bodfish, J. W. (2005). Sensory and motor features in autism: Assessment and intervention. In F. R. Volkmar, R. Paul, A. Klin, & D. J. Cohen (Eds.), *Handbook of autism and pervasive developmental disorders: Vol. 2. Assessment, interventions, and policy* (3rd ed., pp. 831-862). Hoboken, NJ: John Wiley & Sons.

Baranek, G. T., Reinhartsen, D. B., & Wannamaker, S. W. (2001). Play: Engaging young children with autism. In R. A. Huebner (Ed.), *Autism: A sensorimotor approach to management* (pp. 313-351). Gaithersburg, MD: Aspen Publishers.

Barnett, L. A. (1998). The adaptive powers of being playful. In S. Reifel (Series Ed.) & M. C. Duncan, G. Chick, & A. Aycock (Vol. Eds.), *Play and culture studies. Vol. 1. Diversions and divergences in fields of play* (pp. 97-119). Greenwich, CT: Ablex Publishing.

Black, M., Freeman, B. J., & Montgomery, J. (1975). Systematic observation of play behavior in autistic children. *Journal of Autism and Childhood Schizophrenia, 5*, 363-371.

Blanche, E. I. (1997). Doing with—not doing to: Play and the child with cerebral palsy. In L. D. Parham & L. S. Fazio (Eds.), *Play in occupational therapy for children* (pp. 202-218). St. Louis: Mosby.

Bristol, M. M., Cohen, D. J., Costello, E. J., Denckla, M., Eckberg, T. J., Kallen, R., et al. (1996). State of the science in autism: Report to the National Institutes of Health. *Journal of Autism and Developmental Disorders, 26*(2), 121-154.

Brockmeyer, R. D. (2001). My greatest wish: "I must play! I must play! I must play!" In R. A. Huebner (Ed.), *Autism: A sensorimotor approach to management* (pp. 423-442). Gaithersburg, MD: Aspen Publishers.

Buitelaar, J. K. (1995). Attachment and social withdrawal in autism: Hypotheses and findings. *Behaviour, 132*, 319-350.

Bundy, A. C. (1991). Play theory and sensory integration. In A. G. Fisher, E. A. Murray, & A. C. Bundy (Eds.), *Sensory integration theory and practice* (pp. 46-68). Philadelphia: F. A. Davis.

Bundy, A. C. (1993). Assessment of play and leisure: Delineation of the problem. *American Journal of Occupational Therapy, 47*, 217-222.

Bundy, A. C. (1997). Play and playfulness: What to look for. In L. D. Parham & L. S. Fazio (Eds.), *Play in occupational therapy for children* (pp. 52-66). St. Louis: Mosby.

Carpenter, M., Pennington, B. F., & Rogers, S. J. (2002). Interrelations among social-cognitive skills in young children with autism. *Journal of Autism and Developmental Disorders, 32*(2), 91-106.

Charlop, M. H., Schreibman, L., & Kurtz, P. F. (1991). Childhood autism. In T. R. Kratochwill & R. J. Morris (Eds.), *The practice of child therapy* (2nd ed., pp. 257-297). New York: Pergamon Press.

Charlop-Christy, M. H. (2003, April 6). *Social skills development for children with autism*. Paper presented at the Trends in Autism Conference, Claremont, CA.

Charman, T., & Baron-Cohen, S. (1997). Brief report: Prompted pretend play in autism. *Journal of Autism and Developmental Disorders, 27*(3), 325-332.

Charman, T., Swettenham, J., Baron-Cohen, S., Cox, A., Baird, G., & Drew, A. (1997). Infants with autism: An investigation of empathy, pretend play, joint attention, and imitation. *Developmental Psychology, 33*(5), 781-789.

Clark, F. A., Parham, D., Carlson, M. E., Frank, G., Jackson, J., Pierce, D., et al. (1991). Occupational science: Academic innovation in the service of occupational therapy's future. *American Journal of Occupational Therapy, 45*, 300-310.

Cole, M., & Cole, S. (1993). *The development of children* (2nd ed.). New York: W.H. Freeman.

Cross, L. A., & Coster, W. J. (1997). Symbolic play language during sensory integration treatment. *American Journal of Occupational Therapy, 51*(10), 808-814.

Dawson, G., Hill, D., Spencer, A., Galpert, L., & Watson, L. (1990). Affective exchanges between young autistic child and their mothers. *Journal of Abnormal Child Psychology, 18*(3), 335-345.

Deitz, J. C., & Swinth, Y. (1997). Accessing play through assistive technology. In L. D. Parham & L. S. Fazio (Eds.), *Play in occupational therapy for children* (pp. 219-232). St. Louis: Mosby.

Densmore, A. E. (2004, March 13). *Drawing out the social capacities of a child with autism through narrative play therapy*. Paper presented at the Trends in Autism Conference, Claremont, CA.

Desha, L., Ziviani, J., & Rodger, S. (2003). Play preferences and behavior of preschool children with autistic spectrum disorder in the clinical environment. *Physical and Occupational Therapy in Pediatrics, 23*(1), 21-42.

Dissanayake, C., & Crossley, S. A. (1996). Proximity and sociable behaviors in autism: Evidence for attachment. *Journal of Child Psychiatry, 37*(2), 149-156.

Donnelly, J., & Bovee, J. (2003). Reflections on play: Recollections from a mother and her son with Asperger syndrome. *Autism 7*(4), 471-476.

Fensom, L., Kagan, J., Kearsley, R. B., & Zelazo, P. R. (1976). The developmental progression of manipulative play in the first two years. *Child Development, 47*, 232-236.

Field, T. (1979). Games parents play with normal and high-risk infants. *Child Psychiatry and Human Development, 10*(1), 41-48.

Florey, L. L. (1969). Intrinsic motivation: The dynamics of occupational therapy theory. *American Journal of Occupational Therapy, 23*, 319-322.

Florey, L. L., & Greene, S. (1997). Play in middle childhood: A focus on children with behavior and emotional disorders. In L. D. Parham & L. S. Fazio (Eds.), *Play in occupational therapy for children* (pp. 126-143). St. Louis: Mosby.

Fraits-Hunt, D., & Zemke, R. (1996). Games mothers play with their full-term and pre-term infants. In R. Zemke & F. Clark (Eds.), *Occupational science: The evolving discipline* (pp. 217-226). Philadelphia: F.A. Davis.

Fredrickson, B. L. (2003, July-August). The value of positive emotions: The emerging science of positive psychology is coming to understand why it's good to feel good. *American Scientist, 91*, 330-335.

Freud, S. (1955). Beyond the pleasure principle. In J. Strachey (Ed.), *The standard edition of the complete psychological works of Sigmund Freud, Vol. 18* (pp. 3-66). London: Hogarth and the Institute of Psychoanalysis. (Original work published 1920.)

Gaines, E. C. (2002). The relationship between sensory processing and play in children with autistic spectrum disorders. *Dissertation Abstracts International, 63*(4-B), 2055.

Gaylord-Ross, R. J., Haring, T. G., Breen, C., & Pitts-Conway, V. (1984). The training and generalization of social interaction skills with autistic youth. *Journal of Applied Behavior Analysis, 17*, 229-247.

Geist, R., & Kielhofner, G. (1998). *The Pediatric Volitional Questionnaire*. Chicago: Model of Human Occupational Clearinghouse, Department of Occupational Therapy, University of Illinois.

Gibson, E. J. (1988). Exploratory behavior in the development of perceiving, acting, and the acquiring of knowledge. *Annual Review in Psychology, 39*, 1-41.

Goldstein, J. (1995). Aggressive toy play. In A. D. Pellegrini (Ed.), *The future of play theory: A multidisciplinary inquiry into the contributions of Brian Sutton-Smith* (pp. 127-147). Albany, NY: State University of New York Press.

Goode, D. A., & Gaddy, M. R. (1976). Ascertaining choice with alingual, deaf-blind, and retarded clients. *Mental Retardation, 14*(6), 10-12.

Gopnik, A., & Meltzoff, A. (1993). Words and thoughts in infancy: The specificity hypothesis and the development of categorization and naming. *Advances in Infancy Research, 8*, 217-249.

Grandin, T. (1996). Brief report: Response to National Institutes of Health Report. *Journal of Autism and Developmental Disorders, 26*(2), 185-187.

Gray, C. (1994/2000). *The new social story book*. Arlington, TX: Future Horizons.

Greenspan, S. I. (2001). The affect diathesis hypothesis: The role of emotions in the core deficit in autism and in the development of intelligence and social skills. *Journal of Developmental and Learning Disorders, 5*(1), 1-45.

Hahn, H. (1989). The politics of special education. In D. K. Lipsky & A. Gartner (Eds.), *Beyond separate education: Quality education for all* (pp. 225-241). Baltimore: Paul H. Brookes.

Happe, F. G. (1996). Studying weak central coherence at low levels: Children with autism do not succumb to visual illusions; A research note. *Journal of Child Psychology and Psychiatry, 37*(7), 873-876.

Haring, T. G., & Lovinger, L. (1989). Promoting social interaction through teaching generalized play initiation responses to preschool children with autism. *Journal of the Association for Persons with Severe Handicaps, 14*(1), 58-67.

Hayes, S. C., Rincover, A., & Volosin, D. (1980). Variables influencing the acquisition and maintenance of aggressive behavior: Modeling versus sensory reinforcement. *Journal of Abnormal Psychology, 89*(2), 254-262.

Hellendoorn, J., van der Kooij, R., & Sutton-Smith, B. (Eds.). (1994). *Play and intervention*. Albany, NY: State University of New York Press.

Henricks, T. S. (1997). *Play as ascending meaning: Implications of a general model of play.* Paper presented at the annual meeting of The Association for the Study of Play.

Hinojosa, J., & Kramer, P. (1997). Integrating children with disabilities into family play. In L. D. Parham & L. S. Fazio (Eds.), *Play in occupational therapy for children* (pp. 159-170). St. Louis: Mosby.

Hobson, R. P., & Lee, A. (1999). Imitation and identification in autism. *Journal of Child Psychology and Psychiatry, 40*(4), 649-659.

Holloway, E. (1997). Fostering parent-infant playfulness in the neonatal intensive care unit. In L. D. Parham & L. S. Fazio (Eds.), *Play in occupational therapy for children* (pp. 171-183). St. Louis: Mosby.

Huebner, R. A., & Kraemer, G. W. (2001). Sensorimotor aspects of attachment and social relatedness in autism. In R. A. Huebner (Ed.), *Autism: A sensorimotor approach to management* (pp. 209-244). Gaithersburg, MD: Aspen Publishers.

Jarrold, C. (2003). A review of research into pretend play in autism. *Autism, 7*(4), 379-390.

Jarrold, C., Boucher, J., & Smith, P. (1993). Symbolic play in autism: A review. *Journal of Autism and Developmental Disorders, 23,* 281-309.

Jarrold, C., Smith, P., Boucher, J., & Harris, P. (1994). Children with autism's comprehension of pretence. *Journal of Autism and Developmental Disorders, 24,* 433-456.

Jordan, R. (2003). Social play and autistic spectrum disorders: A perspective on theory, implications and educational approaches. *Autism, 7*(4), 347-360.

Kanner, L. (1943). Autistic disturbances of affective contact. *Nervous Child, 2,* 217-250.

Kasari, C., Sigman, M., Mundy, P., & Yirmiya, N. (1990). Affective sharing in the context of joint attention interactions of normal, autistic, and mentally retarded children. *Journal of Autism and Developmental Disorders, 20*(1), 87-100.

Kavanaugh, R. D., & Harris, P. L. (1994). Imagining the outcome of pretend transformations: Assessing the competence of normal children and children with autism. *Developmental Psychology, 30,* 847-854.

Kelly-Byrne, D. (1989). *A child's play life: An ethnographic study.* New York: Teachers College.

Knox, S. H. (1997). *Play and play styles of preschool children* (Unpublished doctoral dissertation, University of Southern California, Los Angeles).

Koegel, R. L., Dyer, K., & Bell, L. K. (1987). The influence of child-preferred activities on autistic children's social behavior. *Journal of Applied Behavior Analysis, 20*(3), 243-252.

Koegel, R. L., Firestone, P. B., Kramme, K. W., & Dunlap, G. (1974). Increasing spontaneous play by suppressing self-stimulation in autistic children. *Journal of Applied Behavior Analysis, 7,* 521-528.

Kuoch, H., & Mirenda, P. (2003). Social story interventions for young children with autism spectrum disorders. *Focus on Autism and Other Developmental Disabilities, 18*(4), 219-227.

Largo, R. H., & Howard, J. A. (1979). Developmental progression in play behavior of children between nine and thirty months. I. Spontaneous play and imitation. *Developmental Medicine and Child Neurology, 21,* 299-310.

Lewis, V., & Boucher, J. (1995). Generativity in the play of young people with autism. *Journal of Autism and Developmental Disorders, 25*(2), 105-121.

Libby, S., Powell, S., Messer, D., & Jordan, R. (1997). Imitation of pretend play acts by children with autism and Down syndrome. *Journal of Autism and Developmental Disorders, 27*(4), 365-383.

McHale, S. M. (1983). Social interactions of autistic and nonhandicapped children during free play. *American Journal of Orthopsychiatry, 53,* 81-91.

Mesibov, G. B. (1984). Social skills training with verbal autistic adolescents and adults: A program model. *Journal of Autism and Developmental Disorders, 14*(4), 395-403.

Miller, H. (1996, June). Eye contact and gaze aversion: Implications for persons with autism. *Sensory Integration Special Interest Section Newsletter, 19*(2), 1-3.

Mook, B. (1994). Therapeutic play: From interpretation to intervention. In J. Hellendoorn, R. van der Kooij, & B. Sutton-Smith (Eds.), *Play and intervention* (pp. 39-52). Albany, NY: State University of New York Press.

Mundy, P., & Crowson, M. (1997). Joint attention and early social communication: Implications for research on intervention with autism. *Journal of Autism and Developmental Disorders, 27*(6), 653-676.

Mundy, P., Sigman, M., & Kasari, C. (1990). A longitudinal study of joint attention and language development in autistic children. *Journal of Autism and Developmental Disabilities, 20*(1), 115-128.

National Institute of Mental Health (1995). *Basic behavioral science research for mental health: A national investment* (NIH Publication No. 95-3682). Washington, DC: U.S. Government Printing Office.

O'Connor, R. D. (1969). Modification of social withdrawal through symbolic modeling. *Journal of Applied Behavior Analysis, 2,* 15-22.

Odom, S. L., & Strain, P. S. (1984). Peer-mediated approaches to promoting children's social interaction: A review. *American Journal of Orthopsychiatry, 54,* 544-557.

Ornitz, E. M. (1974). The modulation of sensory input and motor output in autistic children. *Journal of Autism and Childhood Schizophrenia, 4*(3), 197-215.

Owens, R. E., Jr. (2001). *Language development: An introduction* (5th ed.). Boston: Allyn & Bacon.

Parham, L. D. (1996). Perspectives on play. In R. Zemke & F. Clark (Eds.), *Occupational science: The evolving discipline* (pp. 71-80). Philadelphia: F.A. Davis.

Parham, L. D., & Primeau, L. (1997). Play and occupational therapy. In L. D. Parham & L. S. Fazio (Eds.), *Play in occupational therapy for children* (pp. 2-21). St. Louis: Mosby.

Parten, M. B. (1932). Social participation among preschool children. *Journal of Abnormal Psychology, 27,* 243-269.

Pedersen, J., Livoir-Petersen, M. F., & Scheide, J. T. M. (1989). An ethological approach to autism: An analysis of visual behavior and interpersonal contact in a child versus adult interaction. *Acta Psychiatrica Scandinavica, 80,* 346-355.

Pellegrini, A. D. (1995). Boys' rough-and-rumble play and social competence: Contemporaneous and longitudinal relations. In A. D. Pellegrini (Ed.), *The future of play theory: A multidisciplinary inquiry into the contributions of Brian Sutton-Smith* (pp. 107-126). Albany, NY: State University of New York Press.

Pennington, B. F. (1991). *Diagnosing learning disorders: A neuropsychological framework*. New York: Guilford Press.

Petroski, H. (1999, May-June). Work and play. *American Scientist, 87*(3), 208-212.

Piaget, J. (1962). *Play, dreams, and imitation in childhood*. (C. Gattegno & F. M. Hodgson Trans.) New York: W.W. Norton. (Original work published in 1951.)

Piantanida, D. B. (2004, March 13). Facilitating social skills. Paper presented at the Trends in Autism Conference, Claremont, CA.

Pierce, K., & Schreibman, L. (1995). Increasing complex social behaviors in children with autism: Effects of peer-implemented pivotal response training. *Journal of Applied Behavioral Analysis, 28*(3), 285-295.

Power, T. G. (2000). *Play and exploration in children and animals*. Mahwah, NJ: Lawrence Erlbaum.

Ragland, E. U., Kerr, M. M., & Strain, P. S. (1978). Behavior of withdrawn autistic children: Effects of peer social initiations. *Behavior Modification, 2*(4), 565-578.

Rapin, I. (1991). Autistic children: Diagnosis and clinical features. *Pediatrics, 87*(Supplement), 751-760.

Reilly, M. (1974). *Play as exploratory learning: Studies of curiosity behavior*. Beverly Hills, CA: Sage Publications.

Restall, G., & Magill-Evans, J. (1994). Play and preschool children with autism. *American Journal of Occupational Therapy, 48*(2), 113-120.

Riguet, C. B., Taylor, N. D., Benaroya, S., & Klein, L. S. (1981). Symbolic play in autistic, Down's, and normal children of equivalent mental age. *Journal of Autism and Developmental Disorders, 11*, 439-448.

Ritvo, E. R., & Freeman, B. J. (1978). National Society for Autistic Children definition of the syndrome of autism. *Journal of Autism and Childhood Schizophrenia, 8*, 162-167.

Robinson, A. L. (1977). Play: The arena for acquisition of rules for competent behavior. *American Journal of Occupational Therapy, 31*, 248-253.

Rogers, C. S., Impara, J. C., Frary, R. B., Harris, T., Meeks, A., Semanic-Lauth, S., et al. (1998). Measuring playfulness: Development of the Child Behaviors Inventory of Playfulness. In S. Reifel (Series Ed.) & M. C. Duncan, G. Chick, & A. Aycock (Vol. Eds.), *Play and culture studies. Vol. 1. Diversions and divergences in fields of play* (pp. 121-135). Greenwich, CT: Ablex Publishing.

Rogers, S. J. (2000). Interventions that facilitate socialization in children with autism. *Journal of Autism and Developmental Disorders, 30*(5), 399-409.

Rogers, S. J., Hepburn, S. L., Stackhouse, T., & Wehner, E. (2003). Imitation performance in toddlers with autism and those with other developmental disorders. *Journal of Child Psychology and Psychiatry, 44*(5), 763-781.

Rogers, S. J., & Pennington, B. F. (1991). A theoretical approach to deficits in infantile autism. *Development and Psychopathology, 3*, 137-162.

Romanczyk, R. G., Diament, C., Goren, E. R., Trunell, G., & Harris, S. L. (1975). Increasing isolate and social play in severely disturbed children: Intervention and postintervention effectiveness. *Journal of Autism and Childhood Schizophrenia, 5*(1), 57-70.

Rubin, K. H., Fein, G. G., & Vandenberg, B. (1983). Play. In P. H. Mussen (Series Ed.) & E. M. Hetherington (Vol. Ed.), *Handbook of child psychology. Vol. 4. Socialization, personality, and social development* (4th ed., pp. 693-774). New York: John Wiley & Sons.

Rutherford, M. D., & Rogers, S. J. (2003). Cognitive underpinnings of pretend play in autism. *Journal of Autism and Developmental Disorders, 33*(3), 289-302.

Rutter, M. (1978). Diagnosis and definition of childhood autism. *Journal of Autism and Childhood Schizophrenia, 8*, 139-161.

Schafer, G. E. (1994). Games of complexity: Reflections on play structure and play intervention. In J. Hellendoorn, R. van der Kooij, & B. Sutton-Smith (Eds.), *Play and intervention* (pp. 77-84). Albany, NY: State University of New York Press.

Schreibman, L., & Charlop, M. H. (1989). Infantile autism. In T. H. Ollendick & M. Hersen (Eds.), *Handbook of child psychopathology* (pp. 105-129). New York: Plenum.

Schuler, A. L. (2003). Beyond echoplaylia: Promoting language in children with autism. *Autism, 7*(4), 455-469.

Shafer, M. S., Egel, A. L., & Neef, N. A. (1984). Training mildly handicapped peers to facilitate changes in the social interaction skills of autistic children. *Journal of Applied Behavior Analysis, 17*, 461-476.

Sigman, M., & Ruskin, E. (1999). Continuity and change in the social competence of children with autism, Down syndrome, and developmental delays. *Monographs of the Society for Research in Child Development, 64*, 1-114.

Sigman, M., & Ungerer, J. A. (1984). Attachment behaviors in autistic children. *Journal of Autism and Developmental Disorders, 14*(3), 231-244.

Singer, D. G., & Singer, J. L. (1990). *The house of make-believe: Children's play and the developing imagination*. Cambridge, MA: Harvard University Press.

Spitzer, S. L. (2001). *No words necessary: An ethnography of daily activities with children who don't talk* (Unpublished doctoral dissertation, University of Southern California, Los Angeles).

Spitzer, S. L. (2003). With and without words: Exploring occupation in relation to young children with autism. *Journal of Occupational Science, 10*(2), 67-79.

Spitzer, S. L. (2004). Common and uncommon daily activities in individuals with autism: Challenges and opportunities for supporting occupation. In H. Miller-Kuhaneck (Ed.), *Autism: A comprehensive occupational therapy approach* (2nd ed., pp. 83-106). Bethesda, MD: American Occupational Therapy Association.

Stahmer, A. C. (1995). Teaching symbolic play skills to children with autism using pivotal response training. *Journal of Autism and Developmental Disorders, 25*(2), 123-141.

Stahmer, A. C., Ingersoll, B., & Carter, C. (2003). Behavioral approaches to promoting play. *Autism, 7*(4), 401-413.

Stone, W. L., Ousley, O. Y., & Littleford, C. D. (1997). Motor imitation in young children with autism: What's the object? *Journal of Abnormal Child Psychology, 25*(6), 475-485.

Stone, W. L., Ousley, O. Y., Yoder, P. J., Hogan, K. L., & Hepburn, S. L. (1997). Nonverbal communication in two-and three-year-old children with autism. *Journal of Autism and Developmental Disorders, 27*(6), 677-696.

Strain, P. S. (1980). Social behavior programming with severely handicapped and autistic children. In B. Wilcox & A. Thompson (Eds.), *Critical issues in educating autistic children and youth* (pp. 179-205). Washington, DC: U.S. Department of Education.

Strain, P. S. (1983). Generalization of autistic children's social behavior change: Effects of developmentally integrated and segregated settings. *Analysis and Intervention in Developmental Disabilities, 3*, 23-34.

Sutton-Smith, B. (1971). The playful modes of knowing. In G. Engstrom (Ed.), *Play: The child strives towards self-realization* (pp. 13-25). Washington, DC: National Association for the Education of Young Children.

Sutton-Smith, B. (1994). Paradigms of intervention. In J. Hellendoorn, R. van der Kooij, & B. Sutton-Smith (Eds.), *Play and intervention* (pp. 3-21). Albany, NY: State University of New York Press.

Sutton-Smith, B. (1997). *The ambiguity of play.* Cambridge, MA: Harvard University Press.

Takata, N. (1974). Play as a prescription. In M. Reilly (Ed.), *Play as exploratory learning* (pp. 209-246). Beverly Hills, CA: Sage Publications.

Tanta, K. J. (2004). Promoting peer interaction in children with an autism spectrum disorder. In H. Miller-Kuhaneck (Ed.), *Autism: A comprehensive occupational therapy approach* (2nd ed., pp. 155-170). Bethesda, MD: American Occupational Therapy Association.

Tardif, C., Plumet, M., Beaudichon, J., Waller, D., Bouvard, M., & Leboyer, M. (1995). Micro-analysis of social interactions between autistic children and normal adults in semi-structured play situations. *International Journal of Behavioral Development, 18*(4), 727-747.

Tiegerman, E., & Primavera, L. (1981). Object manipulation: An interactional strategy with autistic children. *Journal of Autism and Developmental Disorders, 11*(4), 427-438.

Trecker, A., & Miller-Kuhaneck, H. (2004). Play and praxis in children with an autism spectrum disorder. In H. Miller-Kuhaneck (Ed.), *Autism: A comprehensive occupational therapy approach* (2nd ed., pp. 193-213). Bethesda, MD: American Occupational Therapy Association.

Tryon, A. S., & Keane, S. P. (1986). Promoting imitative play through generalized observational learning in autisticlike children. *Journal of Abnormal Child Psychology, 14*(4), 537-549.

Ungerer, J. A., & Sigman, M. (1981). Symbolic play and language comprehension in autistic children. *Journal of the American Academy of Child Psychiatry, 20*, 318-337.

Van Berckelaer-Onnes, I. A. (2003). Promoting early play. *Autism, 7*(4), 415-423.

Vygotsky, L. S. (1978). *Mind in society: The development of higher psychological processes* (translated from 1932). Cambridge, MA: Harvard University Press.

Weider, S., & Greenspan, S. I. (2003). Climbing the symbolic ladder in the DIR model through floor time/interactive play. *Autism, 7*(4), 425-435.

Williams, E. (2003). A comparative review of early forms of object-directed play and parent-infant play in typical infants and young children with autism. *Autism, 7*(4), 361-377.

Williams, E., Costall, A., & Reddy, V. (1999). Children with autism experience problems with both objects and people. *Journal of Autism and Developmental Disorders, 29*(5), 367-378.

Williams, E., Reddy, V., & Costall, A. (2001). Taking a closer look at functional play in children with autism. *Journal of Autism and Developmental Disorders, 31*(1), 67-77.

Wing, L. (1995). Play is not the work of the child: Young children's perceptions of work and play. *Early Childhood Research Quarterly, 10*, 223-247.

Wolfberg, P. J. (1999). *Play and imagination in children with autism.* New York: Teachers College Press.

Wolfberg, P. J., & Schuler, A. L. (1993). Integrated play groups: A model for promoting the social and cognitive dimensions of play in children with autism. *Journal of Autism and Developmental Disorders, 23*(3), 467-489.

Wulff, S. B. (1985). The symbolic and object play of children with autism: A review. *Journal of Autism and Developmental Disorders, 15*, 139-148.

Yang, T., Wolfberg, P. J., Wu, S., & Hwu, P. (2003). Supporting children on the autism spectrum in peer play at home and school: Piloting the integrated play groups model in Taiwan. *Autism, 7*(4), 437-453.

Yerxa, E. J., Clark, F., Frank, G., Jackson, J., Parham, D., Pierce, D., et al. (1990). An introduction to occupational science, a foundation for occupational therapy in the 21st century. In J. A. Johnson & E. J. Yerxa (Eds.), *Occupational science: The foundation for new models of practice* (pp. 1-17). New York: Haworth Press.

Ziviani, J., Boyle, M., & Rodger, S. (2001). An introduction to play and the preschool child with autistic spectrum disorder. *British Journal of Occupational Therapy, 64*(1), 17-22.

15

Play in Children with Cerebral Palsy: Doing With—Not Doing To

Erna Imperatore Blanche

KEY TERMS

cerebral palsy
play in treatment
play as motivator
play as context
facilitating play

Several years ago a therapist treated a 3-year-old girl, Sandra, in whom hypotonic cerebral palsy had been diagnosed. Sandra was barely able to maintain her head against gravity, was unable to coordinate reach and grasp, and did not communicate her needs other than by blinking her eyes and making sounds. She liked to participate in baking cookies, was fond of Barbie dolls, and enjoyed the interaction with other children, but she did not enjoy puzzles or any motor activity she was asked to perform during the course of treatment. Sandra demonstrated her dislike by closing her eyes or pretending to be unable to hold her head up.

Treating Sandra was a challenge. Her nontestable cognitive abilities appeared to be significantly higher than her motor skills, so she was somewhat able to control her environment by opening and closing her eyes to express interest. When motivated, she participated in the treatment session by being alert. When the activity was not appealing to her, she closed her eyes or leaned her head against the table. It took the therapist a long time to figure out that physical fatigue was not the main reason for lack of participation. At that point the therapist decided that having a successful session would require careful observation of the activities during which Sandra appeared alert and attending.

During one of the treatment sessions the therapist noticed that Sandra appeared interested in a girl her own age, the sibling of another child who was receiving treatment at the same time. In her hope to actively involve Sandra, the therapist included this little girl in the treatment session. The sibling carried her Barbie dolls into the treatment room, and the therapist, following Sandra's sudden interest, decided to incorporate the dolls and the other little girl into a tea party. The session went well. The children later played simple board games, made a picture, and played with cars. The therapist attended to Sandra's tendency to withdraw from an activity as an indicator of her intrinsic motivation. She also looked for other activities that could be enjoyable, not necessarily activities chosen to address the child's multiple limitations.

When the therapist left that facility, Sandra's mother thanked her, adding that during her treatment sessions she "did with" rather than "did to" Sandra, and that that difference made the experience meaningful for the child. The therapist thought about the mother's words and wondered whether, in reality, she "did with" all the children she treated or whether the desperation of not being able to have Sandra participate in the treatment prompted her to move in that direction. She decided that entering into play with children regardless of their diagnosis was the key and that "doing with" was what she needed to do with all her clients.

Although this story is years old, it captures the pivotal role of intrinsic motivation and enjoyment during the intervention and in the life of individuals with physical disabilities. Current trends in rehabilitation emphasize the importance of satisfaction, well-being, and participation in society as important goals of the intervention process; therefore the role of intrinsic motivation, enjoyment, and active play has become salient. Occupational therapy's focus on intrinsic motivation and play is important not only in the context of the child's present situation, but also as a vehicle to help develop leisure skills that last throughout life. The recent literature on leisure emphasizes play and leisure as a resource in transcending negative life experiences and contributing to the ability to manage stress, increase self-concept and self-esteem, enhance social relationships, and transform (Blanche, 1999; Iwasaki, 2001, 2003; Kleiber, Hutchinson, & Williams, 2002; Specht, King, Brown, & Foris, 2002; Trenberth & Dewe, 2002). Because children with cerebral palsy may have decreased self-esteem and increased social isolation (Magill-Evans & Restall, 1991; Manuel, Balkrishnan, Camacho, Smith, & Koman, 2003), developing play and leisure skills early in life may have a later effect on their social and emotional well-being.

Prevailing views of cerebral palsy (CP) portray the deficit as a sensorimotor disorder that affects the child's interactions with the environment, including full participation in society. However, CP, as well as other physical disabilities, also affects the child's social-emotional development and the family's well-being. Although these issues are related to the physical limitations accompanying CP, they have an important effect later in life on functional activity and engagement in the community. Success in life for individuals with CP is related to psychosocial factors that include others' belief in them, their belief in their own capabilities, and a sense of belonging when others accept them (King, Cathers, Polgar, MacKinnon, & Havens, 2000).

The nature of CP restricts play and overall development in two ways. Reduced interactions affect the use of play as a context for learning and for practicing adaptive behaviors, and limited ability to enter into play restricts the experience of play as a spontaneous, intrinsically motivated, joyous activity that may lead to an increased sense of satisfaction and well-being.

This chapter emphasizes the need to incorporate play into the intervention process and into the lives of children with CP so they can develop a sense of mastery that leads to increased satisfaction and well-being. It stresses the importance of play as a context for learning, an intrinsically rewarding experience, and a source for social-emotional benefits. The first part of the chapter addresses the limitations of CP and its impact on play, and the second part discusses ways to incorporate play into the treatment session and the life of the child. Examples from treatment sessions are used to illustrate each concept. Because play is a spontaneous, intrinsically motivated activity, most successful events described in this chapter were not planned but rather occurred "accidentally" during a treatment session. The successful resolution of the event, however, depended on the therapist's ability first to recognize the potential of that activity, then to follow the child's lead, and last to trust his or her skills to handle the process while suspending the consequences of not following the original plan for the time being. In other words, it required the therapist to enter into play "with" the child.

CHARACTERISTICS OF PLAY

Play is described in different ways. The most frequently cited views of play describe it as an activity that is intrinsically motivated and flexible (Bruner, 1972),

enjoyable (Piaget, 1962), arousing (Ellis, 1973), active, and spontaneous, and during which reality might be temporarily suspended (Singer & Singer, 1977). During the performance of daily occupations, elements of play are intertwined with functional tasks. For an activity to be considered play, it must have some of the characteristics just mentioned. The literature on play often attempts to make a distinction between play and work or play and drudgery. Drudgery, defined as "the enforced engagement in distasteful physical or mental effort to obtain the means of survival" (Pugmire-Stoy, 1992, p. 4), is considered the opposite of play. An activity is experienced as approaching play if it contains a greater share of play characteristics and less of drudgery.

For the child with CP, play and therapy are sometimes mutually exclusive activities. Rast (1986) stated, "In the therapeutic setting, play often becomes a tool used to work toward a goal, despite the fact that the goal-oriented, externally controlled aspects of the therapy situation conflict with the essence of play itself" (p. 30). Pugmire-Stoy (1992) reinforced this point by writing that some of the "so-called 'play'" (p. 4) presented to handicapped children is closer to drudgery. Therefore including the essence of play into the session can be a challenge. As clinicians, therapists tend to use play as a motivator or a context for learning adaptive skills; however, they need to recognize the value of play as a context for fun as much as a context for learning. Only by understanding this context for fun will they be able to promote the child's intrinsic motivation, spontaneity, and feeling of being able to actively direct her or his own actions and have mastery over the environment. Thus a whole new dimension and potential can be added to the therapeutic process and the life of the child with CP.

Play can be summarized as having three roles in the therapy for a child with physical or cognitive impairment. The first role of play is as an important childhood occupation that provides context for learning and adaptation (Bruner, 1972; Bundy, 1992; Munoz, 1986; Reilly, 1974; Robinson, 1977). The literature that uses this view of play often emphasizes the value of assessing developmental levels of play because this provides a window into the child's level of skill development (Casby, 1992; D'Eugenio, 1986; Fewell & Glick, 1993). This role of play is viewed as important because play serves a function of preparation for adult performance.

The second role of play described in the occupational therapy literature is as a reward or motivator for the child to interact with the environment and thus reach treatment objectives. This view of play often describes the use of appropriate toys, activities, and games to encourage active participation, as when a neurodevelopmental treatment (NDT) approach is employed in the treatment of CP (Boehme, 1987; Rast, 1986). Both the first and second views of play regard it as a means to an end or as an experience that serves a purpose: in the first view play is seen as preparing the child for adult work performance, and in the second view play has the immediate purpose of motivating the child to interact within the treatment session. Positioning during play (Diamant, 1992; Finnie, 1975) and adapting toys for the child (Batty, 1989; Langley, 1990) can be considered part of these traditions. In general, these traditional approaches to play in the child with CP fail to explore fully the inherent worth of play and instead reinforce its role in the acquisition of functional skills.

More recent literature challenges the initial emphasis placed on play as a vehicle for learning skills for future performance (Caldwell, 1986) and explores a third role of play by emphasizing the basic characteristics that define the quality of the play experience as an end in itself (Blanche, 2002; Bundy, 1993). Although researchers view play as an occupation that is not exclusively at the service of learning skills or motivating clients, practitioners do not appear to see its value beyond these goals. Couch (1998) explored the role of play in the practice of 224 pediatric occupational therapists and concluded that although they included play as motivator and reinforcer, the focus was not necessarily on developing play skills or engaging in play. In other words, play is still a vehicle for attaining functional skills.

Bundy (1993) described a play-nonplay continuum based on the individual's perception of control, source of motivation, and suspension of reality and urged therapists using a sensory integration approach to evaluate each activity in reference to this continuum. Similarly, activities should be assessed for their potential for play when other approaches (such as NDT) are used in the treatment of a child with CP. An awareness of the basic characteristics of play ensures a better use of play as a context for the acquisition of treatment goals. Fostering these play characteristics in the child with CP is a challenge, however, and thus is seldom observed in treatment.

In an attempt to increase awareness of the importance of play in occupational therapy, Blanche (2002) summarized play as a process-oriented occupation that includes certain characteristics: Play is spontaneous, exciting, energy producing or expending, physically and mentally active, relaxing or somewhat stressful, pleasurable, and considered nonessential. It may include creativity, imagination, and a sense of freedom; may not have a clear purpose; and is performed for oneself. The most important characteristic is the pleasure derived from the process of engaging in the activity rather than the pleasure derived from the product of the activity (Blanche, 1999, 2002). An activity is not considered "play" or "not play" but is analyzed as a process-oriented activity that has more or fewer of the characteristics of play. Therefore, during the intervention an activity that is joyful, spontaneous, exciting, and active has many of the characteristics of play even if it is not imaginative, creative, or relaxing. Analysis

of play in this form allows the therapist to include elements of play even when the therapeutic occupation would not traditionally be considered play. In using this approach to play, a therapist does not have to design an activity as "play or no play" but does have to design it to allow characteristics of play to be present and thus contribute to development of the child's play skills.

Play takes many forms, and the characteristics of play present themselves differently among individuals. Some of the process-oriented experiences associated with play are restoration, ludos (nonserious behaviors such as teasing and joking), increased self-awareness, mastery, adventure, and creativity.

This chapter proposes that the purpose of incorporating play into treatment lies not only in its role in fostering the acquisition of functional skills, but also in its role as an enriching experience in its own right. The role of play in the individual's development of a sense of mastery over the environment has been identified in children without disabilities, as well as in children with CP (Bruner, 1972; Rast, 1986); this increased perception of the self as capable of mastering the environment stems from the pleasure, flexibility, spontaneity, and intrinsic motivation to participate in the decision-making process that are promoted by play. Recent literature emphasizes the importance of a sense of well-being, satisfaction, and increased active participation in society. The inclusion of play with all or some of its characteristics is pivotal in the attainment of these goals. This view of play incorporates play in the treatment session in the context of fun, as well as a context of learning, and includes all treatment activities.

Fostering play in the child with CP involves many factors. First, it requires an understanding of the child's limitations in movement, sensation-perception, and cognition. Second, it demands awareness of the limitations imposed on the child by the physical environment and the adult's predisposition to play. Third, it calls for understanding of the fundamental characteristics of the play experience and the use of activities that may lead to it. The impact of these areas on play is described in the following section. Therapists need to be aware that, regardless of the nature and extent of the limitations of children with CP, they often spontaneously rise above these to seek ways to engage in play.

LIMITATIONS IN CHILDREN WITH CEREBRAL PALSY

The multiple disabilities that accompany CP interfere differentially with the child's participation in everyday tasks such as self-care, schoolwork, and play. Play as a context for learning and as a joyful activity is limited in children with CP. As a context for learning, play is constrained primarily by the child's physical challenges. As an enjoyable, spontaneous, intrinsically motivated activity, play is limited not only by the disability, but also by the restraints imposed by those surrounding the child. These limitations imposed by people and the environment are often more restrictive than the child's physical handicaps. Although the child is frequently able to engage in spontaneous playful interaction that does not require use of the less developed skills, the people in the child's environment often unconsciously interfere with the expressions of these behaviors. Both the inherent and the environmental limitations are described fully in the following subsections.

Limitations in Movement

The movement limitations in children with CP have been extensively described (Bly, 1983; Bobath & Bobath, 1975). The severity of these movement deficits has an impact on play in two ways. First, it affects the child's ability to actively access and explore the environment; second, once the child finds something that interests him or her, the movement deficits limit the potential to enter spontaneously into active play. These two factors impair the child's sense of mastery over the world. Children with severe movement disabilities have great difficulty engaging in activities for their sensorimotor pleasure. Since this is the first expression of play observed in the child (Piaget, 1962), reduced exposure to this form of play may, in turn, further restrict the child's development of motor coordination, as well as perceptual and cognitive development. Because play is an arena that leads to mastery (Bruner, 1972; White, 1959), the inability to enter fully into play early in life may affect the child's perception of having control over the environment and hence the development of intrinsic motivation. Simply stated, these children are used to "being done to" rather than "doing with" and may tend to perceive themselves as spectators rather than actors.

Older children who have movement deficits but no severe limitations in cognitive development are often able to enter into other forms of play through social interactions, fantasy play, and humor. They may use their communication skills to initiate contact with others and feel that they have an impact on the environment. The play of children with less severe movement disorders is often affected more by perceptual and cognitive deficits than by the movement deficit per se. Although they may be able to ambulate and hence increase their accessibility to play materials, perceptual and cognitive limitations may confine their engagement in play. It is important when evaluating the play of these children to identify each limitation's impact on the experience of play.

Sensory Processing Limitations

Sensory and motor deficits presented by children with CP have been often viewed as interrelated (Fetters, 1991; Moore, 1984). Sensory and perceptual deficits may occur secondarily to the movement limitations or may result from primary neurological damage (Moore, 1984). Sensory processing deficits in a child with CP affect play in different ways: first, they have an impact on the child's preference for certain play materials and activities; second, they affect modulation and hence sustained attention; and third, the child fails to benefit from intense sensory experiences either because of being hyporesponsive to the input or because intensity is not provided. For instance, hyporesponsiveness and deficits in tactile discrimination and modulation affect children's ability to obtain information about an object and thus influence their toy preference (Curry & Exner, 1988; Danella, 1973). This preference may mask motor as much as sensory-perceptual restrictions. Research studies and clinical observations have shown that multiply handicapped children exhibit a strong preference for vibratory toys (Danella, 1973) and for hard rather than soft toys (Curry & Exner, 1988). This preference for toys that provide distinct somatosensory inputs may indicate a sensory modulation problem that should be addressed during treatment.

Children who are able to move in space but exhibit vestibular modulation deficits may avoid moving equipment because of a hypersensitivity to movement or a gravitational insecurity. These sensory modulation deficits, added to the postural limitations, affect the child's active participation in treatment and on the playground.

Deficient visual perception may also affect a child's choice of play activity. Children with CP may not choose to play with toys that require refined perception of visual figure ground, spatial relations, or visual discrimination, such as puzzles, nesting toys, and construction materials. Although the therapist may need to address visual perception areas, they are not good choices for recreation or fostering of autonomous play, at least not initially.

Sensory modulation deficits affect the child's ability to maintain an optimal level of arousal so that attention and learning of new concepts can occur. Children with modulation deficits have difficulty engaging in play either because their arousal level is too low, which interferes with active movement and motivation to participate, or because it is extremely high, which interferes with a child's ability to maintain attention on the play activity.

A child who is hyporesponsive to input may receive decreased input even when he or she is exposed to an enriched environment. As a result the child's self-awareness is reduced.

Limitations in Cognitive Abilities

Cognitive impairments are often described as accompanying CP and may be more handicapping than the restrictions in movement. In children with severe spastic quadriplegia, intellectual level has been found to have a greater impact on the acquisition of early cognitive milestones than does severity of physical limitations (Eagle, 1985). Consequently, in a child with severe deficits in both movement and severe cognition, the cognitive limitations affect the development of play to a greater degree than do motor abilities.

Cognitive limitations may affect the ability to enter into make-believe and fantasy play. During fantasy play the child replays the past and anticipates the future. Therefore fantasy play has an impact on development of the capacity to anticipate practical consequences of actions (Singer & Singer, 1977). Children with CP may spontaneously enter into fantasy play, whereas therapists and parents tend to focus on play with objects and may neglect to consider the value of make-believe or pretend play. Fantasy play is an area that should be valued by the adult working with children.

Limitations in Environmental Interactions

In addition to the limitations that are inherent in a diagnosis of CP, the outside environment imposes physical and social restrictions that may be at least as confining as the disorder itself. The physical limitations reduce the child's access to several factors of play: materials, such as appropriate toys; environments, such as recreational facilities; and extracurricular activities that promote play, such as sports, drama, and art. Social barriers may occur when the imposition of others' values and beliefs limits social interactions. Physical limitations to recreational and leisure facilities in the environment are widely recognized. The following section focuses on the limitations that occur in social interactions.

Limitations in Social Interactions

Social constraints on play are evidenced in the child's interactions with adults and peers. The influence of teachers, caregivers, and other adults in the development of play and other activities has been well documented (Caldwell, 1986; Hanzlik, 1989, 1990; Kogan, Tyler, & Turner, 1974; Missiuna & Pollock, 1991; Shevin, 1987). Several external factors contribute to different patterns of activity and diminished play in children with CP.

First, because of the nature of the physical limitations, the child with CP needs more adult intervention to perform simple activities and spends more time interacting with adults than do nondisabled children. Caregivers often tend to overprotect the child, and this adult interaction typically contains little play (Missiuna & Pollock, 1991). Furthermore, the child's free time is reduced because of the need for therapy (Missiuna and Pollock, 1991). These children usually participate in "tightly defined sequencing of objectives" and "tightly defined instructional approaches" (Shevin, 1987, p. 237) that do not allow much flexibility or spontaneity. This happens in the classroom and in other settings.

In addition to the aforementioned factors, children with CP are exposed to attitudes toward play in which play is infrequent and not connected to the development of autonomy and self-direction (Shevin, 1987). Children with CP often demonstrate the intrinsic motivation and potential to enter into play, but they experience physical and environmentally imposed obstacles that result in different daily activity patterns from those of children without disabilities. When activity patterns of children with CP and spina bifida were compared with those of nondisabled children, children with CP and spina bifida were found to spend more time in quiet recreation, dependent activities, and activities of personal care and less time in active recreation, activities away from home, and household tasks. Their activities were less varied and were often accompanied by social interaction (Brown & Gordon, 1987).

In summary, physically challenged children spend larger amounts of time in structured activities that may constrict the sense of freedom necessary to explore the environment and engage in play. They have less opportunity to make decisions about what to do, where to go, whom to be with, and how to do something. As a result, they comonly have a decreased belief that they may be able to act on the environment.

The impact of adult intervention on the experience of play in a child with CP starts early in life. Mother-infant verbal and nonverbal interaction may be the primary component of play. In this interaction with the caregiver, children learn to respond with cognitive, motor, and social adaptations (Hanzlik, 1990). In turn, the caregiver adjusts to and reinforces the child's responses, and thus infants and caregivers mutually contribute to the interaction (Hanzlik, 1990). If the child is unable to respond to these interactions adaptively, there is a risk that deviations will develop. These anomalies in the interactive process may affect the social, cognitive, and physical development of the infant (Hanzlik, 1990).

A professional's emphasis on the child's physical limitations indirectly affects the parent-child interaction because it may cause the caregiver to overfocus on physical development and neglect other facets of development (Kogan et al., 1974), including play. Professionals often teach parents about the importance of therapeutic intervention during the daily routine. This further constrains the parents' time and disposition to engage in spontaneous play (Hanzlik, 1989, 1990). The degree of physical limitation affects the interaction in such a way that over the years, parents gradually become less affectionate during play and therapy sessions, particularly in cases where children make less physical progress (Kogan et al., 1974).

The difficulties and frustrations experienced by a child with CP may cultivate apathy and withdrawal (Mogford, 1977) and thereby negatively affect the child's interaction with other children (Missiuna & Pollock, 1991).

Children with CP have limited opportunities for play with nondisabled children unless it is carefully planned. This occurs because there is still a stigma attached to these children and because their slower responses affect the playful interaction. When these children have the opportunity to play with nondisabled peers, such as when they are placed in mainstream programs, interaction between these groups is seldom encouraged (Shevin, 1987).

It is a paradox that adults who know little about play teach children how to play (Caldwell, 1986). This certainly applies to children with CP. Caregivers, teachers, and therapists need to become more aware not only of the importance of play as a means to an end, but also of ways to foster the child's intrinsic motivation to seek opportunities for play as a pleasurable activity in itself. Playful interaction among children with similar physical difficulties is limited by the presence of multiple disabilities and may need adult facilitation. The following example illustrates this point.

CASE EXAMPLE 1

Sam, Jenny, and Rick

Three parents carry their children, Sam, Jenny, and Rick, into the treatment room and place them on the mat. Sam and Jenny have a diagnosis of spastic quadriparesis, and Rick has spastic athetosis. They are unable to sit independently but can roll and creep. Soon after Sam is placed on the floor, he recognizes Rick and Jenny, smiles, and creeps toward them. His spasticity becomes more evident as he pulls his weight on his arms. When he reaches Jenny he says, "Hi" and looks around for Sarah, his therapist. Jenny, prone, hyperextends her head and smiles in response but is unable to change her position. Rick attempts to catch Sam's attention by vocalizing, but his sounds do not make clear words. Sam stays near them, smiling while he continues to wait for his therapist.

This description illustrates spontaneous interaction among children with CP. Sam approached the other children and initiated a potentially playful interaction. Jenny's and Rick's responses, however, were limited to smiles and vocalizations and did not further evolve into a playful interaction, probably because the required movement adaptations were beyond their capabilities. Children with CP may initiate a playful interaction by reaching, smiling, or bringing a toy over to another individual, but they tend to rely on the other person to expand on this initial interaction. A group of children with similar deficits may have difficulty entering into a playful interaction together.

In summary, the play of a child with CP is restricted by the inherent limitations of the diagnosis and by sociocultural constraints imposed by others in the environment.

Nevertheless, these children possess the intrinsic motivation to enter into alternative forms of playful interaction. When serving these children, therapists must be aware of the nature of the disorders presented by the child and how these disorders interfere with the capacity to play. More important, they need to be aware of adults' responsibility in either facilitating or inhibiting play.

ROLE OF PLAY IN TREATMENT AND EVERYDAY LIFE

As previously discussed, fostering play in a child with CP requires understanding the role of play in everyday life and how it is constrained by factors in both the child and the environment, including adults' values and predisposition to play. Fostering play requires having appropriate play materials, play space, playtime, and playmates (Pugmire-Stoy, 1992). Since these elements are not enough to spark play in a child with CP, the adult needs to view himself or herself as a primary tool in facilitating play in treatment and everyday life.

Play in the Treatment Session

In the United States the preferred approach to treating movement disorder of children with CP is NDT. The goal of NDT is to increase the child's functional ability by facilitating normal postural control and movement patterns. Although some authors believe that play and NDT can be easily combined (Anderson, Hinojosa, & Strauch, 1987; Erhardt, 1993), NDT's focus on postural adjustments during function requires great creativity to avoid inhibiting the possibilities of entering into spontaneous play. The most often described relationship between NDT and play is this:

Play as motivation → NDT treatment → Image on
movement → Ability to play

Play can be used during the treatment session to motivate the child to move by providing a meaningful context and distracting the child from the therapeutic objectives (Anderson et al., 1987; Rast, 1986). Improved movement abilities gained during the NDT session in turn affect the child's potential to engage in exploration and free play outside the treatment session.

In the past, the use of NDT techniques did not provide room for a serious consideration of play in the treatment session. It is interesting to note, however, that although play has long been considered an important topic in occupational therapy for children with CP (Craig & Hendin, 1951; Robinault, 1953), the introduction of NDT principles into the occupational therapy literature did not address the context of play (Fiorentino, 1966; Myzak & Fiorentino, 1961). Interest in play in connection with NDT did not develop until after the NDT approach was firmly established among occupational therapists and probably resulted from the increased interest in play in the occupational therapy literature (Reilly, 1974). The view of play that evolved during the 1970s and 1980s and has since been expanded is described at the beginning of this chapter. From this perspective, play has the following purposes in the treatment of the child with CP:

- As a motivator or reinforcer (often through the use of a toy or as promised playtime at the end of the session)
- As an arena or meaningful context where skills are acquired for future performance
- As an enjoyable, intrinsically motivated, spontaneous, process-oriented activity

Caldwell (1986) proposed that "we have so overweighed our research toward play as a means to an end that we have lost the essence of what play means in the life of the young child" (p. 307). This section addresses all three uses of play but emphasizes the importance of the often neglected third use as the one that restores the essence of play to the life of the child with CP. To embrace this view in treatment, therapists need to be able to distinguish among play as a motivator, play as a context for acquisition of adaptive skills, and play as an intrinsically motivated, process-oriented activity.

Play as Motivator or Reinforcement

When play is used to motivate a child to interact and participate in treatment, it is important to consider all the possibilities that play can offer. First, therapists need to select materials that will encourage play and to determine how to use the materials and space to their maximum potential. Second, they need to be aware that if they are to use play as motivation, they must allow playtime during the session. Third, they need to consider that other forms of play may be more productive than those requiring the child to use fine motor manipulation. Fourth, they need to avoid some common mistakes during treatment.

Play materials

The term "play materials" generally refers to toys. The sensorimotor toys used in therapy are often not conducive to play but have been chosen by therapists to affect motor coordination and other deficit areas. Hence they are seldom regarded as objects for play by the child (Figure 15-1). When asked whether he wanted to play with some coordination toys while waiting for his mom, Sam, a 5-year-old with spastic diplegia, emphasized this point by saying, "No. That's not fun, that's work!" If therapists want to encourage play rather than solely functional motor performance through the use of an educational "toy," they should pay attention to the way they use space and toys. Even when spaces and materials are colorful and attractive, the most difficult challenges for clinicians are finding a toy that addresses both the therapist's goals and the child's motivation and interests and treating the child without having total control over the space in which he or she plays. In the therapeutic setting, clinicians often sacrifice motivation for therapeutic

value and transform play into a vehicle for meeting motor goals. For example, therapists control the toys the child uses and the space the child can explore. Exploration often leads to play, but for a child with CP, the need to use positioning equipment in the home and classroom commonly restricts that possibility (Graham & Bryant, 1993). In treatment, handling of the child should take place during free exploration and should not be limited to a confined space (Figure 15-2). The following case example illustrates that point.

CASE EXAMPLE 2

Mark

The treatment room is large and inviting. There are colorful balls, rolls, and toys on the blue mats. A therapist, Marcie, treats Mark, an attractive 3-year-old boy with spastic diplegia. His mother sits nearby with the younger sibling. Mark lies prone on the mat, his head resting on his arms. Upon a request from the therapist, he raises his head and begins to move slowly toward her. He stops and rests. His muscle tone is low but increases when he attempts to move in space. His movements are slow and ponderous. Suddenly his younger sibling runs by him to get a toy. Mark raises his head eagerly, follows her movements with his head, and chases her by pulling on his arms and creeping in her direction. As he moves, his muscle tone increases and flexion is observed in his body. The therapist calls to him and asks him to stop and instead come to her. Mark stops but ignores the request to creep back. Marcie approaches him and helps him sit on a red bolster. Mark has little control over his movements. His balance is poor, and he tends to use his arms for support.

Marcie places a ring stack in front of Mark and asks the youngster to reach. His attempt to reach is slow and difficult. His trunk is slouched, his head is laterally tilted, and he leans on his hands against the bolster. The therapist wonders whether the activity is too demanding and changes his position. He now sits sideways against the bolster. Marcie shows him a book; she plans to maintain his attention and work on his sitting balance by pointing to the pictures in the book. At first Mark appears interested in the book, but soon he slouches against the bolster and leans his head on his arms as he looks around the room.

In this example Mark indicated little intrinsic motivation to engage in the sensorimotor activities presented to him. However, he did appear interested in the other child moving around him. The therapist's goals included the development of postural control to participate in functional activities. At this point in treatment it might have been more beneficial to use the other child as a playmate

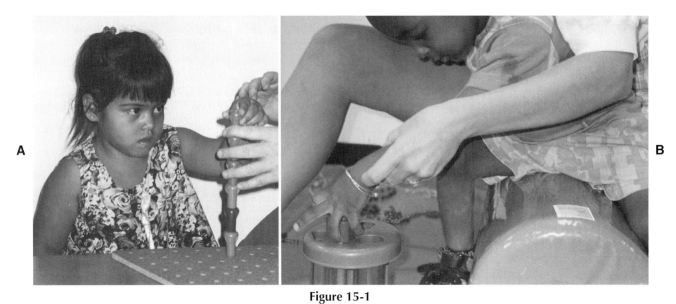

Figure 15-1

The use of coordination toys to facilitate reach, grasp, release, and trunk control. These activities may or may not be considered play by the child.

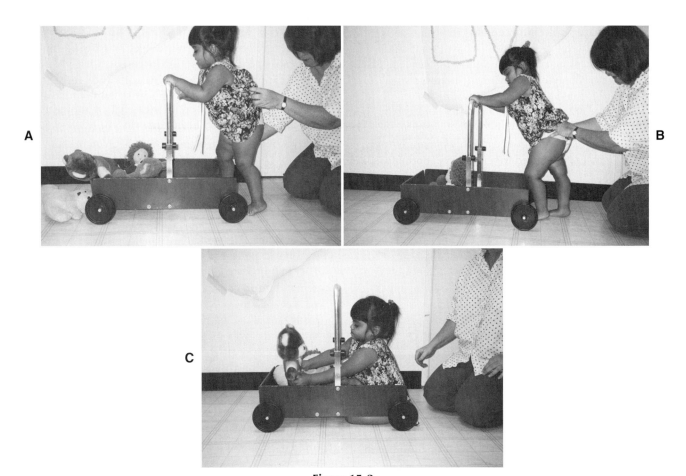

Figure 15-2

A, *A carriage with dolls can motivate the child to move.* **B,** *In some cases (see right knee) adequate body alignment is lost in the enthusiasm of performing the activity.* **C,** *In other cases the child's motivation to play may take momentary priority over the treatment goal.*

to motivate Mark to maintain an erect position. In this case the use of sensorimotor play materials was too demanding and not motivating enough for the child.

If therapists want to encourage genuine play rather than motor performance with an educational "toy," they should pay attention to the toys they provide. The selection of appropriate toys to encourage active participation during treatment has been extensively documented (Ayrault, 1977; Musselwhite, 1986). The choice of toy depends on the purpose of play. Toys are chosen for their educational and therapeutic value or for their recreational value (Tebo, 1986). Therapeutic toys are selected based on the needs of the child, but recreational toys are meant to facilitate independent play and are chosen based on the child's acquired skills and motivation. When choosing a toy, the therapist must consider its inherent features (safety, durability, degree of structure offered by the toy, responsiveness of the toy, and motivational value of the toy), the age appropriateness of the toy, and its therapeutic value (Musselwhite, 1986).

The toys for children with severe movement deficits have to be carefully chosen. Sometimes commercially available toys can be adapted to enhance their responsive nature so that they are easily triggered by the child's limited movements. A child with severe deficits often chooses to play if the toy is colorful and produces dramatic rewards for simple movements (Mogford, 1977). In reference to the therapeutic value of toys, children with fluctuating muscle tone benefit from toys that are heavier and offer resistance because they facilitate proximal stability and increase sensory feedback (Boehme, 1987). Children with hypertonicity need lighter toys that offer some unpredictability because such toys facilitate a greater range of movement and decrease the tendency to remain in a fixed position (Boehme, 1987). Toys that require less precise manipulative skills, such as textured play dough, action toys, stickers, magnetic toys, rice, brushes, and shaving cream or foam may also be appropriate choices for most children (Figure 15-3). Toys that do not have rigid, preset rules and that allow flexibility may increase the motivation to participate and enhance the child's feeling of mastery over the material.

A discussion about play materials would not be complete without the inclusion of the computer as a tool for play. Computers are now part of most households, and web sites serving people with CP have proliferated. Computers offer children with CP the possibility to enter into virtual play and thus engage in playful interactions that are not hindered by their physical limitations. Engagement in virtual play is reported to increase motivation, interest, and self-efficacy in children with CP (Reid, 2002). For people with physical disabilities, the use of computers and virtual play prob-

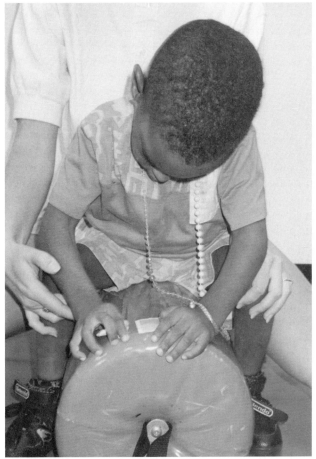

Figure 15-3

This 4-year-old expressed interest in playing with stickers. The therapist accommodated her treatment goals (weight bearing) to include this activity in the treatment session.

ably opens the most promising avenue for enjoyment and full participation in the prevalent culture.

Playtime

Therapists who use playtime for reinforcement need to be careful not to banish it consistently until the end of the session. If play is used to reinforce a specific action, it should be consistently allowed at the appropriate point during the session, not necessarily at the end. In the classroom setting the timing of the free-play activity before lunch, after a class period, or at the end of the day makes it particularly vulnerable to interruption and postponement (Shevin, 1987). The same occurs in the therapeutic session. Playtime allowed only at the end of the session may carry the message of decreased importance and lack of regard for what the child deems important.

Different Forms of Play

Different forms of play include fantasy play, social interactions, and sensation seeking. These are sometimes more powerful sources of motivation than manipulation of toys. The incorporation of other children, who may or may not have a disability, into the treatment session as playmates with the purpose of motivating movement, active participation, and social interaction can often prove to be enriching (Figure 15-4).

Practices to Be Avoided

A habit that should be discouraged is the use of toys as lures to prompt the child to participate. Therapists often display a toy to instigate a specific movement such as reach or ambulation, but when the child is close to the promised toy, the therapist moves it farther away to elicit a more perfect movement or a longer sequence of movement. This practice decreases motivation and active participation on the part of the child.

The therapist should not introduce a toy that requires manipulation while attempting to facilitate a gross motor skill such as balance. Although it is important to facilitate movement within a meaningful context, in everyday life people seldom perform activities that simultaneously require gross motor, fine motor–perceptual, and cognitive effort. When working on the development of gross motor skills, the therapist may find it beneficial to encourage fantasy play, such as pretending and storytelling, rather than forms of play that require fine motor manipulation. Later, after the new gross motor skill is developed, the therapist can incorporate it into forms of play that require reach, grasp, release, and fine motor manipulation.

Another practice to avoid is repeating the same activity several times consecutively. For example, when using construction toys, puzzles, blocks, or action figures, therapists sometimes ask the child to place pieces into a container or put a puzzle together. Once the child performs the activity successfully, the therapist dumps the pieces out and asks the child to repeat the activity. This habit may be effective in facilitating a desired movement, but it takes perceived control away from the child and reinforces the child's perception of lack of mastery over the environment. If play, rather than toys, is used to motivate the child, the therapist should consider alternative forms of play and the use of playmates to enhance the experience.

Play as Context

Play has been described as an activity that provides context to the development of adaptive skills (Munoz, 1986; Rast, 1986; Robinson, 1977; Sparling, Walker, & Singdahlsen, 1984). This view considers play to be useful in serving the development of motor, cognitive, and social skills for future use, rather than as a purely enjoyable experience. The playful activity is still chosen for its educational or therapeutic value. However, this view also recognizes play as a valuable activity with distinct characteristics and not just as a reward or motivation for some other goal.

When thinking about play as a context for developing functional skills, the therapist needs to understand

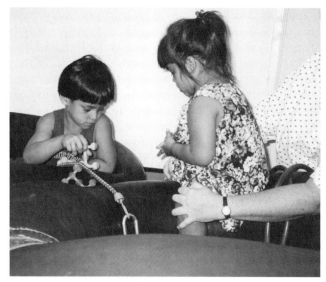

Figure 15-4
Interactive play during a treatment session.

that the child and therapist may have different purposes for activities and therefore may view them differently. Activities that appear to be enjoyable to the adult may not be considered play by the child. Not all functions performed by children are play, but many activities can be spontaneously transformed into play. A therapist may transform a treatment session into play by allowing the child to choose an activity, be spontaneous, and have fun. Activities can be transformed into play by the child's willingness to enter an enjoyable world in which reality is momentarily suspended and the goal of the activity is the performance of it. Even when the therapist's motivation is to incorporate play for the acquisition of specific developmental skills, attention to the child's perception of play increases the probability of the child's full participation. This point is discussed further in the next section.

The use of play as context for NDT techniques can now be discussed in reference to motor control theories based on an ecological approach that views the actor and environment as inseparable in the acquisition of skills (Gliner, 1985). This approach emphasizes the need for a treatment environment that is "critical in eliciting the type of action (movement if you will) that is adaptive" (Fetters, 1991, p. 222). The goal of the therapist is to create an environment with "opportunities for normal, or at least preferred, movement patterns" (Fetters, 1991, p. 222). These motor control theories advocate a less "hands-on" approach to teaching motor problem-solving skills. They suggest that the therapist should elicit self-initiated movement and active exploratory experiences from the child while considering environmental restrictions and musculoskeletal constraints, the child's motivation, opportunities to practice abilities, and the development of effective compensations when necessary (Fetters, 1991; Gliner, 1985). This chapter proposes that, in such a model, play provides a relevant context for the acquisition of skills. Play is a motivating, freely chosen activity during which the therapist can elicit active movement and exploration and the child can develop problem-solving skills and strategies in a task-oriented context and can practice newly acquired skills.

Principles of motivation and environmentally relevant activities are central to theories of occupational therapy and were long ago incorporated in sensory integrative treatment (Ayres, 1972; Gliner, 1985). However, their inclusion in the treatment of motor skills for children with CP is based on more recent motor control theories that emphasize the importance of context-relevant, self-initiated movement as a concern both for occupational therapists and for other professionals working with the child. Box 15-1 summarizes the considerations for using play in treatment for the child with CP. These considerations are discussed in detail in the following sections.

Play as an End in Itself

Incorporating play into the treatment session and the life of the child with CP requires understanding of the characteristics and essence of play. The following basic components of play can be incorporated into treatment:

1. *Spontaneity in starting, changing, or ending an activity.* For the child, spontaneity may lead to increased variability of behavioral responses and may have an impact on creativity (Singer & Singer, 1977).
2. *Intrinsic motivation to initiate, create, or be part of an activity.* Fostering intrinsic motivation may enhance the child's sense of control.
3. *Ability to suspend reality.* This may affect the child's motivation to participate in treatment activities.
4. *Enjoyment of the process rather than focusing on the end product.* This may increase active participation.
5. *Active participation, whether physically, cognitively, or socially.* Active participation affects learning and overall performance.
6. *Increased arousal.* Play can be used to increase arousal level and hence can be incorporated into treatment. Level of arousal has an impact on the child's attention and active interaction with the environment.

These concepts are next described in relation to the use of play as motivator, as context, and as enjoyable activity.

Spontaneity

Freedom to be spontaneous is often inhibited by physical limitations. When therapists evaluate play, they frequently place children in an inviting environment where they are encouraged to play spontaneously. Sheridan (1975) referred to the importance of systematic observations of spontaneous play in children with disabilities. These observations often yield valuable information about a child's ability to self-organize and interact with the environment.

Box 15-1 *Considerations for Play in Treatment*

Play to Motivate Participation
Use of materials and space
- Features of the toys: safety, motivational
- Structure provided, responsiveness
- Age appropriateness
- Therapeutic value: treatment goals
Use of playtime
Use of playmates
Use of multiple forms of play
- Social interaction
- Sensory input
- Fantasy (suspension of reality)

Play as a Context for the Development of Adaptive Skills
Therapist's treatment goal
Child's motivation to participate

Play as an End in Itself
Intrinsic motivation
Spontaneity
Enjoyment
Suspension of reality
Active engagement—sense of control
Increased arousal

Levitt (1975) described the interactions of children with CP in an adventure playground designed to stimulate motor and sensory experiences. In this situation children demonstrated two types of behavior. On the one hand, the opportunity for the children to move spontaneously allowed them to practice movements that were already established in therapy. Some of these behaviors included movement skills that were rarely possible in the school, clinic, or hospital setting. On the other hand, children regressed to lower levels of motor ability if the play activity was overly demanding yet highly interesting (Levitt, 1975). These are important considerations in treatment. The child who engages in spontaneous play may need additional support so that he or she progresses to the next level of motor development rather than regressing to previous ones.

Adults have a pivotal role in encouraging spontaneity. The therapist can incorporate spontaneity into the treatment session by being less directive and providing flexible activities that allow modifications or bending of the rules. Puzzles and coordination toys do not permit a great deal of spontaneous behavior. On the contrary, they follow preestablished patterns and discourage the child from spontaneously choosing to end or prolong the activity as she or he sees fit.

Intrinsic Motivation

Being intrinsically motivated requires having basic ideas of how to interact with objects and space. Because of motor and other limitations, children with CP do not have much freedom to choose and carry out a task. In addition, adults seldom provide these children with the opportunity to offer their opinion or select among several alternatives. Their highly structured daily routines greatly reduce the possibility to express intrinsically motivated behavior. When children with CP are asked to choose between several alternatives, they often respond, "I don't know." Intrinsic motivation may be hindered by several factors: cognitive limitations that affect the development of new ideas, physical limitations that limit the choices, and externally produced limitations set by caregivers and other adults for the child at home, at school, and in therapy.

Findings in motor control research have emphasized the importance of motivation in task performance and the treatment of CP (Giuliani, 1991). The use of sensory integration principles in conjunction with NDT provides a useful frame of reference for facilitating intrinsic motivation. To foster intrinsic motivation during the treatment session, the therapist can provide choices of activities and encourage decision making. Hence, the environment and the therapist need to be flexible to allow intrinsic motivation to emerge.

■ *Clinical Vignette* ■

Erika, a 4-year-old girl with a diagnosis of spastic diplegia, received occupational therapy once a week in a setting that served multiple diagnoses and used several treatment approaches. The treatment goals included facilitation of sitting balance, shoulder flexion against gravity, and bilateral activities. Erika was inquisitive, often asking what the other children were doing and tending to prefer to observe the other children instead of playing with the play dough, puzzles, blocks, and stickers that the therapist presented to increase her perceptual-motor skills.

On one occasion Erika appeared particularly uninterested in the activities she was asked to choose from, and she looked up at the glider and asked the therapist whether they could do that. Although this had not been one of the choices given to Erika, she appeared to have her heart set on doing that activity. The therapist realized that hanging from the glider could trigger increased spasticity in the lower extremities and also that Erika's hands were not strong enough to hold the weight of her entire hanging body. At that point the therapist decided that as long as one of her goals was to facilitate upper extremity movement above Erika's head in conjunction with active trunk extension against gravity, she could try to do just that by holding Erika up in her arms so that Erika could reach for the glider. When the child reached, the therapist, still

problem solving, lowered her hands to Erika's lower extremities and maintained these in abduction to avoid an abnormal extensor pattern. Erika laughed as she moved in space holding onto the glider, and she then "fell" into a pillow. After that she sat on the bolster and continued happily with the perceptual-motor activities provided by the therapist.

This vignette illustrates how the child's intrinsic motivation to perform an activity was respected and encouraged by the therapist. Making this a successful activity required physical and mental effort from the therapist. The activity itself lasted at most a minute; however, the memory of the experience stayed with Erika. In subsequent sessions Erika continued to choose some of the activities that she wanted to perform. Certain of these activities worked well with the treatment goals; other were cut short by the therapist because they facilitated increased tone and abnormal posturing and therefore conflicted with some of the treatment goals. Erika did not mind having some activities eliminated as long as she could choose others.

During the treatment session both functional tasks and playful experiences are important. Work and play are part of people's lives, and both can be incorporated into treatment without always considering one at the expense of other. The vignette about Erika illustrates how therapist and child negotiated an agreement that allowed both work and play.

Suspension of Reality in Fantasy Play

Fantasy play requires the individual to be able temporarily to suspend reality and its consequences. The ability to suspend reality and enter a make-believe world has an important role in the child's development and may contribute to creativity (Singer & Singer, 1977). Fantasy can be used throughout a treatment session to motivate a child or encourage active use of creative thought processes. Clinicians are sometimes unaware of the value of social interaction and fantasy play in assisting treatment sessions. The following case example illustrates that point.

CASE EXAMPLE 3

Johnny

A summer storm starts as Luisa, a physical therapist, is ready to begin the treatment session with Johnny. She is aware that Johnny is extremely sensitive to noise and therefore very frightened of the storm that is coming. At first Luisa hopes that the child will not notice that it is getting darker and that the rain is coming harder. When Johnny expresses his discomfort, she knows that the session may be over unless she figures out how to distract him. Luisa decides to enter into fantasy with the child. She tells him a story that she makes up as the thunder booms and rain is coming down. She explains that this is just a party happening somewhere in the sky. The angels are having fun, and they are getting mighty rowdy. The noise of thunder is interpreted as barrels of soda that they are rolling down to be refilled, and the lightning occurs because the angels are quite mischievous and play with the lights. The entire storm is translated into the angels having a merry old time! Johnny enters into the story by asking about each sound that he hears: "Is that a barrel rolling down?" or "Are they dancing?" The session continues successfully, and Johnny has a good time.

In this example both therapist and child viewed the time as meaningful. For Johnny the meaning was provided by the storytelling, and for Luisa the meaning was derived from the success of the treatment activity. The therapist used fantasy play to shift attention and motivate the child to stay with the activity while she continued to facilitate postural control. Luisa entered into fantasy play as a way to distract Johnny, but she unconsciously incorporated all the elements that make play an end in itself: she was spontaneous, and she respected the child's intrinsic motivation to participate in the making of the story and thus did not control the outcome. The story line suspended reality, and they had fun creating it. Fantasy play could also have been used to encourage a creative thought process by having the child create the story himself. In that case play would have been used as motivator, as context, and as an intrinsically motivated joyous activity in its own right.

Closely related to fantasy and creativity is the use of educational drama and educational art to foster development in physically challenged children. Sparling et al. (1984) reported the use of controlled experience of drama and art with 14 physically challenged children. Their findings suggested that art and drama had a significant effect on cognitive, social, emotional, motor, language, and activities of daily living performance, with drama having a greater effect on the first three areas and art having a greater effect on the last three.

Fantasy play can be used to encourage the child to suspend reality and use creative thought processes. Alternate storytelling is an activity that can be used during the session to encourage active participation by the child. In this situation the child and the therapist take turns making up a story. Each of them needs to adapt to the changes made by the previous person and is required to continue the story. A less demanding incorporation of fantasy play is the use of hats, jewelry, and social games that facilitate the ability to pretend (Figure 15-5). Children with CP often enjoy treating a doll on a ball. This behavior might be viewed as illustrating the major emphasis in their lives.

Fun and Enjoyment

To increase the child's enjoyment of a task, the therapist needs to include activities that are process oriented rather than end product or goal oriented. Whether an activity is process oriented or end product oriented is ultimately determined by the child performing the task. For example, some children find the process of making a picture to be fun, others derive pleasure from the completed task, and still others consider it simply to be drudgery. If the

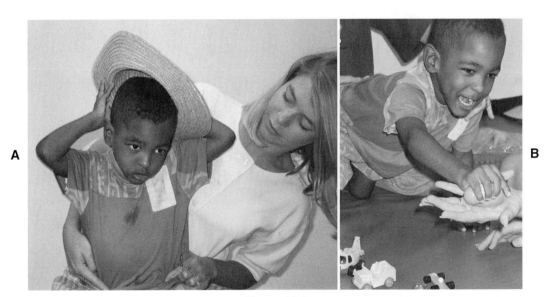

Figure 15-5
A, *Hats can be used during fantasy play to facilitate head control and upper extremity reach.* **B,** *Little people, cars, and other social toys are sometimes less demanding and more motivating for the child. Most functions that can be facilitated with a coordination toy can be performed with action toys.*

process is a chore, the pleasure of the completed picture may not be enough to make the activity fun. It is difficult to find sensorimotor activities that are enjoyable for a child with CP. As previously mentioned, nonstructured materials such as play dough, water, and bubbles allow the child to have fun while manipulating the material. Social play and action toys such as dolls, cups, and cars also permit some freedom and enjoyment (Figure 15-5, *B*). Activities that provide enhanced sensory input, such as playing in the sand or water, swinging, and pounding play dough, are often enjoyable and process oriented (Figure 15-6).

In the treatment of children with CP, therapists tend to provide play activities that address their movement limitations. These activities are seldom considered fun and are seldom chosen by the child. However, a child may choose to repeat an activity because it is fun, and this activity may prove to be a useful context for practicing specific skills. Practicing newly acquired skills improves the child's motor ability and provides a sense of mastery that may increase pleasure derived from the activity.

Increased Arousal

Through the use of sensory input, play can be incorporated into an activity to increase arousal. This input can be used to modify the child's arousal level and hence improve attention. Play is often described as an activity that is sought because of its arousing qualities (Ellis, 1973), as when children twirl and swing. Children with CP may be limited in their search for an arousing experience. In treatment a session can be started with an arousing play experience that has been transformed to meet the treatment goals.

CASE EXAMPLE 4

Brian

Brian, a 5-year-old with spastic hemiplegia, has been treated for most of his life. The treatment goals include improving postural control, hand skills, and visual-motor coordination. On one occasion the treating clinician notices that Brian becomes more cooperative after an arousing play activity that involves tactile input. They call this game "Ninjas." Brian is the Ninja Turtle and the therapist is "Shredder" or "the bad guy." Each carries a long-handled brush that can be used to brush the other's feet. The big treatment balls and bolsters lying around the treatment room become the obstacles that have to be sorted out while a player is running away. Both therapist and child chase each other. During this activity Brian, who is usually inattentive and trips often, is able to maneuver through most obstacles in space, go up and down ramps, and maintain his balance while climbing onto equipment (Figure 15-7). The activity is performed for a short time, but the increased arousal occurring during that time affects Brian's ability to attend and he is able to participate more actively in the subsequent tabletop activities.

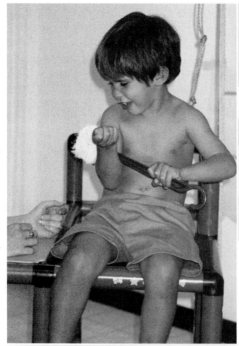
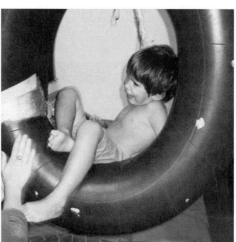

Figure 15-6

*The integration of equipment that provides sensory input, such as, **A,** brushes and, **B,** swings, assists in preparing the child's arousal level and motivation to actively engage in an activity.*

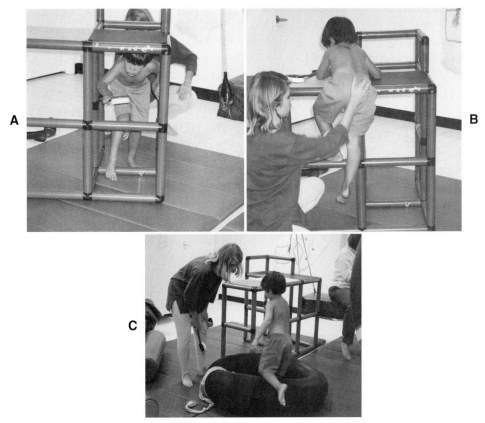

Figure 15-7

A *and* **B,** *Children are often motivated to participate in active games (role playing Ninja Turtles, Power Rangers, etc.) that can be used to facilitate movements in space while negotiating obstacles.* **C,** *The use of tires and large equipment can encourage balance, upper extremity weight bearing, and active movements in space.*

Encouraging Independent Play and Recreational Activities

The ultimate goal of encouraging play during school and treatment sessions is to enhance the child's motivation to engage independently in play. Yet external factors such as the daily routine and the physical environment may have to be modified for play to occur outside the controlled environment. Fostering play outside the structured environment requires understanding the child's preferred play and offering the child the opportunity to have appropriate play materials, play space, playtime, and playmates (Blanche, 2002; Pugmire-Stoy, 1992). To understand the child's preferred play, the therapist observes and interviews the child about preferences in process-oriented occupations. The therapist should ask whether the child enjoys imagination, intense sensory experiences, being exposed to new information, social interactions, or quiet time. Based on the child's preferences, the play materials, play space, playtime, and playmates are chosen. Box 15-2 summarizes the areas

the therapist should consider when fostering play outside the treatment area.

When the therapist is fostering independent play, a selection of novel materials and toys should be available for the child. Toy lending libraries offer the opportunity to have a large selection of toys and games from which the child can choose (Munoz, 1986). Sometimes the materials must be adapted to meet the needs of the child. When independent play is to be facilitated, the selection of play materials should relate to the everyday environment, such as playing in the snow, piling and jumping into leaves, and splashing water (Musselwhite, 1986). Toys for independent play may also need to be more responsive and easier to handle than those used with adult guidance. In summary, the choice of materials should allow the child to explore, master, and control.

The play space includes having a specific space for the child to play. The space and the materials can allow novelty and surprise or may provide a quiet space

Box 15-2   *Fostering Play Outside The Treatment Area*

Play Materials
Type of toys
Toy variety (construction, sociodramatic, etc.)
Need for adaptive toys
Toy lending libraries

Play Space
Consideration of distractions
Seating and positioning
Adapted playgrounds
Backyard activities

Playtime
Individual and with others
• At home
• Play dates
In the community and with others
• Art classes
• Theater productions

Playmates
Non–physically challenged children
Siblings and neighbors
Classmates (in mainstreamed program)

for the child. In some cases the child needs to be offered unfamiliar environments and allowed to explore space freely. In other instances he or she may need positioning equipment to engage in play. Play space includes adapted playgrounds, adapted backyards, and adapted ways to explore the community as an alternative for the child. Children with physical disabilities can enjoy outdoor activities such as gardening, nature walks, picnics, and animal husbandry if a few adaptations are made (Greenstein, Miner, Kudela, & Bloom, 1993). Occupational therapists should assume an active role not only in adapting the child's playground, but in planning community playgrounds (Stout, 1988).

Even when children with CP have busy routines that do not allow free time to engage in spontaneous play, playtime should be scheduled during the day. This may be free time before dinner, scheduled time with a friend, or a recreational activity such as an art class. Some schools plan a theater production in which parents and children participate. Such a program provides a potential opportunity for the parents, teachers, and children to engage in play.

Playing with nondisabled siblings, neighbors, and friends can prove to be an enriching experience for the child with CP and for the playmates. Socially inclined children may enter more easily into play when other children are present. Other children may prefer to observe

peers rather than enter into play with them. Nondisabled children offer better role models of spontaneous play behavior than adults. However, when a child with CP participates in a mainstream special education program, teachers and other adults seldom encourage this interaction (Shevin, 1987).

The closest nondisabled playmates for children with CP are their siblings. The inclusion of siblings in the rehabilitation process can have positive effects on the functional performance in children with CP (Craft, Lakin, Oppliger, Clancy, & Vanderlinden, 1990). Occupational therapists can include siblings in play situations through participation in camp experiences, intervention sessions, and outings.

Role of the Adult in Facilitating Play

Adults play a pivotal role in enhancing or inhibiting the child's capacity to play (Jones & Reynolds, 1992; Musselwhite, 1986; Newson & Head, 1979). In the case of the child with CP, adults may have to take a more directive role in encouraging the child to interact actively with the environment (Newson & Head, 1979). Sometimes, however, the adult may just need to have an inviting role in encouraging play. Therefore, when fostering play, therapists should take into consideration their own readiness to allow play to occur, the role they take in it, and the tactics they use to facilitate play (Musselwhite, 1986). Musselwhite (1986) and Jones and Reynolds (1992) identified several roles taken by the adult during play with the child. These roles can be summarized as follows:
• *The stage manager.* The adult takes the responsibility to provide the time and arrange the physical environment so that it invites play (Jones & Reynolds, 1992). This is the role often taken by preschool teachers and therapists using an sensory integration approach.
• *The mediator.* The adult assists in child-to-child and child–to–physical world interaction by modeling problem-solving skills during play (Jones & Reynolds, 1992). Occupational therapists often use this approach when considering the context of play to resolve a problem.
• *The director.* The adult takes an active role in getting and maintaining the child's attention and interest in play, demonstrates specific skills and behaviors, and controls the playful interaction between two children or between the adult and the child (Jones & Reynolds, 1992; Musselwhite, 1986). This role may be taken by therapists when working with children who are severely limited and when using play as a context for learning adaptive skills.
• *The observer.* The adult does not enter into play but sits back, takes notes, and analyzes the situation (Jones and Reynolds, 1992; Musselwhite, 1986). This role is used by the therapist during the assessment of play skills.
• *The player.* The adult enters into play with the child. The decision to assume this role depends on the

adult's preferred style of interaction, the child's need for challenge, and the child's ability to sustain play (Jones & Reynolds, 1992). Both adult and child may act as equal partners, taking turns in the interaction. The adult may have to initiate an interaction but then actively encourages the child to participate and respond (Musselwhite, 1986). The biggest risk of adopting this role is the hazard of taking over the interaction, especially if this role is adopted from the beginning and the child is not given a chance to develop his or her own play. Adopting the role of player may enhance the content of play and enrich the relationship between adult and child (Jones & Reynolds, 1992). Therapists need to strive for the player role when inviting the child to enter into play as a spontaneous, intrinsically motivated behavior.

Adults in the environment of children with CP may inhibit play for several reasons: because they do not believe it is important, because they do not know what to do to enter into play with the child, or because they are overeager to facilitate it. In a study of children's participation in an adventure playground, Levitt (1975) described the adult's behavior as overly eager to have the child enjoy the visit. When adults are overeager to foster a successful experience, they may act too fast and not allow the child to explore a given situation fully.

When Nothing Works

The treatment sessions described in this chapter illustrate how difficult it can be to have genuine play during treatment. When the activity is unsuccessful, the following questions can guide the clinical reasoning process:

1. In reference to the therapists' own style and views of play:
   a. How do they value play? What are their biases about the child's play?
   b. What is their style of play? Do they prefer creativity, adventure, mastery, ludos, or restoration types of activities?
   c. Are they cueing into the child's verbal and nonverbal messages about interest and motivation? Even when these motivations are weakly expressed, or their expression is severely limited?
   d. Once they have cued into the child's motivations, are they willing to be flexible enough to change the process (not the goals) of the therapeutic interaction?
   e. Are they willing to work with someone else's idea? Are they open to surprise?
   f. Are they accepting of multiple outcomes—which may not be what was initially planned?
2. What roles are they taking when facilitating play (i.e., stage manager, director, observer, or facilitator)?
3. Is the activity at the child's motor and cognitive developmental level?
4. Is the appropriate amount of sensory input being provided to the child? Is low arousal level affecting muscle tone and drive to explore the environment?
5. Is the activity structured in such a way that the meaning is eliminated, for example, in repetition of manipulative tasks?

SUMMARY

Play for the child with CP can be used as motivation, as context to promote competence, and as spontaneous, enjoyable activity. This chapter emphasizes the importance of understanding the characteristics of play and the role of the adult in promoting play for the child with CP. For that to occur, play must be considered not only a means to an end, but also an end in itself.

Review Questions

1. This chapter discusses the roles of play in normal development. Consider how these roles are relevant to the child with cerebral palsy.
2. Consider how limitations in movement, sensory processing, cognition, and environment may have an impact on the play of the child with CP. How may treatment address each of these types of limitation?
3. Contrast the ways in which play is used in treatment as a motivator, as a context for skill acquisition, and as a process-oriented activity.
4. Describe considerations that are needed in the selection of toys for children with severe movement deficits.
5. How may the therapist encourage spontaneity and enjoyment in the play of the child with cerebral palsy?
6. What are the roles that adults may take on when facilitating play? Under what circumstances are the roles typically assumed?

REFERENCES

Anderson, J., Hinojosa, J., & Strauch, C. (1987). Integrating play in neuro-developmental treatment. *American Journal of Occupational Therapy, 41*(7), 421-426.

Ayrault, E. W. (1977). *Growing up handicapped—A guide for parents and professionals to helping the exceptional child* (pp. 97-107). New York: Seabury Press.

Ayres, A. J. (1972). *Sensory integration and learning disorders.* Los Angeles: Western Psychological Services.

Batty, J. (1989, Feb. 23). Making disabled children smile is as easy as flipping a switch. *OT Week.*

Blanche, E. I. (1999). *Play and process: The experience of play in the life of the adult.* Ann Arbor, MI: University of Michigan.

Blanche, E. I. (2002). Play and process: Adult play embedded in the daily routine. In J. Roopnarire (Ed.), *Conceptual, social-cognitive, and contextual issues in the field of play. Vol. 4.* (pp. 249-278). Westport, CT: Ablex Publishing.

Bly, L. (1983). *The components of normal movement during the first year of life and abnormal motor development* (monograph). Chicago, IL: Neurodevelopmental Treatment Association.

Bobath, K., & Bobath, B. (1975). *Motor development in the different types of cerebral palsy*. London: William Heineman Medical Books.

Boehme, R. (1987). *Developing mid range control and function in children with fluctuating muscle tone*. Milwaukee, WI: Boehme Workshops.

Brown, M., & Gordon, W. A. (1987). Impact of impairments on activity patterns of children. *Archives of Physical Medicine and Rehabilitation, 68*, 828-832.

Bruner, J. S. (1972). The nature and uses of immaturity. *American Psychologist, 27*, 687-708.

Bundy, A. C. (1992). Play: The most important occupation in children. *Sensory Integration Special Interest Section Newsletter, 15*, 1-2.

Bundy, A. C. (1993). Assessment of play and leisure: Delineation of the problem. *American Journal of Occupational Therapy, 47*, 217-222.

Caldwell, B. (1986). The significance of parent-child interaction in children's development. In A. W. Gottfried & C. Caldwell Brown (Eds.), *Play interactions—The contributions of play materials and parental involvement to children's development*. Proceedings from the eleventh Johnson and Johnson Pediatric Round Table (pp. 305-310). Lexington, MA: Lexington Books.

Casby, M. W. (1992). Symbolic play: Development and assessment considerations. *Infants and Young Children, 4*(3), 43-48.

Couch, K. J. (1998). The role of play in pediatric occupational therapy. *American Journal of Occupational Therapy, 52*(2), 111-117.

Craft, M. J., Lakin, J. A., Oppliger, R. A., Clancy, G. M., & Vanderlinden, D. W. (1990). Siblings as agents for promoting the functional status of children with cerebral palsy. *Developmental Medicine and Child Neurology, 32*(12), 1049-1057.

Craig, H. L., & Hendin, J. (1951). Toys for children with cerebral palsy. *American Journal of Occupational Therapy, 5*(2), 50-51.

Curry, J., & Exner, C. (1988). Comparison of tactile preferences in children with and without cerebral palsy. *American Journal of Occupational Therapy, 27*, 457-463.

Danella, E. A. (1973). A study of tactile preference in multiply-handicapped children. *American Journal of Occupational Therapy, 27*(8), 457-463.

D'Eugenio, D. (1986). Infant play: A reflection of cognitive and motor development. In *Play: A skill for life—A monograph project of the Developmental Disabilities Special Interest Section of the American Occupational Therapy Association* (pp. 55-66). Rockville, MD: American Occupational Therapy Association.

Diamant, R. (1992). *Positioning for play—Home activities for parents of young children*. Tucson, AZ: Therapy Skill Builders.

Eagle, R. S. (1985). Deprivation of early sensorimotor experience and cognition in the severely involved cerebral-palsied child. *Journal of Autism and Developmental Disorders, 15*(3), 269-283.

Ellis, M. J. (1973). *Why people play*. Englewood Cliffs, NJ: Prentice Hall.

Erhardt, R. (1993). Cerebral palsy. In H. Hopkins & H. Smith (Eds.), *Willard and Spackman's occupational therapy* (8th ed., pp. 430-458). Philadelphia: J. B. Lippincott.

Fetters, L. (1991). Cerebral palsy: Contemporary treatment concepts. In M. Lister (Ed.), *Contemporary management of motor control problems—Proceedings of the II STEP Conference*. (pp. 219-224). Fredericksburg, VA: Bookcrafters.

Fewell, R. R., & Glick, M. (1993). Observing play: An appropriate process for learning and assessment. *Infants and Young Children, 5*(4), 35-43.

Finnie, N. (1975). *Handling the young cerebral palsied child at home*. New York: E.P. Dutton.

Fiorentino, M. R. (1966). The changing dimension of occupational therapy. *American Journal of Occupational Therapy, 20*(5), 251-252.

Giuliani, C. A. (1991). Theories of motor control: New concepts for physical therapy. In M. Lister (Ed.), *Contemporary management of motor control problems—Proceedings of the II Step Conference* (pp. 29-35). Fredericksburg, VA: Bookcrafters.

Gliner, J. (1985). Purposeful activity in motor learning theory: An event approach to motor skill acquisition. *American Journal of Occupational Therapy, 39*(1), 28-34.

Graham, M., & Bryant, D. (1993). Developmentally appropriate environments for children with special needs. *Infants and Young Children 5*(3), 31-42.

Greenstein, D., Miner, N., Kudela, E., & Bloom, S. (1993). *Backyards and butterflies—Ways to include children with disabilities in outdoor activities*. Ithaca, NY: New York State Rural Health and Safety Council.

Hanzlik, J. R. (1989). The effect of intervention on the free-play experience for mothers and their infants with developmental delay and cerebral palsy. *Physical and Occupational Therapy in Pediatrics, 9*(2), 33-51.

Hanzlik, J. R. (1990). Interaction between mothers and their infants with developmental disabilities: Analysis and review. *Physical and Occupational Therapy in Pediatrics, 9*(4), 33-47.

Iwasaki, Y. (2001). Contributions of leisure to coping with daily hassles in university students' lives. *Canadian Journal of Behavioural Science, 33*(2), 128-141.

Iwasaki, Y. (2003). The impact of leisure coping beliefs and strategies on adaptive outcomes. *Leisure Studies, 22*, 93-108.

Jones, E., & Reynolds, G. (1992). *The play's the thing . . . Teachers' roles in children's play*. New York: Teachers College Press.

King, G., Cathers, T., Pogar, J., MacKinnon, E., & Havens, L. (2000). Success in life for older adolescents with cerebral palsy. *Qualitative Health Research, 10*(6), 734-749.

Kleiber, D., Hutchinson, S., & Williams, R. (2002). Leisure as a resource in transcending negative life events: Self-protection, self-restoration, and personal transformation. *Leisure Sciences, 24*, 219-235.

Kogan, K. L., Tyler, N., & Turner, P. (1974). The process of interpersonal adaptation between mothers and their cerebral palsied children. *Developmental Medicine and Child Neurology, 16*, 518-527.

Langley, M. B. (1990). A developmental approach to the use of toys for facilitation of environmental control. *Physical and Occupational Therapy in Pediatrics, 12*(4), 69-91. (Special issue on rehabilitation technology.)

Levitt, S. (1975). A study of gross motor skills of cerebral palsied children in an adventure playground for handicapped children. *Child: Care, Health and Development, 1*, 29-43.

Magill-Evans, J., & Restall, G. (1991). Self-esteem of persons with cerebral palsy: From adolescence to adulthood. *American Journal of Occupational Therapy.* 45(9), 819-825.

Manuel, J., Balkrishnan, R., Camacho, F., Smith, B., & Koman, A. (2003). Factors associated with self-esteem in pre-adolescents and adolescents with cerebral palsy. *Journal of Adolescent Health, 32,* 456-458.

Missiuna, C., & Pollock, N. (1991). Play deprivation in children with physical disabilities: The role of the occupational therapist in preventing secondary disability. *American Journal of Occupational Therapy, 45*(10), 882-888.

Mogford, K. (1977). The play of handicapped children. In B. Tizard & D. Harvey (Eds.), *Biology of play* (pp. 170-184). London: Spastics International.

Moore, J. (1984, May). The neuroanatomy and pathology of cerebral palsy. Selected proceedings from Barbro Salek Memorial Symposium. *Neurodevelopmental Treatment Association Newsletter,* pp. 3-58.

Munoz, J. P. (1986). The significance of fostering play development in handicapped children. In *Play: A skill for life—A monograph project of the Developmental Disabilities Special Interest Section of the American Occupational Therapy Association* (pp. 1-11). Rockville, MD: American Occupational Therapy Association.

Musselwhite, C. R. (1986). *Adaptive play for special needs children.* San Diego, CA: College-Hill Press.

Mysak, E., & Fiorentino, M. R. (1961). Neurophysiological considerations in occupational therapy for the cerebral palsied. *American Journal of Occupational Therapy, 15*(3), 112-117.

Newson, E., & Head, J. (1979). Play and playthings for the handicapped child. In J. & E. Newson (Eds.), *Toys and playthings* (pp. 140-158). New York: Pantheon Books.

Piaget, J. (1962). *Play, dreams and imitation in childhood.* (C. Gattegno & F. M. Hodgson, Trans.). New York: W.W. Norton. (Original work published in 1951).

Pugmire-Stoy, M. C. (1992). *Spontaneous play in early childhood.* Albany, NY: Delmar Publishers.

Rast, M. (1986). Play and therapy, play or therapy. In *Play: A skill for life—A monograph project of the Developmental Disabilities Special Interest Section of the American Occupational Therapy Association* (pp. 29-41). Rockville, MD: American Occupational Therapy Association.

Reid, D. T. (2002). Benefits of a virtual play rehabilitation environment for children with cerebral palsy on perceptions of self-efficacy: A pilot study. *Pediatric Rehabilitation, 5*(3), 141-148.

Reilly, M. (1974). Defining a cobweb. In M. Reilly (Ed.), *Play as exploratory learning—Studies of curiosity behavior* (pp. 57-116). Beverly Hills, CA: Sage Publications.

Robinault, I. P. (1953). Occupational therapy technics for the pre-school hemiplegic—Toys and training. *American Journal of Occupational Therapy, 7*(5), 205-207.

Robinson, A. (1977). Play: The arena for acquisition of rules for competent behavior. *American Journal of Occupational Therapy, 25,* 281-284.

Sheridan, M. D. (1975). The importance of spontaneous play in the fundamental learning of handicapped children. *Child: Care, Health and Development, 1,* 3-17.

Shevin, M. (1987). Play in special education settings. In J. H. Block & N. R. King (Eds.), *School play—A source book* (pp. 219-251). New York: Teachers College Press.

Singer, D., & Singer, J. (1977). *Partners in play—A step by step guide to imaginative play in children.* New York: Harper & Row.

Sparling, J. W., Walker, D. F., & Singdahlsen, J. (1984). Play techniques with neurologically impaired preschoolers. *American Journal of Occupational Therapy, 38*(9), 603-612.

Specht, J., King, G., Brown, E., & Foris, C. (2002). The importance of leisure in the lives of persons with congenital physical disabilities. *American Journal of Occupational Therapy, 56*(4), 436-445.

Stout, J. (1988). Planning playgrounds for children with disabilities. *American Journal of Occupational Therapy, 42*(10), 653-657.

Tebo, S. E. (1986). Evaluating play selection and its possible effects on play behaviors of children with severe mental impairment. In *Play: A skill for life—A monograph project of the Developmental Disabilities Special Interest Section of the American Occupational Therapy Association* (pp. 13-25). Rockville, MD: American Occupational Therapy Association.

Trenberth, L. & Dewe, P. (2002). The importance of leisure as a means of coping with work related stress: an exploratory study. *Counselling Psychology Quarterly, 15*(1), 59-72.

White, R. W. (1959). Motivation reconsidered: The concept of competence. *Psychological Review, 66,* 297-333.

INTERNET RESOURCES

1. Suggestions for toys and play materials:
   http://www.cerebralpalsytoysandplayaids.com/index.html

2. Focus on promoting opportunities for inclusion through the use of technology. Provides access guides for recreational activities, sports, entertainment, and travel:
   http://www.infinitec.org/who.htm
   http://www.in.finitec.org/play/index.html

3. United Cerebral Palsy of New York City—tips about assistive technology:
   http://www.ucpnyc.org/info/assist/playandrecreation.cfm#1

4. Suggestions for toys and toy material:
   www.lekotek.org

16

Accessing Play Through Assistive Technology

JEAN CROSETTO DEITZ AND YVONNE SWINTH

KEY TERMS

play deprivation
assistive technology
toy and environmental adaptations
augmentative communication
alternative communication
environmental control systems
mobility devices
adaptive sports equipment
virtual reality

Clinical Vignettes

Adrienne, a 3-year-old with spinal muscular atrophy, whips across her preschool playground in a shiny yellow car with black roll bars. She's chasing Jason, who rides a red tricycle. Her teacher holds a remote control, a safety feature designed so that she can stop the car with a flick of a switch and, if necessary, redirect the car.

Dante, a toddler with cerebral palsy, hits a big red switch to activate a tape player. He smiles and attempts to sing as his favorite song plays.

Jennifer, a high school student with juvenile arthritis, plays a video adventure game with a friend. They are taking a break during an annual staff meeting. Jennifer is an expert at using her computer to design graphics for the high school yearbook.

All of these children lack most of the motor skills of their typically developing peers. However, technology helps to equalize the environment, allowing them to participate in play and leisure activities, both alone and with others. It provides them with opportunities to participate in play or leisure activities and socialize in the same settings as their peers without disabilities.

Although there are many definitions of play, most include the concept that play is "an activity voluntarily engaged in for pleasure" (Simon & Daub, 1993, p. 118). Play is one of the primary occupations of childhood, and Simon and Daub (1993) contended that through play "the child learns to explore, develop, and master physical and social skills" (p. 118) and to adapt within his or her environment and culture. According to Piaget (1952), play and cognitive development are interdependent, with play fostering the child's competence in his or her world; for some children, however, the ability to play is compromised because of a disability. The result may be frustration, unsuccessful experiences, and ultimately learned helplessness.

Brinker and Lewis (1982) maintained that an important competence of young infants is the "ability to detect and utilize co-occurrences" (p. 1). Since infants with impairments in body functions or structures (World Health Organization, 2001) have difficulties in using these co-occurrences, further impairments may result. This in turn may lead to limitation in performance in areas of occupation (American Occupational Therapy Association [AOTA], 2002).

According to Cotton (1984), play helps a child learn to cope with frustration, anxiety, and failure. An example of repeated failure when there is no chance of success is an 8-year-old boy with severe motor impairments trying to move the pieces in a chess game. No matter how hard he tries, success is never achieved. If the same child is equipped with a computer, software for playing chess, and an alternative access system he can use successfully, he can compete as an equal with able-bodied peers, experiencing and learning to cope with anxiety when questioning the advisability of a given move and with the frustration of thinking a move is ideal and then experiencing failure when an opponent announces checkmate. Although

395

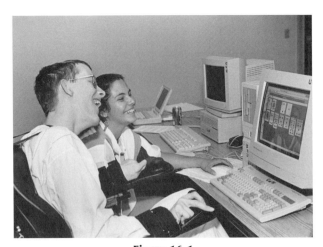

Figure 16-1

Teens use a computer to play cards. (Courtesy Mary Levin, DO-IT Project, University of Washington, Seattle, WA.)

some efforts bring realistic frustration and failure for the child, not every effort brings failure. Practice has the potential of leading to favorable moves and experiences of success. These experiences can help the child learn the joy and benefit of involvement and acquire skills in coping effectively with realistic frustration (Figure 16-1).

Missiuna and Pollock (1991) distinguished between primary and secondary forms of play deprivation experienced by children with physical disabilities. According to these authors, primary forms of play deprivation refer to those play experiences the child is denied because of impairments. For example, consider the child with a visual impairment who will not have the opportunity to play with mixing colors when painting. Regardless of the intervention, this primary form of play deprivation will remain unchanged. By contrast, secondary forms of play deprivation occur when no analogous forms of play are substituted for play experiences the child is denied because of impairment. In the previous example, a toy or device that allows the child to mix sounds instead of colors could allow the child to control the play and participate in a creative process. The failure to have access to such alternative forms of play is believed to be related to learned helplessness and dependence. According to Missiuna and Pollock, children who are unable to experience normal childhood play because of impairments "may encounter secondary social, emotional, and psychological disabilities" (1991, p. 883), many of which could be avoided through the use of alternative play experiences. Often, in such cases, assistive technology can enable children with disabilities to engage, either independently or with their peers, in alternative forms of play.

Leisure can be defined as "intrinsically motivating activities for amusement, relaxation, spontaneous enjoyment or self-expression" (Swinth & Tanta, 2003, p. 3). Although many attributes of play and leisure are the same, there are some differences. These differences should

be considered in the planning of occupational therapy evaluation and intervention to address this area of occupational performance. One difference between play and leisure is that play is often considered a key part of the development of children, whereas leisure is often engaged in simply for enjoyment and self-expression. Like play, there may be primary and secondary leisure deprivation. For example, an adolescent with tetraplegia cerebral palsy who does not have the opportunity to play tennis is experiencing primary leisure deprivation because of the impairment itself. Secondary leisure deprivation occurs only if this adolescent cannot participate in another form of leisure that enables competition, teamwork, and opportunities for socialization with peers. This alternative may be facilitated through technology that increasingly is being used by individuals, with and without disabilities.

WHAT IS ASSISTIVE TECHNOLOGY?

An assistive technology device is "any item, piece of equipment, or product system, whether acquired commercially off the shelf, modified, or customized, that is used to increase, maintain, or improve functional capabilities of individuals with disabilities" (H.R. Rep. No. 100-819, 1988). According to the American Occupational Therapy Association position statement on assistive technology, "the intent is to use technology as a tool to optimize the individual's participation in areas of occupation" (AOTA, 2004, p. 678). Assistive technology devices are available on a continuum ranging from low to high technology. There is no clear distinction between low and high technology, but in general, as assistive technology becomes more complex, it is considered high technology. This typically includes computers, alternative or augmentative communication systems, environmental control systems, and power mobility devices. By contrast, low-technology solutions tend to be less complex (e.g., simple devices to stabilize toys, large fasteners on doll clothes, or nonelectronic communication aids). If selected with care, technology, whether low or high, can empower children with disabilities so they can maximize their potential to engage in play activities and other developmentally appropriate occupations.

ASSESSMENT MODELS AND FRAMEWORKS FOR ASSISTIVE TECHNOLOGY DECISION MAKING

The assistive technology assessment process should be multifaceted, systematic, dynamic, and thoughtful. Numerous models or frameworks have been used to guide this process, and the therapist, working with a team, should consider adopting or adapting one or more of these to guide decision making within his or her setting. Three of the most common of these are the Human Activity Assistive Technology (HAAT) model (Cook & Hussey,

2002), the Wisconsin Assistive Technology Initiative (WATI) framework (Wisconsin Assistive Technology Initiative [WATI], 2004), and the Student, Environment, Tasks, Tools (SETT) framework (Zabala, 2005).

According to the HAAT model (Cook & Hussey, 2002), the process starts with the need or desire of a child to perform an activity and involves careful consideration of four primary interrelated factors: human, activity, assistive technology, and context. According to this model, human includes physical, cognitive, and psychosocial factors; activity is determined by life roles and defines the goal of the assistive technology system; and assistive technologies, including instructions and training, are extrinsic enablers that have the potential to improve occupational performance. All of these are embedded in the context that includes the setting (e.g., home, school, community), the social contexts (e.g., peers, family members, strangers), the cultural context (e.g., beliefs, values), and the physical contexts (e.g., light, sound, heat).

The W.A.T.I. Assessment Package also provides a framework to guide the assessment process. According to this framework, the assessment process is systematic and made up of three parts: information gathering, decision making, and trial use (Wisconsin Assistive Technology Initiative, 2004, p. 12). The first part, information gathering, is composed of gathering information about factors such as the "child's abilities, difficulties, environment, and tasks" (WATI, 2004, p. 16) and scheduling a meeting with the team. The second part, decision making, involves problem identification, prioritization of tasks for solution generation, generation of possible solutions, selection of a solution, and development of an implementation plan. The third part, trial use, includes implementation of the planned trials and a follow-up process (WATI, 2004, p. 17). The W.A.T.I. Assessment Package (2004) includes detailed worksheets to assist the team with question identification, gathering of information about the child and environment, and solution generation.

The SETT framework considers, as a first part of the assessment process, the child, the environments, and the tasks necessary for active participation (Zabala, 2005). Under each of these topics questions are posed. For example, under the Student category are the questions, "What does the student need to do?" and "What are the student's special needs and current abilities?" Under the Environments category are questions such as "What materials and equipment are currently available...?" "What supports are available to the student and the people working with the student on a daily basis?" and "How are the attitudes and expectations of the people in the environment likely to affect the student's performance?" Under the Tasks category are questions such as "What is everyone else doing?" "What are the critical elements of the activities?" and "How might the activities be modified to accommodate the student's special needs?" (Zabala, 2005,

pp. 5-6). The topic of Tools is addressed only after the team has addressed the first three categories. An example of a question in the Tools category is "What no tech, low tech, and high tech options should be considered for inclusion in an assistive technology system for a student with these needs and abilities doing these tasks in these environments?" (Zabala, 2005, p. 6). This question highlights the complexity of the decision-making process and the necessity of considering student, environment, and task data when exploring potential intervention solutions.

Regardless of the approach selected or developed by the team, the assessment process should focus on the child and his or her unique characteristics and interests; the social, physical, and cultural contexts in which the child participates, would like to participate, or needs to participate; and the activity demands. These considerations also should include any concerns, issues, and feedback from family members and caregivers. Once these are understood, an intervention can be planned. This may include the use of toys with universal design features or assistive technologies to support the child's participation in context. Because of the changing needs of children, this assessment and intervention process, once commenced, is ongoing.

EXAMPLES OF TOYS WITH UNIVERSAL DESIGN FEATURES AND ASSISTIVE TECHNOLOGIES FOR ENHANCING PLAY

The specific toys with universal design features and toy adaptations and devices described in the following sections are used as examples to provide a framework for understanding issues related to occupational therapy evaluation and intervention in this area of practice. The clinician should be reminded that numerous other options exist. New technologies are being developed daily, and when considering the use of assistive technology, the clinician is responsible for being knowledgeable about current toys and devices.

Enhancement of Play Through Careful Selection of Toys with Universal Design Features or Through Simple Toy and Environmental Adaptations

Occupational therapists often select toys with universal design features or use simple toy and environmental adaptations to enable children with disabilities to play (Lane & Mistrett, 2002). Typically these solutions are low cost, low maintenance, readily available, and limited only by the imaginations of the therapist and those working with the child with a disability. Increasingly, toys are being developed that are switch operated, brightly colored, and noise producing, features that make them usable and appealing to children with varied abilities. An example is a stacking toy that flashes bright lights and makes sounds when the child successfully puts a brightly colored ring on a pole. These features make this commercial toy especially suited for use by a child who has low vision or is blind. A recent collaborative project through the Elks Therapy Program for Children, toy manufacturers, and toy retailers has resulted in a web site (www.goodtogrowtoys.com) that contains resources regarding toys for children with disabilities. This project includes a large number of toy evaluations that help family members and professionals make decisions regarding appropriate toys for children with disabilities. Information regarding the project can be obtained from the web site. Additional examples of toys and adaptations can be found by touring toy stores and web sites.

Children with disabilities and their families have designed some of the best low-technology solutions. Examples of low-technology solutions are Velcro fastenings on doll clothes so that the child can engage in symbolic play (make-believe), jigs and other stabilizers (e.g., Dual-Lock [Don Johnson, Inc.]) on wheelchair lap tray surfaces and on the backs of toys to stabilize play materials, and handles on pieces of puzzles and board games. For children with fine motor difficulties, some play materials can be enlarged or handles with special grips can be designed. Adaptations or careful selection of riding toys can enable a child with a disability to participate in play with his or her peers that would not be possible with many of the traditional toys such as tricycles, scooters, and bicycles. For example, for a child with lower extremity limitations, riding toys propelled by arm movements rather than leg movements could be considered; for a child with poor trunk stability, a tricycle seat could be adapted to provide additional support; and for a child experiencing difficulty with keeping his or her feet on the pedals of a tricycle, straps could be added.

Creative ideas on simple adaptations specific to outdoor activities for children with disabilities are provided in the book *Backyards and Butterflies* (Greenstein, 1993). According to the author, most of the ideas in her book were developed by rural parents to enable their children to enjoy and participate in outdoor activities. The solutions presented apply predominantly to the home environment and are relatively inexpensive, homemade assistive technology solutions. Included are creative designs for a wheelchair-accessible plant table, adapted handles for gardening supplies (hoses, trowels, etc.), special carriers for garden tools, adapted fishing poles, accessible bird feeders, spill-proof containers for holding wildflowers, easily accessible insect houses, custom-made horseback riding aids, adaptations for large toys with wheels (i.e., tricycles, bicycles, wagons), and safe and accessible swings and slides. In addition, this resource deals with accessibility in the berry patch, caring for animals, and backyard design including such factors as porches, ramps, fences, and picnic tables. Although these solutions were contributed predominantly by parents in rural environments, many are equally applicable to children living in cities.

Other simple technology solutions involve the use of toys with switches. Typically, these toys run on batteries and when activated produce action, sound, visual effects, or tactile sensations (e.g., vibrations). Examples of toys with switches are monkeys that clang their cymbals; dogs that bark, wag their tails, and roll over; trains that travel around tracks chugging and periodically whistling; and a variety of busy boxes. Some switch-activated toys can be purchased in toy stores and do not require adaptation, others can be purchased with switches designed for children with disabilities (e.g., from Ablenet, Inc., or Enabling Devices), and still others must be adapted. An example of the former is a voice-activated, head-mounted water gun. Jean Isaacs described use of this toy by her 10-year-old son, Forrest, who uses a wheelchair for mobility and has limited motor control (Isaacs, 1994). Once the gun was strapped to Forrest's head and the microphone was positioned, he was able to participate independently in a water gun party, soaking peers by looking at them and making a sound.

When a battery-operated toy, game, or appliance does not have a switch that can be operated by a child with a disability, it typically can be easily adapted using the Battery Device Adapter (Ablenet, Inc.). This device is cost effective and can be used to connect a battery-operated device to a switch matched to the child's abilities. A list of addresses of the manufacturers of products and other resources mentioned in this chapter can be found in the Internet Resources at the end of this chapter.

Numerous books and articles are available to assist therapists and parents with the process of selecting, using, and making switches (Cole & Swinth, 2004; Glennen & Church, 1992; Johnston, 2003; Parette, Strother, & Hourcade, 1986; Williams & Matesi, 1988; Wright & Nomura, 1991). In addition, the document "Playing with Switches: Birth Through Two" can be downloaded from the Let's Play! Project at http://letsplay.buffalo.edu. This is an excellent resource that provides a basic discussion of such topics as switches and toys; examples of reactive toys and switches; switch characteristics and considerations; positioning options; and switch interfaces. This web site also identifies companies having switches, adapted toys, and switch interface resources for children with disabilities.

Appropriate application of toys with switches has several advantages. First, compared with higher technology solutions, they are relatively simple and in many cases make it possible for the child to access developmentally appropriate toys. More important, involvement with this type of toy is useful for the chronologically or developmentally young child because it enables the experience of co-occurrence between the child and the environment. Drawing on Piaget's work, Brinker and Lewis postulated that co-occurrences act on the child in four ways. First, co-occurrences orient the organism to attend to the environment. Second, they arouse the organism and help to modulate its state. Third, the detection of co-occurrences leads to a positive affective tone. Fourth, through the operation of memory, they become the aliments for subsequent intentional actions and ultimately for the development of mental structure (1982, p. 3).

Sullivan and Lewis (1993, 2000) described a contingency curriculum and proposed that contingency learning results in promotion of attention to the external environment, a positive emotional response, and a basis for means-end problem solving. Based on their work, Shull, Deitz, Billingsley, Wendel, and Kartin (2004), using single-subject research methods, examined the effects of an evaluation and intervention process involving switch-operated devices for a 6-year-old girl with profound multiple disabilities in a preschool environment. Because this child's impairments included profound mental retardation and cortical blindness, the stimuli chosen to be activated by a switch were a hair dryer blowing warm air and then music. This is congruent with Langley's (1990) emphasis on the importance of matching the type of stimulus to the child's abilities. This child was successful in using switches, and her state modulation was noted to improve when she was participating in these activities.

The use of switch-activated toys and devices is highly appropriate for children starting in substage 3 (4 to 8 months) of the sensorimotor period, during which time children repeat acts involving objects outside of themselves. In the early stages toys and switches can be carefully selected and designed so that gross, random movements produce a result. For example, a large switch, sensitive to lower extremity movement, could be placed under the feet of a child with a severe motor impairment. When the child moves the lower extremities, the switch would activate a music box. As the child matures and develops a beginning understanding of cause and effect, more complex toys can be employed that are activated by more complex access systems such as multiple switch arrays or joysticks. As the child develops, toys should be changed often and should be selected for providing variety. Examples are a tape recorder that plays favorite songs or stories and a remote control car that can be driven at a variety of speeds and in a variety of directions. Through playing with switch-operated toys, children may develop basic skills in such areas as object permanence, cause-effect relationships, and directionality. In addition, they begin to learn that the surrounding environment can be controlled. Since many children with limited motor control are unable to manipulate toys independently at the appropriate stage in development, switch toys can provide a viable alternative, allowing them to play and explore similarly to their peers who are not disabled (Swinth, 1998). The complexity of play with switch toys can be expanded by using them with other materials. For example, a switch-operated toy car can be used to knock down a block tower or bowling pins or to deliver an item to another person, or water and blue and yellow food coloring can be placed in the bowl of a toy electric mixer so the child can create green water (Figure 16-2).

Use of toys with switches has limitations, and therapists are cautioned to avoid misuse. First, for most children developmentally beyond 18 months to 2 years, many of the toys that can be activated with switches are repetitious and become boring after the first few times of use unless combined with other materials. Second, many of these toys typically provide limited opportunities for creativity. Third, use of a variety of switch toys can become costly. Therefore, switch toys are most appropriate for use with children in the early stages of development or as transitional toys leading to play facilitated through higher technology solutions involving computers, communication augmentation systems, environmental control systems, and power mobility (Figure 16-3).

Enhancement of Play Through Computers

Computer use for play or leisure is becoming increasingly common in most school and some home environments. Children who are typically developing, as well as those with disabilities, are being introduced to computers at younger ages. The computer, combined with thoughtfully selected access systems and software, can enhance play or leisure experiences in three ways. First, it can provide simulations of experiences that would be difficult, if not impossible, for the child to engage in without the computer. For example, a child with severe motor impairments may never be able to experience the excitement of a game of chase and capture on the playground or in the neighborhood.

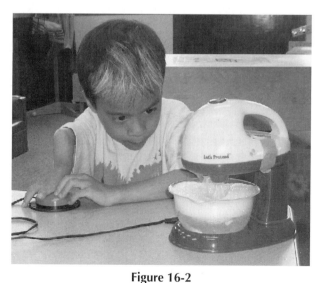

Figure 16-2

The child uses a switch to activate a toy mixer with soap and water in a mixing bowl.

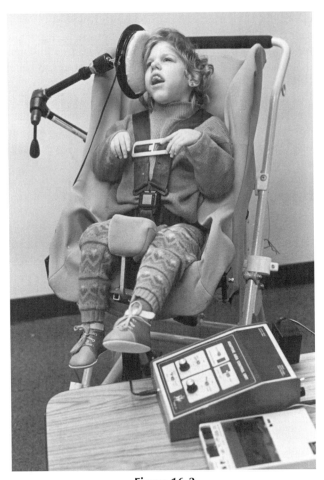

Figure 16-3

The child uses a switch to activate a tape recording of her favorite music. (Courtesy Bruce Terami.)

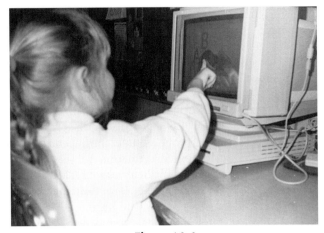

Figure 16-4

The child uses a computer with a Touch Window (Don Johnston Incorporated) to play a simple game.

However, the chasing and capturing can be simulated through computer games, with resultant excitement and intense involvement. Second, the computer and related software provide a variety of play or leisure opportunities unique to the modality (e.g., interactive stories with audiovisual flexibility, adventure challenges, or mysteries involving problem solving). Provided the child with the disability can access the computer, he or she can engage in these play or leisure activities as an equal with peers and adults. Third, the computer and related software can be used to facilitate play between children with and without disabilities, as demonstrated by Spiegel-McGill, Zippiroli, and Mistrett (1989). These researchers used a single-subject alternating treatments design to study the effect of three play conditions (microcomputer play, remote-controlled robot play, play without technology) on the amount of time each of four preschoolers with disabilities interacted with a peer who was socially competent and without disabilities. All of the children were in an integrated preschool. Findings from this study suggested that microcomputers facilitated social interaction for the

two children with significant social and language deficits and physical disabilities. For the two children with only mild social interaction deficits, however, the microcomputer did not appear to enhance social interaction with peers without disabilities.

One of the primary benefits of the computer as an assistive device to enhance play is that it is highly adaptable in terms of both methods of access and types of play activities available through software. Relative to method of access, advances in general input device–emulating interfaces enable alterations to meet the needs of a specific child with a disability (Cook & Hussey, 2002). This may involve both computer hardware and software. Setups may be in the hard disk drive or in a peripheral device such as an adapted keyboard (Cook & Hussey, 2002). Since some children with disabilities are not successful with a standard keyboard or mouse, computer access systems often must be selected and modified to meet individual needs. Categories of computer access include (1) physical keyboard adaptations, such as changes to standard keyboards and expanded or miniature keyboards; (2) virtual keyboards such as Morse code input, voice input, and on-screen keyboards; and (3) mouse emulators such as the Headmaster Plus (Prentke Romich Company), the HeadMouse Extreme (Madenta Communications, Inc.), and the Touch Window (Don Johnston Incorporated) (Figure 16-4). It is important to remember that these alternative access systems are not necessarily compatible with all software selected to enhance play. Some access systems work only with specially designed programs, whereas others are compatible with most standard programs. This latter group, known collectively as keyboard and mouse emulators, allows input from a source other than the standard keyboard or mouse to be interpreted as input from either of these sources. Before an access system is purchased, compatibility with software the child is likely to use should be evaluated.

In addition to being adaptable in terms of access, the computer is ideal because of its adaptability to the types of play activities available through software. These programs range from extremely simple and appropriate for use with very young children to highly complex and challenging for precocious teens. An example of the former is *Baby Smash* (http://bugau.yhps.tn.edu.tw/site/many_kidsplay/down/mac/babysmash.html). When using *Baby Smash* a child can hit any key on the computer keyboard, or use a switch setup, to add graphics (e.g., lightning bolts, circles) to the computer screen while the computer concurrently plays music or makes a sound. In one study by Swinth, Anson, and Deitz (1993), 60% of 20 typically developing 6- through 8-month-old infants demonstrated ability to use a hand switch to access the computer and successfully play an adapted version of the latter cause-effect program. Adaptations involved shortening the time the music played after switch activation so that infants had to reactivate the switch to continue playing. Glickman, Deitz, Anson, and Stewart (1995) studied whether the switch control site (head versus hand) influences the age at which young children can activate a computer to play a cause-effect game. They found that using the head switch was more challenging; less than half of the children from 12 through 17 months were successful with this task. This research suggests that placing the switch outside the child's visual field may make the task more challenging. As a result, therapists should work to keep the switch within the child's visual field if possible.

Examples of highly complex programs are *SimCity Classic* (free online) and *The 3D Adventures of Nancy Drew* (Her Interactive, Inc.). *SimCity Classic* allows participants to create and run their own city, including houses, roads, people, and so on. The Nancy Drew adventures involve the older child or young teen in unraveling mysteries by using problem solving and creative thinking. Because these games require deductive reasoning, involve abstract and hypothetical situations, and necessitate organizing and systematizing, they are appropriate for preteens and teens at Piaget's formal operations stage of development.

Between the extremes are a variety of programs for children with diverse interests and at various developmental levels. Programs such as *KidPix Deluxe 3* (Broderbund) allow a child to use the computer as a crayon or paintbrush to "color" or "paint" a picture or to create with sound art; in *Let's Go to the Circus!* (Voyager), an interactive cartoon, the child engages in activities such as creating a clown face, dressing characters for a parade, and solving problems; and public domain programs such as checkers and solitaire allow a child to play board and card games, either alone or with a peer. For the preteen or teen with low cognitive skills, there are games with a high interest level that involve basic choice making and turn taking. An example of such a game is *Shop 'til You Drop*

(Don Johnson, Inc.). The variety of programs available for use on the same computer make it possible for software to continue to meet a child's needs as he or she develops and interests and capabilities change.

Many web sites offer simple computer games and activities for children from 6 months of age through adolescence. Some of these can be accessed through single-switch systems or adapted keyboards. Many of the activities from these web sites (e.g., Fisher-Price and Disney) are based on common characters encountered by children and adolescents (e.g., Dora, Blue's Clues, Simpsons). There also are online web sites where teenagers can go to play games such as chess or checkers with a friend living in another location.

An additional benefit of the computer is that the Internet allows a school-age child or teen to access more of the world. This capability is particularly beneficial for individuals with severe motor or sensory (e.g., blind, deaf) impairments. Randy Hammer, who is blind, exemplifies effective use of the Internet by a teenager for educational and recreational purposes (Hammer, 1994). Hammer described using the Internet with a screen reader to browse through the newspaper, selecting articles to read for enjoyment. In addition, he described using telnet to access chat systems and "talk to people in California about the earthquakes there" or "ask people in Kansas City about the Chiefs' chances in the Superbowl" (Hammer, 1994, p. 25). He stated that chat systems provide a way to "make new friends" (Hammer, 1994, p. 25).

Enhancement of Play Through Augmentative and Alternative Communication Systems

Communication, both verbal and nonverbal (e.g., gestures, signs), is an important part of play for children. If communication is compromised by impairments, this can limit children's opportunities to engage in play and other relevant occupations. When this occurs, the use of augmentative or alternative communication systems should be considered and the final selection should reflect the child's communication needs. Carefully selected augmentative or alternative communication systems can make it possible for children with communication impairments to take part in a variety of play and leisure activities, such as participating in a game of Simon Says with neighborhood children, engaging in the necessary interactions required for playing a board game with a friend, and sharing stories with peers at lunch.

Augmentative communication and alternative communication do not require oral language skills (Swinth, 2005). The distinction between augmentative and alternative communication is that the former supplements, enhances, or supports oral communication, whereas the latter replaces it (Lewis, 1993). The possibilities for alternative or augmentative communication are numerous. Many children start with simple communication boards or a picture exchange system (PECS). The former typically are boards displaying pictures, letters, words, or word symbols, which the child uses to communicate by pointing or looking at the desired picture or symbol. PECS allows a child to initiate "a communicative act for a concrete outcome within a social context" (Frost & Bondy, 1994). For example, a child using the PECS might give a picture of a desired item or activity to another child or adult in exchange for that item or the opportunity to engage in the activity. There are also simple systems such as the Cheap Talk (Abilitation) that can be programmed to contain multiple messages. For example, a girl who is playing a board game with her peers could have prerecorded messages in her Cheap Talk that say things like "My turn," "I get to go up," and "Please draw a card for me." The ability to communicate allows the child to participate more fully in the activity.

More complex, high-technology solutions involve computerized systems that are operated through special software. Some high-technology solutions, referred to as dedicated systems, involve microcomputers that can be operated only as communication aids (Lewis, 1993). Examples of these are the Pathfinder Plus (Prentke Romich Co.) and the Vantage Plus (Prentke Romich Co.). In other cases portable microcomputers are adapted for use as augmentative or alternative communication aids. In either situation, choices of access and output methods are available. For access, both direct selection (e.g., pointing directly to the desired symbol) and scanning may be considered. For some children direct selection is facilitated with special aids such as mouthsticks or light beam pointers. Scanning, by contrast, is an indirect selection process in which the user is presented with communication aid symbols (i.e., letters, pictures) until the user indicates that the selected symbol is the desired choice. Output methods for high-technology systems vary and can be spoken (i.e., taped speech, synthesized speech), printed, or a combination of both spoken and printed.

Use of communication systems can be frustrating for both the receiver and the speaker for three primary reasons. First, these systems can be difficult to learn to use; second, synthesized speech can be hard to understand; and third, communication using any type of system takes longer than speaking. As a result, selection of an alternative or augmentative communication system for a child or teen should take into consideration both the needs of the user and the anticipated communication partners. For example, if communication partners are likely to be very young children or individuals with poor reading skills or vision, a system with spoken output might be preferable to one that exclusively provides printed output. By contrast, if the primary communication partner has a hearing impairment, printed output may be preferred. It is also important to teach communication partners (even very young children) strategies to facilitate interaction with the individual employing a communication system. With children this can be incorporated with play in such a way that communication via the system augments play, and play using the system ultimately enhances communication skills. Therefore play should be considered in the choice of the type of communication augmentation system for a child and the words and phrases to be included in that system.

In addition to communication devices for use in multiple situations, commercial communication toys that can enhance the play of children with disabilities should be considered. An example of such a device is JokeMaster Jr (Excalibur Electronics, Inc.). The nose on the clownlike face is a switch that when activated results in the telling of a classic children's joke. To hear the joke again, the child presses one of the eyes; to hear a new joke, the child presses the nose again.

Enhancement of Play Through Environmental Control Systems

As previously noted, one of the ways children play is by interacting within their environments. For children with disabilities, such opportunities can be severely limited. However, with the use of environmental controls, possibilities for an increased variety of play and leisure activities become available. Environmental control systems can be simple, involving minor adaptations to one appliance in the home, or they can be complex, involving elaborate control systems and multiple appliances. Whether simple or complex, such systems can make it possible for children to engage in activities such as turning lights on and off, activating a stereo or television, talking on the telephone, and helping to cook in the kitchen. When environmental controls are considered, it is first necessary to determine what parts of the environment it is appropriate and possible for the child to control and what parts of the environment the child desires to control. This requires evaluating the child's environment and daily routine, as well as the child's functional capabilities and motivation. For instance, it is important to know whether the child enjoys music, stories on tape, cookie baking, or television programs. Typically, young children start with single-switch systems that allow them to participate in such activities as "helping mom" mix cookie dough by being in charge of turning the mixer on and off. As the child progresses developmentally, more complex environmental control systems, many of which are microprocessor controlled, can be employed to allow the child or teen to operate multiple appliances (e.g., television, computer, stereo, lights) using a single system. Such systems, whether simple or complex, can help children increase their functional independence and their ability to participate in a broader range of play and leisure activities than would be possible without environmental controls.

Enhancement of Play Through Mobility Devices

Movement is integrally tied to play at all stages of development. Children in the sensorimotor stage of development move (crawl, creep, walk, and run) for the pure pleasure of the experience and as a means of exploring their environments. As the children grow older, movement continues to be an important component in their play. On playgrounds, preschoolers can be observed chasing each other, negotiating playground equipment, and riding toys with wheels. As children reach school age, games requiring movement become more complex in terms of skills required and rules for participating. At all stages of development, if a child's movement is compromised by impairments, alternative methods of mobility are needed for engagement in play and leisure activities.

Both theoretical and research literature supports the introduction of power mobility to very young children with motor impairments (Butler, 1986; Butler, Okamoto, & McKay, 1983, 1984; Campos, Kermoian, & Zumbahlen, 1992; Deitz, Swinth, & White, 2002; Douglas & Ryan, 1987; Kermoian, 1997, 1998; Wright & Kohn, 1993). First, it is an attainable skill for young children that can partially compensate for gross motor movement limitations. Second, it appears to be associated with an increase in self-initiated behaviors, especially those related to spatial exploration and to the sense of independence and competence. Most of the theoretical and research literature relates to children who are typically developing or have disabilities that primarily affect their mobility. By contrast, the work of Deitz and colleagues (2002) focused on the effects of a power mobility riding toy on the participation behaviors of two young children with spastic quadriplegia and developmental delay. Findings indicated that both children were successful in using the power mobility riding toy during gym and recess and that use of the toy had a reliable and clinically important effect on initiation of movement occurrences.

The lack of self-initiated mobility experiences early in life has potential negative consequences. Butler (1986) observed that onset of a passive, dependent pattern "coincided with failure of the normal development of locomotion about 12 months of age, and was increasingly manifested as inhibited locomotion progressively interfered with normal childhood activities" (p. 325). Therefore it seems desirable to explore alternative mobility options as soon as a child's impairment impedes his or her mobility. Some options involve low technology (see Case Example 1 on p. 406), whereas others require high technology. The GO-BOT and Mini-BOT (based on the original Transitional Power Mobility Aid, the Maddak Inc. award winner at the 1994 American Occupational

Therapy Association National Conference [Javernick, 1994]) are examples of the latter. The Mini-BOT, with the ABS Stander (Mobility4kids), can be used by a child as small as 24 inches in height, and even smaller children can be accommodated with specialized positioning devices. Using up to four switches or a joystick, a child can experience self-initiated exploratory mobility and can physically interact with the environment. Advantages of this mobility device are its small size and design features that facilitate access to preschool tabletops and positioning on a level with peers. Wright and Kohn (1993) described use of this device in a mainstreamed preschool classroom by a 3-year-old child with a diagnosis of spinal muscular atrophy, type II. This child had a power wheelchair but would not use it in the classroom because "it positioned her above the level of her peers, and she could not access table top activities" (Wright & Kohn, 1993, p. 29). By contrast, after the first day the Transitional Power Mobility Aid was introduced into the child's classroom, the child moved independently from one tabletop activity to another and her teachers reported an increase in her interactions with peers. This suggests that an important consideration in choice of a mobility device is positioning of the child, both in relation to aspects of the environment that the child wants to access and in relation to peers (Figure 16-5).

A variety of power mobility devices have been designed for children and teens, and new options are being developed regularly. To facilitate play and leisure involvement, the power mobility device should have design features that enable activities in which the child or teen currently wants to engage and potential future activities. For example, a child whose primary concern is vertical positioning might prefer a mobility device such as the Playman Robo (Permobil), which resembles a small forklift. The child can control the vertical position of the seat from an on-floor position to 9 inches of added vertical access above the normal seat position. This ability to control the vertical position of the seat enables the child to play on the floor with peers, to be positioned appropriately at school desks and dining tables, and to access play materials on shelves of varying heights. However, this advantage should be balanced against potential limitations. Its predecessor, the Turbo, was noted as having a relatively large turning radius and a slow maximum speed (Deitz, Jaffe, Wolf, Massagli, & Anson, 1991). In making a final selection, the child, family, and interdisciplinary team should weigh these and other variables and often must establish priorities, since one device typically does not meet all needs.

Another option that has been used successfully for young children, either as a transitional mobility device or as a toy, is an electric car (Figure 16-6), available in toy stores or from sources such as Mobility4kids. These have the advantages of being relatively low in cost, being

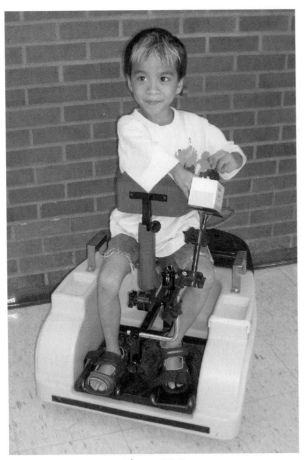

Figure 16-5
A child uses GO-BOT in the preschool classroom.

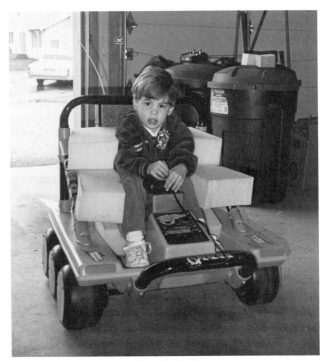

Figure 16-6
A child drives a toy car in the family garage.

easy to transport in the trunk of a large car, being adaptable in terms of positioning and controls, and looking like a toy. The use of a toy as a transitional mobility device not only facilitates play, but also may help the child and family progress to the use of another type of mobility aid. Disadvantages of electric cars are that they tend to be noisy and are less durable than power wheelchairs. However, as mobility toys for use in large spaces (e.g., playgrounds, gyms), electric toy cars allow children with disabilities to join peers in typical childhood games involving moving, bumping, turning, and chasing (see Case Example 3 on p. 406).

As the child gets older, the types of play and leisure activities in which he or she wants to engage should be taken into consideration when manual or power wheelchairs are selected. Some manual and power chair users, especially in the teen years, choose to participate in wheelchair competitive sports such as tennis, basketball, and racing. For manual chair users, participation in these activities can be enhanced by use of lightweight and ultra-lightweight sport wheelchairs weighing from approximately 40 pounds to less than 25 pounds. Many designs allow adjustment of wheel positions and seat heights, making it possible to optimize biomechanical efficiency (Masse,

Lamontagne, & O'Rianin, 1992). An added advantage of these chairs is that they are highly portable, in most cases fitting easily in a car trunk. This makes it possible for a teen with a disability to travel to recreational events (e.g., football games, movies, parties) with peers without requiring special accommodations for transportation.

Enhancement of Play and Leisure Through Adaptive Sports Equipment

Often it is important for children and teens with disabilities to be able to participate in outdoor leisure activities with their families and peers. This can be facilitated through the use of adaptive sports equipment combined with special instruction. Recreational programs for people with disabilities are typically staffed by volunteers and provide equipment, instruction, and transportation for children and teens. As a result of these programs and specialized equipment, children and teens with disabilities can bicycle, water ski, snow ski (both Alpine and Nordic), and sail. For biking there are three major classes of adaptation: (1) hand-powered three wheelers for individuals with lower extremity impairments; (2) foot-powered three wheelers for individuals with balance difficulties; and (3) tandems (either regular tandems or tandems with recumbent seats that provide additional trunk stability and that allow either foot or hand pedaling) for people with sensory or motor impairments or developmental disabilities. Tandems have the advantage that another person can travel on the same bicycle as the individual with the disability, thus allowing participation in the leisure activity while compensating for the individual's impairment (e.g., eyes to see the road, additional strength and endurance to pedal, judgment about traffic).

Adaptive equipment is available for both downhill and cross-country skiers with disabilities. Examples are sit-skis, bi-skis, and mono-skis for people with lower extremity impairments. A variety of adapted poles are suited to individual needs. For example, an individual with a lower extremity amputation can often use one ski aided by adapted poles that circle the forearm like Lofstrand crutches and have small skis on the tips. Similarly, adaptive equipment such as the Kan-Ski (Quickie Designs, Inc.), a wide single ski on which the participant sits, makes it possible for a person with mobility and balance impairments to water ski. The Shake-A-Leg Foundation, operating in several locations in the United States, has been instrumental in adapting sailboats and related facilities to accommodate the needs of people with disabilities, especially those who are normally wheelchair bound. In addition, they provide instruction and support for those interested in participating in recreational or competitive sailing. Other leisure activities such as golf, water skiing, swimming, river rafting, canoeing, hiking, camping, cycling, horseback riding, bowling, basketball, and tennis are offered through adapted programs offered by specialized organizations and local park and recreation departments.

Assistive devices such as those described make it possible for children and teens to participate in a wide range of sports activities. To assist children and teens and their families in exploring options, occupational therapists should be familiar with recreational programs in their communities that provide equipment, evaluation, training, and outings for people with disabilities. In addition, they must be sensitive and responsive to family interests and needs. For example, if a family has a history of downhill skiing and a child is born with spina bifida, it is important to make the family aware of adaptive ski equipment and specialized instruction for people with lower extremity limitations. Instead of either giving up a favorite leisure activity or leaving the child at home, the family can include the child in their winter outings by using adapted equipment (Figure 16-7).

Adapted Cars and Specialized Drivers' Education

Most teenagers look forward to obtaining a driver's license, one of the activities within our society that signals passage to maturity. Driving enlarges the world teens can access independently. For many this skill is perceived as increasing competence and independence and becomes a gateway to a variety of developmentally appropriate

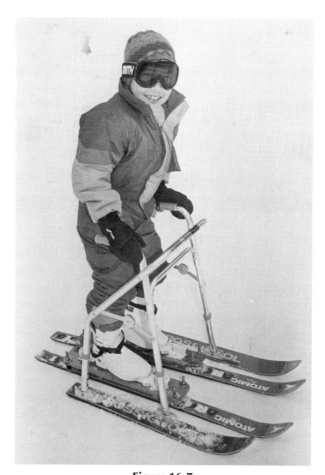

Figure 16-7
A child uses adapted equipment for skiing. (Courtesy Outdoors for All Foundation.)

leisure activities. Therefore, it is important for the sensitive therapist to consider the value that driving has for an older teen with a disability. Driving may require adaptations for vehicles such as ramp and lift systems, reduced-effort steering, and hand controls for accelerating and braking. Drivers' education that is modified to meet individual needs should be considered. If the resources are available and the teenager is able to drive with appropriate adaptations, independent driving may allow the teen to pursue such activities as attending sports events, meeting with peers at community restaurants, and participating in school or church functions. Given the need of teens to establish their independence, the value of driving as opposed to being transported by a parent should not be minimized.

CASE EXAMPLES

The case examples presented in this section involve the use of assistive technology to enhance play experiences for children with disabilities. These vignettes are intended as realistic examples, rather than model solutions, of the application of assistive technology to enhance play and leisure involvement for children and teens at a variety of developmental levels. Many of these vignettes also reflect consideration of multiple factors in the selection and design of assistive technology solutions that are sensitive to the needs of the child or teen and the characteristics of his or her environment. Both low- and high-technology solutions are presented.

CASE EXAMPLE 1

Lynn: 3½ to 7½ Months

Lynn was born with a congenitally dislocated hip and as a result was in a spica cast (extending from waist to ankles) from 3½ to 7½ months of age. As she began to reach for toys, she was frustrated when her attempts resulted in pushing the toys out of her range. Two solutions were effective. First, when prone, Lynn was positioned facing the corner of her crib, within reach of the bumper guard. Toys were positioned between Lynn and the bumper guard. Thus, when Lynn's early attempts to reach a toy resulted in pushing the toy away, the toy was stopped by the bumper guard and stayed within the radius of her reach. The second solution involved rigging a sturdy line from one end of Lynn's crib to the other and then tying a toy to the line in such a way that when Lynn was supine, she could reach the toy but not the ribbon attaching the toy to the line. This was important to avoid injury caused by the ribbon's wrapping around a body part. Typically 10 or more toys were attached to the line at the foot of Lynn's crib. One toy was slid into position for play, and when Lynn tired of that toy, her mother, in the course of doing her housework, slid the present toy to the head of the crib and moved the next toy within reach. This allowed Lynn to play independently for short periods of time and met her needs until she was 6 months old. At that time, when in a prone position, Lynn would try futilely to move forward using her arms. The spica cast was like an anchor. Lynn's unsuccessful attempts resulted in temper tantrums and inconsolable crying. In an attempt to allow Lynn to move independently, she was strapped to a scooter board, positioned so that her shoulders and arms were free. Using this device she happily and independently explored her home environment. These low-technology, low-cost solutions facilitated involvement in developmentally appropriate activities and assisted with state regulation while Lynn was immobilized by her cast. When the spica cast was removed, no further intervention was required and Lynn quickly learned to crawl like other infants her age.

CASE EXAMPLE 2

Suni: 10 Months

Suni, a child with cerebral palsy resulting in quadriplegia, appeared to be cognitively normal. At 10 months of age she was demonstrating an awareness of and interest in her surroundings. When she tried to use her upper extremities to manipulate toys, however, she appeared to be frustrated by her lack of control. As a result, Suni's parents and therapists decided it was time to introduce Suni to simple cause-effect computer games to provide her with play opportunities she could control and with a modality for developing prerequisite computer skills for later use in school. When positioned properly, Suni had adequate upper extremity control to use a touch window as long as refined or accurate motor movements were not required. At the developmental center, Suni appeared to enjoy computer play and did not exhibit the frustration she displayed when attempting to manipulate toys. Through a grant, her parents were able to purchase a computer system for home. Suni's parents reported that playing computer games with Suni became a favorite family activity. Suni appeared to enjoy the mutual interaction, and her siblings reported that they liked being able to play "with" her, rather than doing something "to" her.

The early introduction of assistive technology provided Suni with some control over her environment during play and gave her opportunities to interact with family members and peers during this process. In addition, computer play helped Suni develop some of the prerequisite skills for using the computer for later schoolwork, since it was anticipated that Suni would be more functional at word processing than at writing with a pencil.

CASE EXAMPLE 3

Julia: 5 Years

Julia, a 5-year-old with spinal muscular atrophy, had limited motor control of her upper extremities and no voluntary control of her lower extremities. She attended a regular preschool, where she was the only child with a disability. Julia enjoyed interacting with her peers but became frustrated when her highly mobile classmates moved away from her and she could not follow independently. She had a travel wheelchair, and although her parents and therapists were working on obtaining funding for a power wheelchair, it was anticipated that it would be an additional 9 months before Julia would receive her new chair.

While waiting for funding and for processing of paperwork for Julia's new wheelchair, Julia's therapists and her parents began to look for a transitional method for mobility that would allow her to participate in active play both in the classroom and on the playground. One therapist recommended obtaining and adapting a battery-operated ride-on toy car because it was an age-appropriate toy that Julia could control independently. After being provided with information by the therapist, the family obtained the car and materials necessary for adapting it to meet Julia's needs. These adaptations included the addition of a remote control device with an emergency shutoff button that could be used by the adult supervising Julia while she played in the car, adjustable speed settings for different environments (e.g., slow for the classroom, fast for the playground), a large ball on top of the joystick for Julia to grasp, a foam insert to provide additional trunk control and stability, and a seat belt for safety and support.

Julia quickly adjusted to her car. Since it was low to the ground and she had some control of her upper extremities, she was able to transfer in and out of it independently. Her therapist added a bar on one side of the car that Julia could grasp for stabilization during transfers. Julia appeared to enjoy the car most at recess when she joined her peers who were "driving trikes." The group members would ride in circles, bump into each other, and play chase. Before getting her car, Julia could only observe these activities. It was noted that during car play, Julia began to initiate more interactions with her peers and her peers tended to interact more with her. Nine months later, Julia received her power wheelchair and made the transition to a public school kindergarten class. In that setting Julia used her power wheelchair for mobility during playground games.

CASE EXAMPLE 4
Jamal: 8 Years

It was late summer and Jamal was recovering from a left upper extremity amputation above the elbow. Because of the severity of his injury, plans for fitting and training with a prosthesis were not scheduled for another month. Jamal, an active 8-year-old, was frustrated and bored during this phase and decided that he would like to join his siblings and peers when picking blackberries, playing with Legos, and riding bicycles. He was experiencing difficulty with berrypicking because he could not hold a container for berries and pick at the same time. The therapist cut a large hole in the top of a small plastic bleach bottle, leaving the handle intact; thoroughly cleaned the bottle; and

showed Jamal how he could strap the bottle to his waist using his belt. This freed his hand for picking berries.

Jamal had given up playing with interlocking blocks, his favorite quiet activity, because of inability to stabilize the vehicle or building he was constructing when he attempted to add additional pieces. Jamal's father, working with the therapist, constructed a solid, flat work surface for Jamal and his friends that was covered with base plates so that the object Jamal was building could be attached to the surface and would not slide around each time a new block was added. Jamal's parents also had Jamal's bicycle braking system adapted for right-hand control of both the front and back wheels. These assistive technology solutions helped Jamal engage in play and leisure activities both alone and with his peers during a transitional period. It was anticipated that he would continue to use the interlocking block building surface and bicycle adaptations even after being fitted with the prosthesis.

CASE EXAMPLE 5
David: 12 Years

David, a 12-year-old boy with cerebral palsy and severe quadriparesis, used a power wheelchair for mobility and a Pathfinder (Prentke Romich Company) for communication. David was fully included in all classes at his school and interfaced his Pathfinder with a computer to complete his academic assignments. David, like his sixth-grade peers, began to notice girls and soon had a "girlfriend" who often called him at home. To David's dismay someone always had to hold the phone for him and he could only listen and provide occasional verbalizations. David complained to his parents and therapists that he wanted to talk on the phone "like his friends." As a result, David's family and therapists worked together to develop a system for phone talking. This involved adapting a telephone headset so that it would not interfere with the placement of David's optic light and so that the phone mouthpiece extended toward his light talker. David and his family also put the phone numbers he used most frequently on automatic dial and adapted the latter so David could activate it independently. David still had to be set up on the system, but once set up, he was free to make private phone calls and join in the common preteen leisure activity of talking on the phone.

CASE EXAMPLE 6

Karl: 14 Years

Karl, a freshman in high school who had sustained a head injury during elementary school, valued participation in intramural sports on Tuesdays. Although reminded before leaving for school on Tuesday, by the afternoon Karl would forget the day of the week and take the bus home immediately after school. As a result, he regularly missed out on a favorite activity. So that Karl would remember this variation in his schedule, he was supplied with a watch with an alarm feature. Before school on Tuesdays, Karl's mother would remind Karl about intramural sports. Karl would set his alarm for a preprogrammed time (2 minutes after the dismissal bell at the end of the day). The alarm served as a sufficient reminder that the schedule was different on Tuesdays. This method was chosen rather than having the teacher assume responsibility for reminding Karl because it gave Karl more responsibility for his leisure time activities.

CASE EXAMPLE 7

Dawn: 17 Years

Teenage students with physical disabilities frequently voice frustration that emphasis is placed on therapy and assistive technology to aid in movement around school and participation in academic classes, but little attention is given to extracurricular activities. Dawn, a high school sophomore who had cerebral palsy with triplegia, expressed this concern. When questioned about her desires, Dawn indicated that she was interested in basketball even though she could not play. She decided that the next best thing would be to take statistics for the boys' basketball games. Working with her parents and her therapist, she developed a plan. First, she talked to the basketball coach and found out what would be required to assume the role of "official stats person." The coach was supportive and willing to work with Dawn and her therapist. Because Dawn required use of either a manual chair or an electric scooter for mobility, transportation to and from away games, as well as accessibility to all gyms, was addressed. Next, Dawn and her therapist worked together to develop a "statistics sheet" on the laptop computer that Dawn used with a word prediction program for all written work. During her sophomore year Dawn kept statistics for the junior varsity team; during her junior year she advanced to the varsity team. During her senior year the team went to the state championships and the school ensured that an accessible bus was available

so that Dawn could go as well. She reported that she enjoyed her new circle of friends from basketball and that she wanted to explore other possible ways to get involved in extracurricular activities.

IMPORTANCE OF WORKING AS A TEAM

Most children requiring technology to enable or enhance play experiences also need technology to maximize their participation in other areas of occupational performance (e.g., education, activities of daily living). As a result, these children benefit from integrated technology solutions assessed, developed, and implemented through a team process, with strong parent-professional partnerships (Judge, 2002). According to Carney and Dix (1992), using the interdisciplinary team model fosters a "whole child" approach that takes into consideration intellectual, physical, sensory, and psychosocial factors. In complex situations teams should be composed of a variety of individuals, including but not limited to occupational therapists, rehabilitation engineers, teachers, speech-language pathologists, physical therapists, psychologists, vision specialists, physiatrists, and aides. Most important, the family or care providers and, if possible, the child should be active members of the team. Burnett and Dutton (1994) stated, "Parents can bring a broad knowledge of what has and has not worked for their child in the past, a wealth of experience, a set of family goals and values, and an understanding of how the child communicates" (p. 4). They further contended that parents must be fully involved in the team and the decision-making process and that this involvement increases the likelihood that technology strategies will be carried out at home. For children within the school system, this same level of involvement is important for teachers who are directly involved with these children (Swinth, 1994).

Often, because of the challenges of daily demands related to self-care and school, play and leisure are forgotten. Direct communication with the child or the teen regarding his or her desires related to play and leisure is important. For the chronologically or developmentally young child, this may involve presenting two alternatives and allowing a choice. By contrast, a child who is older and cognitively able can be involved directly in selecting types of play and leisure activities, describing or demonstrating challenges encountered in attempting to engage in those activities, and arriving at possible solutions. Solutions should be sensitive and responsive to preferences of the child and family concerning comfort for the child and the caregiver, energy conservation for the child or teen, the environments in which the child lives (including cultural and ethnic factors), and the flexibility of the device. The assessment process primarily should occur in the child's natural environments and choice of device should be evaluated relative to use in multiple settings, such as the home, school, playground, and community (Judge, 2002) and in relation to compatibility with technology devices likely to be selected for future use or for use in other occupations. For example, for a preschool child who has been using a variety of switch-activated toys, the team might decide that computer games would provide developmentally appropriate and varied play experiences. Because of the cost of computers, when making a selection, the team would need to consider not only the child's immediate play needs, but also potential future uses of the computer (e.g., word processing, drawing).

Attention should be directed to cost and funding issues, the durability of the selected technology in relation to anticipated frequency and length of use, and the availability of repair options and ease of repair. Provisions should be made for training the child, caregivers, and teachers to use the technology; for monitoring progress; and for providing thorough, periodic reevaluation (Cook & Hussey, 2002). The latter is necessary because children change developmentally, their needs may change as a result of disease processes, and they may develop new ideas about what they want to do.

Equally important is the need for therapists to keep abreast of new technology options and the function, capability, and durability of these options. Resources in this process are continuing education programs, vendors, colleagues, individuals who use technology, and ABLEDATA, a comprehensive information source for assistive technology sponsored by the National Institute on Disability and Rehabilitation Research. Regardless of the resources used, therapists are responsible for maintaining current knowledge of technology options and regularly sharing this information with children, their families, and other team members.

DIRECTIONS FOR THE FUTURE

Technology for helping children with disabilities access play is constantly being updated. For example, Bookworm (AbleNet) allows children with disabilities to "read" common children's books, and IntelliTools Classroom Suite can be used to develop a variety of activities for play and interaction with peers. It is hoped that the future will bring more computer games involving creativity. For example, a 5-year-old child may lack the motor capability to engage in imaginative play with a dollhouse equipped with a family, a dog, and furniture. If a program existed for creative dollhouse play, this child could engage in similar imaginative play using the computer. An elaborate dollhouse could be depicted on the screen and surrounded by a variety of options such as a family (including individuals with disabilities), furniture for the living room, furniture for the bedroom, and so forth. By clicking on specific options, the child could move objects to the desired rooms and then arrange the furniture or people. By clicking on a specific section of the dollhouse, a room could be enlarged to allow more detailed play within that room. A paint palette also could be included so that the child could reupholster the couch, dye the mother's hair, or refinish the woodwork. Clicking on kitchen cupboards would open doors to reveal dishes and food. With additional clicks these could be removed from the cupboards and arranged for a dinner party. Clothes for the family could be found in drawers and closets. Switching to another program, the child could build a spaceship with Legos. The possibilities are endless, and the final advantage is that after minutes or hours of play with tiny pieces (e.g., blocks, dollhouse furniture), putting away the toys is like magic, involving only a click.

Virtual reality, "a looking-glass technology that transports the user into an imaginary, three-dimensional universe created with software" (*The New York Times*, April 13, 1994, p. B6), is a technology whose potential for use with children with disabilities is being explored. This technology was originally developed for training pilots and astronauts. In pediatric rehabilitation, virtual reality has been used to help children learn to operate power mobility devices. For example, at the Oregon Research Institute, Christopher, a 5-year-old child with cerebral palsy, participated in wheelchair driver's education in a virtual world. Securely strapped into a power mobility device and wearing a special headset, he used the joystick to "negotiate challenging terrain: grassy fields, pools of mud, long panes of ice" (*The New York Times*, April 13, 1994, p. B6). Others are using virtual reality technology to enable children with disabilities to participate in soccer, basketball, picture painting, and dance (Reid, 2004). Relative to the latter, Reid (2004) proposed a model of playfulness and flow in virtual reality interactions that draws on the work of scholars such as Czikszentmihalyi (1975) and Bundy (1997). Preliminary research, relating to this model and using a projected virtual reality system, suggests that virtual reality experiences may influence a child's beliefs about his or her abilities and a relationship exists between volition and playfulness (Reid, 2004). Qualitative interviews were conducted with 19 children with cerebral palsy who participated in virtual reality play. Some indicated that even though they knew the experiences were not real, the experiences were real to them in their minds and they saw themselves as being soccer players or participants in other activities (Reid, 2004). Although this work is preliminary, it suggests opportunities to extend play experiences for children with disabilities, allowing them to take on roles and explore environments (e.g., the woods, the mountains, an ocean beach, the streets of a city) otherwise not open to them. The extent to which this technology will open doors to more play and leisure options for children and teens with disabilities is limited only by funding constraints and the creativity and motivation of software developers (Figure 16-8).

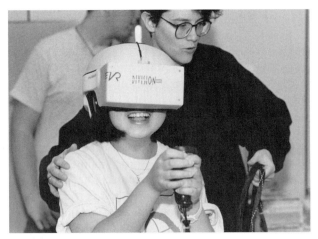

Figure 16-8

A teen uses a virtual reality system to "chase sharks." (Courtesy Mary Levin, DO-IT Project, University of Washington, Seattle.)

Review Questions

1. What is assistive technology, and how can it be used to facilitate the participation of a child with a disability in play and leisure activities? Explain why this is important.

2. Discuss three frameworks to guide the assistive technology assessment process, and apply one of these to a case example.

3. Discuss how simple toy and environmental adaptations can be made to enhance the play of children with a variety of disabilities.

4. Describe several ways that computer use can enhance the play of children and teens with disabilities.

5. Differentiate between augmentative and alternate communication, and describe how each can contribute to the play and leisure experiences of children with disabilities.

6. What types of activities can environmental control systems and mobility devices make possible for children with disabilities? Provide specific examples of each.

7. Discuss equipment adaptations that can enhance the potential of children and teens to engage in sports.

8. Relative to assistive technology and play or leisure, explain the role and responsibilities of the therapist on the interdisciplinary team.

REFERENCES

American Occupational Therapy Association (2002). Occupational therapy practice framework: Domain and process. *American Journal of Occupational Therapy, 56,* 609-639.

American Occupational Therapy Association. (2004). Assistive technology within occupational therapy practice. *American Journal of Occupational Therapy, 58,* 678-679.

Brinker, R. P., & Lewis, M. (1982). Discovering the competent handicapped infant: A process approach to assessment and intervention. *Topics in Early Childhood Special Education, 2,* 1-15.

Bundy, A. (1997). Play and playfulness: What to look for. In L. D. Parham & L. S. Fazio (Eds.), *Play in occupational therapy for children* (pp. 52-66). St. Louis: Mosby.

Burnett, S., & Dutton, D. (1994). Responsiveness to consumers. *Technology Special Interest Section Newsletter, 4*(2), 3-4.

Butler, C. (1986). Effects of powered mobility on self-initiated behaviors of very young children with locomotor disability. *Developmental Medicine and Child Neurology, 28,* 325-332.

Butler, C., Okamoto, G., & McKay, T. (1983). Powered mobility for very young disabled children. *Developmental Medicine and Child Neurology, 25,* 472-474.

Butler, C., Okamoto, G., & McKay, T. (1984). Motorized wheelchair driving by disabled children. *Archives of Physical and Medical Rehabilitation, 65,* 95-97.

Campos, J., Kermoian, R., & Zumbahlen, M. (1992). Socioemotional transformations in the family system following infant crawling onset. In N. Eisenberg & R. Fabes (Eds.), *New directions for child development: No. 55. Emotion and its regulation in early development* (pp. 25-40). San Francisco: Jossey-Bass.

Carney, J., & Dix, C. (1992). Integrating assistive technology in the classroom and community. In G. Church & S. Glennen (Eds.). *The handbook of assistive technology* (pp. 207-240). San Diego: Singular Publishing Group.

Cole, J., & Swinth, Y. L. (2004). Comparison of the touch-free switch to a physical switch, children's abilities and preferences: A pilot study. *Journal of Special Education Technology, 19*(2), 19-30.

Cook, A. M., & Hussey, S. M. (2002). *Assistive technologies: Principles and practice.* St. Louis: Mosby.

Cotton, N. (1984). Childhood play as an analog to adult capacity to work. *Child Psychiatry and Human Development, 14,* 135-144.

Cziksentmihalyi, M. (1975). *Beyond boredom and anxiety.* San Francisco: Jossey-Bass.

Deitz, J., Jaffe, K. M., Wolf, L. S., Massagli, T. L., & Anson, D. (1991). Pediatric power wheelchairs: Evaluation of function in the home and school environments. *Assistive Technology, 3,* 24-31.

Deitz, J., Swinth, Y., & White, O. (2002). Powered mobility and preschoolers with complex developmental delays. *American Journal of Occupational Therapy, 56,* 86-96.

Douglas, J., & Ryan, M. (1987). A preschool severely disabled boy and his powered wheelchair: A case study. *Child: Care, Health and Development, 13,* 303-309.

Frost, L. A., & Bondy, A. S. (1994). *PECS: The picture exchange communication system training manual.* Cherry Hill, NJ: Pyramid Educational Consultants.

Glennen, S., & Church, G. (1992). Adaptive toys and environmental controls. In G. Church & S. Glennen (Eds.), *The handbook of assistive technology* (pp. 173-205). San Diego: Singular Publishing Group.

Glickman, L., Deitz, J., Anson, D., & Stewart, K. (1995). The effect of switch control site on computer skills of infants and toddlers. *American Journal of Occupational Therapy, 50,* 545-553.

Greenstein, D. (1993). *Backyards and butterflies.* Ithaca, NY: New York State Rural Health and Safety Council.

Hammer, R. (1994). Overcoming challenges via the Internet. *Windows on Computing, 15,* 25-26.

H.R. Rep. No. 100-819, 100th Congress, 2d Session (1988).

In virtual reality, tools for the disabled. (1994, April 13). *The New York Times*, p. B6.

Isaacs, J. (1994). Forrest pumps: A sound-activated water gun works without adaptations. *Exceptional Parent, 24,* 40-41.

Javernick, J. (1994, Sept. 1). Maddak Inc. awards OT practitioners' creativity. *O.T. Week, 8,* 62.

Johnston, S. (2003). Making the most of single switch technology: A primer. *Journal of Special Education Technology, 18,* 47-50.

Judge, S. (2002). Family-centered assistive technology assessment and intervention practices for early intervention. *Infants & Young Children, 15,* 60-68.

Kermoian, R. (1997). Locomotion experience and psychological development in infancy. In J. Furumasu (Ed.), *Pediatric powered mobility: Developmental perspectives, technical issues, clinical approaches* (pp. 7-21). Arlington, VA: Rehabilitation Engineering and Assistive Technology Association of America.

Kermoian, R. (1998). Locomotor experience facilitates psychological functioning: Implications for assistive mobility for young children. In D. Gray, L. Quatrano, & M. Lieberman (Eds.), *Designing and using assistive technology: The human perspective* (pp. 251-268). Baltimore: Paul H. Brookes.

Lane, S., & Mistrett, S. (2002). Let's play! Assistive technology interventions for play. *Young Exceptional Children, 5,* 19-27.

Langley, M. B. (1990). A developmental approach to the use of toys for facilitation of environmental control. *Physical & Occupational Therapy in Pediatrics, 10,* 69-91.

Lewis, R. B. (1993). *Special education technology.* Pacific Grove, CA: Brooks Cole Publishing.

Masse, L. C., Lamontagne, M., & O'Rianin, M. D. (1992). Biomechanical analysis of wheelchair propulsion for various seating positions. *Journal of Rehabilitation Research and Development, 29,* 12-28.

Missiuna, C., & Pollock, N. (1991). Play deprivation in children with physical disabilities: The role of the occupational therapist in preventing secondary disability. *American Journal of Occupational Therapy, 45,* 882-888.

Parette, H., Strother, P., & Hourcade, J. (1986). Microswitches and adaptive equipment for severely impaired students. *Teaching Exceptional Children, 19,* 15-18.

Piaget, J. (1952). *The origins of intelligence in children.* New York: International Universities Press.

Reid, D. (August, 2004). A model of playfulness and flow in virtual reality interactions. *Presence, 13,* 451-462.

Shull, J., Deitz, J., Billingsley, F., Wendel, S., & Kartin, D. (2004). Assistive technology programming for a young child with profound disabilities: A single-subject study. *Physical & Occupational Therapy in Pediatrics, 24*(4), 47-62.

Simon, C. J., & Daub, M. M. (1993). Knowledge bases of occupational therapy, Section 2A: Human development across the life span. In H. L. Hopkins & H. D. Smith (Eds.), *Occupational therapy* (pp. 95-130). Philadelphia: J. B. Lippincott.

Spiegel-McGill, P., Zippiroli, S. M., & Mistrett, S. G. (1989). Microcomputers as social facilitators in integrated preschools. *Journal of Early Intervention, 13,* 249-260.

Sullivan, M., & Lewis, M. (1993). Contingency, means-end skills, and the use of technology in infant intervention. *Infants & Young Children, 5,* 58-77.

Sullivan, M., & Lewis, M. (2000). Assistive technology for the very young: Creating responsive environments. *Infants & Young Children, 12,* 34-52.

Swinth, Y. (1994, September). The role of the special education team in selecting and implementing assistive technology. *School System Special Interest Section Newsletter, 1,* 1-3.

Swinth, Y. (1998). Assistive technology in early intervention: Theory and practice. In J. Case-Smith (Ed.), *Pediatric occupational therapy and early intervention* (2nd ed., pp. 277-298). Woburn, MA: Butterworth-Heinemann.

Swinth, Y. (2005). Assistive technology: Low technology, computers, electronic aids for daily living, and augmentative communication. In J. Case-Smith (Ed.), *Occupational therapy for children* (5th ed., pp. 615-656). St. Louis: Elsevier.

Swinth, Y., Anson, D., & Deitz, J. (1993). Single-switch computer access for infants and toddlers. *American Journal of Occupational Therapy, 47,* 1031-1038.

Swinth, Y. L., & Tanta, K. J. (2003). Play and leisure skill development in school-based practice. In Y. Swinth (Ed.), *Occupational therapy in school-based practice: Contemporary issues and trends* (online course). American Occupational Therapy Association.

Williams, S., & Matesi, D. (1988). Therapeutic intervention with an adapted toy. *American Journal of Occupational Therapy, 42,* 673-676.

Wisconsin Assistive Technology Initiative. (2004). *The W.A.T.I. assessment package.* Retrieved July 17, 2005, from http://www.wati.org/Materials/assessments.html.

World Health Organization. (2001). *International classification of functioning, disability and health (ICF).* Geneva, Switzerland: Author.

Wright, C., & Kohn, J. G. (1993). A transitional powered mobility aid for a toddler with quadrimembral limb deficiency and a preschooler with spinal muscular atrophy. *Journal of the Association of Children's Prosthetic-Orthotic Clinics, 28,* 28-29.

Wright, C., & Nomura, M. (1991). *From toys to computers: Access for the physically disabled child.* Available from C. Wright, P. O. Box 700242, San Jose, CA 95170.

Zabala, J. S. *The SETT framework revisited—SETTing the stage for success: Building success through effective selection and use of assistive technology systems.* Retrieved July 18, 2005, from http://swebuky.edu/~jszaba0/SETT2.html.

INTERNET RESOURCES

This list is provided to assist therapists in locating available resources. It is not exhaustive, nor does it represent an endorsement of companies or products.

Abilitation
www.abilitations.com

ABLEDATA (Information source for assistive technology)
http://www.abledata.com/

AbleNet, Inc.
http://www.ablenetinc.com/

Broderbund
http://www.broderbund.com/

Don Johnston Incorporated
http://www.donjohnston.com/

Dragonfly Toy Company Special Needs Store
http://www.dragonflytoys.com/

Enabling Devices
http://enablingdevices.com/home.aspx

Excalibur Electronics, Inc.
http://www.excaliburelectronics.net

Good to Grow: Helping *all* Kids Develop Through Play
http://www.goodtogrowtoys.com

Her Interactive, Inc.
http://www.herinteractive.com/prod/index.shtml

IntelliTools, Inc.
http://www.intellitools.com/

Madenta Communications Inc.
http://www.madenta.com/

Mobility4kids
http://mobility4kids.com/

Permobil Inc.
http://www.permobil.com/default.aspx?id=4

Play Sheets. Let's Play! Project.
http://letsplay.buffalo.edu/

Prentke Romich Company
http://www.prentrom.com/

Resources for Assistive Technology in Education
http://sweb.uky.edu/~jszaba0/JoyZabala.html

Riverdeep, Inc.
http://rivapprod2.riverdeep.net/portal/page?_pageid=336,
1&_dad=portal&_schema=PORTAL

RJ Cooper & Associates: Software and Hardware for Persons
with Special Needs
http://www.rjcooper.com/index.html

Shake-A-Leg, Inc.
http://www.shakealeg.org/

Sunburst Communications
http://store.sunburst.com/

Tots-n-Tech
http://www.asu.edu/clas/tnt/

Toys and Playtime Tips for Children with Special Needs
http://www.fisher-price.com/US/special_needs/default.asp

Voyager, Matra-Hachette Multimedia (no web address
available)
1 Bridge Street
Irvington, NY 10533-9919

Wisconsin Assistive Technology Initiative
http://www.wati.org/

17

Facilitating Play in Early Intervention

SHELLY J. LANE AND SUSAN MISTRETT

KEY TERMS

early intervention
universal design
sensorimotor play
symbolic play
functional play
constructive play
dramatic play
games-with-rules

Previous chapters in this text have already established that play and childhood are concepts so closely aligned that to consider one without the other is impossible. Research indicates a clear connection between early play experiences and cognitive (Russ, Robins, & Christiano, 1999; Singer, Singer, Plaskon, & Schweder, 2003), social (Klugman & Smilansky, 1990; Krafft & Berk, 1998), and physical development (Marcon, 2003). As early as 1948, the United Nations Declaration of the Rights of the Child declared play to be a basic right of children that takes its place along with other rights such as nutrition, housing, health care, and education. More than just a recreational activity, play is the way for children to explore, learn and develop; it is their primary occupation (Parham & Primeau, 1997).

Perhaps more to the point, play is the foundation for development in early childhood, from birth to 3 years. As the first months and years of development unfold for children, it is apparent that play is the central focus of their universe. They move between exploration and play as they attain the developmental milestones that are associated with self-care, gross and fine motor skills, and cognitive and communication abilities. The language of play is at the heart of development. Young children play with their food long before they learn the skill of eating, playing with their fingers becomes a pastime in and of itself, exploration of body parts and playing with feet and toes can keep them engaged for long minutes, and language evolves as they play with the production of sound. Play is the primary occupation in these early years. It is not balanced with the other occupations of self-care and "work" but instead forms the core for development of these other occupations.

PLAY IN EARLY INTERVENTION

Unfortunately, many infants and toddlers with disabilities have too few opportunities to play. The motor control needed for playing with finger foods or toes is challenged by the presence of spasticity or athetosis; the production of sound is delayed by the same motor issues and conditions. Play with peers is absent because the child with a disability may not have the necessary social skills to enable him or her to play and interact. This "play deprivation" has been shown to negatively affect the development of physical, cognitive, communication, and social skills that lay the foundation for other occupational performance (Lindquist, Mack, & Parham, 1982; Missiuna & Pollock, 1991). The child's natural tendency to play may also be forestalled by a prevailing paradigm in early intervention programs that emphasizes therapeutic interventions instead of play (Bergen, 1991). A dichotomy therefore exists between the development of children without disabilities, which is play based using exploration and discovery learning, and the development of children with disabilities, which becomes skill based, using professional direction for therapeutic intervention. Mastering specific skills is one of the benefits of play, but other outcomes include the intermingling of emotional, intellectual, social, and physical development, which requires an accumulation of experiences (Zigler, Singer, & Bishop-Josef, 2004). These additional outcomes are lost when intervention is directed toward skill development and not play.

This dichotomy in developmental trajectory between children with and without disability highlights what should be the uniqueness of the intent of early intervention (EI) and presents interesting challenges. EI must emphasize the benefits of play to a child's overall development as opposed to specific skill attainment. In many ways this parallels the DIR model developed by Greenspan and Weider (2001). In their model "D" is developmental levels, "I" is individual differences, and "R" is relationships. This model is one in which parent-child interaction is the key to the developmental progression of the child. The DIR model of intervention emphasizes following the child's lead by reading and following cues; it is not prescriptive for skills the child is seen as lacking. With young children, these interactions encapsulate playfulness. As an extension of this model of interaction, we suggest that play must be emphasized for play's sake, not solely, or even primarily, as an enticement or reward in therapy.

The challenges presented to practitioners are several. First, practice must become playful. Practitioners must validate the importance of play, embrace play as worthy of their time and energy, and address it as an important goal in and of itself. Practitioners must also be knowledgeable about both typical play and play for children with disabilities. Second, practitioners must come to grips with the fact that in EI the parent is the primary agent of change, not the practitioner. Practitioners serve as consultants, advisors, facilitators, or guides for parents, not as experts to whom parents turn over their children. Third, any move toward change must take place as an integral part of the context of everyday family life. Giving parents home therapy programs takes them away from their roles as parents and caregivers and turns the home environment into a clinic. Providing parents with a basis for and ideas about play and interaction with their child, which fit within their natural environments, increases the number of activities in which children with disabilities can interactively engage. This significantly increases the number of developmental and learning opportunities for these children (Dunst, Bruder, Trivette, Raab, & McLean, 1998; Dunst, Hamby, Trivette, Raab, & Bruder, 2000). If parents and caregivers increase their capacity to understand and promote successful play activities, a more compelling issue is addressed: what play opportunities can offer children that direct therapeutic intervention cannot.

Getting to this point of being truly play focused and family-caregiver-parent centered, providing play opportunities within real-life contexts that truly meet the child's and family's needs, can be difficult when children have significant disabilities. With a typically developing child it may be enough to introduce a toy, demonstrate its potential, and be available to scaffold for the child as he or she explores and plays. For the child with disabilities additional supports are often needed. Other authors in this book (see Chapters 15, 16, and 18) have suggested the use of assistive technology (AT) as a means to promote play. AT provides an appropriate platform for the promotion of play in EI as well.

UNIVERSAL PLAY

The need for play in early childhood is universally acknowledged. Understanding the universality of play as the occupation of all young children sets play in a developmental context. All children need opportunities not only to play but to play inclusively with other children. Universal design (UD) defines an inclusive approach that uses multisensory, multimodal experiences as a vehicle to discovering and learning (Division for Early Childhood [DEC], 2005). This design implies a choice—some element of the experience is beneficial to everyone. Individuals with wide-ranging abilities (cognitive, physical, social communicative), levels of interest, levels of maturity, learning styles, and cultural identities can access the materials and experience and have fun doing it. UD must be an important consideration when the therapist is identifying toys and environments for play opportunities. Instead of specialized toys for children with disabilities and mass manufactured toys for able-bodied children, universally designed toys can be selected to enable all children to play with the same toys. The end product of this approach is that children with and without disabilities play together, and in the long run all developmental needs of young children with disabilities are addressed.

The "universal" in UD does not imply one optimal solution for everyone. Rather, it reflects an awareness of the unique nature of each child and the need to accommodate differences, creating learning experiences that suit the child and maximize his or her ability to progress. UD can greatly increase a toy's general usability by more children. Beyond designing for children with visual impairments or for children who use toys on their wheelchair tray, the makers of UD toys also consider differences in strength, intellectual ability, and interest. For this purpose, toys should have built-in adaptable features. Children and families do not like the medical or specialized appearance of toys designed for children with disabilities. They are seen as "stigmatizing," promoting a negative self-concept. Changes are needed in the way therapists think about the design of toys (to look at play stages, not ages) and identify age-appropriate toys that provide successful play opportunities for all children. Toys should include strong esthetic qualities, as well as accessible, usable, flexible features.

A Model in Support of Universal Play

Infused across all aspects of the universal play approach to EI are the strategies that fuel it. A play focus is only as good as the strategies that underlie how to initiate, sustain, and expand a playful interaction. Inherent in family-centered services are the strategies that include the family at the core of intervention. Essential to the choice of AT supports are the strategies that go into the appropriate choice of AT and its application.

Figure 17-1 provides an overview of the process to be presented in this chapter. The provision of play opportunities to young children with disabilities requires that practitioners engage in a paradigm shift that allows validation of the importance of play. Furthermore, they must be knowledgeable about play stages. Practitioners learn to recognize the available supports for, and barriers to, play for children with disabilities and to develop strategies to address these barriers. These strategies include AT and play materials as tools and weave play into the family context and child environments.

In spite of the well-established importance of play as the primary way children learn, play is often absent or minimal in the lives of young children with disabilities. A growing concern about this absence has caused a number of researchers to call for investigation into the enhancement of play opportunities for children with disabilities (Fewell & Kaminski, 1988; Lane & Mistrett, 2002; Linder, 1993; Sutton-Smith, 1994). The following section discusses three play barriers that have a considerable impact on young children with disabilities.

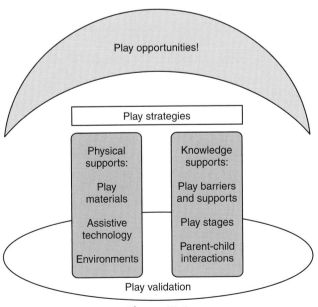

Figure 17-1

Model to support universal play.

BARRIERS TO PLAY FOR YOUNG CHILDREN WITH DISABILITIES
Disabilities as a Play Barrier

For children with disabilities, learning to play can be as difficult to accomplish as developing the ability to eat, bathe, walk, or talk, putting them at a distinct disadvantage when it comes to development. Mobility problems make it difficult, if not impossible, to play hide-and-seek; visual impairments impede a child's ability to find and explore toys on a tray; cognitive disabilities limit the development of pretend play. In fact, any of these disabilities, physical, cognitive, and sensory, pose barriers to spontaneous engagement in play and playful activities (Lane & Mistrett, 1997). Overall, play repertoires of children with disabilities are more limited, play is more often passive and sedentary (Florey, 1971), fewer initiations occur during play (Brodin, 1999), and play occurs less frequently (Li, 1981). In addition, children with disabilities more often engage in solitary play (Bergen, 1991; Jennings, Connors, Stegman, Sankaranarayan, & Mendelsohn, 1985), or play in which social interaction is frequently delayed or distorted, and pretend is often significantly limited (Bergen, 1991; Missiuna & Pollock, 1991). These play deficits can result in serious delays in the attainment of developmental milestones (Brinker & Lewis, 1984; Lindquist, Mack, & Parham, 1982; Missiuna & Pollock, 1991).

A child's disability therefore results in a mismatch between a natural drive to play and the child's ability to play. This mismatch should be as disturbing as any barrier to development. If play is indeed critical to child development, children with disabilities, who are lacking in successful play opportunities, are at increased risk for developmental delays. Yet little research exists regarding the process by which play is best introduced into the lives of these young children.

Service Delivery Framework in Early Intervention as a Barrier

A second barrier to play may be embedded in the very programs designed to support young children. EI programs, established by laws (Education for All Handicapped Children Act Amendments of 1986; Individuals with Disabilities Education Act [IDEA] Amendments of 1990, 1997, and 2004) to provide services to young children and their families, have the goals of enhancing the development of infants and toddlers with disabilities and minimizing their potential for developmental delay. To do so, these programs are charged to enhance the capacity of families to meet the special needs of their infants and toddlers with disabilities (IDEA, 2004) within their natural environments. Most recent data indicate that 80% of EI services are provided in the home (U. S. Department of Education, 2002) where the parents are the primary caregivers, the "experts" regarding their children (Baird & Petersen, 1997). This emphasis underscores that these first years are a period of time in which children's development is intrinsically tied to their interactions with parents and caregivers.

Unfortunately, the role of play in development has been undervalued in EI programs. Primary intervention efforts to date reflect a child-focused, direct teaching framework in which the child's development has been assumed to be linked to participation in intervention-designed instructional activities (McBride & Peterson, 1997; McWilliam, Tocci, & Harbin, 1995; Sandall, McLean, & Smith, 2000). In this prevalent model of skill-based intervention, the provider works directly with the child and is the key agent of change even in the home environment; little is done to promote parent-child relationships in natural environments. The parent is encouraged to implement the intervention activities at home (i.e., as a carryover aide). Research (Fewell & Wheeden, 1998; Mahoney, Boyce, Fewell, Spiker, & Wheeden, 1998) indicates, however, that the effectiveness of intervention is fundamentally dependent on parent-child interactions that are characterized by high parental responsiveness and moderate to low directiveness. In fact, these studies support a high correlation between the manner in which parents interact with their children and the rate of developmental growth during the early years of life (Beckwith & Cohen, 1989; Bradley, 1989). These findings suggest that EI programs might find more success in promoting development by encouraging parents to become more responsive to their children (Spiker, Boyce, & Boyce, 2002) in daily activities. EI providers, however, have had little training on how to implement relationship-focused interactions (Mahoney & Wheeden, 1997; McBride & Peterson, 1997), such as play.

Parents of Children with Disabilities as a Barrier

Parents may unconsciously act to create additional barriers to play. Research suggests that mothers of children with disabilities play less with, and are more controlling of, their children than are mothers of typically developing children (Hanzlik, 1989; Hanzlik & Stevenson, 1986; Kogan & Tyler, 1973). Parents' safety concerns may also act to limit the play activity of their children. Perceptions of their child's inability to handle situations safely may actually limit access to play situations and environments and further impede development (Rogers, 1988b). Many parents have expressed their helplessness in being unable to play if their child has a disability (Hamm, Mistrett, & Ruffino, in press; Mistrett, 2000). They are often unaware of how to respond in ways that increase their child's playful interactions. Nonetheless, their ability to be responsive is critical to promote development through the active engagement of their child (Kim & Mahoney, 2004).

Given the barriers to play, children with disabilities may depend more on adults to provide physical supports in planning for interactive engagement and selecting usable toys. Play for children with disabilities can be facilitated through technology-based supports (Behrmann, Jones, & Wilds, 1989; Daniels, Sparling, Reilly, & Humphry, 1995; Swinth, Anson, & Deitz, 1993). Children with disabilities do not need separate experiences but can flourish with their typical peers when accessible or universally designed toys, within nurturing and supportive environments, are suggested to families by knowledgeable practitioners.

STRATEGIES FOR UNDERSTANDING PLAY AND PLAY STAGES
Play Stages

Attempts to define play generally include the following as essential characteristics: intrinsic motivation, self-direction, freedom to suspend reality, freedom from external rules, and active engagement (Florey, 1971; Musselwhite, 1986; Pellegrini & Boyd, 1993; Takata, 1971; Wright & Nomura, 1985). These characteristics can be applied to play contexts in which toys are present. Piaget identified a developmental sequence of play stages that included sensorimotor, symbolic, and game play. Sensorimotor play predominates during the first 2 years of life and is characterized by practice and repetition. Symbolic play may be seen in the first year of life but blossoms during the second and third years. Although Piaget maintained that early play is strictly object oriented, other investigators have suggested that social play is apparent in young infants in such games as peekaboo and lays the groundwork for later social skills (Brown & Bergen, 2002; Parten, 1932). Smilansky (1968) elaborated on the original Piaget categories and labeled them as follows: (1) functional play—simply repetitive muscle movements with or without objects; (2) constructive play—manipulation of objects to construct or to "create" something; (3) dramatic play—the substitution of an imaginary situation to satisfy the child's personal wishes and needs; and (4) games-with-rules—the acceptance of prearranged rules and the adjustment to these rules. In each stage play progresses from undifferentiated exploration or manipulation to more specific object manipulation (Vondra & Belsky, 1989).

The progression from exploration to object manipulation can provide practitioners with an expanding framework from which to view early play. Findings from the Let's Play! Projects have led Mistrett and Goetz-Ruffino to propose sensory exploration and functional play as separate play stage levels within the sensorimotor play stage (Universal Design for Play, U.S. Department of Education, 2003-2005). Initially objects are explored in nondifferentiated ways through the senses and simple manipulation. In functional play the child progresses to understanding how a toy is used (e.g., pressing buttons on a phone), combining two or more objects (e.g., pouring sand into buckets with a shovel), and beginning self-imitative play (e.g., pretending to drink from a cup) (Belsky & Most, 1981). The child then begins to demonstrate an ability to plan, coordinate, and create within the constructive and pretend (dramatic) play stages, moving again from simple to complex interactions.

The development of play in children with disabilities generally follows the same sequence as that in typically developing children, but developmental pace is often delayed and the quality of play may be reduced (Gowen, Johnson-Martin, Goldman, & Hussey, 1992; Johnson & Ershler, 1985). Children with disabilities engage in more manipulative play, and pretend play may be significantly delayed (Rogers, 1988a; Sigmon & Ungerer, 1984) because of sensory, cognitive, and physical limitations. In defining the play stages most relevant to children from ages birth to 3 years, Table 17-1 offers descriptions of play stages found to be applicable to EI.

When practitioners can describe observable behaviors associated with a child's play stage to the family, a clearer understanding of the child's development emerges. With this approach the family is focused on what the child can do and what interests him or her at a certain stage, emphasizing developmental play sequence. Changes in play behaviors can be noted when families apply strategies to playful interactions. When families understand "what comes next," they can feel more secure in their own ability to gradually apply new strategies and take note of ongoing changes in play behaviors.

Constructing Play Environments

Infants and toddlers grow and learn through sensory and motor explorations by interacting with people and things in their natural environment and watching what happens (DEC, 2005). A number of conditions within the play environment can influence how young children play (Quilitch & Risley, 1973; Smith & Connolly, 1980). These include the way in which the environment is arranged, the quantity, variety, and complexity of toys available, and the presence of peers and adults. The arrangement and design of the environment must be planned to promote interactive play. According to Winter, Bell, and Dempsey (1994), play environments for children with disabilities need access (physical entry), activity (engagement in play), and variability (ability to make choices). The caregiver uses space, relationships, materials, and routines as resources for constructing an interesting, secure, and enjoyable environment that encourages play, exploration, and learning. The setting should attract and encourage the child to interact with other children and with objects. The floors, ceiling, lighting, walls, and furniture all contribute to the child's education about the world.

Practitioners must offer families strategies that reinforce their ability to create enticing environments. When children feel comfortable in their surroundings, they will venture to explore materials and events around them. Inviting play environments include the following features:

- The environment should make children feel safe and secure; both caregivers and children should be relaxed for play to occur.
- The room arrangement should be interesting and allow children to find things easily; how materials are arranged will encourage independence and playful interactions.
- Spaces should engage children's large and small muscles, captivate their senses, and activate their curiosity (Lally & Stewart, 1990). Children should be able to adapt the environment to suit their play.

Table 17-1
Play Stages

Play Stage	Description
Sensorimotor play	Sensory exploration level: The young child uses his or her senses to "explore" objects in the same undifferentiated way with repetitive movements. She or he may repeat movements with two objects (bang cup and spoon together) for sensory response.
	Functional play level: The child manipulates objects in a functional manner (e.g., pressing keys on a keyboard, activating a busy box), and then combines objects (puts balls into and out of containers). Self-directed imitation begins (holds cup to mouth).
Constructive play	The child begins to sort and build with various objects. Materials are used in simple and then more complex ways. Creative expression begins to emerge.
Pretend play	The child begins to create situations (drives a car to a gas station, gives "medicine" to a "sick" friend). The child engages in pretend play in which objects take on new purposes (boxes become cars).

When universal play principles are applied to environments, the space created does not segregate or stigmatize or prevent individuals from using it independently but does benefit all children, including those who have needs that are traditionally not considered.

Selecting Play Materials

Recognizing the child's and family's need for more successful play opportunities, a knowledgeable practitioner will be able to guide parents to identify commercial toys with accessible, adjustable, and flexible features. This is where the principles of UD come into play. However, locating well-designed toys for children with disabilities to use is often difficult for families. Given that children with disabilities often use toys to guide the play activity itself (Brodin, 1999), how a child is able to interact with a toy is of vital importance in influencing whether or not the toy will lead to development (Woodroffe & Willatt, 1976). Frustration can ensue when toys are too difficult to operate; the toys then become an obstacle, not a facilitator of play (Bradley, 1985).

Families are often at a loss when they need to purchase toys. They find it difficult to select toys that their child will like and can use. Often they turn to specialty toy catalogues designed for children with disabilities, which do not allow the parents and children to touch or see the actual item. These toys are considerably more expensive and often less well made. They may look very different from off-the-shelf toys, which points out the differences of the children who will use them. These specialized toys may further widen the gap between the lives of families with children with disabilities and other families.

It is the role of practitioners to guide families in the selection of UD toys that are planned and constructed for all children, including those with disabilities. Although there are no specific features to look for in UD toys, certain elements embedded into the design of toys will allow more children to successfully interact and play with the toy. In the design of a flexible, adjustable, usable toy, multiple options must be present. These inclusive design features address three primary principles: presentation appeal, usability, and engagement in play.

1. Multiple ways of presentation
   a. The design appeals to children's sensory (sound, vision, touch) abilities and preferences. A simple design makes a toy's use easy to understand.
   b. The toy is appealing to children. It may have multiple colors, textures, dimensions, and sounds. The toy's combination of colors, sounds, textures, and movement is appropriate (e.g., not too much, not too little).
   c. The toy's use is easy to understand. Its important parts are highlighted (e.g., knobs, buttons, connectors, areas). The toy's feedback will encourage continued interaction.

2. Multiple ways of use
   a. All children can use equivalent ways for playing with the toy. Physical effort is minimized; a variety of actions can be used to play with toys. The toy can be used in different positions. It can adjust to the child.
   b. The toy is easy to use. It is easy to pick up, hold, and manipulate. The parts (buttons, knobs, pieces, controls) are of adequate size and shape. An appropriate amount of effort (e.g., force, number of turns) is required. It accepts a variety of movements and is stable if intended to be.
   c. The toy is adjustable. It can be used in a variety of positions. The toy's features (e.g., height, volume, softness, speed) can be changed.

3. Multiple ways to play
   a. The toy appeals to children at varying developmental levels and abilities. It encourages use for more than one purpose. The toy holds a child's interest and encourages exploration and discovery. It is fun!
   b. The toy can be played with in different ways. It is adjustable for age and developmental levels and promotes use in more than one way. The child can choose to play with the toy alone or with other children. The toy encourages the child to be active (physically or mentally).
   c. The toy is fun to play with, and there is no right or wrong way to play. Its use promotes discovery (movement, cause and effect, sorting, etc.) and encourages imagination. It will be used over and over again.

Toys with embedded UD features can be used by all children playing together, including those with sensory (vision, hearing), cognitive (thinking, planning), and physical (fine or gross motor) disabilities. UD features must be identified because they act to provide appealing and accessible play materials, as well as space components that support children's abilities to successfully interact and engage in play.

Using Assistive Technology Supports

Technology is increasingly regarded by parents and professionals as holding great promise for more fully including children with disabilities in all activities of daily life, including play (DuBois, 1997; Lane & Mistrett, 2002; Sullivan & Lewis, 2000; Swinth, 1998). Technology supports have been found to be useful in reinstating play by providing children with disabilities access to appropriate toys and play materials (Levin & Enselein, 1990; Mistrett & Lane, 1995).

Children with significant disabilities may require appropriately adapted toys for their developmental level within a stimulating and supportive environment

(Brodin, 1996) to reap the benefits of play. Such toy adaptations can support other design features, such as those described previously.

Knowledgeable practitioners must be able to provide information on technology supports that individual children may need to play successfully. Some children with significant or multiple disabilities may require additional supports to minimize effort and maximize interactions. However, young children and their families may not be ready for highly specialized devices (Horn & Warren, 1987) or may find them "inappropriate" because children are in an ever-changing state of development in their early years. They may, in fact, act instead to further isolate children by calling attention to the disability with an unusual or specialized appearance (Mullick & Seinfeld, 1999). Thus some children reap greater benefits from commercial, off-the shelf options simply because the parents are more likely to use them. As already noted, it is important to begin with toys with UD features that will minimize the need for extensive adaptation to be usable by a wide range of individual children. For example, children who require switch-adapted toys should be able to choose from commercial toys with electronic elements so that they can play with other children using the same toys.

In addition to supporting the use of play materials, AT supports can assist children to further participate in play activities through movement and communication. Movement refers to body positioning and mobility. For young children with significant physical disabilities, the issue may be uncontrolled body movement or, alternatively, an inability to initiate or sustain appropriate positioning or movement. During play, children must be able to move about to explore their environments. Children with sensory impairments may require supports to safely move through and interact within environments. Some may have difficulty changing and maintaining different positions when they play. The positions that a child can use greatly influence the level and quality of play. For example, a toddler who cannot sit up independently will require support to be comfortably and safely maintained in that position and to engage in a play activity.

Interactive communication between infants and caregivers starts much earlier than the onset of a child's speech and is critical to the normal development of language and social abilities. Some children may need supports to express their needs and preferences in ways that are easily understood. Devices that use recorded single or multiple messages to incorporate language into play and other daily activities provide a way for a child to use a voice to communicate. Other devices can act as a switch interface to control a toy and be used to include a message that is heard when the toy is activated. Knowing how to use this AT effectively can enhance opportunities for pretend play for nonverbal young children.

When Is Universal Design Assistive Technology?

Regardless of where AT devices can be found, an item can be defined as AT by the way it is used (Edyburn, 2000). An understanding that AT can "assist" a young child to move, play, communicate, and interact can be the basis for making the federal definition of AT more relevant to young children who are in the process of developing functions and engaging in these activities. A toy with UD features such as large labeled buttons or a tricycle with a molded seat providing postural support can be seen as AT if they can "assist" a child's capabilities to participate in natural developmental opportunities (Brodin, 1999; Mistrett, 2004). Low-tech and UD items may be more advantageous to the dynamic state of development in the early years and better support the young child's functional capabilities; therefore they more appropriately correspond to the federal definition of AT.

When children are able to use play materials effectively, their play repertoires and levels of interactive engagement are extended (Behrmann, 1984; Lane & Mistrett, 1996; Wright & Nomura, 1985). Early successful play experiences with accessible toys can be effective in forestalling the development of learned helplessness and learning deficits (Behrmann, Jones, & Wilds, 1989; Butler, 1986; Douglas, Reeson, & Ryan, 1988; Kinsley & Lagone, 1995; Langley, 1990; Robinson, 1986).

Encouraging Child-Parent Interactions

Understanding how children play is crucial for planning successful play experiences. Because young children may not be able to initiate and play in different ways because of the barriers their disability presents, parents and caregivers may be called on to understand the nuances and scope of play far more than parents whose children without disabilities just seem to "know what to do." If play is understood to result from a child's active engagement with the world, strategies that promote play are those that respond to a child's play in ways that encourage more interactivity. As noted previously, it is through increased interactions that children develop. Parents must modify how they interact with their children to be less directive and more responsive (Greenspan & Weider, 2001). Strategies that promote adult responsivity have been seen to encourage children's use of "pivotal developmental behaviors" such as initiation, practice, exploration, and attentiveness (Mahoney & MacDonald, 2005). Responsive interaction strategies will provide parents with concrete actions to use when promoting "active learning"; they have been used successfully in programs developed for young children with disabilities (Greenspan & Weider, 2001; Mahoney, Boyce, Fewell, Spiker, & Wheeden, 1998; McCollum & Hemmeter, 1997; Spiker, Boyce, & Boyce, 2002). Strategies provide small steps that parents can take toward becoming more responsive to their child, such as "imitate what the child does," "follow the child's lead," or "use mirroring play to join the child's activity." With this approach parents focus on concrete behaviors instead of trying to attain abstract goals such as interacting "more responsively." Not only do the children actively learn, but so do their parents as they engage in responsive interactions with their children.

CASE STUDIES

Helping families to facilitate interactive play requires the practitioner to apply knowledge on play stages, setting up the environment for interactive play, selecting and using materials and supports, and suggesting interactive strategies most appropriate for individual children and families.

CASE EXAMPLE 1

Sammy

Born third in a family of four children, Sammy is a young child with significant developmental delays as a result of periventricular leukomalacia (PVL), which causes him to be very irritable, often crying for hours at a time. This condition prevents him from playing. His parents consider a sedative for Sammy to reduce his crying and the stress on the rest of the family. With the help of their EI therapists, they try several calming techniques, including body weights and heated pads, but nothing seems to help. Finally, a semireclined infant seat with a low-intensity vibration feature is found. When Sammy is placed in the seat and the vibration is turned on, he immediately stops crying and begins to look around. With this AT support, Sammy is able to begin to notice, interact with, and respond to the people and objects around him.

Because Sammy has not interacted with toys until this time, an overhead gym is placed over the chair with two visually interesting toys hanging from it. The toys are lowered with links until they touch his hands. Now he can not only see them, but feel them and watch his hands touch them. Sammy begins to move his hands against the suspended objects, watching what is happening. His parents respond with encouragement and begin to take turns with making the toys move. As Sammy plays more with the toys in this setup, other toys and household items are used and hung at various heights for him to reach toward and kick. As he begins to grab, hold onto, and drop the toys, the links prevent them from rolling out of his sight and reach. As a result of this supportive play environment, Sammy becomes more engaged in the daily activities of his family and shows increased independence during playtime. Box 17-1 describes Sammy's play stage, along with the toys, AT supports, and interactive behaviors that were sought in intervention.

Box 17-1 *Sammy: Sensory Exploration Play*

Toys
Variety of surfaces, textures, sounds, colors, tastes
Rattles
Mirrors
Kick gyms
Universal toys with sensory appeal

Assistive Technology Supports
Child positioning devices
Toy positioning strategies; overhead gym, angled, links
Reactive toys

Interactive Behaviors
Be present and encourage initiations and interactions.
Respond to interactions with facial and vocal enthusiasm.
Take one turn and wait.
Expect your child to interact.
Play sounds back and forth.

CASE EXAMPLE 2

Antone

Antone is a 27-month-old child who lives with his parents and two older sisters. His diagnosis, athetoid cerebral palsy, significantly limits his motor and communication abilities. Although he has a special wheelchair and supports that help him to sit up, he does not like to stay in it too long. He prefers using his right hand and arm. At his preschool, a favorite outside activity for the other children is blowing bubbles and catching them. He is able to only watch excitedly as the other children play. His parents and teachers are looking for ways to increase his level of participation.

Having the ability to blow bubbles would involve Antone in critical elements of the play activity. He could continue to use his wheelchair outside; the tray would be attached. Several blowers are considered that would address his abilities (use of right hand) and minimize what is hard for him (using two hands to dip the wand into the bottle; blowing). Two potential solutions are found. A commercial battery-operated blower "bucket" is activated by pushing the handle down so that bubbles will fly out from the top of the blower for 3 to 5 seconds. Antone can then reactivate it to make more bubbles. A second solution is a switch-activated bubble maker from a specialty catalogue. Using this, he can make bubbles as long as he activates the switch. The commercial blower is thought to be the better solution as it is novel for all the children, requires minimal setup, and because of its batteries, can be further adapted for switch use if necessary.

Strategies to promote participation are discussed between the EI interventionists and family. The best placement of the blower on his tray can be determined upon use and its base can be stabilized with Velcro on the tray. Independent participation is the goal and will be determined by the amount of bubbles he makes for the children to chase! In Box 17-2 toys, AT support, and expectations for Antone's play are described.

Box 17-2 *Antone: Functional Play*

Toys
In and out containers
Busy boxes
Balls
Ride-on toys
Sand and water toys

Assistive Technology Supports
Sitting, standing supports
Table, tray supports
Toy stabilizing materials
Choice making, communication devices

Interactive Strategies
Parallel the child's play to join the activity.
Follow the child's lead.
Communicate less so the child does more.

CASE EXAMPLE 3

Caroline

Born with significant visual limitations, Caroline is legally blind. Her family and doctors feel that she is able to distinguish light from dark and appears to respond to high-contrast patterns. All other developmental areas appear slightly delayed, most likely the result of her visual limitations. Caroline is an only child and spends 3 days a week at a neighborhood preschool. Her teacher consults with a teacher of the visually impaired (TVI) twice a week because she wants Caroline to participate in all activities to the maximum extent. A favorite activity in the classroom is the building center, where a variety of materials are available. The teacher wants to know how to structure the area so that Caroline can participate in building with the other children; she needs help to make choices, locate materials, and begin to build different structures. The teacher wonders if

Caroline will require specialized equipment or adaptations to play materials.

As the teacher and EI interventionist observe the available materials and room setup, they find that Caroline can use many of the common classroom materials; magnet, bristle, Duplo, and other blocks that "stay" together are found to work best. Strategies are discussed that will increase her independence in play and include putting like building materials in open bins, placed on a shelf she can reach. They also find that offering a defined area for Caroline to build in, such as a shallow tray, box lid, or Duplos base, helps her to build successfully on either the table or the floor and encourages other children to join her.

Caroline is in the constructive play stage in this intervention. The toys, AT supports, and strategies for interaction used are shown in Box 17-3.

Box 17-3 *Caroline: Constructive Play*

Toys
Blocks of various materials
Shape sorters
Puzzles, pegboards
Climbing apparatus; tunnels
Creative expression tools and materials

Assistive Technology Supports
Positioning and mobility supports
Bases for confinement
Computer construction software with adapted input: trackballs, touch windows, switch access
Communication system to suggest building activity, turn taking, etc.

Interactive Strategies
Sustain repetitive play.
Join perseverative play (make it interactive).
Translate the child's actions, feelings, intentions into words.
Match the child's interactive pace.

CASE EXAMPLE 4

Abby

Abby is an active child, 32 months of age, who moves quickly from one activity to another, plays with a toy for only seconds before she moves to the next one, and does not seem to be interested in playing with other children. She is able to vocalize some sounds and appears to be most focused when watching TV for short amounts of time. Abby is often unaware that these behaviors annoy her siblings—she is rarely asked to join in play activities anymore.

The EI interventionist and family observe Abby carefully and note her preference for visual toys and screen interactions. They looked for a software program that will present a familiar story or play items on the family computer. They also want a minimal number of keys to control the program because a full keyboard might distract Abby from interacting with the screen. The home computer is located on a desk in a common hallway; her chair used for mealtime is just the right height. A single switch is connected to a computer interface and mounted with Velcro on the monitor. This way the controller and screen reaction are closely connected.

The family and EI interventionist select a software program that depicts the same "little people" that are part of farm, garage, and playground play sets in the house. Abby's interest in the computer program is immediate. She quickly understands what pressing the switch will control and focuses intently on the action on the screen, waiting before pressing the switch again. The little people figures are placed near the computer so that she and her brother could find the one on the screen and pretend to do the same actions. They are encouraged to repeat the same activities off screen with the figures and play sets.

Abby's intervention focuses on pretend play. The description of this intervention can be seen in Box 17-4.

Box 17-4 *Abby: Pretend Play*

Toys
Play sets (farm, zoo, garage)
Dolls, stuffed animals
Puppet theaters
Real-life props: kitchen sets, toolboxes, doctor kits, shopping carts, furniture, boxes
Dress-up clothes

Assistive Technology Supports
Positioning and mobility supports
Puppets on switch toys
Choice-making devices
Single- and multiple-message recording devices
Adaptive materials to make toys easier to use
Computer programs depicting new and familiar situations, storybooks, etc.

Interactive Strategies
Translate the child's actions, feelings, and intentions into words.
Sustain action sequences.
Imitate the child's actions and communications.
Act as a playful partner or audience.

SUMMARY

The role of the EI practitioner in promoting development through play cannot be overstated. A play-based approach founded on family-centered principles can facilitate play opportunities throughout a child's day. With support for the family's ability to observe and recognize play behaviors and to implement the strategies, opportunities for overall development are improved. As a result, parents gain confidence in how (1) the child's natural environments can be arranged to be conducive to active play, (2) toys with UD features can be identified so that children can successfully play with them alone and together, and (3) responsive interactions can be implemented to promote active engagement in play. Together these elements act to maximize the use of the materials and ensure successful play experiences for children. With improved engagement, they will rise to meet new challenges through play.

Review Questions

1. Consider the potential barriers to play faced by children with disabilities and their families. Why is it important to address these barriers? How can using assistive technology and play supports ensure optimal social participation and occupational performance?
2. What information might you provide to a family of a child with a neuromotor deficit (for instance, cerebral palsy) regarding the selection of toys and play materials?
3. What are the pros and cons in the promotion of play for children with disabilities in using "off-the-shelf" toys with universal design?

REFERENCES

Baird, S., & Petersen, J. (1997). Seeking a comfortable fit between family-centered philosophy and early intervention practice: Time for a paradigm shift. *Topics in Early Childhood Special Education, 17*(2), 139-164.

Beckwith, L., & Cohen, S. E. (1989). Maternal responsiveness with pre-term infants and later competency. *New Directions for Child Development, 43*, 75-87.

Behrmann, M., & Lahm, E. (1984). Babies and robots: Technology to assist learning. *Rehabilitation Literature, 45*(7), 194-201.

Behrmann, M., Jones, J. K., & Wilds, M. L. (1989). Technology intervention for very young children with disabilities. *Infants and Young Children, 1*, 66-77.

Bergen, D. (1991, April). *Play as the vehicle for early intervention for at-risk infants and toddlers.* Paper presented at the Annual Meeting of the American Educational Research Association, Chicago.

Belsky, J., & Most, R. (1981). From exploration to play: A cross-section study of infant free play behavior. *Developmental Psychology, 17*(5), 630-639.

Bradley, R. H. (1985). Social-cognitive development and toys. *Topics in Early Childhood Special Education, 5*(3), 11-30.

Bradley, R. H. (1989). HOME measurement of maternal responsiveness. In M. H. Bornstein (Ed.), Maternal responsiveness: Characteristics and consequences (pp. 63-74). San Francisco: Jossey-Bass.

Brinker, R. P., & Lewis, M. (1984). Discovering the competent handicapped infant: A process approach to assessment and intervention. *Topics in Early Childhood Special Education, 2*(2), 1-16.

Brodin, J. (1996, November). *Play in children with profound mental retardation.* Paper presented at a teacher training course and at a parent education course for Ministry of Education, Salta, Argentina.

Brodin, J. (1999). Play in children with severe multiple disabilities: Play with toys—A review. *International Journal of Disability, Development and Education, 46*(1), 25-34.

Brown, M., & Bergen, D. (2002). Play and social interaction of children with disabilities at learning/activity centers in an inclusive preschool. *Journal of Research in Childhood Education, 17*, 26-37.

Butler, C. (1986). Effects of powered mobility on self-initiated behaviors of very young children with locomotor disability. *Developmental Medicine and Child Neurology, 28*, 325-332.

Daniels, L. E., Sparling, J. W., Reilly, M., & Humphry, R. (1995). Use of assistive technology with young children with severe and profound disabilities. *Infant-Toddler Intervention, 5*, 91-112.

Division for Early Childhood (DEC). (In review, 2005). *Division for Early Childhood companion to the NAEYC and NAECS/SDE Early Childhood Curriculum, Assessment, and Program Evaluation: Building an effective, accountable system in programs for children birth through age 8.*

Douglas, J., Reeson, B., & Ryan, M. (1988). Computer microtechnology for a severely disabled preschool child. *Child: Care, Health and Development, 14*, 93-104.

DuBois, S. (1997). Playthings: Toy use, accessibility and adaptation. In B. Chandler (Ed.), *The essence of play: A child's occupation* (pp. 107-128). Bethesda, MD: American Occupational Therapy Association.

Dunst, C. J., Bruder, M. B., Trivette, C. M., Raab, M., & McLean, M. (1998). *Increasing children's learning opportunities through families and communities. Early Childhood Research Institute: Year two progress report.* Asheville, NC: Orelena Hawks Puckett Institute.

Dunst, C. J., Hamby, D., Trivette, C. M., Raab, M., & Bruder, M. B. (2000). Everyday family and community life and children's naturally occurring learning opportunities. *Journal of Early Intervention, 23*(3), 151-164.

Education for All Handicapped Children Act Amendments of 1986, P.L. 99-457, 20 U.S.C. § 1400 et seq.

Edyburn, D. L. (2000). Assistive technology and students with mild disabilities. *Focus on Exceptional Children, 32*(9), 1-23.

Fewell, R., & Wheeden, C. A. (1998). A pilot study of intervention with adolescent mothers and their children: A preliminary examination of child outcomes. *Topics in Early Childhood Special Education, 18*(1), 18-25.

Fewell, R. R., & Kaminski, R. (1988). Play skills development and instruction for young children with handicaps. In S. L. Odom & M. B. Karnes (Eds.), *Early intervention for infants and children with handicaps: An empirical base* (pp. 145-158). Baltimore: Paul H. Brookes.

Florey, L. (1971). An approach to play and play development. *American Journal of Occupational Therapy, 15*(6), 275-280.

Gowen, J. W., Johnson-Martin, N., Goldman, B. D., & Hussey, B. (1992). Object play and exploration in children with and without disabilities: A longitudinal study. *American Journal on Mental Retardation, 97*(1), 21-38.

Greenspan, S., & Weider, S. (1991). *ICDL training videotapes on the DIR® model and floor time techniques.* Baltimore, MD: Interdisciplinary Council on Developmental and Learning.

Greenspan, S., & Weider, S. W. (2001). Floor time techniques and the DIR model. Baltimore, MD: Interdisciplinary Council on Developmental and Learning.

Hamm, E., Mistrett, S. G., & Ruffino, A. G. (in press). Play outcomes and satisfaction with toys and technology in young children with special needs. *Journal of Special Education Technology.*

Hanzlik, J. R. (1989). The effect of intervention on the free-play experience for mothers and their infants with developmental delay and cerebral palsy. *Physical and Occupational Therapy in Pediatrics, 9*(2), 33-51.

Hanzlik, J. R., & Stevenson, M. B. (1986). Interactions of mothers with their infants who are mentally retarded, retarded with cerebral palsy or non-retarded. *American Journal of Mental Deficiency, 90*, 513-520.

Horn, E. M., & Warren, S. F. (1987). Facilitating the acquisition of sensorimotor behavior with a micro-computer mediated teaching system: An experimental analysis. *Journal of the Association for the Severely Handicapped, 12*, 205-215.

Individuals with Disabilities Education Act Amendments of 1990, P.L. 101-476, 20 U.S.C. § 1400 et seq.

Individuals with Disabilities Education Act Amendments of 1997, P.L. 105-17, 20 U.S.C. § 1400 et seq.

Individuals with Disabilities Education Act Amendments of 2004, P.L. 108-446, 20 U.S.C. § 1400 et seq.

Jennings, K. D., Connors, R. E., Stegman, C. E., Sankaranarayan, P., & Mendelsohn, S. (1985). Mastery motivation in young preschoolers: Effect of a physical handicap and implications for educational programming. *Journal of the Division of Early Childhood, 19*(2), 162-169.

Johnson, J. E., & Ershler, J. L. (1985). Social and cognitive play forms and toy use by non-handicapped and handicapped preschoolers. *Topics in Early Childhood Special Education, 5*(3), 69-82.

Kim, J., & Mahoney, G. (2004). The effects of mother's style of interaction on children's engagement: Implications for using responsive interventions with parents. *Topics in Early Childhood Special Education, 24*(1), 31-38.

Kinsley, T. C., & Lagone, J. (1995). Applications of technology for infants, toddlers and preschoolers with disabilities. *Journal of Special Education Technology, 12*(4), 312-324.

Klugman, E., & Smilansky, S. (1990). *Children's play and learning: Perspectives and policy implications.* New York: Teachers College Press.

Kogan, K. L., & Tyler, N. (1973). Mother-child interactions in young physically handicapped children. *American Journal of Mental Deficiency, 77*(5), 492-497.

Krafft, K. C., & Berk, L. E. (1998). Private speech in two preschools: Significance of open-ended activities and make-believe play for verbal self-regulation. *Early Childhood Research Quarterly, 13*, 637-658.

Lally, J. R., & Stewart, J. (1990). *A guide to setting up play environments.* California Department of Education: Center for Child and Family Studies. Retrieved on April 14, 2005, from http://clas.uiuc.edu/fulltext/cl03267/cl03267.html#pubinfo.

Lane, S. J., & Mistrett, S. G. (1996). Play and assistive technology issues for infants and young children with disabilities: A preliminary examination. *Focus on Autism and Other Developmental Disabilities, 11*(2), 96-104.

Lane, S. J., & Mistrett, S. G. (1997). Can and should technology be used as a tool for early intervention? In J. Angelo (Ed.), *Assistive technology for rehabilitation therapists* (pp. 191-120). Philadelphia: F.A. Davis.

Lane, S. J., & Mistrett, S. G. (2002). Let's play! Assistive technology interventions for play. *Young Exceptional Children, 5*(2), 19-27.

Langley, M. B. (1990). A developmental approach to the use of toys for facilitation of environmental control. *Physical and Occupational Therapy in Pediatrics, 10,* 69-91.

Levin, J., & Enselein, K. (1990). *Fun for everyone.* Minneapolis: Ablenet.

Li, A. K. F. (1981). Play and the mentally retarded. *Mental Retardation, 19,* 121-126.

Linder, T. W. (1993). *Transdisciplinary play-based assessment: A functional approach to working with young children.* Baltimore: Paul H. Brookes.

Lindquist, J. E., Mack, W., & Parham, D. L. (1982). A synthesis of occupational behavior and sensory integration concepts in theory and practice, Part 2: Clinical applications. *American Journal of Occupational Therapy, 36,* 433-437.

Mahoney, G., Boyce, G., Fewell, R., Spiker, D., & Wheeden, A. (1998). The relationship of parent-child interaction to the effectiveness of early intervention services for at-risk children and children with disabilities. *Topics in Early Childhood Special Education, 18*(1), 5-17.

Mahoney, G., & MacDonald, J. (2005). *What is responsive training?.* Retrieved on April 26, 2005 from http://www.responsiveteaching.org/RTCurriculum/Strategies.htm.

Mahoney, G., & Wheeden, C. A. (1997). Parent-child interaction: The foundation for family-centered early intervention practice; A reponse to Baird and Peterson. *Topics in Early Childhood Special Education, 17*(2), 165-184.

Marcon, R. (2003). Research in review: Growing children; The physical side of development. *Young Children, 58,* 80-87.

McBride, S. L., & Peterson, C. (1997). Home based intervention with families with children with disabilities: Who is doing what? *Topics in Early Childhood Special Education, 17*(2), 209-233.

McCollum, J. A., & Hemmeter, M. L. (1997). Parent-child interaction intervention when children have disabilities. In M. J. Guralnick (Ed.), *The effectiveness of early intervention* (pp. 549-576). Baltimore: Paul H. Brookes.

McWilliam, R. A., Tocci, L., & Harbin, G. (1995). *Services are child oriented and families like it that way—But why? Findings.* Chapel Hill, NC: Early Childhood Research Institute: Service Utilization, Frank Porter Graham Child Development Center, University of North Carolina.

Missiuna, C., & Pollock, N. (1991). Play deprivation in children with physical disabilities: The role of the occupational therapist in preventing secondary disability. *American Journal of Occupational Therapy, 45*(10), 882-888.

Mistrett, S. (2004). Assistive technology helps young children with disabilities participate in daily activities. *Technology in Action, 1*(4), 1-4.

Mistrett, S. G. (2000). *Let's Play! Project final report.* (Final Report to OSERS, No. H024B50051). Buffalo, NY: State University of New York at Buffalo, Center for Assistive Technology.

Mistrett, S. G., & Lane, S. J. (1995). Using assistive technology for play and learning: Children, from birth to 10 years of age. In W. C. Mann, & J. Lane (Eds.), *Assistive technology for persons with disabilities.* Rockville, MD: American Occupational Therapy Association.

Mullick, A., & Steinfeld, E. (1997, Spring). Universal Design: What it is and isn't. *Innovation, the Journal for Industrial Designers Society of America.*

Musselwhite, C. (1986). *Adaptive play for special needs children: Strategies to enhance communication and learning.* San Diego: College-Hill Press.

Parham, L. D., & Primeau, L. A. (1997). Play and occupational therapy. In L. D. Parham & L. A. Fazio (Eds.), *Play in occupational therapy for children* (pp. 2-21). St. Louis: Mosby.

Parten, M. (1932). Social participation among preschool children. *Journal of Abnormal and Social Psychology, 27,* 243-269.

Pellegrini, A. D., & Boyd, B. (1993). The role of play in early childhood development and education: Issues in definition and function. In B. Spodek (Ed.), *Handbook of research on the education of young children* (pp. 105-121). New York: Macmillan.

Quilitch, H. R., & Risley, T. R. (1973). The effects of play materials on social play. *Journal of Applied Behavior Analysis, 6,* 573-578.

Robinson, L. M. (1986). Designing computer intervention for very young handicapped children. *Journal of the Division for Early Childhood, 10*(3), 209-215.

Rogers, S. J. (1988a). Cognitive characteristics of handicapped children's play: A review. *Journal of the Division for Early Childhood, 12*(2), 161-168.

Rogers, S. J. (1988b). Characteristics of social interactions between mothers and their disabled infants: A review. *Child: Care, Health and Development, 14,* 301-317.

Russ, S. W., Robins, A. L., & Christiano, B. A. (1999). Pretend play: Longitudinal prediction of creativity and affect in fantasy in children. *Creativity Research Journal, 12,* 129-139.

Sandall, S., McLean, M., & Smith, B. (Eds). (2000). *DEC recommended practices in early intervention/early childhood special education.* Reston, VA: Division of Early Childhood.

Sigmon, M., & Ungerer, J. A. (1984). Cognitive and language skills in autistic, mentally retarded, and normal children. *Developmental Psychology, 20*(2), 293-302.

Singer, D. G., Singer, J. L., Plaskon, S. L., & Schweder, A. E. (2003). A role for play in the preschool curriculum. In S. Olfman (Ed.), *All work and no play: How educational reforms are harming our preschoolers* (pp. 59-101). Westport, CT: Greenwood Publishing Group.

Smilansky, S. (1968). *The effects of sociodramatic play on disadvantaged preschool children.* New York: John Wiley & Sons.

Smith, P. K., & Connolly, K. (1980). *The ecology of preschool behavior.* Cambridge, UK: Cambridge University Press.

Spiker, D., Boyce, G. C., & Boyce, L. K. (2002). Parent-child interactions when young children have disabilities. *International Review of Research in Mental Retardation, 25*, 35-70.

Sullivan, M. W., & Lewis, M. (2000). Assistive technology for the very young: Creating responsive environments. *Infants and Young Children, 12*(4), 34-52.

Sutton-Smith, B. (1994). Paradigms of intervention. In J. Hellendoom, R. V. D. Kooij, & B. Sutton-Smith (Eds.), *Play and intervention* (pp. 3-21). Albany, NY: State University of New York Press.

Swinth, Y. (1998). Assistive technology in early intervention: Theory and practice. In J. Case-Smith (Ed.), *Pediatric occupational therapy and early intervention* (2nd ed., pp. 277-298). Boston: Butterworth-Heinemann.

Swinth, Y., Anson, D., & Deitz, J. (1993). Single-switch computer access for infants and toddlers. *American Journal of Occupational Therapy, 47*, 1031-1038.

Takata, N. (1971). The play milieu—A preliminary appraisal. *American Journal of Occupational Therapy, 15*(6), 281-284.

U.S. Department of Education (2002). *Twenty-fourth annual report to Congress on the implementation of the Individuals with Disabilities Education Act*. Washington, DC: U.S. Government Printing Office.

Vondra, J., & Belsky, J. (1989). Infant play at one year: Characteristics and early antecedents. In J. Lockman & A. Hazen (Eds.), *Action in social context: Perspectives on early development*. New York: Plenum Press.

Winter, S. M., Bell, M. J., & Dempsey, J. D. (1994). Creating play environments for children with special needs. *Childhood Education*, 28-31.

Woodroffe, S. E., & Willatt, B. J. (1976). Play materials and toys in education of young children. *Australian Pediatric Journal, 12*, 1-5.

Wright, C., & Nomura, M. (1985). *From toys to computers*. San Jose, CA: Authors.

Zigler, E. F., Singer, D. G., & Bishop-Josef, S. J. (2004). *Children's play: The roots of reading*. Washington, DC: Zero to Three Press.

INTERNET RESOURCES

Resources on Play

Boundless Playgrounds
http://www.boundlessplaygrounds.org/

Center for Creative Play
http://www.centerforcreativeplay.org/

Children's Museum Boston
http://www.bostonkids.org/index2.html

Ingrid's Therapy/Play Site
http://www.goodtogrowtoys.com/

Lekotek
http://www.lekotek.org/

Playing for Keeps
http://www.playingforkeeps.org/

Resources for Information on Assistive Technology and Young Children

ATA Center/Play Information
http://www.ataccess.org/resources/wcp/endefault.html

CEC Division for Early Childhood: AT Wheel for Young Children
http://www.dec-sped.org/

Center for Best Practices in Early Childhood
www.wiu.edu/thecenter/

Family Center on Technology and Disability
www.fctd.info

Let's Play! Projects
http://letsplay.buffalo.edu

Pacer Center—KITE project
http://www.pacer.org/kite/index.htm

Tots 'n Tech
http://tnt.asu.edu/

University of Miami—Mailman Center
http://pediatrics.med.miami.edu/mailman/assist_tech.htm

18

Storytelling, Storymaking, and Fantasy Play

Linda S. Fazio

Practitioners, regardless of discipline, have long used play in therapeutic exchanges with children. Therapeutic play is generally thought to be goal directed and purposive. According to Knox (1993), "for play to be used successfully in treatment, the child should feel responsible for choosing or directing the play episode" (p. 265); this is of particular importance when "the goal is to increase competence in play development" (p. 265). Theoretical and interpretative motivation for the use of play in therapy has varied among disciplines. Historically, occupational therapists have been accustomed to the use of play concepts and modalities in their work with children. It was not at all uncommon for the pediatric occupational therapist to be introduced to a child as the "play lady." That therapist and child engaged in a positive therapeutic play experience may, in fact, be the essence of pediatric occupational therapy.

Occupational therapy practice in pediatric psychiatry has been much less common than in other areas of pediatrics, as continues to be the case. However, programs that exist both clinically and in private practice are rich in their eclectic use of developmental, social-transitional, sensory-integrative, and behavioral approaches to treatment. Much of the work with pediatric psychosocial intervention before the 1980s was strongly influenced by Freudian psychoanalytical interpretation in all the disciplines, and it still is today in those disciplines allied with more traditional psychiatry.

The occupational therapist is accustomed to examining the "occupations" of the patient and to looking at these "occupations" not only as the mode to determine progress, or lack of it, but also as the actual determinant of therapeutic milieu. For the child, of course, play and the accoutrements of play are central. Another attribute of many occupational therapists that perhaps has caused some identity problems for the profession, although a strong plus for the patient, has been their insatiable need and ability to see the potential for attaining therapeutic goals in virtually every activity they encounter. This ability to create rich and exciting therapeutic environments with few restraints and, at times, without consideration of other disciplines' boundaries may cause laypeople not to distinguish the occupational therapist from the teacher, the counselor, the social worker, the recreation therapist, or the "play-lady volunteer"! Over the course of time other disciplines have recognized the value of occupational therapy's rich toolbox and have borrowed selected media and modalities for their therapeutic purposes. Whatever the circumstance initiating the choice of therapeutic environment and modality, it is to the child's best interest that therapists are dedicated. In today's world of print and visual media, interactive computer software, and a wonderful array of games and toys, therapists must be even more alert to the myriad choices for therapy. Often, though, it is the traditional modalities that are the most novel and for that reason offer the most appeal for the child. It is to one of these traditional modalities that this chapter is devoted, that of the *story*.

STORY AS A PLAY TECHNIQUE FOR THERAPEUTIC INTERVENTION

Stories and storytelling are familiar to every child and every adult regardless of culture, socioeconomic circumstances, or tradition. Jay O'Callahan, a professional storyteller quoted in Baldwin (1995), noted that the tradition of storytelling by parents has suffered in the competition with television. He encouraged parents to read stories and then tell them. "Parents make wonderful storytellers because they have strong bonds with the listener and they know their child's needs better than anyone else" (p. 32). Parents do, of course, frequently tell stories to their children; often these take the form of short, on the spot anecdotes told to teach a moral lesson with regard to "what might happen, if" or "when I was a little girl, Grandma used to." These are ways to pass on family values and traditions and are perhaps more effective than any other teaching tool a parent may use.

A therapeutic story is not much different. It serves to assist in the resolution of a problem or issue and sometimes incorporates a moral lesson, although it is perhaps less spontaneous than a parental story and is selected as a modality to bring about a therapeutic goal or goals. Baldwin recounted a story told by a therapist who worked with terminally ill children. Her patient, an 11-year-old boy named Jonathan, had leukemia. His wish was to have his ashes scattered over Lake Michigan. When the child died, his parents and younger brother, Charlie, age 5, went out on the lake to scatter the ashes. "A monarch butterfly flew down and Jonathan's mother said, 'Look! That's Jonathan!' The next day they were out on their boat and again a monarch butterfly flew down to them, and this time Charlie said, 'Look! That's Jonathan.' Later, they were sitting on the beach and a gray moth flew up from the sand. Charlie shouted, 'Look! That's Jonathan but he's wearing a different shirt.'" (p. 34). This story, told for the benefit of the younger brother, had healing benefit for the family unit and for each family member.

Stories may involve parents and families in other ways. Kral (1986) discussed the use of stories to assist in widening the range of options available to a parent, or perhaps a teacher, in dealing with a child. Parents of children with problems often generate "solutional" stories spontaneously when together in a group. Shared stories of how they deal with a child's difficult behaviors prompt other stories and therefore offer potential solutions. Therapists are all familiar with the stories they tell each other regarding their patients, and they have all benefited from these exchanges. Most often the benefit gained has been in the creation of scenarios that they can try with their own patients, but perhaps more important, therapists are able to encourage a sense of security and professional empowerment in their abilities to use their therapeutic skills.

Kral also discussed social-emotional therapy for children in the school setting. Whereas direct skill-based approaches are often used to treat behavioral problems related to school, indirect methods can be particularly effective because they make use of the child's strengths and abilities, rather than perhaps assuming that none exist. The telling of stories is such an indirect method. A widely used "alert program for self-regulation," How Does Your Engine Run, is an example of a behavioral approach to positive changes in children that employs the somewhat indirect use of metaphor (e.g., how does your "engine" run today?) (Shellenberger & Williams, 1994).

Frequently, in storytelling and storymaking, the therapist functions as a translator or guide in what may be considered a potentially confusing sea of communication, where the child's interpretation may be inaccurate or skewed. The telling of stories can be used to elicit the child's interpretation of an event or series of events that may have been disturbing, to share the meaning the child attaches to such events, to determine how the child incorporates this meaning into his or her emotional action plan, and, in shared group storytelling, to provide a nonthreatening sounding panel for how this "action plan" is perceived to be culturally and socially appropriate. The latter is what Bruner (1990) describes as the way "felicity conditions a method of negotiating and renegotiating meanings by the mediation of narrative techniques" (p. 67).

Children learn a language as a tool with which to mediate interactions within their environment. Whether this language is verbal or nonverbal, it is, as John Austin described, learning "how to do things with words" (1962, Preface). This communicative environment includes spoken and nonspoken language, and the child is expected to learn how to negotiate and operate within it. Hassibi and Breuer (1980) noted that "behavioral or psychological normalcy is a value-laden concept, varying broadly in its application from community to community and subject to changes in interpretation in different times" (p. 1). Not all of the elements of a communicative environment may be present, or their appropriate combinations and sequential orderings may not be such that the child receives the kinds of experiences suited to his or her needs (Robertson & Barford, 1976). This is an even more complicated task for children who receive and encode communications in alternative or obscure ways, such as those experienced by cognitively, visually, or hearing impaired children.

Bruner (1990) made a claim that very early in a child's development, before language actually develops, there is an ability to grasp "folk psychology." This is an initial understanding of how the group of which the child is a part interprets events; in the child's development it is a "feature of praxis before the child is able to express or comprehend the same matters by language" (p. 74). It appears that very young children, perhaps before age 4 years, have some understanding of the way their particular social-cultural group ascribes meaning to the actions of those around them and particularly to the circumstances in which actions occur because someone has held a false belief. Children younger than 4 years seem to be capable of withholding information and giving false information, as in, for example, the often heard explanation, "I didn't do it! She did it" to cover an accident or some occurrence that the child wishes not to share with the parent or caregiver. The point here is that a child learns a complicated series of communicative gymnastics necessary to give and to acquire the social and emotional necessities he or she needs as a member of a functioning sociocultural group. For whatever reason it appears that the cognitively or emotionally disabled child may not develop those protolinguistic competencies necessary to attend to all the meaning variables required for successful adult interactions within a folk group.

Praxis begins with ideation or forming an idea of what to do; this bears a direct relationship to the process of knowing how to do it. A. Jean Ayres (1985) described ideation as a cognitive process that involved understanding that possibilities might take place in relation to actions of self, objects, or people. Ideation allows the child to begin to plan what to do. Guided imaging, in the form of a therapist- and child-created story, allows the child to sample and create "just-right" challenges without risk. This is a particularly important experience when there is a gap between forming the idea and knowing how to translate the idea into action, as is often true for the cognitively and emotionally disabled child.

One of the functions of play, according to Florey (1981), is the organizing effect on behavior realized through the conceptualization of possibilities. This process of conceptualizing can be guided for the disabled child through therapeutic storytelling and storymaking. There is little risk if the possibilities, ideas, or actions generated by a child in a story format are proved ineffective or unrealistic. Through this process the therapist can assist the child in developing more appropriate possibilities, ideas, and actions.

The therapist can also function as a translator or guide to the child's interpretation of how actual events transpired and to the meanings attached to them. The therapist or other children in a mutual storytelling group can serve as interpreters of social and cultural appropriateness of actions. The process of hearing the child's story can provide a window for the therapist to view the child's world and his or her perceived impact on it.

Children often perceive the world in strongly structured categories or dichotomies; furthermore, they are persistent in their attachment to these dichotomies of good and bad, lie or truth, for or against. Russo and Jaques (1976) described the case of a child who relied so heavily on the stubborn use of categories that when they became frustrating or painful, "he could not realistically reconsider the situation, but resorted to sulking, crying, and temper tantrums not reacting to the realistic environment but to the world created by his own faulty and pervasive generalizations" (p. 395). Stories were used to assist the child in developing insights regarding his inability to deal with the gray areas of his experiences as he approached the developmental phases of adolescence. Through mutual stories practice was gained in the general classification of the child's experiences and

the abstraction of different scenarios with resultant repercussions and potential outcomes.

According to Gardner (1976), children have no great interest in developing insights into their own or others' behavior. In Gardner's interpretation, conscious awareness of unconscious processes is a form of therapy best reserved for adults, although it can also be useful for adolescents. The development of the therapist's insights into the child's frustrations and resulting behaviors is, of course, critical to the advancement of therapy.

Dorothy Singer's work in play therapy and the use of stories has relied heavily on the interpretation of the symbolic play of children (Singer, 1986, 1988; Singer & Singer, 1990). "A major component, then, of pretend play is the capacity of young children actually to experience symbolic or imagery-laden thought" (Singer & Singer, 1990, p. 189). The child's capacity to use imagery or fantasy as a coping skill can be encouraged through storytelling therapies. Use of fantasy can help a child explore feelings and ideas, assist a child in the resolution of conflicts, and bring about cognitive change.

For the young child, life is probably a "story." Young children have an ability to humanize objects in their environment and to endow them with human feeling and emotion. The following illustration is a brief excerpt from a group storytelling transcription in which a snow dome was used to initiate the stories (Figure 18-1):

Jean: I think that little deer is shaking; it must be very cold in that snow.

Kent: That's not real snow; it's fake, plastic probably. It's probably really warm in that ball.

Nancy: Yeah; I'd like it in there; it's so cozy and nobody could bother you unless you wanted to let them in. I wouldn't let any of you in!

Kent: So, who cares; if you let someone in, the dome would have to be broken and you wouldn't be safe anymore, would you?

Jean: Soooo; that's why she's not going to let you in, dummy.

When therapists attempt to understand how stories affect therapeutic outcomes, they must consider what Bandler and Grinder (1975) described as the surface and deep meaning of stories. "Surface meaning" refers to the more obvious storyline or literal interpretation. For the previous illustration the "surface story" involved the small deer in the dome. Deep meaning exists at the core of the story, its implicit meaning. Deep meaning can be interpreted differently by each individual. For Nancy the dome may have offered safety and security. For Kent, the aggressive realist, it was a barrier to be broken. And for Jean, the creative philosopher, it was an opportunity to defend her friend. Fairy tales such as *Sleeping Beauty*,

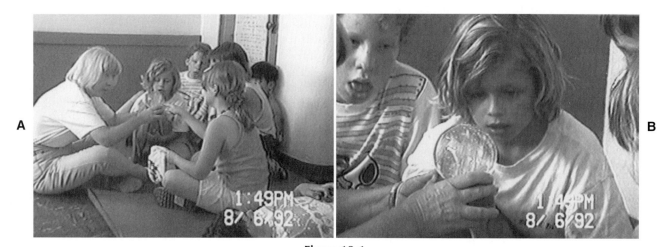

Figure 18-1

A, *Mutual storymaking that spontaneously occurred during a videotaped treatment session. The therapist is using a snow dome to facilitate the storymaking process.* *B*, *"I think that little deer is cold."*

Cinderella, and *The Ugly Duckling* are skillfully crafted stories of charming people, parties, and kindnesses, but also of evil and harmful people. These observations represent the surface structure of the stories. The deep structure exhibits intricacies of courage, love, sacrifice, and trust. It is often through this deep structure that the therapist works. However, therapy using surface structure can be equally effective. This is particularly the case within the dimensions of much of occupational therapy pediatric practice that involves the goals of improved social interactions, verbal expressions of feelings, encouragement of developmentally appropriate fantasy, and creativity. Such behaviors as taking turns, being kind to others, listening, using words to describe feelings, using self-control, being a group member, cooperating with others, empathizing with others, and understanding the impact of one's own actions and words on others are all sensitive to surface story construction. In general these stories fall into the categories of "What?" "What if?" and "How?"

The remainder of this chapter presents descriptions of frequently used storytelling and storymaking techniques.

MUTUAL AND SERIAL STORYTELLING

The mutual storytelling technique was originally proposed by Richard Gardner (1971) as a way to use children's stories for therapeutic purposes. The process of mutual storytelling is one in which the child begins a story as the therapist listens. The intent, as proposed by Gardner, is that the therapist look for unspoken psychodynamic meaning in the story. The therapist then responds to the story by telling one of his or her own. In the original use of this method the therapist's story contains the same characters and occurs in a similar setting, but the therapist introduces healthier, more adaptive solutions to whatever problems or conflicts the child may have introduced. The

psychodynamic supposition is that the child's unconscious receives the potential solutions and incorporates them in the conscious. In this technique the potential solutions are subtle; the child is not told how to handle a problem(s) and therefore does not actively resist the solution. The novelty of this technique also stimulates the child's interest and perhaps contributes to receptivity.

In my experience children are very much interested in this process and some equate it with video and computer games in which the central figure in a story, with the assistance of the child, may select from several adventure scenarios. Verbally telling a story that is in fact based on the child's own experience allows the child to fit this selection of scenarios to his or her own circumstances and ferret out potential solutions.

The following is a partial transcription from one of my therapy sessions with Jeff, a 9-year-old boy who was identified by teachers as having a behavior problem, with possible attention deficit disorder. The therapy was after school in a practice office set up for work with children and adolescents (comfortable sofa, table lamps, carpet, computer with selected game software, and relaxation monitoring software; cabinets with board games, dolls, and toys; dollhouse; music tapes and tape player; VCR and monitor and video tapes).

Therapist: Hello, sir *(hug)*...how are you?

Jeff: Okay, I guess *(moves around room; looks out of window)*...my mom's not waiting today, she has to take Karen to the dentist...anyway she's mad at me.

Therapist: *(sitting on sofa)* I'm tired today, how about entertaining me?

Jeff: *(joining therapist on sofa)* Okay, I'll tell you a joke. What did the cow say when he jumped over the moon?

Therapist: I don't know.

Jeff: Uh…I don't know either…*(laughing)* that's the joke, get it?

Therapist: (laughing) You're too smart today; how about telling me a story?

Jeff: I don't know any stories.

Therapist: Oh, it doesn't have to be fancy. Tell me about your day. *(Therapist puts feet up and closes eyes.)*

Jeff: Okay, but I'll just tell you some of it.

Therapist: Okay, I'm listening.

Jeff: Keep your eyes closed, but don't go to sleep; I'll know. I'm going to tell it like I'm another boy, okay?

Therapist: Okay.

Jeff: I went to get in line for the lunchroom but the teacher says, "No, you stay at your desk, Jason" (that's my name) and I sit down but I'm mad and I let her know, I look as mad as I can. Like this…open your eyes. Keep your eyes open because you need to see what happens next *(moves from sofa to small chair near center of room)*…this is my desk…I get even more mad because the kids are going to the lunch room and I can't go…so I get up to go anyway and my desk falls over…like this *(knocks over the chair)*…okay, that's it, that's the end.

Therapist: Okay, my turn now?

Jeff: Okay, I'm tired, I'm going to sleep during yours *(relaxes on sofa with eyes closed).*

Therapist: Okay, I'll tell mine very quietly so I don't wake you. There was a boy named Jeff…

Jeff: No, the boy's name is Jason.

Therapist: I forgot, go back to sleep. There was a boy named Jason and he went to Mrs. _____'s third grade; he was a pretty nice boy; he took care of his rabbit, Oreo; and he tried to be nice to his sister most of the time.

Jeff: (giggles) I don't think so!

Therapist: Shhhh, you're asleep. Sometimes at school, though, Jason had some problems. Seems he had some trouble listening to what the teacher said…and when she got upset with him…he got very mad! Jason's therapist knew how to solve the problem… This boy needs bigger ears, or maybe just more smaller ones…what do you think, is this a good story, or what?

Jeff: (giggles) Bigger ears, so big they look like balloons over his head.

Therapist: …very big ears; and when the teacher talked to Jason the ears turned toward her just like radar! But, you know what?

Jeff: Everybody laughed?

Therapist: Well, that too; but even more interesting, Jason still didn't listen to the teacher… so the therapist said, big ears just won't do it…we have to think of something else. What about better eyes? Maybe that

will do the trick. So the next time the teacher asked Jason a question, he looked straight at her with his really sharp eyes and watched very carefully as quietly as he could so his eyes could do their work and what do you know, it was easier to hear her…isn't that funny?

Jeff: Yeah, hearing with your eyes; that is too very weird…I like it! Bionic eyes.

Therapist: And something else that's weird…when Jason looked at the teacher and let his eyes really listen…he didn't mind doing what she said…and he didn't feel so bad anymore…he was even smiling a lot! End of story! Well, what do you think?

Jeff: Not too bad, not too bad…for you, anyway *(laughs).*

Therapist: (hugs his shoulders and falls back against pillows) A compliment, from you…I can't stand it! Think the eye thing will help Jason smile more?

Jeff: I don't know…I have to think about it.

Therapist: Try it out for him…would you? Let me know what you think next week?

This was one of a number of individual sessions with Jeff. In addition, he was a member of a small group of children (boys and girls) who were seen weekly. Activities were most often board games, arts and crafts, and community outings. Individual therapy would not have been as effective without this peer-based reinforcement of individual goals.

On occasion serial storytelling was used with the group. Oaklander (1978) referred to this kind of mutual storytelling as a "story collage" (p. 94). This version of storytelling consisted of each member having the opportunity to initiate a story of his or her choice; each member then took turns to continue the story. Rules were agreed on regarding the courtesy extended to each group member (e.g., no interruptions, no derogatory comments). The therapist did not usually enter into the storytelling but instead offered a summary of her interpretation of the "moral" of the story (it was mutually decided that each story was to have a beginning, a middle, an end, and a moral). Over time Jeff did manage his negative behaviors more effectively (as reported by his teacher and his mother); he remained emotionally and socially engaged in the therapy sessions and was more relaxed and spontaneous. Continuing, shared treatment goals were negotiated among Jeff, his mother, his teacher, and the therapist. The addition of storytelling to the therapeutic milieu offered a novel and creative avenue of play for Jeff and for the therapist.

Storytelling is not always easy for the child or for the therapist. It is useful to work with the child's real situations, often in a "Tell me about your day," "How was the soccer game?" approach. Gardner (1971) suggested using a tape recorder and a microphone. The child has a personal tape labeled with his or her name, and no one else is permitted to hear it. A "guest of honor" or "television program" format is used, and rules are established by the therapist (no stories that you've heard, read, or seen on television). Sometimes if the child is intimidated by the idea of telling a story, the therapist may begin and then suggest that the child continue with little bits of the story. For example, the therapist may offer, "Once upon a time in a distant land there lived a…" as the child fills in the gaps.

Focusing on a moral ("What can we learn from this story?") offers a therapeutic potential. Use of this moral to help the child change behaviors or for the adolescent to gain insight requires integration and translation to treatment goals and objectives.

Therapists with a strong interest in the psychodynamic model of practice can find much psychodynamic and symbolic meaning in the child's stories and may seek to translate this meaning for the child through using the child's characters and setting to create stories with psychoanalytic interpretation. This may have therapeutic potential for the adult and perhaps for the adolescent, but the use of more surface-oriented stories providing the child with workable behavioral adaptations seems to be more effective with younger children. The telling of a story by a child can certainly provide catharsis for anger, frustration, and sadness and can also provide a sharing of "just feeling good."

The therapist bridges a challenging situation when working in the pediatric cognitive-psychosocial domain. He or she must be able to experience the child's world and the child's interpretation of that world, while providing the benefit of the adult's experience in creating multiple options that are more adaptive and functional than the self-defeating ones that the child may have chosen or that the child's disability may have imposed. This is certainly a therapy benefiting from the therapist's positive life experience. However, if the therapist loses sight of the task and pleasure of being a child, the therapy is not effective.

PERSONALIZED STORYMAKING

Making stories to fit a particular child's situation is not unlike what has been described previously except that it is not necessarily initiated by the child's story but is rather the therapist's construction based on the circumstance and perceived emotions of the child. Robertson and Barford (1976) saw this kind of storymaking as appealing to the child's realm of fantasy and offering, vicariously, a means of acting out feelings that cannot be expressed in reality. Their work with children in hospital settings not only provides a release for the child's feelings but also encourages the child to get well. When a child is experiencing a long-term and painful illness, the use of fantasy

scenarios to help in alleviating pain and to maintain focus on wellness is useful. The therapist's use of fantasy scenarios can be broadened to include cartoons, comic books, television, and action figures.

Adults live their lives based on a personal story they have composed for themselves or, sometimes, based on stories others have composed for them. Adults' stories include a past, present, and future. Smith (1989) believed that adults' personal stories have three components: experiences, concepts, and themes. "Experiences are the people, places, and events that are a part of our history… Concepts are beliefs or ideas we have about ourselves and others that we use to screen and interpret experiences and to guide our behavior and themes are general, abstract principles that summarize and consolidate experiences and concepts…themes give unity to personal stories" (p. 7). These, then, would be the components that therapists would use to construct personal stories. The selection of themes would be based on mutually agreed upon therapeutic goals.

FANTASY, GUIDED AFFECTIVE IMAGERY, RELAXATION, AND THE USE OF METAPHORS
Fantasy and Imaging

What is meant by "imagery"? Images appear to be associated with the right hemisphere of the brain and its functions, which include the ability to construct visual and auditory "pictures," spatial representation, and fantasy. Generating images, imaging, and imagination, according to Sherrod and Singer (1984), are not necessarily the same things. Images may be thought of as internalized representations of sensory information with no actual stimulation. Thus people are able to recreate a picture or image of their living rooms or a significant other in their mind's eye. When people manipulate these images in their mind's eye, to imagine, for example, that maybe the sofa would be better in front of the window, this is imaging. Imagination requires the generation of images and manipulating them with a level of sophistication that may include generating thoughts about alternative scenarios and the actual creation of a script or story for action. It is this capacity for imagination that is observed in the play of a child when he or she includes dolls and toys in acting out various daily activities (eating pretend lunches, diapering a doll, or driving a truck to the store). There is some support for the idea that children's imaginary companions are a result of their capacity for eidetic imagery. According to Piaget and Inhelder (1971), a characteristic of children with imaginary playmates may be that they enjoy imaginative play with more positive outcomes than negative ones.

Daydreams are a familiar representation of imaging and the processes of imagination known to most of us (Singer, 1988; Starker, 1982). In Mihaly Csikszentmihalyi's (1984) work with the daydreams and fantasies of children and adolescents, he described the process as a form of information processing having to do with the self, whatever the person is currently concerned about, and general problem solving. When working with children and adolescents therapists must ask at what point in development the ability to image actually makes an appearance. Piaget (1962) believed that images make an appearance in the later part of the sensorimotor period of life, between the ages of 18 and 24 months, or at approximately the time that object permanency fully emerges. During the preoperational stage, about the age of 2 or 3 years, some pretend or make-believe play begins to develop. Between the ages of 4 and 6 years, true symbolic play or the substitution of one object for another in play can be observed quite frequently (Piaget & Inhelder, 1971). It is at this point in development that children can express imaging not only through language, but also through drawings, vocalizations, and movement (e.g., an elephant walks and sounds like this).

Later, during the stage of concrete operations, approximately ages 7 through 12 years, children begin to move away from imaginative, make-believe play, favoring more rule-bound games in groups. The ability to image is, of course, still there, and many children at this stage begin to develop very sophisticated language and graphic representations of fantasy and imaging. The child begins to move into the stage of formal operations at around 12 years of age, and continuing into adolescence and adulthood the ability to image and daydream is at its peak (Singer, 1986; Singer & Singer, 1990). Adolescents may spend a great deal of time daydreaming about future plans and "trying out" different potential life roles.

With a cognitively delayed child it may be difficult to determine exactly how the child receives, manipulates, and incorporates fantasy and imaging. One of the best measures may be to elicit verbal descriptions of events and to note if the descriptions contain images, or to ask for drawings that represent fantasy and imaging. Singer (1973, 1986) suggested the use of visual–spatial ability tests or, more simply, asking the child such direct questions as "What's your favorite game?" "What do you do when alone?" or "Do you have an imaginary playmate?" (1973). The therapist can also observe the free play and activity of the child and note whether imaginative play occurs. Noting the child's ability to manipulate imagery is important when selecting types of stories and storytelling techniques for therapeutic purposes.

Jones and Ponton (2002) explored the need children seem to have for fantasy and make-believe. According to these authors the extremes of good and powerful superheroes versus figures portraying evil were commonplace in the fantasies of most children. In my experience, when children retell stories they have seen on television or in the movies, they minimize the "evil" capacity of truly horrific characters (at least horrific in the adult's interpretation).

Vampires may be expressed as "mean bloodsuckers" by a child, complete with gleeful demonstrations of neck biting, but they are seldom treated with fear or disdain. If there are rats in the same story, they are usually treated with more real interest!

McIlwraith and Schallow (1982-1983) found a positive correlation between extensive and unmonitored television viewing and dysphoric, hostile, ruminative fantasies. They did not, however, find that television viewing substituted for or replaced self-produced fantasies. In my work television and movie characters certainly influence the stories children choose to tell, including events recently witnessed on the news, although the children's stories never seem to reproduce exactly the events or stories they have observed. Instead, these characters and events only seem to provide impetus or color for the stories. Applebee (1978) provided analysis of children's stories and determined that children ages 2 to 5 years had difficulty separating fact and fantasy. The stories of boys at these ages tended to venture farther from home than did the stories of girls at similar ages.

Guided Affective Imagery and Relaxation Techniques

Guided affective imagery, historically, was a psychoanalytically oriented technique that was used with children as young as age 6. The topics presented to the child through imagery were not directly linked to the presenting problem but were indirect scenarios of similar content (Leuner, Horn, & Klessman, 1983). The technique continues to be used in this way, particularly in European psychiatry. Rosenstiel and Scott (1977) indicated several major points that must be considered in the use of imagery: (1) the scenes used in imagery must be geared to the cognitive abilities of the child; (2) the therapist should select the natural imagery of the child as a basis for the therapeutic exchange because the use of familiar characters allows the child more comfort with this technique; and (3) the therapist must be alert to the child's breathing patterns and changes in facial expressions to note any anxiety that may be created by the particular images selected.

The use of guided imagery is closely linked to relaxation techniques and may be considered an extension of basic muscle relaxation and the generation of relaxing, peaceful images. This characteristic of the technique may be the most useful, particularly when it is coupled with a therapeutic story. The child (or children in small groups) is encouraged to sit comfortably or to lie down. The room may be darkened. Relaxing images may include a place the child has described as particularly pleasant (e.g., grandmother's kitchen, riding in the car). The scene may be set with an object such as a snow dome or music box (Fazio, 1992).

Sometimes it may be more effective to use a scene with which the child has no association. Steps in the process involve relaxation, setting the scene, and telling the story (by the therapist, the child, or a combination of both). Frequently, if a state of relaxation occurs, the child prefers that the therapist tell the story. The use of imagery can be effective as a way to retell a child's story with alternative solutions to problems being presented by the therapist. The therapist can assist the child in imaging how the solutions can be carried out and what the outcomes may be, or may not be. Used in this way, guided affective imagery creates a very focused, calming way to present alternative solutions to problems presented by the child, or interpreted by the therapist. If the child has difficulty (depending on developmental age) keeping his or her eyes closed and "creating pictures" in his or her head, it can be useful to encourage this process by suggesting that the child create a film strip or video or see himself or herself on a stage or screen. Most children can relate to this and have little difficulty creating images of themselves doing or saying things that the therapist suggests. Singer (1993) referred to "mind play" in describing therapeutic imagery. This is a term that children can relate to.

In the use of basic relaxation the therapist asks the child to relax his or her muscles, usually through a sequential tightening and relaxing of muscle groups; eyes are closed. The child is then asked to image a quiet, pleasant, peaceful scene. Deep breathing is demonstrated and modeled by the therapist. The child may be seated comfortably or lying down. Lusk (1992) provided an excellent resource for relaxation and imagery scripts that may be adapted for adults, adolescents, or children. Relaxation training has been used fairly widely with children of all ages and in a variety of settings. Singer (1993) referred to the work of Setterlind in using relaxation training in a physical education program for normal children aged 10 through 18 years. These children were found to experience an increase in measures of positive self-insight, self-control, and self-influence.

Martin and Williams (1990), in describing therapeutic work using guided imagery with adolescents and adults, note that it may be effective to substitute a positive image when the client is experiencing an anxiety-producing negative situation, or to substitute an exaggerated image that carries far worse consequences than the client's fears. For children the therapist can provide images of potential coping mechanisms in the form of a person or persons who the child believes can handle anything. Often this is an actual person the child knows, and sometimes it is a fantasy figure the child admires. The child can then image himself or herself modeling the admirable behavior. Sometimes an image can be created to make a potentially threatening person or situation less threatening in the child's eyes (e.g., the doctor trying to ride the child's tricycle or badly executing a skateboarder's maneuvers).

The work of Achterberg and Lawlis (1984) in helping cancer patients to create "cancer-destroying" images is similar to the approaches described above. Figure 18-2 represents drawings by children experiencing chronic illness. The "illness" was most often represented by small, menacing figures of bugs, scorpions, and spiders who were subdued by the child. In these drawings one child "used a long, really sharp knife to cut them down," and the other "formed a radiation screen that made them unconscious, and then dead."

Kazdin (1988), Spivack and Shure (1982), and Meichenbaum and Goodman (1971) described combinations of therapeutic techniques that are based in cognitive therapy. Children are instructed in how to make positive "I" statements that are repeated out loud. The therapist can then reinforce these statements through stories that are different from the child's situation but require similar strengths, followed by stories with the child as the central character, using his or her positive statements to achieve desired goals. Sometimes imagery may provide an experience for a child from which he or she may be excluded in real life because of physical or cognitive limitations or social isolation.

The following transcription provides an example of how a guided affective imagery session can be used for the rehearsal of alternative ways to cope with a potentially anxiety-producing situation. Kim is a 12-year-old girl who has been referred to therapy by her parents because of negative and failing school behaviors and difficulty in making friends. Kim is seated in a lounge chair with feet up; the therapist is seated nearby. The transcription begins after general muscle relaxation is accomplished:

Therapist: You're very relaxed now; feeling a little sleepy and heavy...I'm going to slowly count to 10 and as I do, I want you to see the numbers in your head like soft clouds. With each count you're one step closer to your special place...one...two...three...feeling more and more relaxed *(counting continues slowly with reinforcement phrases)* you're in the place you like best...feeling very relaxed, and very safe; take a minute to look around you...feeling very good to be here...Now you're ready to think about the performance you'd like to do for the talent show...staying very relaxed...your hands are resting in your lap; your face is relaxed, no tightness anywhere. See yourself backstage, waiting to go on. How do you look?

Kim: I look okay; I'm wearing a black, short dress. But I'm nervous; I feel sick.

Therapist: Freeze the picture and focus on relaxing; make your stomach very, very tight; so tight. Now let out your breath very slowly. Breathe deep and relax your stomach. Go back to your picture. You look good; can I start the tape?

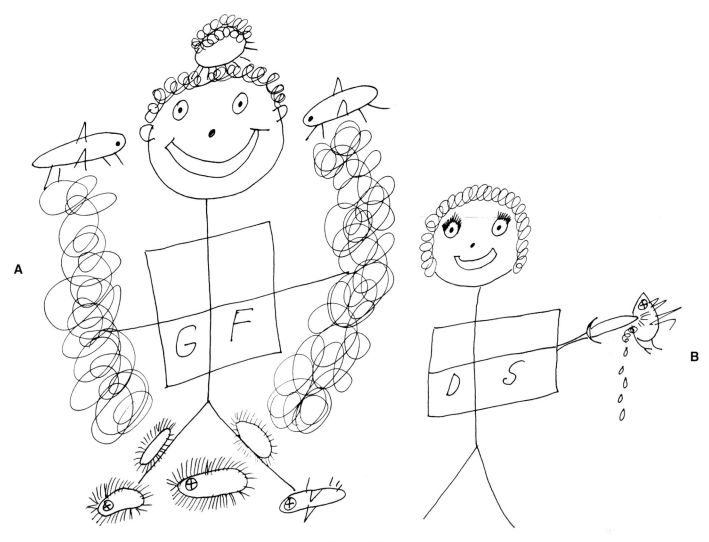

Figure 18-2

Drawings by chronically ill children. **A,** *The child explained the drawing by saying, "This is a germ fighter; radiation comes out of his fingers and kills germs; the germs look like centipedes, ugly flies, and even tarantulas!"* **B,** *The child's description of the drawing was, "This is a disease saver sword-girl; the sword sticks into bacteria until they die!"*

Kim: Go ahead, I think I'm ready.

Therapist: Sing the song in your head; make it real; move around, lift your hands; it's just you and the song in your safe, secure place. Take as much time as you need.

The imagery ended with counting in the reverse and reinforcement of feeling relaxed, safe, and secure. There were several sessions like this, followed by an actual dress rehearsal for the therapist. Kim performed at the talent show, the first school event in which she had participated.

Sessions of this kind were conducted with other children and included the rehearsal of numerous actions and events, including taking a test, kicking a soccer ball, talking to a girl, and reading out loud in class. Barell (1980) and Finke (1989) supported the idea that "there is a subtle tendency for movements to be initiated automatically whenever such movements are imaged" (pp. 215-216). Imaging may be particularly facilitative when the coordination of hands and feet is desirable in an action or series of actions. Rosenberg (1987) suggested similar links between imaging an activity or action and carrying it out. Performers and athletes frequently talk about "psyching" themselves out and imaging an activity before actually doing it.

Metaphorical Forms in Storytelling

Metaphors can assume many forms: proverbs, fairy tales, poems, parables, and numerous combinations and variations of these. The use of metaphorical stories to transmit a lesson or selected "words of wisdom" is in every culture's repertoire of subtle teaching tools. Even very young children understand metaphors and, if not, seem particularly challenged to figure them out. They are, after all, puzzles to be unraveled.

Metaphors, when used in therapy, are indirect; they are most effective when they reflect the primary elements of the client's problem and one or more solutions to the problem, but the content of the metaphorical form is very different from the actual problem (Dolan, 1986; Frey, 1993; Gordon, 1978; Mills & Crowley, 1986). Burns (2005) offered the practitioner and parent what he described as the art and skill of crafting and telling stories using metaphors. In his book *101 Healing Stories for Kids and Teens: Using Metaphors in Therapy*, he offered healing and teaching stories to include areas of caring for yourself, changing patterns of behavior, managing relationships, developing life skills, and many others. From these, therapists can go on to generate their own stories or can alter these to offer personalized stories for the children they serve. Lankton and Lankton (1989) also offered structured metaphors to be used in accomplishing therapeutic goals for children and adults. For these authors therapeutic goals and related metaphors for adults are organized in terms of attitudes, behavior, family structure change, self-image, identity organization and role development, and discipline and enjoyment, and for children and adolescents as learning self-control, sadness and grief, overcoming fears, and other areas of concern.

Religious teachings rely heavily on metaphor through proverbs and parables and may be preferred by parents. Fairy tales and metaphorical stories are an excellent way to engage a therapeutic group because they can relate to a wide variety of problems and concerns. Films geared toward adolescent audiences such as *Pretty in Pink* (Deutch, 1986) and *Rumble Fish* (Coppola, 1983) can be extremely useful as an impetus for group therapy interactions. Adolescents can easily identify with the actors and stories in these contemporary fairy tales. Many cartoons, for all ages, also meet this purpose. Mills and Crowley (1986) referred to the use of clay, paint, drawing, and puppetry to assist in the production of therapeutic metaphors.

Nursery Rhymes and Songs for Young Children

"The itsy bitsy spider climbs up the water spout…down came the rain and washed the spider out…out came the sun and dried up all the rain…and the itsy bitsy spider climbed up the spout again"…and again, and again, and again! Accompanied by hand motions and facial expressions, this little song speaks to anyone who has ever worked hard to achieve a goal, regardless of age or circumstances.

Comic book characters such as Spiderman and Batman present metaphorical messages that appear to be universal considering their popularity and appeal. Frey (1993) noted that "universal metaphors focus on issues that are common to human existence, such themes as anger, embarrassment, irrational thoughts, or procrastination" (p. 228). Hart (2003) described Japanese comic figures such as the manga villains. These characters have broad popularity with children and adolescents across cultures.

Coupling beauty with evil is the trademark of the manga witches. What better metaphor for the confusion between good and evil that most adults fear but many young children seem to accept? Frey suggested that the use of goals separates the use of metaphors in therapy from other settings. Therapeutic metaphors may "offer new choices, show different ways of perceiving a situation, and tap a variety of dormant beliefs, attitudes, and values of the child" (p. 223).

Oaklander (1978) suggested combining fantasy and drawing. When using the idea of a special place in facilitating relaxation, some children like to extend this to drawings or paintings using favored colors, shapes, and people. These drawings can be used to encourage the sharing of personal "special places" with other children in therapy or with siblings or other family members. A series of drawings can be produced and bound in a scrapbook or, if drawing is not the child's forte, magazine photos, actual photos, found objects, and construction paper can be used to produce a "special places and special things" collage.

Singer (1993) supported the use of motoric imagery, such as "repeating a word such as 'monkey' and demonstrating what a monkey can do" (p. 215). This facilitates a child's cognitive functioning by coupling enactment with a story to assist in comprehension and memory tasks.

Stories Combined with Other Media

Younger children may find it difficult to involve themselves in storytelling activities without some accompanying opportunity for action. This may also be true for older children, particularly those who are attention deficit disordered, developmentally disabled, or emotionally disabled. However, storytelling can also be a calming activity. After school or after sports, therapy sessions can frequently be effective because the child is exhausted and ready for a snack and a story.

It is easier to engage some children to tell stories themselves if they can relate the story through a doll or puppet. They may find it particularly hard to tell stories about themselves or family members. Constructing a hand puppet that represents the child can be useful, first as a way to help the child "see" the self and then as a tool to enhance "self" stories. These puppets are placed in a special place and are not used by other children. They can be taken down whenever the child wishes. An autistic child was observed using her hand puppet in self-talk. The therapist was able to use this observed opportunity to assist the child in a similarly fashioned communication with another child in therapy. The children continued to play together through their puppets and in later sessions often wore the puppets on their hands, but they frequently played together without the benefit of the puppets' "doing the communication."

Sitting on the floor, telling a serial story through puppets, is an excellent way to engage several children in a group play activity. Such an activity with puppets may be easier to initiate if it is designed around a commonly known fairy tale. Numerous puppets of fairy tale characters are available in toy stores, or they can be constructed by the children and the therapist. The therapist can initiate the story with each child taking a turn to continue it. The therapist can then construct the ending based on his or her interpretation of the most therapeutic outcome. Through the children's selective memory, personal interpretation, and creativity, the stories are seldom the ones the therapist might have expected! Bettelheim (1976) pointed out that "the child will extract different meaning from the same fairy tale, depending on his interests and needs of the moment" (p. 12).

Older children are usually able to engage in this kind of activity without benefit of puppets. They particularly enjoy the telling of "fractured fairy tales" (an approach you may recall from the *Rocky and Bullwinkle* television cartoons). The intent seems to be who can be the funniest and most outrageous. The perceptive therapist can learn a great deal about the child's real concerns, hopes, and fears from these stories and can return to these issues in further therapeutic exchanges. Richard Gardner's *Fairy Tales for Today's Children* (1974), *Modern Fairy Tales* (1977), and *Stories About the Real World* (1972) are good resources for stories that put a contemporary twist on a familiar tale. Adolescents find these stories entertaining and an opportunity to compare their observations of the world with those of other group members. No one ever quite agrees on the choices the hero or heroine may make, and this initiates excellent content for group communication and interaction. The therapist is responsible for maintaining these sessions as a safe environment for children to try out their perceptions of the world and examine their positions in it. This is one of the most challenging tasks for the therapist: avoiding a free-for-all without setting overly demanding limits. Usually the children and the therapist agree on the rules for the group sessions. For the therapist to maintain a safe environment and to protect the therapeutic integrity of the group, it must be maintained at no more than four or five children, depending on the diagnosis and dynamics of each child.

Games to enhance the telling of stories can be a novel way to elicit personal narratives. The Ungame, Storytelling Card Game, and even picture Lotto cards can be used to initiate stories. The therapist may also consider constructing his or her own storytelling "grab bag." This consists of phrases (typed or printed on small cards) that were selected to be personally meaningful to the child or children; the cards can be blindly selected from the bag or box to help the child focus on issues that can be developed in a mutual story with the therapist. Children might also type their own cards on the computer to create boxes or bags of their own. A box of "happy" or "positive" phrases (selected by the child) can be comforting when the child comes to therapy after a school day full of what may seem to be insurmountable problems.

Singer (1993) described the use of exercises or games to assist children in gaining control over the circumstances in their lives. Such games and exercises are also useful in facilitating the child's ability to use his or her imagination in a playful and pleasurable way. *Put Your Mother on the Ceiling* by deMille (1973) is an example. His exercises included imaginative ways to deal with images of school, pain, parents, and so forth; the game is not malicious but offers a safe way (the child's imagination) to deal with difficult events. The child can learn that controlled imagination and fantasy can be a fun way to help with real problems that may not be of the child's making.

Pantomime is another resource for developing alternate ways to tell stories. This can be particularly engaging for a child who is less comfortable with verbal communication or for children who tend to rely on verbal communication. For these children an opportunity to "act out" a story may offer an emotional release of energy that is therapeutically more facilitative. *The Magic If* by Kelly (1973) offers stories suitable to pantomime.

Maurice Sendak is a masterly creator of stories that speak to children's fears and concerns. The reading of Sendak's *Where the Wild Things Are* (1963) offers an opportunity for children to relate to the character's struggle to tame the menacing "monsters" (whatever they might be for each child). Coupling this story with guided imaging of the child's own particular "monsters" helps the story to be individually therapeutic. Many fairy tales are initiated with a "journey," and this can become a significant metaphor for children and for adults. Starting out on a quest or adventure seems to indicate an opportunity to change the way things are, to make them better, and to start over. And, even though we may not really believe that the hero and heroine live happily ever after, it is comforting to hear this ending to a story. Children, particularly, are optimistic that their personal stories will have a happy ending. Who is to say that incorporating that idea into one's belief system will not positively affect the outcome? "Once upon a time," "set out on a very long journey," and he or she "lived happily ever after" are phrases people have come to expect in stories, and ones that are comforting to them.

Bettelheim (1976) described the realities that are expressed in the conventional fairy tale. Life is often a struggle, but if a person maintains a steadfast path, a positive end is likely to be accomplished. In Bettelheim's interpretation, more contemporary stories for children often avoid these more existential issues, but in fact children may benefit from suggestions in symbolic form as to how they may deal with the "slings and arrows" of daily living. The reality is that problems cannot be avoided, but they can be handled in a positive manner that gains positive outcomes for a child.

The production of art forms is another approach to the use of stories in therapy. Kramer (1971) proposed that the "production of art contributes to the development of psychic organization that is able to function under pressure without breakdown or the need to resort to stultifying defensive measures" (p. xiii). Kramer also described what she termed "pictographic communication" or the use of "graphic symbols to relieve immediate anxiety and restore confidence" (p. 60). Occupational therapists, because of their occupation-based perspective, see play as incorporating the very widest dimensions for activity selection. The playroom typically includes such a broad assortment of potentially playful media that therapy and stories can be enhanced in multiple ways through toys, arts and crafts, and computers, to name but a few.

The scripting of stories, personal or otherwise, can be accomplished with computer word processing or with drawing programs for creating visual stories. Adolescents particularly enjoy this kind of storymaking. Scripting followed by videotaping can be an excellent group process activity and can take on the form of a club when this kind of rule-bound, adult rehearsal activity is deemed developmentally and therapeutically appropriate.

The reading of existing children's stories is an excellent therapeutic activity, whether used independently or as an entry into storymaking. The therapist can read to the child, or the child to the therapist, or stories can be created in response to illustrations. The therapist can also suggest stories that the parent may share with the child at home (Figure 18-3). Subject matter can be selected from an array of children's stories to best meet the therapeutic needs of the child, whether to assist with issues of perceived or real rejection by other children; failure in school; serious illness or death of a parent, grandparent, sibling, friend, or pet; divorce of parents; or foster home placement. Oaklander (1978) noted that children may not respond as well to stories that specifically try to get at children's feelings but are rather more engaged by stories that are told to entertain the child. As mentioned previously, the symbolic or metaphorical interpretations prompted by the supposedly innocuous story may be the most meaningful to the child. A children's book that is both entertaining and therapeutic in format and style is *A Terrible Thing Happened* by Margaret Holmes (2000). This story helps children resolve feelings after witnessing a violent or traumatic event. The children's book *Maybe Days: A Book for Children in Foster Care* by Wilgochi and Wright (2002) offers a story to help children in foster care with questions, feelings, and concerns they may have about current and future dilemmas of foster care and family.

Smith (1989) referred to the multiplicity of messages that may be found in existing children's stories: "having a purpose, pursuing one's dreams, overcoming fears, learning to act decisively, coping with inevitable loss; sharing, generosity, and compassion; and understanding conse-

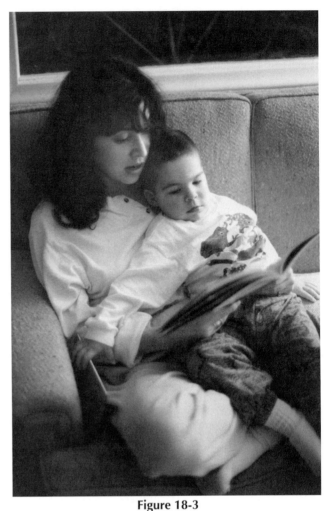

Figure 18-3

The therapist can suggest specific stories that the parent might read to the child at home. (Courtesy Shay McAtee.)

quences and identifying alternatives" (p. 62). These are but a few of the themes that may be constructed from existing stories for children. Smith included reviews of picture books that are appropriate for children from 2 to 8 years of age (pp. 269-285). Appendix 18-A at the end of this chapter is a list of children's books and stories, with brief descriptions, to assist therapists in developing their own libraries.

SUMMARY

This chapter is intended to stimulate the reader's interest in a form of play that has been with people from the beginning and one that is so obvious that therapists may have neglected it as they craft therapeutic play experiences. Stories, whether read or told, another's or one's own, independently constructed or shared, can be selected and adapted to the therapeutic goals of any child. Therapists should browse through the children's section of their local bookstores, enjoy old and new stories, and admire the beautiful illustrations. Many of the stories will seem appropriate to the therapist's experiences or those of someone they know. Many of them will seem to tell a metaphorical story of a child in the therapist's practice. Practitioners can take them to their therapy settings and share them with a child.

Review Questions

1. Describe what is meant by the term "imagery."
2. How is imagery expressed developmentally?
3. Provide examples of scripts that may be appropriate for use in guided affective imagery and relaxation.
4. Suggest some fairy tales from your experience that provide potential therapeutic scenarios.
5. Describe how toys, games, and dolls may be used to enhance the therapeutic gains of storytelling and storymaking.

REFERENCES

Achterberg, J., & Lawlis, G. F. (1984). *Imagery and disease.* Champaign, IL: Institute for Personality and Ability Testing.

Applebee, A. N. (1978). *The child's concept of story.* Chicago: University of Chicago Press.

Austin, J. (1962). *How to do things with words.* Cambridge, MA: Harvard University Press.

Ayres, A. J. (1985). *Developmental dyspraxia and adult onset apraxia.* Los Angeles: Sensory Integration International.

Baldwin, B. (1995, August). The lost art of storytelling. *Better Homes and Gardens,* 32-36.

Bandler, R., & Grinder, J. (1975). *The structure of magic I.* Palo Alto, CA: Science and Behavior Books.

Barell, J. (1980). *Playgrounds of our minds.* New York: Teachers College Press.

Bettelheim, B. (1976). *The uses of enchantment: The meaning and importance of fairy tales.* New York: Knopf.

Bruner, J. S. (1990). *Acts of meaning.* Cambridge, MA: Harvard University Press.

Burns, G. (2005). *101 healing stories for kids and teens.* Hoboken, NJ: John Wiley & Sons.

Coppola, F. (Director) (1983). *Rumble Fish* (film). Universal City, CA: Hot Weather Films.

Csikszentmihalyi, M. (1984). *Being adolescent: Conflict and growth in the teenage years.* New York: Basic Books.

deMille, R. (1973). *Put your mother on the ceiling.* New York: Viking Press.

Deutch, H. (Director) (1986). *Pretty in Pink* (film). Hollywood, CA: Paramount Studios.

Dolan, Y. (1986). Metaphors for motivation and intervention. In S. deShazer & R. Kral (Eds.), *Indirect approaches in therapy* (pp. 1-10). Rockville, MD: Aspen.

Fazio, L. (1992). Tell me a story: The therapeutic metaphor in the practice of pediatric occupational therapy. *American Journal of Occupational Therapy, 46*(2), 112-119.

Finke, R. A. (1989). *Principles of mental imagery.* Cambridge, MA: M. I. T. Press.

Florey, L. L. (1981). Studies of play: Implications for growth, development and for clinical practice. *American Journal of Occupational Therapy, 35*(8), 519-524.

Frey, D. E. (1993). Learning by metaphor. In C. Schaefer (Ed.), *The therapeutic powers of play* (pp. 223-239). Northvale, NJ: Jason Aronson.

Gardner, R. A. (1971). *Therapeutic communication with children, the mutual storytelling technique.* New York: Science House.

Gardner, R. A. (1972). *Dr. Gardner's stories about the real world.* Englewood Cliffs, NJ: Prentice Hall.

Gardner, R. A. (1974). *Dr. Gardner's fairy tales for today's children.* Englewood Cliffs, NJ: Prentice Hall.

Gardner, R. A. (1976). Mutual storytelling technique. In C. Schaefer (Ed.), *The therapeutic use of child's play,* (pp. 314-321). New York: Jason Aronson.

Gardner, R. A. (1977). *Dr. Gardner's modern fairy tales.* Philadelphia: George F. Stickley.

Gordon, D. (1978). *Therapeutic metaphors.* Cupertino, CA: Meta.

Hart, C. (2003). *Manga mania villains.* New York: Watson-Guptill.

Hassibi, M., & Breuer, H. Jr. (1980). *Disordered thinking and communication in children.* New York: Plenum Press.

Holmes, M. (2000). *A terrible thing happened.* Washington, DC: Magination Press.

Jones, G., & Ponton, L. (2002). *Killing monsters: Why children need fantasy, super heroes, and make-believe violence.* New York: Basic Books.

Kazdin, A. E. (1988). *Child psychotherapy: developing and identifying effective treatments.* New York: Pergamon Press.

Kelly, E. (1973). *The magic if.* New York: Drama Book Specialists.

Knox, S. (1993). Play and leisure. In H. Hopkins & H. Smith (Eds.), *Willard and Spackman's occupational therapy* (8th ed., pp. 260-268). Philadelphia: J.B. Lippincott.

Kral, R. (1986). Indirect therapy in the schools. In S. deShazer & R. Kral (Eds.), *Indirect approaches in therapy* (pp. 56-63). Rockville, MD: Aspen.

Kramer, E. (1971). *Art as therapy with children.* New York: Schocken Books.

Lankton, C., & Lankton, S. (1989). *Tales of enchantment: Goal-oriented metaphors for adults and children in therapy.* New York: Brunner/Mazel.

Leuner, H., Horn, G., & Klessman, E. (1983). Guided affective imagery with children and adolescents. New York: Plenum Press.

Lusk, J. (1992). *30 scripts for relaxation, imagery and inner healing.* Duluth, MN: Whole Person Associates.

Martin, M., & Williams, R. (1990). Imagery and emotion: clinical and experimental approaches. In P. J. Hampson, D. F. Marks, & J. T. E. Richardson (Eds.), *Imagery: Current developments* (pp. 268-306). London: Routledge.

McIlwraith, R. D., & Schallow, J. R. (1982-1983). Television viewing and styles of children's fantasy. *Imagination, Cognition and Personality, 2,* 323-331.

Meichenbaum, D. H., & Goodman, J. (1971). Training impulsive children to talk to themselves: A means of developing self-control. *Journal of Abnormal Psychology, 77,* 115-126.

Mills, J., & Crowley, R. (1986). *Therapeutic metaphors for children*. New York: Brunner/Mazel.

Oaklander, V. (1978). *Windows to our children*. Moab, UT: Real People Press.

Piaget, J. (1962). *Play, dreams and imitation in childhood*. New York: W.W. Norton.

Piaget, J., & Inhelder, B. (1971). *Mental imagery in the child*. New York: Basic Books.

Robertson, M., & Barford, F. (1976). Story making in psychotherapy with a chronically ill child. In C. Schaefer (Ed.), *The therapeutic use of child's play* (pp. 323-328). New York: Jason Aronson.

Rosenberg, H. S. (1987). Creative drama and imagination. New York: Holt, Rinehart & Winston.

Rosenstiel, A. K., & Scott, D. S. (1977). Four considerations in using imagery techniques with children. *Journal of Behavior Therapy and Experimental Psychiatry, 8*, 287-290.

Russo, S., & Jaques, H. (1976). Semantic play therapy. In C. Schaefer (Ed.), *The therapeutic use of child's play* (pp. 391-398). New York: Jason Aronson.

Sendak, M. (1963). *Where the wild things are*. New York: Harper & Row.

Shellenberger, S., & Williams, M. (1994). *How does your engine run? The alert program for self-regulation*. Albuquerque, NM: TherapyWorks, Inc.

Sherrod, L. R., & Singer, J. L. (1984). The development of make-believe play. In J. H. Goldstein (Ed.), *Sports, games and play* (pp. 1-38). Hillsdale, NJ: Lawrence Erlbaum.

Singer, D. (1986). The development of imagination in early childhood: Foundations of play therapy. In R. van der Kooij & J. Hellendoorn (Eds.), *Play—play therapy—play research* (pp. 105-131). Lisse, The Netherlands: Swets & Zeitlinger.

Singer, D. (1988). The conscious and unconscious stream of thought. In D. Pines (Ed.), *Energy synthesis in science* (pp. 142-180). New York: John Wiley & Sons.

Singer, D. (1993). *Fantasy and visualization: The therapeutic powers of play* (pp. 189-216). Northvale, NJ: Jason Aronson.

Singer, D., & Singer, J. L. (1990). *The house of make believe: Play and the developing imagination*. Cambridge, MA: Harvard University Press.

Singer, J. L. (1973). *The child's world of make-believe*. New York: Academic Press.

Smith, C. A. (1989). *From wonder to wisdom*. New York: New American Library.

Spivack, G., & Shure, M. B. (1982). The cognition of social adjustment: Interpersonal cognitive problem solving thinking. In B. B. Lakey & A. E. Kazdin (Eds.), *Advances in clinical child psychology, Vol. 5* (pp. 323-372). New York: Plenum Press.

Starker, S. (1982). *Fantastic thoughts: All about dreams, daydreams, hallucinations and hypnosis*. Englewood Cliffs, NJ: Prentice Hall.

Wilgochi, J., & Wright, M. (2002). *Maybe days: A book for children in foster care*. Washington, DC: Magination Press.

APPENDIX 18-A

Books, Stories, and Storytelling Games

The following list of children's books, stories, and story-telling games is included to assist therapists in developing libraries of "storytelling" and "storymaking" resources (alphabetical by title).

BOOKS AND STORIES

The Aesop for Children. 2005. New York: Barnes & Noble Books.
A new edition of a classic collection with beautiful illustrations.

Alligator Baby, by R. Munsch and illustrated by M. Martchenko. 1997. New York: Scholastic Books.
A new baby in the family!

The Brothers Lionheart, by Astrid Lindgren. 1985. New York: Penguin Books.
Originally published in Swedish, this is a story of a brother who courageously defends his younger brother against the treacherous Lord Tengil.

A Children's Treasury of Mythology. 2005. New York: Barnes & Noble Books.
A new edition of classic myths of adventure and quest with beautiful illustrations.

Country Angel Christmas, by Tomie dePaola. 1995. New York: G. P. Putnam's Sons.
The smallest child, and seemingly incapable one, is often excluded from plans and activities, but this story illustrates that there is something worthwhile for everyone to do.

Croco'Nile, by Roy Gerraud. 1994. New York: Farrar, Straus & Giroux.
Tale told of an Egyptian brother and sister; the value of compassion and friendship (beautifully illustrated).

Curious George, by H. A. Rey. 1993. Boston: Sandpiper-Houghton Mifflin Books.
A series of titles about the little monkey who always manages to get into trouble with only the best of intentions.

Daddy, Daddy Be There, by Candy Dawson Boyd, illustrated by Floyd Cooper. 1995. New York: Philomel Books.
Highlights important relationships between children and fathers: "Daddy, daddy be there, Tell me I am smart. Tell me I am special, Tell me I am able."

The Emperor's New Clothes, by Hans Christian Andersen, retold by Anthea Bell, illustrated by Dorothee Duntze. 1986. Croton-on-Hudson, NY: North-South Books.
Classic story to demonstrate that common sense wins over vanity and envy.

Fairy Tales for Today's Children, by R. Gardner. 1980. Cresskill, NJ: Creative Therapeutics.
The Princess and the Three Tasks, Hans and Greta, The Ugly Duck, and Cinderelma.

The Girl, the Fish, and the Crown, adapted and illustrated by Marilee Heyer. 1995. New York: Viking Press.
Adaptation of a Spanish folktale of a selfish young girl who comes to know the value of compassion and generosity.

Goldilocks and the Three Bears, retold and illustrated by Lorinda Bryan Conley. 1981. New York: G. P. Putnam's Sons.
The story everyone is familiar with, beautifully illustrated.

Grandma's Shoes, by Libby Hathorn, illustrated by Elvira. 1994. New York: Little, Brown.
A little girl copes with her grandmother's death by slipping into the woman's shoes and enjoying some special memories.

Great Children's Stories, The Classic Volland Edition. 2005. New York: Barnes & Noble Books.
A new edition of a classic collection that includes such favorites as Mother Goose with beautiful illustrations.

Hansel and Gretel, retold by Rika Lesser, illustrated by Paul O. Zelinsky. 1984. New York: Dodd, Mead Publishers.
A familiar story reflecting step-family dynamics and sibling unity.

I Won't Go to Bed! by A. Baruffi. 2005. New York: Sterling.
One of the "I'm going to read series" for children first learning to read.

It's a Spoon, Not a Shovel, by Caralyn Buehner, illustrated by Mark Buehner. 1995. New York: Dial Books.
This is an interactive, "What's the best answer?" book for teaching manners.

It's Kwanzaa, by Linda and Clay Goss. 1995. New York: G. P. Putnam's Sons.
This little book celebrates African heritage through stories and illustrations. Good to stimulate cultural sharing in groups.

The Juniper Tree and Other Tales from Grimm, translated by Lore Segal, illustrated by Maurice Sendak. 1973. New York: Farrar, Straus & Giroux.
These are classic Grimm stories with the added beauty of Sendak's illustrations. Published in a two-volume collector's edition.

Just a Secret, by G. Mayer and M. Mayer. 2005. New York: Golden Books.
A fun book for young children about making and keeping secrets.

Leo the Late Bloomer, by Robert Kraus, illustrated by Jose Aruego. 1973. New York: E. P. Dutton.
It sometimes takes awhile to catch up developmentally, but you may shine when you do!

The Little Engine That Could, by Watty Piper, illustrated by George and Doris Hauman. 1954. New York: Platt & Munk.
Classic story of perseverance.

Love You Forever, by R. Munsch, illustrated by S. McGraw. 2004. Buffalo, NY: Firefly Books.
Mrs. Cole on an Onion Roll and Other School Poems, by Kalli Dakos, illustrated by JoAnn Adinolfi. 1995. New York: Simon & Schuster Books for Young Readers.
All kinds of things that can happen at school, good and bad; prompts children to share school experiences.

Mufaro's Beautiful Daughters. An African Tale, by John Steptoe. 1987. New York: Lothrop, Lee & Shepard Books.
Pride frequently goes before a fall; kindness wins out at last—at least in this story. (Caldecott Honor book.)

Multicultural Fables and Fairy Tales, by Tara McCarthy. 1993. New York: Scholastic, Inc.
Stories and accompanying activities to help children formulate their own fables and morals.

My Favorite Things, by R. Rodgers and O. Hammerstein II, illustrated by James Warhola. 1994. New York: Simon & Schuster Books for Young Readers.
"When the dog bites, when the bee stings, when I'm feeling sad, I simply remember my favorite things and then I don't feel so bad!"

Night of the Gargoyles, by Eve Bunting, illustrated by David Wiesner. 1994. New York: Clarion Books.
This has the potential of being scary, but even scary things can be funny.

Nightmare in My Closet, by Mercer Mayer. 1968. New York: Dial Press.
Recognition of a child's fear of "What's hiding in the closet?"

One-Hundred-And-One Read-Aloud Classics, edited by Pamela Horn. 1995. New York: Black Dog and Leventhal Publishers.
Great collection of stories!

Pippi, by Astrid Lindgren. 1992. Stockholm, Sweden: Raben & Sjogren.
The tales of Pippi Longstocking make for great reading. It happens that this edition is written in a cartoon format captioned in Swedish. Neither I nor my clients have been able to read it, but they've told some wonderful stories based on the pictures. The stories are, of course, published in many languages, including English.

Reynard the Fox, adapted from classic folk tale, and illustrated by Alain Vaes. 1994. Atlanta: Turner Publishing.
Reynard the fox, trickster and deceiver, gets his in this story and discovers the secrets of being just and good.

Sad Underwear and Other Complications, by Judith Viorst, illustrated by Richard Hull. 1995. New York: Atheneum Books, Simon & Schuster.
One of a series of poetry collections that examine a wide variety of feelings and problems (potential and real) from a child's point of view. Such chapters as Fairy Tales, Stuff You Should Know, Pals and Pests, and Knock Knocks.

Smoky Night, by Eve Bunting, illustrated by David Diaz. 1994. San Diego: Harcourt Brace.
The Los Angeles riots prompted this story for children about the value of cooperation no matter what one's background or nationality. (Caldecott Medal.)

Spinning Tales Weaving Hope, edited by E. Brody, J. Goldspinner, K. Green, R. Leventhal, and J. Porcino, 1992. Philadelphia: New Society Publishers.
Topics included are living with ourselves and others and protecting our environment.

The Steadfast Tin Soldier, a Hans Christian Andersen tale retold by Tor Seidler, illustrated by Fred Marcellino. 1992. New York: Harper Collins.
A timeless story of love, vanity, patience, and virtue.

Stellaluna, by Janell Cannon. 1993. San Diego: Harcourt Brace.
This is a lovely little story about a somewhat frail and unattractive little bat who is trying to figure out what it means to be a bat and, in the process, learns about friendship. (American Booksellers Book of the Year in 1994.)

Stephanie's Ponytail, by R. Munsch, illustrated by M. Martchenko. 2005. Buffalo, NY: Annick Press.
A story about the trials and tribulations of a little girl with a wonderful ponytail.

The Story of the Three Kingdoms, by W. D. Myers, illustrated by Ashley Bryan. 1995. New York: Harper Collins.
"From that day on the People held their heads high, never forgetting to sit by the fire and tell their stories. Never forgetting that in the stories could be found wisdom and in wisdom, strength." (Preface.)

Stranger in the Mirror, by Allen Say. 1995. Boston: Houghton Mifflin.
This is a story about a young Asian boy, his and others' perception of aging, and the physical differences between people.

Talking Walls, by M. Burns Knight, illustrated by Anne Sibling O'Brien. 1992. Gardiner, ME: Tilbury House.
Introduction to many cultures through the concept of "walls"; illustrates the impact of walls on people who build them and are divided or unified by these partitions. Older children find this one stimulating.

Tanya and Emily in a Dance for Two, by Patricia Lee Gauch, illustrated by Satomi Ichikawa. 1994. New York: Philomel Books.
This book celebrates cooperation, individual strengths and skills, and the importance of spirit and discipline.

The Teacher from the Black Lagoon, by M. Thaler. 2005. New York: Scholastic.
A popular story for young children on encounters with "difficult" teachers.

Tell Me A Story, adapted by Amy Friedman, illustrated by Jillian Hulme Gilliland. 1993. Kansas City: Andrews & McMeel.
Nineteen folk tales and legends from around the world.

Time for Bed, by Mem Fox. 1993. San Diego, CA: Gulliver Books, Harcourt Brace.
A picture book of animals preparing their babies for sleep. Good for when a child needs to be quietly cuddled.

A Tooth Fairy's Tale, by David Christiana. 1994. New York: Farrar, Straus, & Giroux.
A beautifully illustrated tale of hope, dedication, and perseverance.

The Ugly Duckling, by Hans Christian Andersen, retold by Marianna Mayer, illustrated by Thomas Locher. 1987. New York: Macmillan.
Beauty is truly in the eye of the beholder.

The Velveteen Rabbit, by Margery Williams, illustrated by William Nicholson. 1975. New York: Avon Books.
"What is REAL?" asked the Rabbit. The Skin Horse replied "Real isn't how you are made, it's a thing that happens to you. When a child loves you for a long, long time."

The Waiting Day, by Harriett Diller, illustrated by Chi Chung. 1994. New York: Green Tiger Press, Simon & Schuster.
A ferryman in ancient China works furiously to please his customers, but an apparently idle beggar teaches him a lesson in how to appreciate the beauty of "what is."

Where the Wild Things Are, by Maurice Sendak. 1963. New York: Harper & Row.
Monsters aren't necessarily much different from you!

GAMES FOR GENERATING COMMUNICATION AND SELF-STORIES

Stop, Relax and Think. Childswork, Childsplay. The Center for Applied Psychology. 1-800-962-1141.
A board game to help impulsive children learn to focus and think before they act. The feelings cards ask the child to respond to a situation with how he or she might feel in that situation. Recommended for ages 6 to 12.

The Storytelling Card Game. Richard Gardner. 1988. Creative Therapeutics, 155 County Road, Cresskill, NJ, 07626-0317.
Twenty-four picture cards; twenty are scenes free of humans or animals, and four are blank; fifteen human figurines for the board game with arrow spinner.

The Ungame. Talicor, Incorporated. Post Office Box 6382, Anaheim, CA, 92816.
This is a noncompetitive game, appropriate for older children and adults, that explores a wide range of human experience through "draw" cards. Structured on two levels, one that is relatively superficial, and one with potentially more sensitive statements or questions. Examples: "If you could relive one year of your life, what year would it be? Why?" "Complete the sentence: Something I really like about myself is _____."

Glossary

Achievement 1. Performance that is linked to public expectancies or standards of excellence. 2. Something accomplished, especially by ability or special effort; connotes final accomplishment of something noteworthy; an attainment.

Adaptation 1. A change or response to stress of any kind; may be normal, self-protective, and developmental. 2. A change in the fit between organism and environment that is beneficial to the organism. 3. A change in routine, materials, or equipment that enables a person with a disability to function independently or to participate more fully in an activity.

Adaptive equipment Any structure, design, instrument, contrivance, or device that enables a person with a disability to function independently or to participate more fully in an activity.

Adaptive response A successful or appropriate reaction to an environmental challenge.

Adaptive sports equipment Any structure, instrument, contrivance, modification, or device that enables a person with a disability to participate in a sport.

Alternative communication Modes of transferring messages or information from one person to another in place of oral communication; alternative media may be verbal or nonverbal, direct or remote.

Arousal modulation The central nervous system's regulation of its own level of excitation; the regulation of neural systems that influence the organism's level of wakefulness, alertness, attention to environmental information, and readiness to respond to stimuli.

Assistive technology Mechanisms, devices, or methods of "doing something" with added assistive adaptations to enhance performance and independence.

Associative play Ludic activity that requires participation in relatively simple social interactions with peers, with no division of labor or product; from Parten's classification of social play in early childhood. See also **Cooperative play, Parallel play.**

Auditory Pertaining to the sense of hearing.

Auditory defensiveness A type of sensory integrative disorder in which there is a tendency to react with distress to ordinary sounds; a tendency to overreact to sounds that are not disturbing or uncomfortable for most people.

Augmentative communication Modes of transferring messages or information from one person to another to supplement, enhance, or support oral communication; alternative media may be verbal or nonverbal, direct or remote.

Autism A pervasive developmental disorder with onset in infancy or early childhood, characterized by impaired social interaction, impaired communication, and a remarkably restricted repertoire of activities and interests; thought to result from brain dysfunction. The term "autism" may be used to refer to pervasive developmental disorders (also called autism spectrum disorders) in general, or specifically to a particular diagnosis within the autism spectrum, called "autistic disorder."

Autotelic Intrinsically motivated; done for its own sake.

Behavioral flexibility The capacity to create new strategies for action in response to changing situations.

Bundy's model of playfulness Graphic depiction of playfulness as determined by three elements, each in a continuum: intrinsic motivation, internal control, and freedom to suspend reality. A summation of each of the three elements determines the degree to which playfulness is present in a given transaction.

Caregiver-child interactions Interchanges between children and their caregivers during the course of daily activities, which influence cognitive and language outcomes.

Centering the family in care See **Family-centered care**.

Cerebral palsy A motor function disorder caused by a permanent, nonprogressive brain defect or lesion present at birth or shortly thereafter. The disorder is usually associated with premature or abnormal birth and intrapartum asphyxia, causing damage to the nervous system.

Classical theories of play Theories of play that originated before World War I, specifically in the late nineteenth and early twentieth centuries. Prominent classical theorists of play include Schiller, Spencer, Lazarus, Patrick, Groos, and Hall.

Competence The state of being adequate to meet the demands of a task or situation.

Connected knowing A way of understanding a person as a person by entering the other person's perspective to discover the premises for his or her point of view.

Constructive play Activity that involves the manipulation of objects to construct or to "create" something, and is performed for the pleasure or satisfaction of doing the activity.

Contemporary theories of play Theories of play that emerged during the midtwentieth to early twenty-first centuries. Prominent contemporary theorists of play include Bateson, Bruner, Burghardt, Ellis, Erikson, Huizinga, Mead, Piaget, and Sutton-Smith.

Cooperative play Ludic activity that requires participation in highly organized and complex peer interactions for a purpose, such as making something or engaging in a game with rules; from Parten's classification of social play in early childhood.

Creativity The ability to be original in thought or expression.

Dramatic play Imitative activity in which a child fantasizes and acts out various domestic and social roles and situations, such as rocking a doll or pretending to teach school. It is the predominant form of play among preschool children. See also **Sociodramatic play**.

Dysphasia   A type of disorder in which a child has difficulty with speech or language that cannot be attributed to a specific medical condition, developmental disability, or lack of environmental models or opportunity.

Dyspraxia   A type of disorder in which a child has difficulty with praxis that cannot be attributed to a medical condition, developmental disability, or lack of environmental opportunity. See also **Praxis.**

Early intervention   Programs that provide services to young children and their families to enhance the development of infants and toddlers with disabilities and to minimize their potential for developmental delay.

Educational reform   The removal or correction of schooling practices deemed to be inappropriate or ineffective.

Effectance motivation   An inherent drive to have an effect on the environment; to take pleasure in being a cause of some action or event.

Environment   The physical, social, symbolic, or cultural context in which occupation (including play) occurs.

Environmental control system   Any structure, design, instrument, contrivance, or device that enables a person with a disability to effect changes in the surroundings in which daily routines take place and thereby gain more functional independence. Environmental control systems may consist of simple switches that operate appliances or turn on lights, or they may be complex microprocessor-controlled systems that enable the person to operate multiple appliances.

Environmental supportiveness   The extent to which the environment facilitates or impedes engagement in play and other activities.

Evolutionary biology of play   The study of patterns of play behavior across species, with emphasis on the adaptive functions of these behavioral patterns.

Exploration   Behavior that involves investigation of the environment. In arousal modulation theories, exploration is usually interpreted as the organism's attempt to reduce stimulation by becoming familiar with properties of the environment. In this view, exploration is characterized by serious affect and investigation of a novel environment. This is distinct from play, which involves stimulus-seeking behaviors, a relaxed attitude in a familiar environment, and experimentation with different actions on the object.

Facilitating play   Creating conditions that are favorable to engagement in play or to increased level of complexity of play activities

Family   A group of two or more individuals who provide the primary nurturing environment within which the child physically develops, matures, and learns. The family is an interactional system that can be described through its members, organization, and behavior; it has routines and traditions that give cohesion and stability; it has its own rules and boundaries that let members know how to behave; and it moves through a life cycle over time.

Family adaptations   Changes in family routines and activities that are beneficial to all family members or to the well-being of the family as a whole. See also **Adaptation**.

Family-centered care   A philosophy in which the child is viewed by the therapist as a member of a family unit; the family is instrumental in the retrieval of information for assessment and in the dissemination of intervention.

Family Observation Guide   A format for gathering information about family characteristics, child characteristics, and family and child play preferences, as part of a clinical assessment.

Family play   Ludic, leisure, or recreational activity that is performed by the family as the primary unit, rather than by individual family members in isolation. Family play is strongly influenced by the values, culture, and setting of the family; it may arise spontaneously or be highly organized and preplanned.

Family story   A narrative formulated by a child's family members that conveys their understandings, concerns, and values in relation to the child.

Fantasy   1. The usually pleasant process of subjectively creating free and unrestrained thoughts or emotional inventions. 2. A mental image. 3. Subjectively solving complex problems by imagining them in concrete symbols and images.

Fantasy play   Private, internal imaginative activity that may involve daydreaming or interior monologue. Fantasy play is thought to be the result of a developmental process in which the overt, action-oriented imaginative play of early childhood is transformed into private imagery and covert language during middle childhood.

Follow-up   The act of maintaining or reestablishing contact to evaluate, produce, or sustain benefits of intervention.

Framing   1. The giving and receiving of social cues that mark a given situation as playful; an essential aspect of playfulness, according to Bundy; see also **Metacommunication.** 2. The therapeutic process of considering a circumstance or set of circumstances within the person's emotional and social life, usually to create realistic and positive outcomes; may use a narrative approach to redefine a person's life situation. 3. Changing the conceptual or emotional viewpoint in relation to which a situation is experienced and placing it in an alternative frame that fits the "facts" of a concrete situation equally well, thereby changing its entire meaning (also called reframing).

Freedom to suspend reality   The ability to create new play situations and to interact with objects, materials, space, and people in ways that are fluid, flexible, and not bound to the constraints of "real life." See also **Bundy's model of playfulness.**

Fun   That which provides mirth and amusement; enjoyment; playfulness.

Functional play   Presymbolic activity in which an infant uses an object in a functionally appropriate way relative to his or her body, thereby demonstrating awareness of how the object is conventionally used, for example, raising an empty cup to the lips as if to drink.

Game   1. A amusement or pastime; an activity characterized by play. 2. A competitive activity involving skill, chance, or endurance on the part of two or more persons who play according to a set of rules, usually for their own amusement or for that of spectators.

Games with rules   Play activities that require an individual to abide by explicit, socially sanctioned regulations governing conduct, action, or procedure; highest level in Piaget's hierarchy of games.

Gravitational insecurity   A type of sensory integrative disorder in which the individual feels irrational fear, anxiety, or distress in relation to movement or a change of position; a tendency to react negatively and fearfully to movement experiences, particularly those involving a change in head position and movement backward or upward through space.

Guided affective imagery The therapist's process of aiding and assisting the client's production of images to create alternative solutions to problems.

Habits Skills that are performed so routinely that they have become automatic; allow efficiency in daily occupations.

Ideation The ability to conceptualize a new action to be performed in a given situation; a cognitive process that involves generating an idea of what to do; requires understanding the possibilities for actions in relation to objects and other people in the environment; generally precedes motor planning, which addresses the plan for how to do the action.

Imagery The formation of mental concepts, figures, ideas; a product of the imagination.

Imaginary play See **Imaginative play**.

Imaginative play Ludic activity that involves symbolism; may consist of relatively simple symbolic games or complex sociodramatic play; may be solitary or highly social; may be a precursor to fantasy in later childhood and adolescence. See also **Symbolic play.**

Imitation 1. The act of following, copying, or mimicking another person or group of people in action or manner; often seen within the context of childhood play. Piaget distinguished imitation from play; imitation involved accommodation to reality whereas play was assimilation, a joyful exercising of existing schemata. 2. A dimension of the Revised Knox Preschool Play Scale that addresses the ways children gain an understanding of the social world; includes factors of imitation, imagination, dramatization, music, and books.

Institutionalization State of living for an extended period of time in a residential setting for large groups of individuals who receive routine care from workers. Historically, people who are institutionalized tend to be those who are orphaned, disabled, or abandoned or otherwise lack families that are available, capable, or willing to care for them adequately. When care provided to infants and children is not optimal, institutionalization is associated with delays in all areas of development—physical growth, language, intellect, motor skills, and social-emotional development—as well as with abnormal stress reactions and increased risk of infectious disease.

Internal control The extent to which an individual is in charge of his or her actions and, to some extent, the outcome of an activity; an essential element of play in Bundy's model of playfulness.

Interview The process of orally gathering clinically relevant information from the child and his or her family via conversation or a schedule of questions.

Intrinsic motivation A prompt to action that comes from within the individual and is not prompted by outside influences; drive to action that is rewarded by the doing of the activity itself rather than some external reward. Intrinsic motivation is widely accepted as an essential ingredient of play.

Knox Preschool Play Scale See **Revised Knox Preschool Play Scale**.

Leisure 1. Freedom from the demands of work or duty. 2. Free or unoccupied time; a block of time in which there is no external pressure to generate a product. 3. Unhurried ease. 4. Play, particularly play in adulthood; leisure in this sense is usually associated with a conviction that it is necessary for individual life satisfaction and maintenance of social order and that there are legitimate times, spaces, and practices associated with leisure. 5. A nonobligatory activity that is intrinsically motivated and engaged in during discretionary time, that is, time not committed to obligatory occupations such as work, self-care, or sleep.

Life story A narrative that connects together the experiences that have occurred over one's life.

Ludic Of or pertaining to play; playful; usually connotes an activity or experience that is highly autotelic, spontaneous, and flexible.

Making meaning The act of uncovering or creating purpose or special significance through engagement in occupation or activity.

Mastery The state of being competent; having adequate skills to exert some degree of control over one's environment and situation.

Material management A dimension of the Revised Knox Preschool Play Scale that addresses the manner in which children handle materials and the purposes for which materials are used; process through which children learn control and use of material surroundings; contains factors of manipulation, construction, interest or attention to specific types of activities, purpose or goal, and attention span.

Metacommunication A message about communication; term coined by Gregory Bateson in relation to the message "This is play," a signal that subsequent behavior is playful, not instrumental.

Metaphor A figure of speech in which a term or phrase is applied to something that it does not literally denote to suggest a resemblance, as: "He isn't my cup of tea." Metaphor is used in some psychosocial therapies to carry indirect, potentially therapeutic meaning.

Meyer's philosophy of occupation The idea that health and adaptation to the complex demands of society require a rhythmic temporal pattern in occupations and a dynamic balance of work, rest, play, and sleep; developed by psychiatrist and prominent founder of occupational therapy, Adolph Meyer, in the early part of the twentieth century.

Middle childhood The period of development that extends approximately from 6 through 11 years of age; 6- through 8-year-olds are considered to be in the early period of middle childhood, whereas middle to late childhood encompasses the ages 8 through 11 years.

Mobility device 1. Any structure, instrument, contrivance, equipment, or mode of transportation or action that enables individuals with disabilities to move independently from one location to another in the environment. 2. Adaptive orthotic equipment that enables upper extremity function to accomplish certain activities of daily living.

Motivational properties Those elements or characteristics of environments and objects that prompt interest and action.

Motor planning The process of mentally organizing a novel action; a cognitive process that precedes observable motor performance; involves the organization of timing and sequencing of actions.

Mutual storytelling   A form of therapeutic storytelling in which the child and the therapist each share in the development of a story. The therapist uses the child's responses in directing the story toward positive therapeutic outcomes. This technique was developed by a psychiatrist, Richard Gardner.

Narrative   1. A story that conveys the personal meanings that an individual imbues on life events. 2. Technique of presenting information in the form of a story.

Narrative methods   Technique for obtaining information about an individual's unique life experiences using a conversational style rather than formal question-and-answer exchange.

Neonatal intensive care unit (NICU)   An acute-care section of a hospital containing sophisticated technological equipment and highly specialized medical intervention for the management and care of newborn infants who are premature, ill, or at risk for medical or developmental problems.

Neuroregulatory ability   The capacity of an infant to maintain or regain a stable, well-modulated balance among autonomic, motor, state, and attentional systems; involves interaction with the environment, for example, signaling and responding to caregivers in a manner that reduces infant stress.

Nonprescriptive stance   An intervention approach in which the therapist sensitizes caregivers to their child's unique capacities by taking into consideration individual differences in infant and child behavior, parent attributes, and cultural patterns of caregiving, without framing the child's characteristics as clinical indicators of a pathological condition or disability.

Novelty   Something new, unusual, or unexpected.

Object play   Ludic manipulation of tangible things.

Observation-based assessment   Clinical evaluation method that involves watching a child's behavior carefully, either in a clinical setting or in the everyday contexts of the child's life.

Occupation   The intentional engagement of an individual in an activity within the ongoing stream of human behavior; occupation is thought to influence health, either positively or negatively. Play is a special kind of occupation.

Occupational accuracy   The extent to which a therapeutic activity is clearly aligned with and targeted on treatment goals.

Occupational appeal   The attractiveness of a therapeutic activity to the person engaging in it.

Occupational behavior   1. A lifespan developmental continuum of play and work. 2. A frame of reference for occupational therapy practice, founded by Mary Reilly, emphasizing mastery, achievement, and ultimately health through engagement in play and work occupations.

Occupational intactness   The degree to which an activity used in intervention is whole; the degree to which an intervention activity preserves the natural conditions under which it typically occurs in relation to the patient's experiences of choice, social situation, time, and space.

Occupational justice   The principle or ideal of being just or fair, specifically in relation to availability of opportunities to engage in occupations that support health and well-being.

Occupational role of player   The expected pattern of behavior associated with occupancy of a distinctive position in society, specifically the position of being an infant or young child whose responsibility it is to acquire skills and habits in play that are essential for competence in later life roles.

Occupational scaffolding   Guidance, task modification, or assistance provided by an adult that enables a child to participate as much as possible in a particular occupation; perceived by the child as play even in occupations that conventionally are classified as work, for example, a household chore.

Occupational science   An academic discipline that is designed to provide a knowledge base on the nature of the human as an occupational being and to be useful for the clinical practice of occupational therapy.

Parallel play   Ludic activity in which the young child is beside peer(s) and engages in a similar activity, but does not interact with peer(s); from Parten's classification of social play in early childhood.

Parent-infant play   Self-initiated, intrinsically motivated, and often spontaneous interactions and exchanges between caregiver and infant that bring satisfaction and pleasure to both.

Participation   1. The act of taking or performing a part in an activity or event. 2. The active sharing of a social exchange or event with others. 3. A dimension of the Revised Knox Preschool Play Scale that addresses the amount and manner of interaction with persons in the environment and the degree of independence and cooperation demonstrated in play activities; contains factors of type or level of social interaction, cooperation with others, and language.

Pediatric Interest Profiles   Three age-appropriate profiles of play and leisure interests and participation that can be used with children and adolescents who have disabilities, as well as those who do not have disabilities.

Peer relations   Interactions and exchanges between persons who are considered to be "age mates," or companions, or associates at roughly the same level of development; may relate to any domain of development or achievement, such as same-age preschoolers or college classmates of varying ages.

Personalized storymaking   1. The process of creating stories about one's real-life events and actions. 2. The process of inserting oneself as the main character in existing stories or fairy tales and projecting different outcomes.

Play   1. An attitude or mode of experience that involves intrinsic motivation, emphasis on process rather than product and internal rather than external control, and an "as-if" or pretend element; takes place in a safe, nonthreatening environment with social sanctions. 2. Any spontaneous or organized activity that provides enjoyment, entertainment, amusement, or diversion.

Play as context   A view of play that emphasizes its dependence on situational conditions, such as freedom from perceived threat, illness, hunger, or heightened stress.

Play as end goal   The use of indicators of play quality, quantity, or complexity to establish intervention goals or to document intervention outcomes.

Play as means   The use of play as a critical ingredient in the process of providing an intervention, in order to achieve therapeutic goals.

Play as motivator   The use of play as a means for enticing the child to engage in an activity that he or she would not otherwise choose to do.

Play as therapeutic medium   See **Play as means**.

Play deficit   1. A condition in which a child's play skills are immature for the child's chronological age. 2. A mismatch between play skills and play preferences, such that the child chooses to do activities for which he or she lacks skills; this leads to frustration and poor self-esteem. 3. Limited involvement in play because of very low playfulness.

Play deprivation   A condition or circumstance in which the child is prevented from engaging in developmentally appropriate play opportunities; may be environmentally imposed or a result of illness or injury.

Play environment   1. The physical, symbolic, social, and cultural surroundings where play typically occurs. 2. Physical, symbolic, social, or cultural surroundings that are designed to support engagement in play.

Play experience   Subjective state characterized by perceived intrinsic motivation, internal control, and freedom to suspend reality, while engaging in an activity.

Play history   1. An interview schedule in which a caregiver or child is asked to furnish information about the child's past and current interests and patterns of participation in play. 2. A specific assessment instrument developed by Takata that enables the therapist to develop a play diagnosis and prescription based on a caregiver's history of the child's play.

Play in the therapy session   See **Play as means.**

Play in treatment   The strategic use of play as a means of intervention or as an end goal of intervention. See **Play as end goal** and **Play as means.**

Play interests   A tendency to pay special attention to, or seek out, certain kinds of ludic activities.

Playfulness   1. The tendency to seek out opportunities for play, or to respond to overtures of play with interest and pleasure. 2. A behavioral or personality trait characterized by flexibility, manifest joy, and spontaneity.

Playground design   The practice of planning environments, usually outdoors, that are intended to provide a safe place for child play involving physical activity, sensory exploration, and object manipulation in a community context.

Practice games   Ludic activities that involve the doing of actions purely for the pleasure of exercising them, without elements of make-believe or socially shared rules; term coined by Piaget to denote the most primitive type of game playing. This type of play is also called **sensorimotor play** and dominates the first 2 years of infancy.

Praxis   The ability to conceptualize, organize, and execute nonhabitual motor tasks.

Preexercise theory   A classical theory of play attributed to Groos, who explained play as the primary vehicle through which instinctive behavior is expressed and gradually refined into mature behaviors. Play is viewed as a product of an evolutionary biological process and is associated with the learning of behaviors critical to adaptation in adulthood.

Preparation for treatment   The process of setting up activities or environmental features before an intervention session to optimize child engagement.

Pretend play   Ludic activity that involves symbolic games and suspension of reality. See also **Freedom to suspend reality, Symbolic play.**

Pretense-symbolic   A dimension of the Revised Knox Preschool Play Scale that addresses the ways children learn about the world through imitation and make-believe; contains factors of imitation and dramatization. This dimension replaces the imitation dimension of earlier versions of this scale.

Revised Knox Preschool Play Scale   An assessment instrument that utilizes observations of play in natural environments of children from birth through approximately 5 years of age. Observations are organized into four broad categories of child abilities: space management, material management, imitation or pretense symbolic play, and social participation. Earlier versions of this instrument are also known as the Play Scale and the Preschool Play Scale. See also **Material management, Participation, Space management.**

Rhetorics of play   Persuasive discourses that represent particular attitudes and assumptions regarding the essence of play.

Rough-and-tumble play   Ludic activity that occurs in early childhood and consists of play fighting in the form of very active wrestling and chasing with peers, older children, and adults. This type of play is a very common behavioral pattern of young animals, especially primates, and is the kind of play that is most similar across humans and nonhumans.

Rules   1. Symbols or mental representations that codify experience; concepts acquired in play. 2. Socially sanctioned, explicit regulations governing conduct, action, procedure, or arrangement; see also **Rules of games.**

Rule learning   The process by which the child acquires symbols or mental representations of experience; takes place during play, particularly in what Reilly called the exploratory behavior phase of play; involves ludic exploration of the properties and patterns of body actions, objects, materials, and social interactions. Rule learning entails the generation of actions or subroutines of behavior that correspond to stored mental representations; for example, dumping and pouring are behavioral subroutines associated with substances that have the properties of liquids.

Rules of games   Socially sanctioned, explicit regulations governing conduct, action, procedure, or arrangement during a competitive activity involving skill, chance, or endurance on the part of two or more persons.

School-based occupational therapy   Occupational therapy assessment and intervention services that are provided within the context of the school environment and under the jurisdiction of the school system.

Self-report measures   A common strategy for assessing play or leisure among older children and adolescents, usually in the form of checklists or questionnaires.

Sensorimotor play   Purely autotelic experiences focusing on motion and sensations, without the elements of make-believe or socially shared rules; predominates during the first 2 years of life. Also called practice games or practice play. See also **Autotelic.**

Sensory integration   1. The organization of sensory input for use. 2. A frame of reference for occupational therapy practice, founded by A. Jean Ayres, that focuses on the neurological organization of sensory information for functional engagement in occupations.

Sensory modulation   A person's ability to self-regulate physiological or behavioral responses to sensory stimuli in a manner that is adaptive.

Skills   Consolidations of rule-based subroutines of behavior that produce goal-directed behavior; for example, the subroutines of grasping the handle of a pitcher, pouring, and holding a glass are combined in the skill of pouring a drink. Skills, when practiced repeatedly until automatic, become habits.

Social-emotional context of infancy   The situations and circumstances that involve infant-caregiver interactions with mutual feelings of enjoyment and connectedness, as during routine caregiving and other types of interactions such as synchronized exchanges of smiles, sounds, and gazes.

Social participation   See **Participation**.

Social skills   Routinized behaviors that enable a person to successfully negotiate interchanges and relationships with others, for example, the communication and emotional capacities needed to establish bonds with family members, converse with others, share activities with others, and establish and maintain friendships.

Social play   Participation in ludic activities with other people; this initially occurs in relation to primary caregivers and later takes place with siblings or peers.

Space management   A dimension of the Revised Knox Preschool Play Scale that addresses the ways children learn to manage their bodies and the space around them through experimentation and exploration; contains factors of gross motor activity, territory or area used in play, and exploration.

Spatial negotiation skills   Routinized behaviors that enable a person to successfully navigate through space and manipulate objects effectively in space; examples include transporting objects, clambering over a variety of surfaces, going in and out of circumscribed places, and using an object as a tool to affect another object.

Storymaking   The creation of a narrative that recasts and projects past experiences into an anticipated future. Storymaking may be used in occupational therapy with the intent of helping the recipient to create ideas for future life scenarios.

Storytelling   The development of a narrative, either true or fictitious, in prose or verse, designed to amuse or interest the hearer or reader. When used in therapy, storytelling may have the additional intent of providing the recipient with alternatives in thought or behavior.

Suspension of reality   The degree to which an individual in play chooses to assume identities, act out events, or control materials in ways that diverge from the usual constraints of real life; an essential element of play in Bundy's model of playfulness.

Symbolic play   The stage of play that predominates during the second and third years of life.

Symbolism   The representation of an idea, action, or object by the use of another, as in systems of writing, poetic language, or dreams.

Synactive Model of Neurobehavioral Organization   A model developed by Als that describes a newborn's emerging behavioral organization and how development proceeds via a continuous balancing of infant-environment interactions and the interplay among five neurobehavioral subsystems within the infant.

Tactile   Of or pertaining to the sense of touch; involves processing by sensory receptors in the skin and by structures throughout the central nervous system, including specialized areas in the diencephalon and cerebral cortex.

Tactile defensiveness   A type of sensory integrative disorder in which there is a tendency to have strong negative emotional responses to ordinary touch sensations.

Temporal negotiation skills   Routinized behaviors that enable a person to organize actions within time. Examples include the entrainment of biotemporal rhythms with familial or cultural temporal rhythms, such as establishing a sleep routine; recognition of temporal sequences of events, as in anticipation of morning routines; and appropriate timing and sequencing of actions to attain a goal, such as producing a simple song on a toy instrument.

Test of Environmental Supportiveness (TOES)   A test developed by Bundy to assess the extent to which elements of a particular environment support a player's motivations for play; meant to be administered in conjunction with the Test of Playfulness.

Test of Playfulness (ToP)   An assessment instrument developed by Bundy to operationalize play and playfulness in young children via observational ratings. Based on Bundy's model of playfulness.

Therapeutic use of self   The therapist's conscious or unconscious utilization of personal traits and interactions as a tool to facilitate treatment goals; may include strategies such as initiating an activity, providing emotional support and assistance, giving positive feedback and encouragement, exhibiting a playful attitude, and giving assurance of safety.

Therapist design skill   The ability of the occupational therapist to create activities that are tailored to meet the unique needs and goals of each child.

Therapist's story   A narrative formulated by a therapist that conveys his or her interpretations and concerns in relation to the child, based on professional knowledge and clinical experience.

Toy and environmental adaptations   See definition 3 for **Adaptation**.

Universal design   An inclusive approach to creating new forms of objects and environments that are appealing and helpful to a wide range of consumers, including those with a variety of disabilities. Toys and play equipment with universal design features are likely to be easily manipulated, flexible in use, tolerant of error, and simple to activate with easily perceived operating mechanisms such as switches or buttons.

Vestibular sensation   Information regarding one's head position and motion in relation to gravity. The vestibular sensory system classically is viewed as a type of proprioception. The word "vestibular" in this sense refers to the vestibule of the inner ear, where the receptors of this system are located; vestibular processing in the central nervous system primarily involves the brainstem and indirectly influences many other parts of the brain. Vestibular sensation interacts closely with vision and with proprioception arising from muscles to regulate posture, balance, and visual field stability.

Vestibular-bilateral and sequencing disorders   A type of sensory interactive disorder characterized by poor postural mechanisms, inadequate coordination of the two sides of the body, and difficulties with motor sequencing; thought to be related to dysfunction in central processing of vestibular sensations.

Virtual reality   A technology that allows users to interact with a computer-simulated environment, usually visual in nature, but sometimes incorporating auditory and tactile information.

Index

Symbols: *f*, figure; *b*, box; *t*, table.